PROFESSIONAL NURSING CONCEPTS

Competencies for Quality Leadership

FOURTH EDITION

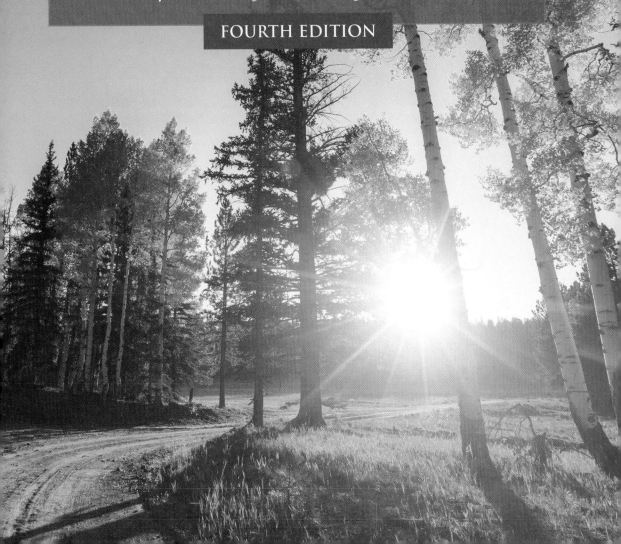

Anita Finkelman

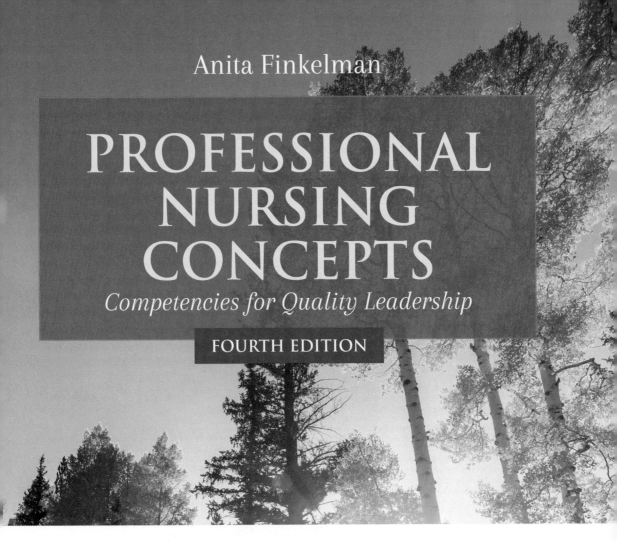

PROFESSIONAL NURSING CONCEPTS

Competencies for Quality Leadership

FOURTH EDITION

ANITA FINKELMAN, MSN, RN
Visiting Lecturer, Nursing Department
Recanati School for Community Health Professions
Faculty of the Health Sciences
Ben-Gurion University of the Negev
Beersheba, Israel

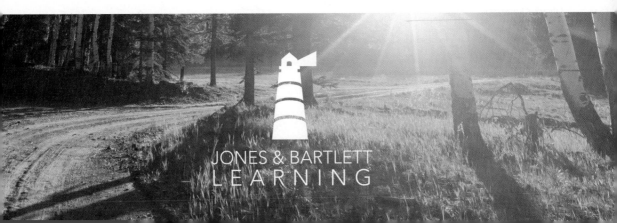

JONES & BARTLETT
LEARNING

World Headquarters
Jones & Bartlett Learning
5 Wall Street
Burlington, MA 01803
978-443-5000
info@jblearning.com
www.jblearning.com

Jones & Bartlett Learning books and products are available through most bookstores and online booksellers. To contact Jones & Bartlett Learning directly, call 800-832-0034, fax 978-443-8000, or visit our website, www.jblearning.com.

12795-9

Production Credits

VP, Product Management: David D. Cella
Director, Product Management: Amanda Martin
Product Manager: Rebecca Stephenson
Product Assistant: Anna-Maria Forger
Senior Vendor Manager: Sara Kelly
Senior Marketing Manager: Jennifer Scherzay
Product Fulfillment Manager: Wendy Kilborn
Composition and Project Management: S4Carlisle Publishing Services

Cover Design: Kristin E. Parker
Rights & Media Specialist: Wes DeShano
Media Development Editor: Troy Liston
Cover Image (Title Page, Part Opener, Chapter Opener): © Galyna Andrushko/Shutterstock
Printing and Binding: LSC Communications
Cover Printing: LSC Communications

Library of Congress Cataloging-in-Publication Data

Names: Finkelman, Anita, author.
Title: Professional nursing concepts : competencies for quality leadership / Anita Finkelman.
Description: Fourth edition. | Burlington, MA : Jones & Bartlett Learning, [2019] | Includes bibliographical references and index.
Identifiers: LCCN 2017035478 | ISBN 9781284127270
Subjects: | MESH: Nursing | Nursing Care | Nurse's Role | Leadership | United States
Classification: LCC RT82 | NLM WY 100 AA1 | DDC 610.7306/9--dc23 LC record available at https://lccn.loc.gov/2017035478

6048

Printed in the United States of America
22 21 20 19 18   10 9 8 7 6 5 4

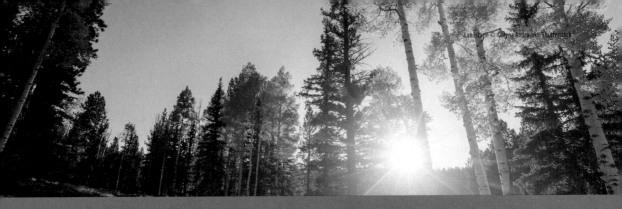

Contents

Section 2: The Healthcare Context

Section 3: Core Healthcare Professional Competencies

Section 4: The Practice of Nursing Today and in the Future

Chapter 14 The Future: Transformation of Nursing Practice through Leadership 461

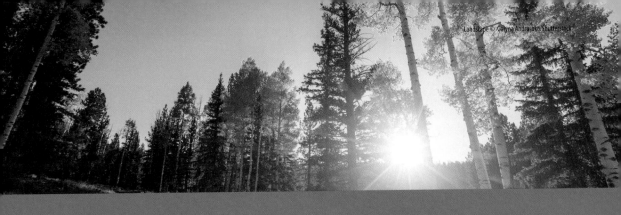

Acknowledgments

I thank my family for all of their support of my writing: Fred, Shoshannah, and Deborah. Thank you to Elisabeth Garofalo for her role as developmental editor; Amanda Martin for her guidance in the ongoing editions of this text; Emma Huggard for her hands-on management of the project; Wes Deshano for his guidance regarding copyright; the editing team; all the team at JBL who have participated in this project; and the production team. I also want to recognize all students and faculty I have worked with who taught me so much about what students need to know to practice competently and guidance faculty need to provide effective learning experiences for students in the classroom, simulation, and clinical settings.

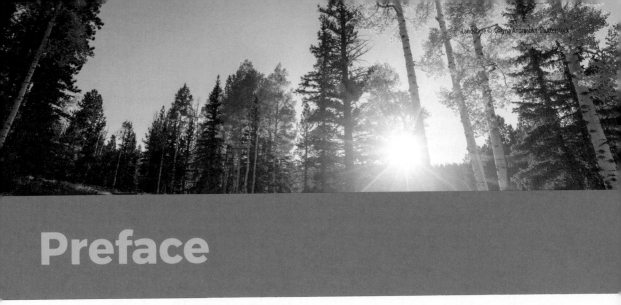

Preface

The development of this text is motivated by the need to provide students who are beginning their nursing education or working toward their baccalaureate degree for career development with background information about the nursing profession and the critical healthcare delivery issues that affect our profession. This goal has been the same for all of its editions, but it is even more imperative today as we have experienced changes due to healthcare legislation and as we experience more changes with a new presidential administration. Change is part of health care, and we need to understand where we came from and update ourselves so we can effectively engage in the change process that lies ahead of us. We hear much about healthcare reimbursement in the news, and this is important—but we cannot ignore that we have a healthcare system that needs repair and improvement. Thus, this fourth edition continues to emphasize quality improvement and the nurse's role in quality improvement, ensuring patient-centered care.

Nursing students today are asked to cover much information in their courses and develop clinical competencies in a short period of time. It is critical that each student recognize that nursing does not happen in isolation, but rather it is part of the entire healthcare experience. Nurses need to assume critical roles in this experience through their unique professional expertise and leadership. They are also members of the interprofessional healthcare team; they must work with others to provide and improve care in a healthcare environment that provides a healthy workplace and a positive patient experience.

This text consists of 14 chapters, divided into four sections. **Section 1** focuses on the profession of nursing. In these chapters, students will learn about the dynamic history of nursing and how the profession developed; the complex essence of nursing (knowledge and caring); nursing education, accreditation, and regulation; and how to succeed as nursing students.

Section 2 explores the healthcare context in which nursing is practiced. Health policy and political action are very important today in health care and in nursing. Students need to know about ethical and legal issues that currently apply to their practice and issues that might apply in the future as registered nurses. Students typically think most about caring for the acutely ill, but the health context is broader than this and includes health promotion, disease prevention, and illness across the continuum of care in the community. Though nursing is practiced in many different settings and healthcare organizations, the final chapter in this section focuses on acute care organizations, providing students with an in-depth exploration of one type of healthcare organization.

Section 3 moves the discussion to the core healthcare professions competencies that are expected for all healthcare professions. Each chapter in this section focuses on one of the core competencies. Though this section covers these competencies in depth, the competencies are relevant to all the content in this text. The five competencies are (Institute of Medicine, 2003):

1. Provide patient-centered care.
2. Work in interprofessional teams.
3. Employ evidence-based practice.
4. Apply quality improvement.
5. Utilize informatics.

Section 4 brings us to the end of this text, although not to the end of learning. The chapter in this section focuses on the transformation of nursing practice through leadership, connecting the key concepts in the text.

This fourth edition also includes three appendices. The first focuses on quality improvement measurement and analysis methods, providing students with a quick reference for information about quality improvement that can be used throughout the nursing program and to develop their expertise in quality improvement. The other appendices provide students with important information related to staffing and healthy work environments, as well as finding the right job.

Each chapter includes objectives, an outline of the chapter to help organize students' reading, key terms that are found in the chapter and defined in the Glossary, content with headers that apply to the chapter outline, and chapter highlights. A new chapter feature is the Stop and Consider statement found after each major section in a chapter. This statement asks the student to take a break from reading and to reflect on some aspect of the content

just covered. This is not meant to be a question or a summary statement of the preceding content. The end-of-chapter section, Engaging in the Content, includes a number of features to augment student learning. This section expands on features found in the third edition. Discussion Questions, Critical Thinking Activities, and Case Studies provide a variety of methods to examine the chapter content. Some of these may be done by individual students, and others by student teams, either in the classroom or online. The *Electronic Reflection Journal* directs students to develop a log or diary over the course of using the text. The journal can be maintained in students' computers or tablets and updated throughout the course; it can also be expanded as students progress in their nursing program, encouraging them to keep a professional journal for reflection. This process provides students with opportunities to reflect on content, supporting the development of professional self-awareness. Each chapter has two Case Studies with questions. A new feature in this edition is Working Backward to Develop a Case, which allows students to be creative in applying chapter content by using the questions provided to develop a case scenario. Individual students or student teams may develop the case scenario and then exchange the case scenario with other students to use in a traditional case experience—reviewing the scenario and responding to the questions. Above all, this text is patient centered—its content and learning activities for students. Nurses care for and about patients.

Special Note: The Affordable Care Act of 2010 (ACA) is discussed in this text because it has been a major factor in healthcare delivery since 2010. Due to the change in presidential administrations and possible changes in healthcare policy and laws that guide healthcare policy, some of the information in this text about the ACA may change. This is a good example of the need for nurses to remain vigilant to changes in healthcare policy because these changes usually affect nurses and nursing practice.

Information up through June 2017 is accurate, but after this date, the information about ACA may be reflective of past healthcare policy. It is important to understand health policy from past to current policy, and with the ACA and subsequent policy we have a living experience of this need.

Reference

Institute of Medicine. (2003). *Health professions education: A bridge to quality.* Retrieved from http://www.iom.edu/Reports/2003/Health-Professions-Education-A-Bridge-to-Quality.aspx

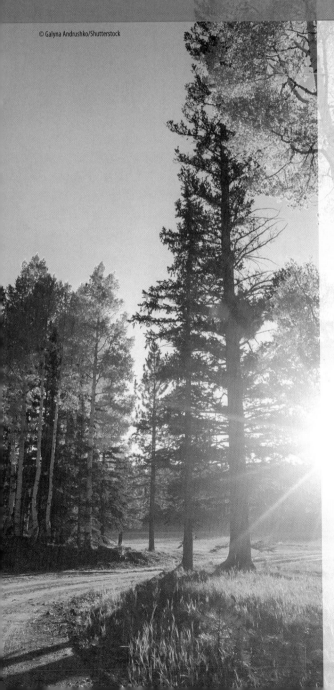

Section 1

The Profession of Nursing

The first section of this text introduces the nursing student to the profession of nursing. The Development of Professional Nursing: History, Development, and the Nursing Profession *chapter reviews the history and development of the nursing profession and what it means for nursing to be a profession. The* Essence of Nursing: Knowledge and Caring *chapter discusses the essence of nursing, focusing on the need for knowledge and caring and how nursing students develop throughout the nursing education program to be knowledgeable, competent, and caring. The* Nursing Education, Accreditation, and Regulation *chapter examines nursing education, accreditation of nursing education programs, and regulation of the practice of nursing. The* Success in Your Nursing Education Program *chapter provides information about the nursing student experience.*

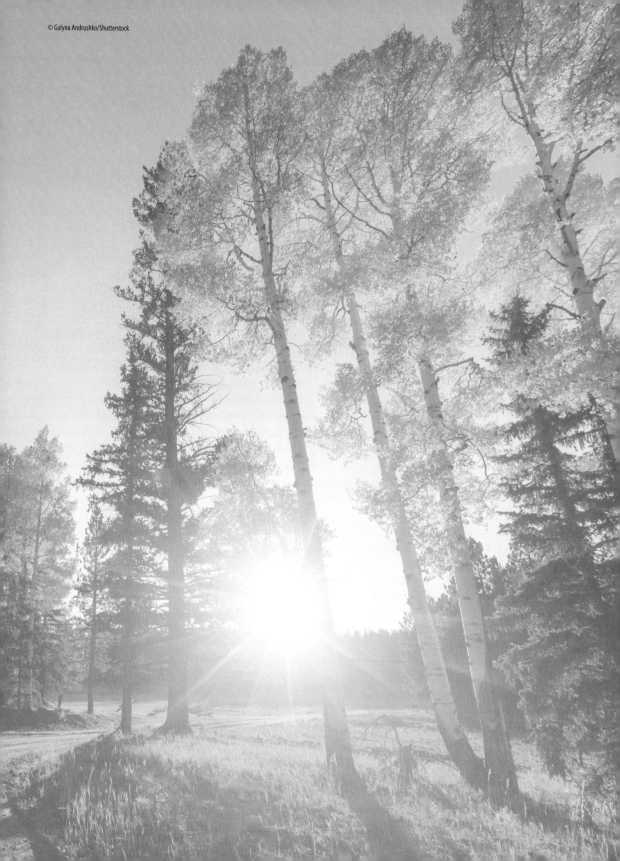

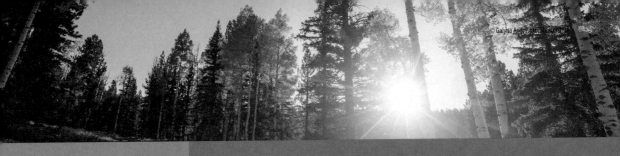

Chapter 1

Professional Nursing: History and Development of the Nursing Profession

CHAPTER OBJECTIVES

At the conclusion of this chapter, the learner will be able to:

- Examine key figures, events in nursing history, and critical nursing historical themes within the sociopolitical context of the time.
- Discuss critical professional concepts, professionalism in nursing, and relevance of

standards and professional organizations to the nursing profession.
- Describe the current and past image of nursing and related critical issues.

CHAPTER OUTLINE

KEY TERMS

Accountability
Autonomy
Code of ethics
Colleagueship

Nursing
Professional organization
Professionalism
Responsibility

Scope of practice
Social policy statement
Standards

Introduction

This text presents an introduction to the nursing profession and critical aspects of nursing care and the delivery of health care. To begin the journey to graduation, licensure, and then practice, it is important to understand several aspects of the nursing profession. What is professional nursing? How did it develop? What factors influence the view of the profession? This chapter addresses these questions.

From Past to Present:
Nursing History

It is important for nursing students to learn about nursing history. Nursing's history provides a framework for understanding how nursing is practiced today and the societal trends shaping the profession. The characteristics of nursing as a profession and what nurses do today have their roots in the past, not only in the history of nursing, but also in the history of health care and society in general. Today, health care is highly complex; diagnostic methods and therapies have been developed that offer many opportunities for prevention, treatment, and cures that did not exist even a few years ago. Understanding this development is part of this discussion; it helps us to appreciate where nursing is today and may provide stimulus for changes in the future. "Nursing is conceptualized as a practice discipline with a mandate from society to enhance the health and well-being of humanity" (Shaw, 1993, p. 1654).

The past portrayal of nurses as handmaidens and assistants to physicians has its roots in the profession's religious beginnings, but over time this view of nurses changed. The following sections examine the story of nursing and explore how it developed as a profession.

The History Surrounding the Development of Nursing as a Profession

When nursing history is described, distinct historical periods typically are discussed: early history (AD 1–500), rise of Christianity and the Middle Ages (500–1500), Renaissance (mid-1300s–1600s), and the Industrial Revolution (mid-1700s–mid-1800s). In addition, the historical perspective must include the different regions and environments in which the historical events took place. Early history focuses on Africa, the Mediterranean, Asia, and the Middle East. The focus then turns to Europe, with the rise of Christianity and subsequent major changes that span several centuries. Nursing history expands as British colonists arrive in America, and a new country and environment helped to slowly develop the nursing profession, which at the time was not a profession. Throughout all these periods and locations, wars had an impact on nursing. As a consequence of the varied places and times in which nursing has existed, major historical events, different cultures and languages, varying views on what constitutes disease and illness, roles of women, political issues, and location and environment have influenced these professions. Nursing has probably existed for as long as humans have been ill; someone always took care of the sick. This does not mean that there was a formal nursing position; rather, in most early cases, the nurse was a woman who cared for ill family members. This discussion begins with this group and then expands to the development and implementation of a formal nursing position and then later to multiple roles and different healthcare settings and recognition of nursing as a profession.

Early History

Early history of nursing focused on the Ancient Egyptians and Hebrews, Greeks, and Romans. During this time, communities often had women who assisted with childbearing as a form of nursing care, and some physicians had assistants. The Egyptians had physicians, and sick persons looking for magical answers would go to them or to priests or sorcerers.

Hebrew (Jewish) physicians kept records and developed a hygiene code that examined issues such as personal and community hygiene, contagion, disinfection, and preparation of food and water (Masters, 2005). This occurred at a time when hygiene was very poor—a condition that continued for several centuries. Disease and disability were viewed as curses and related to sins, which meant that afflicted persons had to change or follow the religious statutes (Bullough & Bullough, 1978).

Greek mythology recognized health issues and physicians in its gods. Hippocrates, a Greek physician, is known as the father of medicine. He contributed to health care by writing a medical textbook that was used for centuries, and he developed an approach to disease that would later be referred to as epidemiology. Hippocrates wrote the Hippocratic Oath (Bullough & Bullough, 1978), which is still recited by new physicians and also influenced the writing of the Nightingale Pledge (see **Exhibit 1-1**). The Greeks viewed health as a balance between body and mind—a different perspective from earlier views of health that focused on curses and sins.

Throughout this entire period, the wounded and ill in the armies required care. Generally, during this period—which represents thousands of years and involved several major cultures that rose and fell—nursing care was provided, but not nursing as it is thought of today. People took care of those who were sick and those going through childbirth, representing an early nursing role.

Rise of Christianity and the Middle Ages

The rise of Christianity led to more structured nursing care, but still it was far from professional nursing. Women continued to carry most of the burden of caring for the poor and the sick. The church set up a system for care that included the role of the deaconess, who provided care in homes. Women who served in these roles had to follow strict rules set by the church. This role eventually evolved into that of nuns, who began to live and work in convents. The convent was considered a safe place for women. The sick came to the convents for nursing care and also received spiritual care (Wall, 2003). The establishment of convents and the nursing care provided there formed the seed for what, hundreds of years later, would become the Catholic system of hospitals that still exists today.

Men were also involved in nursing at this time. For example, men in the Crusades cared for the sick and injured. These men wore large red crosses on their uniforms to distinguish them from the fighting soldiers. The "red cross" later became the symbol for the International Committee of the Red Cross.

Altruism and connecting care to religion were major themes during this period. Even Nightingale continued with these themes in developing her view of nursing. Disease was common and spread quickly, and medical care had little to offer in the way of prevention or cure. Institutions that were called hospitals were not like modern hospitals; they primarily served travelers and sometimes the sick (Kalisch & Kalisch, 1986, 2005).

The Protestant Reformation had a major impact on some of the care given to the sick and injured. The Catholic Church's loss of power in some areas resulted in the closing of hospitals, and some convents closed or moved. The hospitals that remained were no longer staffed by nuns, but rather by women from the lower classes who often had major problems, such as alcoholism or were former prostitutes. This is what Florence Nightingale found when she entered nursing.

Renaissance and the Enlightenment

The Renaissance had a major impact on health and the view of illness. This period was one of significant advancement in science, though by today's standards, it might be viewed as limited. These early discoveries led to advancements that had never been imagined.

This is the period, spanning many years, of Columbus and the French and American Revolutions when education became more important. Leonardo da Vinci's drawings of the human anatomy, which were done to help him understand the human body for his sculptures, provided details that had not been recognized before (Donahue, 1985). The 18th century was a period of many discoveries and changes (Dietz & Lehozky, 1963; Masters, 2005; Rosen, 1958), including the following:

- Jenner's smallpox vaccination method was developed during a time of high death rates from smallpox.
- Psychiatry became a medical specialty area, through the influence of Freud and others.
- The pulse watch and the stethoscope were developed, changing how physical assessment was conducted.
- Pasteur discovered the process of pasteurization, which had an impact on food and milk contamination.
- Lister used some of Pasteur's research and developed approaches to antiseptic surgery; as a result of this work, Lister is known as the father of surgery.
- Koch studied anthrax and cholera, both major diseases of the time, demonstrating that they were transmitted by water, food, and clothing.

- As a result of this work, he became known as the father of microbiology.
- Klebs, Pasteur, Lister, and Koch all contributed to the development of the germ theory.

Industrial Revolution

The Industrial Revolution brought changes in the workplace, but many were not positive from a health perspective. The crowded factories of this era were hazardous and served as breeding grounds for disease. People worked long hours and often under harsh conditions. This was a period of great exploitation of children, particularly those of the lower classes, who were forced to work at very young ages (Masters, 2005). No child labor laws existed, so preteen children often worked in factories alongside adults. Some children were forced to quit school to earn wages to help support their families. Cities were crowded and very dirty, with epidemics erupting about which little could be done. There were few public health laws and services to alleviate the causes.

Colonization of America and the Growth of Nursing in the United States

The initial experiences of nursing in the United States were not much different from those described for Britain and Europe. Nurses were of the lower class and had limited or no training; hospitals were not used by the upper classes, but rather by the lower classes and the poor. Hospitals were dirty and lacked formal care services.

Nursing in the United States did move forward, as described in **Exhibit 1-2** demonstrating nursing activities and changes that occurred over time. Significant steps were taken to improve nursing education and the profession of nursing. The first nursing schools—or, as they were called, training schools—were modeled after Nightingale's school. Some of the earlier schools were in Boston, New York, and Connecticut. The same approach was taken in these schools as in Britain. Stress was placed on moral character and subservience, with efforts to move away from using lower-class women with dubious histories (Masters, 2005). Limitations regarding what women could do on their own continued to be a major problem—for example, women could not vote and had limited rights.

In the early 1900s, this situation began to change when women obtained the right to vote, but only with great effort. The Nurses' Associated Alumnae, established in 1896, was renamed the American Nurses Association (ANA) in 1911. At the same time, the first nursing journal, *American Journal of Nursing* (*AJN*), was created through the ANA. The *AJN* was published until early 2006, when the ANA replaced it with *American Nurse Today* as its official journal. The *AJN*, the oldest U.S. nursing journal, still exists today, but a company that is not associated with ANA publishes it. Its content has always focused on issues facing nurses and their patients. Additional information about significant nursing professional activities is discussed in this chapter and other chapters throughout this text.

Although some nurse leaders were ardent suffragists, Nightingale was not interested in these ideas, even though women in Britain did not have the right to vote. Nightingale felt that the focus should be on allowing (a permissive statement indicative of women's status) women to own property and then linking voting rights to this ownership right (Masters, 2005). There was, however, communication across the ocean between U.S. and British nurses. They did not always agree on the approach to take on the road to professionalism; in fact, nurses did not always agree on this issue within the United States. Nurse leaders and practicing nurses helped nursing to grow into a profession during times of war (American Revolution, Civil War, the Spanish–American War, World War I, World War II, Korean War, Vietnam War, and modern wars today). The website *Experiencing War: Women at War* offers information about some of the nurses who served in these wars, providing nursing care leadership and further developing the nursing profession.

In the 1930s, the Great Depression also had an impact on the nursing field, "resulting in widespread unemployment of private duty nurses and the closing of nursing schools, while simultaneously creating the increasing need for charity health services for the population" (Masters, 2005, p. 28). This meant that there were fewer student nurses to staff the hospitals. As a consequence, nurses were hired, albeit at very low pay, to replace them. Until that time, hospitals had depended on student nurses to staff the hospitals, and nurses who had completed training (term then used for nursing education) served as private-duty nurses in homes. Using students to staff hospitals continued until the university-based nursing effort grew; however, during the Depression, there was a greater need to replace nursing students with nurses when schools closed. On one level, this could be seen as an improvement in care, but the obstacle of low pay was difficult to overcome, resulting in a long history of low pay scales for nurses.

In the 1940s and 1950s, other changes occurred in the U.S. healthcare system that had a direct impact on nursing. Certainly, scientific discoveries were changing care, but important health policy changes occurred as well. The Hill-Burton Act (1946) established federal funds to build more hospitals; as a result of this building boom, at one point in the 1980s, there were too many hospital beds. In turn, many nurses lost their jobs in hospitals because their salaries represented the largest operating expense and there were not enough patients to fill the beds. There is some belief that this decision still affects fluctuating problems of nursing shortage either at the national level or in specific states and healthcare organizations, though its scope has varied over the past few years. When more nurses are needed, some of the nurses who are laid off move into new jobs or careers or leave the workforce so they are not available when the need for nurses increases again. The latter half of the 20th century represented a period of rapid change in healthcare reimbursement due to the growth of health insurance; greater attempts to manage care, particularly to reduce costs; and the establishment of Medicare and Medicaid. Such rapid changes are now being seen again in the 21st century with the passage of the Patient Protection and Affordable Care Act of 2010 (ACA) and possible future changes to this law. During these times, typically more nurses and other healthcare providers are needed. The *Healthcare Delivery System: Focus on Acute Care* chapter discusses some of these issues in more detail. The *Health Policy and Political Action: Critical Actions for Nurses* chapter examines the most significant issue in current healthcare delivery—namely, the ACA. In addition in 1922, 1946, and then in 2010, critical reports were published describing the status of nursing education, as discussed later in this text in content about nursing education.

Little has been said in this description of nursing history about the role of men and minorities in nursing; groups that had limited involvement in the profession's early history. This lack of diversity—men and minorities—has been a long-term problem for the profession. Segregation and discrimination also existed in nursing, just as they did in the society at large. The National Association of Colored Graduate Nurses closed in 1951 when the ANA began to accept African American nurses as members. Nevertheless, concern remains about the limited number of minorities in health care. The Sullivan Commission's report on health profession diversity, *Missing Persons: Minorities in the Health Professions* (L. Sullivan, 2004), is an important document offering recommendations to improve diversity in the health professions. The American Association of Colleges of Nursing (AACN, 2004) responded to this critical report by recommending the following actions:

- Health profession schools should hire diversity program managers and develop strategic plans that outline specific goals, standards, policies, and accountability mechanisms to ensure institutional diversity and cultural competence.

- Colleges and universities should provide an array of support services to minority students, including mentoring, resources for developing test-taking skills, and application counseling.
- Schools of nursing granting baccalaureate degrees should provide and support bridging programs that enable graduates of 2-year colleges to succeed in the transition to 4-year institutions. Graduates of associate degree nursing programs should be encouraged to enroll in baccalaureate nursing programs and supported after they enroll.
- AACN and other health profession organizations should work with schools to promote enhanced admissions policies, cultural competence training, and minority student recruitment.
- To remove financial barriers to nursing education, public and private funding organizations should provide scholarships, loan forgiveness programs, and tuition reimbursement to students and institutions.
- Congress should substantially increase funding for diversity programs within the National Health Service Corps and Titles VII and VIII of the Public Health Service Act.

These recommendations and efforts to improve the number of minorities in all health professions have had some impact, but more improvement is required. This topic also relates to the problem of healthcare disparities, as noted in other chapters.

The number of men in nursing has increased over the years but still is not where it should be. Men served as nurses in the early history period, such as noted earlier in the chapter in the Crusades and monks provided care in monasteries. After this period, however, men were not accepted as nurses because nursing was viewed as a woman's role. The poet Walt Whitman was a nurse in the Civil War. Thus, there were men in nursing, though few, and some were well known—but perhaps not for their nursing (Kalisch & Kalisch, 1986). Early in the history of nursing schools in the United States, men were not accepted. This may have been influenced by the gender-segregated housing for nursing students and the model of apprenticeship that focused on women (Bullough, 2006). In part, this female dominance was also the result of nursing's religious roots, which promoted sisters as nurses. This made it difficult for men to come into the system and the culture—it was a women's profession.

After the major wars—such as World Wars I and II, Korean War, and Vietnam War—medics came home and entered nursing programs, and they continue to do so. In 1940, the ANA did recognize men by having a session on men in nursing at its convention. When schools of nursing began to transition to academic settings, more men applied to nursing programs. Men in nursing have to contend with male-dominated medicine, which has influenced men becoming nurses. There was a time when male nurses were also able to get commissions in the military when women could not, and this increased their numbers in the military (Bullough, 2006). These changes did have an impact, but the increase in salaries and improvement in work conditions had the strongest effect on increasing the number of men in nursing.

In 2001, Boughn conducted a study to explore why women and men choose nursing. The results of this study indicated that female and male participants did not differ in their desire to care for others. Both groups had a strong interest in power and empowerment, but female students were more interested in using their power to empower others, whereas male students were more interested in empowering the profession. The most significant difference was found in the expectations of salary and working conditions, with men expecting more. Why would not both males and females expect higher salaries and better working conditions? Is this still part of the view of nursing and nurses from nursing's past?

Luther Christman was a well-known nurse leader who served as a nurse for many years, retiring at the age of 87, and after retirement, he continued to be an active voice for the profession and for men in nursing until his death in 2011. According to

Sullivan, Christman stated that "men in medicine were reluctant to give up power to women and, by the same token, women in nursing have fought to retain their power. Medicine, however, was forced to admit women after affirmative action legislation was enacted" (2002, p. 10). "Sadly," Christman reported, "nursing, with a majority of women, was not required to adhere to affirmative action policies" (Sullivan, 2002, p. 12). There is an organization for men in nursing, the American Assembly for Men in Nursing (AAMN), and men are also members of other nursing organizations. In 2010, the AAMN began a campaign to increase the number of men in the profession by increasing enrollment of men in nursing programs from current 10% to 20% (American Assembly for Men in Nursing, 2017). The campaign is called "20 $\times$ 20: Choose Nursing."

There is no question that the majority of nurses are White females, and this needs to change. There has been an increase in the number of male and minority nurses, but not enough. There is a greater need to actively seek out more male and minority students (Cohen, 2007). Men and minorities in nursing should reach out and mentor student nurses and new nurses to provide them with the support they require as they enter a profession predominantly composed of White women. More media coverage would also be helpful in publicizing the role of men and minorities in nursing; for example, when photos are distributed to the media, photos should emphasize the diversity of the profession.

Men are a very small percentage of the total number of registered nurses (RNs) living and working in the United States, although their numbers continue to grow (U.S. Department of Health and Human Services [HHS], Health Resources and Services Administration [HRSA], & Bureau of Health Professions [BOHP], 2010). Before 2000, 6.2% of RNs were men; by 2008, this percentage had increased to 9.6%. Male and female RNs are equally likely to have a baccalaureate degree, but male RNs are more likely to also have a non-nursing degree. By 2013, men represented 10.7% of the RN workforce, which was not a major increase from 2008, but an increase nevertheless (Farmer, 2015). The AACN noted that in 2014–2015, enrollment of men in nursing programs improved: 11.8% in baccalaureate programs, 10.8% in master's programs, 9.6% in research-focused doctoral programs (PhD), and 11.7% in doctor of nursing practice (DNP) programs (AACN, 2015a). The AACN also notes that 41% of men in the nursing workforce are in nurse anesthetist positions.

Nurse Leaders: History in the Making

The best place to begin to gain a better understanding of nursing history is with a description of its leaders—that is, the nurses who made a difference to the development of the profession. Florence Nightingale is viewed as the "mother" of modern nursing throughout the world. Most nursing students at some point say the Nightingale Pledge, which helps all new nurses connect the past with the present. The Nightingale Pledge is found in **Exhibit 1-1**. It was composed to provide nurses with an oath similar to the physician's Hippocratic Oath. The oath was not written by Nightingale but emphasized her view of nursing, and it is easy to also see the influence of the culture at the time this was written.

Volumes have been written about Nightingale. She has become the almost-perfect vision of a nurse; however, although Nightingale did much for nursing, many who came after her provided even greater direction for the profession. A focus on Nightingale helps to better understand the major changes that occurred in the profession and in nursing leaders. In 1859, Nightingale wrote, "No man, not even a doctor, ever gives any other definition of what a nurse should be than this—'devoted and obedient.' This definition would do just as well for a porter. It might even do for a horse. It would not do for a policeman" (Nightingale, 1992, p. 20). This quote clearly demonstrates that she was outspoken and held strong beliefs, though she lived during a time when this type of forthrightness from a woman was extraordinary.

Nightingale was British and lived and worked in London in the Victorian era during the Industrial Revolution. During this time, the role of women—especially women of the upper classes—was clearly defined and controlled. During this time, women did not work outside the home and maintained a monitored social existence. Their purpose was to be a wife and a mother, two roles that Nightingale never assumed. Education of women was also limited. With the support of her father, Nightingale did obtain some classical education, but there was never any expectation that she would "use" the education (Slater, 1994). "Nightingale grew up knowing what was expected of her life: Women of her class ran the home and supervised the servants. Although this was

---

Exhibit 1-1 The Original Nightingale Pledge

I solemnly pledge myself before God and in the presence of this assembly, to pass my life in purity and to practice my profession faithfully. I will abstain from whatever is deleterious and mischievous, and will not take or knowingly administer any harmful drug. I will do all in my power to maintain and elevate the standard of my profession, and will hold in confidence all personal matters committed to my keeping and all family affairs coming to my knowledge in the practice of my calling. With loyalty will I endeavor to aid the physician, in his work, and devote myself to the welfare of those committed to my care.

Composed by Lystra Gretter in 1893 for the class graduating from Harper Hospital, Detroit, Michigan.

not her goal, the household management skills that she learned from her mother were put to good use when she entered the hospital environment. Because of her social standing, she was in the company of educated and influential men, and she learned the "art of influencing powerful men" (Slater, 1994, p. 143). This skill was used a great deal by Nightingale as she fought for reforms.

Nightingale held different views about the women of her time. She had "a strong conviction that women have the mental abilities to achieve whatever they wish to achieve: compose music, solve scientific problems, create social projects of great importance" (Chinn, 2001, p. 441). She felt that women should question their assigned roles, and she herself wanted to serve people. When she reached her 20s, Nightingale felt an increasing desire to help others and decided that she wanted to become a nurse. Nurses at that time came from the lower classes, and, of course, any training for this type of role was out of the question. Her parents refused to support her goal, and because women were not free to make this type of decision by themselves, she was blocked. Nightingale became angry and then depressed. When her depression worsened, her parents finally relented and allowed her to attend nurse's training in Germany. This venture was kept a secret, and people she knew were told that she was away at a spa for 3 months' rest (Slater, 1994). Nightingale was also educated in math and science, which would lead her to use statistics to demonstrate the nurse's impact on health outcomes. Had it not been for her social standing and her ability to obtain some education, coupled with her friendship with Dr. Elizabeth Blackwell, nurses might well have remained uneducated assistants to doctors, at least for a longer period of time than they did.

An important fact about Nightingale is that she was very religious—to the point that she felt God had called on her to help others (Woodham-Smith, 1951). She also felt that the body and mind were separate entities, but both needed to be considered from a health standpoint. This view later served

as the basis of nursing's holistic view of health. Nightingale's convictions also influenced her views of nurses and nursing practice. She viewed patients as persons who were unable to help themselves or who were dying. She is quoted as saying, "What nursing has to do . . . is to put the patient in the best condition for nature to act upon him" (Seymer, 1954, p. 13). Nightingale also recognized that a patient's health depends on environmental factors such as light, noise, odors, and heat—something that we examine more closely today in nursing and in health care by also using alternative and complementary methods. In her work during the Crimean War, she applied her beliefs about the body and mind by arranging activities for the soldiers, providing them with classes and books, and supporting their connection with home—an early version of what is now often called holistic care. Later, this type of focus on the total patient became an integral part of psychiatric–mental health nursing and then nursing in general. Nightingale's other interest—in sanitary reform—also grew from her experience in the Crimean War. She worked with influential men to make changes. Although she did not agree with some of the new theories, she did support the value of education in improving social problems and believed that education should also include moral, physical, and practical aspects (Widerquist, 1997). Later, nurses based more of their interventions on science and evidence-based practice.

The many important discoveries noted earlier such as the work done by Lister and Pasteur had an impact on nursing over the long term and changed the sociopolitical climate of health care—for example, public health policy and services. Nightingale, however, did not agree with the new theory of contagion, but over time, the nursing profession accepted these new theories, which remain critical components of patient care today. Nightingale stressed, however, that the mind–body connection—putting patients in the best situation for healing—ultimately made the difference. Discovering methods for preventing disease and using this information in disease prevention is an important part of nursing today. Public/community health is certainly concerned with many of the same issues that led to critical new discoveries so many years ago, such as contamination of food and water and preventing disease worldwide.

During the Industrial Revolution, Nightingale and enlightened citizens tried to reform some of working conditions that were leading to health and public problems. Indeed, as Nightingale stated in *Notes on Nursing* and *Notes on Hospitals* (1992, 1859), "there are five essential points in securing the health of houses: pure air, pure water, efficient drainage, cleanliness, and light." She strongly supported more efforts to promote health and felt that this was more cost-effective than treating illness—important healthcare principles today. These ideas are good examples reflecting the influence of the environment and culture in which a person lives and works on personal views and problems.

Nightingale wrote four small books—or treatises, as they were called—thus starting the idea that nurses need to publish and share what they do and what they learn about patient care. The titles of the books were *Notes on Matters Affecting the Health, Efficiency, and Hospital Administration of the British Army* (1858a), *Subsidiary Notes as to the Introduction of Female Nursing into Military Hospitals* (1858b), *Notes on Hospitals* (1859), and *Notes on Nursing* (1860, republished in 1992). The first three focused on hospitals that she visited, including military hospitals (Slater, 1994). Nightingale collected a lot of data. Her interest in healthcare data analysis helped to lay the groundwork for epidemiology, highlighting the importance of data in nursing, particularly in a public health context, and also established an initial foundation for nursing research and evidence-based practice. These early initiatives also relate to the current quality improvement efforts requiring measurement and analysis of large quantities of data. An interesting fact is that *Notes on Nursing* was not written for nurses, but rather for women who cared for ill family members. As late as 1860, Nightingale had not completely given up

on the idea of care provided by women as a form of service to family and friends. This text was popular when it was published because, at the time, family members provided most of the nursing care.

Nightingale's religious and upper-class background had a major impact on her important efforts to improve both nursing education and nursing practice in the hospital setting. Nurses were of the lower class; usually had no education; and were often alcoholics, prostitutes, and women who were down on their luck. Nightingale changed all that. She believed that patients needed educated nurses to care for them, and she founded the first organized school of nursing. Nightingale's school, which opened in London in 1860, accepted women of a higher class—not alcoholics and former prostitutes, as had been the case with previous generations of nurses. The students were not viewed as servants, and their loyalty was to the school, not to the hospital. This point is somewhat confusing and must be viewed from the perspective that important changes were made; however, these were not monumental changes, but a beginning. For example, even in Nightingale's school, students were very much a part of the hospital; they staffed the hospital, representing free labor and worked long hours. This approach developed into the diploma school model, considered an apprenticeship model. Today, diploma schools have less direct relationships with hospitals, and in some cases, they have transitioned to associate degree programs and, in other cases, baccalaureate degrees. There are few schools of nursing today that are diploma schools (see the *Nursing Education, Accreditation, and Regulation* chapter).

Nightingale's students did receive some training, which had not been provided in an organized manner prior to her efforts. Her religious views also had an impact on the rigid educational system she proposed and implemented. She expected students to have high moral values. Training was still based on an apprenticeship model and continued to be for some time in Britain, Europe, and the United States. The structure of hospital nursing was also very rigid, with a matron in charge. This rigidity persisted for decades and, in some cases, may still be present in some hospital nursing organizations.

Nurses in Britain began to recognize the need to band together, and they eventually formed the British Nurses Association. This organization took on the issue of regulating nursing practice. Nightingale did not approve of efforts made to establish state registration (licensure) of nurses, mostly because she did not trust the leaders' goals (Freeman, 2007). There were no known standards for nursing, so how one became a registered nurse was unclear. Many questions were raised regarding the definition of nursing, who should be registered, and who controlled nursing. Some critics agree that Nightingale did make changes, but the way she made the changes also had negative effects, including delaying the development of the profession (particularly supporting nurses' subordinate position to physicians), failing to encourage nursing education offered at a university level, and delaying licensure (Freeman, 2007). Despite this criticism, Nightingale still holds an important place in nursing history as a major leader for the profession.

The vignettes in **Exhibit 1-2** describe some of the contributions made by nursing leaders, emphasizing that Nightingale is not the only important nursing leader. People do not operate in a vacuum, of course, and neither did the nurses highlighted in this exhibit. Many factors influenced nurse leaders, such as their communities, the society, their education, and the time in which they practiced.

Exhibit 1-2 A Glimpse into the Contributions of Nurses in the United States

This list does not represent all the important nursing leaders but does provide examples of the broad range of their contributions and highlights specific achievements. These glimpses are written in the first person, but they are not direct quotes.

Dorothea Dix (1840–1841)

I traveled the state of Massachusetts to call attention to the present state of insane persons confined within this Commonwealth, in cages, stalls, pens! Chained, naked, beaten with rods, and lashed into obedience. Just by bettering the conditions for these persons, I showed that mental illnesses aren't all incurable.

Linda Richards (1869)

I was the first of five students to enroll in the New England Hospital for Women and Children and the first to graduate. Upon graduation, I was fortunate to obtain employment at the Bellevue Hospital in New York City. Here I created the first written reporting system, charting and maintaining individual patient records.

Clara Barton (1881)

The need in America for an institution that is not selfish must originate in the recognition of some evil is adding to the sum of human suffering or diminishing the sum of happiness. Today, my efforts to organize such an institution have been successful: the National Society of the Red Cross.

Isabel Hampton Robb (1896)

In 1896, I organized the Nurses' Associated Alumnae of the United States and Canada and served as the first president. Later this organization became the American Nurses Association (ANA). I also founded the American Society of Superintendents of Training Schools for Nurses, which later became the National League of Nursing Education (NLNE) and then changed its name to the National League for Nursing (NLN). Through these professional organizations, I was able to initiate many improvements in nursing education.

(Continues)

Exhibit 1-2 *(continued)*

Sophia Palmer (1900)

I launched the *American Journal of Nursing* and served as editor-in-chief of the journal for 20 years. I believe my forceful editorials helped guide nursing thought and shape nursing practice and events.

Lavinia L. Dock (1907)

I became a staunch advocate of legislation to control nursing practice. Realizing the problems that students faced in studying drugs and solutions, I wrote one of the first nursing textbooks, *Materia Medica for Nurses*. I served as foreign editor of *American Journal of Nursing* and coauthored the book, *The History of Nursing*.

Martha Minerva Franklin (1908)

I actively campaigned for racial equality in nursing and guided 52 nurses to form the National Association of Colored Graduate Nurses.

Mary Mahoney (1909)

In 1908, the National Association of Colored Graduate Nurses was formed. As the first professional Black nurse, I gave the welcome address at the organization's first conference.

Mary Adelaide Nutting (1910)

I advocated for university education for nurses and developed the first program of this type. Upon accepting the chairmanship at the Department of Nursing Education at Teachers College, Columbia University, I became the first nurse to be appointed to a university professorship.

Lillian Wald (1918)

My goal was to ensure that women and children, immigrants and the poor, and members of all ethnic and religious groups would realize America's promise of life, liberty, and the pursuit of happiness. The Henry Street Settlement and the Visiting Nurse Service in New York City championed public health nursing, housing reform, suffrage, world peace, and the rights of women, children, immigrants, and working people.

Mary Breckenridge (1920)

Through my own personal tragedies, I realized that medical care for mothers and babies in rural America was needed. I started the Frontier Nursing Service in Kentucky.

Elizabeth Russell Belford, Mary Tolle Wright, Edith Moore Copeland, Dorothy Garrigus Adams, Ethel Palmer Clarke, Elizabeth McWilliams Miller, and Marie Hippensteel Lingeman (1922)

We were the founders of the Sigma Theta Tau International Honor Society of Nursing. Each of us provided insights that advanced scholarship, leadership, research, and practice.

Susie Walking Bear Yellowtail (1930–1960)

I traveled for 30 years throughout North America, walking to reservations to improve health care and Indian health services. I established the Native ANA and received the President's Award for Outstanding Nursing Healthcare.

Virginia Avenel Henderson (1939)

I am referred to as the first lady of nursing. I think of myself as an author, an avid researcher, and a visionary. One of my greatest contributions to the nursing profession was revising Harmer's *Textbook of the Principles and Practice of Nursing*, which has been widely adopted by schools of nursing.

Lucile Petry Leone (1943)

As the founder of the U.S. Cadet Nurse Corps, I believe we succeeded because we had a saleable package from the beginning. Women immediately liked the idea of being able to combine war service with professional education for the future.

Exhibit 1-2 *(continued)*

Esther Lucille Brown (1946)

I issued a report titled *Nursing for the Future*. This report severely criticized the overall quality of nursing education. Thus, with the Brown report, nursing education finally began the long-discussed move to accreditation of nursing education programs.

Lydia Hall (1963–1969)

I established and directed the Loeb Center for Nursing and Rehabilitation at Montefiore Hospital in the Bronx, New York. Through my research in nursing and long-term care, I developed a theory (core, care, and cure) that the direct professional nurse-to-patient relationship is itself therapeutic and nursing care is the chief therapy for the chronically ill patient.

Martha Rogers (1963–1965)

I served as editor of *Journal of Nursing Science*, focusing my attention on improving and expanding nursing education, developing the scientific basis of nursing practice through professional education, and differentiating between professional and technical careers in nursing. My book, *An Introduction to the Theoretical Basis of Nursing* (1970), marked the beginning of nursing's search for a theoretical base. Later, my work led to a greater emphasis on research and evidence-based practice.

Loretta Ford (1965)

I co-developed the first nurse practitioner program in 1965 by integrating the traditional roles of the nurse with advanced medical training and the community outreach mission of a public health official.

Madeleine Leininger (1974)

I began, and continued to guide, nursing in the recognition that the culture care needs of people in the world will be met by nurses prepared in transcultural nursing.

Florence Wald (1975)

I devoted my life to the compassionate care for the dying. I founded Hospice Incorporated in Connecticut, which is the model for hospice care in the United States and abroad.

Joann Ashley (1976)

I wrote *Hospitals, Paternalism, and the Role of the Nurse* during the height of the women's movement. My book created controversy with its pointed condemnation of sexism toward, and exploitation of, nurses by hospital administrators and physicians.

Luther Christman (1980)

As founder and dean of the Rush University College of Nursing, I was linked to the "Rush Model," a unified approach to nursing education and practice that continues to set new standards of excellence. As dean of Vanderbilt University's School of Nursing, I was the first to employ African American women as faculty at Vanderbilt University, and I became one of the founders of the National Male Nurses Association, now known as the American Assembly for Men in Nursing.

Hildegard E. Peplau (1997)

I became known as the "Nurse of the Century." I was the first nurse to serve the ANA as executive director and later as president, and I served two terms on the Board of the International Council of Nurses. My work in psychiatric–mental health nursing emphasized the nurse–patient relationship.

Linda Aiken (2007)

My policy research agenda is motivated by a commitment to improving healthcare outcomes building an evidence base for health services care and management and providing direction for national policy makers, resulting in greater recognition of the role that nursing care has on patient outcomes. Nurses need to be actively engaged in research to improve care.

Patricia Benner (current)

I have long been involved in nursing education and developed many initiatives to improve nursing education and thus nursing

(Continues)

Exhibit 1-2 *(continued)*

practice. In 1982, I published a major book that discussed the process that nurses go through from novice to expert. In 2010, I led an extensive study on the current status of nursing education, the first such study since the 1922 Goldmark report and the 1948 Brown report. My report, *Educating Nurses: A Call for Radical Transformation* (2010), noted many areas of nursing education that need improvement.

Beatrice Kalisch and Phillip Kalisch (current)

We have worked together to recognize the importance of the image of nursing as a profession. In doing this, we have examined the many roles of nurses and issues that impact their work, such as workforce shortages. In our examination we have included different media as sources such as films, television, fiction, and press coverage. The profession should not ignore its professional image.

National Academy of Nursing Living Legends

The National Academy of Nursing selects exemplar nursing leaders for recognition of their leadership in health care in the United States and globally. The organization's website provides information on these leaders and their contributions.

Themes: Looking into the Nursing Profession's History

The discipline of nursing slowly evolved from the traditional role of women, apprenticeship, humanitarian aims, religious ideals, intuition, common sense, trial and error, theories, and research and was influenced by medicine, technology, politics, social issues, war, economics, and feminism (Brooks & Kleine-Kracht, 1983; Gorenberg, 1983; Keller, 1979; Jacobs & Huether, 1978; Kidd & Morrison, 1988; Lynaugh & Fagin, 1988; Perry, 1985). It is impossible to provide a detailed history of nursing's evolution in one chapter, so only critical historical events are discussed.

Writing about nursing history itself has its own interesting history (Connolly, 2004). Historians who wrote about nursing prior to the 1950s tended to be nurses, and they wrote for nurses. Although nursing throughout its history has been influenced by social issues of the day, the early publications about nursing history did not link nursing to "the broader social, economic, and cultural context in which events unfolded" but, instead, emphasized the "profession's purity, discipline, and faith" (Connolly, 2004, p. 10). Part of the reason for this narrow view of nursing history is that the discipline of history had limited, if any, contact with the nursing profession. This began to change in the 1950s and 1960s, when the scholarship of nursing history began to expand, though very slowly. In the 1970s, one landmark publication, *Hospitals, Paternalism, and the Role of the Nurse* (Ashley, 1976), addressed social issues as an important aspect of nursing history. The key issue considered in this text was feminism in the society at large and its impact on nursing. As social history became more important, increased examination of nursing, its history, and influences on that history took place. In addition, nursing is tied to political history today. For example, it is very difficult to understand current healthcare delivery concerns without including nursing (such as the impact of the current reports on quality care). All of these considerations have an impact on health policy, including legislation at the state and national levels.

Schools of nursing often highlight their own history for students, faculty, and visitors. This might be done through exhibits about the school's history and, in some cases, a mini-museum. Such materials provide an opportunity to identify how the school's history has developed and how its graduates have affected the community and the profession. The purpose of this chapter is to explore some of the broad issues of nursing history, but this discussion should not replace the history of each school of nursing as the profession developed.

Nursing's past represents a movement from a role based on family and religious ties and the need to provide comfort and care (because this was perceived as a woman's lot in life) to educated professionals serving as the "glue" that holds the healthcare system together. From medieval times through Nightingale's time, nursing represented a role that women played in families to provide care. This care extended to anyone in need, but after Nightingale highlighted what a woman could do with some degree of education, physicians/doctors recognized that women needed to have some degree of training. Education was introduced, but mainly to serve the need of hospitals to have a labor force. Thus, the apprenticeship model of nursing was born.

Why would nursing perceive a need for greater education? Primarily because of advances in science, increased knowledge of germs and diseases, and increased training of doctors, nurses needed to understand basic anatomy, physiology, pathophysiology, and epidemiology to provide better care. Slowly it was recognized that to carry out doctors' orders efficiently, nurses required some degree of understanding of causes and effects of environmental exposures and of disease causation. Thus, the move from hospital nursing schools to university education occurred.

Critics of Nightingale suggest that although the "lady with the lamp" image—that is, a nurse with a light moving among the wounded in the Crimea—is laudable, it presented the nurse as a caring, take-charge person who would go to great lengths and even sacrifice her own safety and health to provide care (Shames, 1993). The message sent to the public was that nurses were not powerful. They were caring, but they would not fight to change the conditions of hospitals and patient care. Hospitals "owned" nurses and considered them cheap labor. Today, some hospitals still hold the same view, though they would never admit it publicly. This view of healthcare delivery suggests that doctors are defined by their scope of practice in treating diseases, whereas nurses are seen as promoting health, adding to the view of the lesser status of nursing (Shames, 1993). This view also has led to problems between the two professions as they argue over which profession is better at caring for patients. The view that nurses are angels of mercy rather than well-educated professionals reinforces the idea that nurses care but really do not have to think; this view may be perpetuated by advertisements that depict nurses as angels or caring ethereal humans (Gordon, 2005). Most patients—especially at 3 a.m., when few other professionals are available—hope that the nurse is not just a caring person, but also a critical thinker who uses clinical reasoning and judgment and knows when to call the rest of the team. As discussed in this text, there is increasing evidence to support this view of the professional nurse and needed competencies, such as the report *Healthcare Education: A Bridge to Quality* (Institute of Medicine [IOM], 2003) and *The Future of Nursing. Leading Change, Advancing Health* (IOM, 2010). These reports and others have had a major impact on the image of the profession and provide recommendations for improving care and the roles and responsibilities of nurses as healthcare professionals and emphasize the need for nursing leadership and graduate education.

Stop and Consider #1

Nursing has existed a long time but in many different forms.

Professionalism:

Critical Professional Concepts and Activities

Today, nursing is an applied science, a practice profession. To appreciate the relevance of this statement requires an understanding of **professionalism** and how it applies to nursing. Nursing is more than just a job; it is a professional career requiring commitment. **Table 1-1** describes some differences in attitudes when comparing an occupation/job and a career/profession.

But what does this really mean, and why does it matter? As described previously in this chapter, getting to where the nursing profession is today was not easy, nor did it happen overnight. Many nurses contributed to the development of nursing as a profession; it mattered to them that nurses be recognized as professionals.

Nursing as a Profession

The current definition of **nursing**, as established by the ANA is "the protection, promotion, and optimization of health and abilities, prevention of illness and injury, alleviation of suffering through the diagnosis and treatment of human response, and advocacy in the care of individuals, families, communities, and populations" (2015a, p. 89). **Exhibit 1-3** provides a historical perspective on the development of a definition for nursing.

The Essence of Nursing: Knowledge and Caring chapter contains a more in-depth discussion of the nature of nursing, but a definition is needed here as a framework for further understanding of nursing as a profession. Is nursing a profession? What is a profession? Why is it important that nursing be recognized as a profession? Some nurses may not think that nursing is a profession, but this is not the position taken by recognized nursing organizations,

Table 1-1 Comparison of Attitudes: Occupation Versus Career

	Occupation	Career
Longevity	Temporary, a means to an end	Lifelong vocation
Educational preparation	Minimal training required, usually associate degree	University professional degree program based on foundation of core liberal arts
Continuing education	Only what is required for the job or to get a raise/promotion	Lifelong learning, continual effort to gain new knowledge, skills, and abilities
Level of commitment	Short-term, as long as job meets personal needs	Long-term commitment to organization and profession
Expectations	Reasonable work for reasonable pay; responsibility ends with shift	Will assume additional responsibilities and volunteer for organizational activities and community-based events

Reproduced from Wilfong, D., Szolis, C., & Haus, C. (2007). *Nursing school success: Tools for constructing your future.* Sudbury, MA: Jones & Bartlett Learning.

Exhibit 1-3 Definitions of Nursing: Historical Perspective

The following list provides a timeline of some of the definitions of nursing.

Florence Nightingale

Having "charge of the personal health of somebody . . . and what nursing has to do . . . is to put the patient in the best possible condition for nature to act upon him." (Nightingale, 1859, p. 79)

Virginia Henderson

"The unique function of the nurse is to assist the individual, sick or well, in the performance of those activities contributing to health or its recovery (or to peaceful death) and that he would perform unaided if he had the necessary strength, will or knowledge. And to do this in such a way as to help him gain independence as rapidly as possible." (Henderson, 1966, p. 21)

Martha Rogers

"The process by which this body of knowledge, nursing science, is used for the purpose of assisting human beings to achieve maximum health within the potential of each person." (Rogers, 1988, p. 100)

American Nurses Association

"Nursing is the protection, promotion, and optimization of health and abilities, prevention of illness and injury, facilitation of healing, alleviation of suffering through the diagnosis and treatment of human responses, and advocacy in the care of individuals, families, communities, and populations." (ANA, 2015b, p. 89; also published in earlier ANA standards)

International Council of Nursing

"Nursing encompasses autonomous and collaborative care of individuals of all ages, families, groups and communities, sick or well and in all settings. Nursing includes the promotion of health, prevention of illness, and the care of ill, disabled and dying people. Advocacy, promotion of a safe environment, research, participation in shaping health policy and in patient and health systems management, and education are also key nursing roles." (ICN, 2002)

Data from Nightingale, F. (1859). *Notes on nursing: What it is and what it is not* (commemorative ed.). Philadelphia, PA: Lippincott; Henderson, V. (1966). *The nature of nursing: A definition and its implications for practice, research, and education.* New York, NY: Macmillan; Rogers, M. (1988). Nursing science and art: A prospective. *Nursing Science Quarterly, 1,* 99; American Nurses Association. (2015). *Nursing scope and standards of practice.* Silver Spring, MD: Author; International Council of Nurses. (2002; retrieved on 2017). Definition of nursing. Retrieved from http://www.icn.ch/who-we-are/icn-definition-of-nursing/

nursing education, and state boards of nursing that are involved in licensure of nurses. Each state has its own definition of nursing that is found in the state's nurse practice act, but the ANA definition noted here encompasses the common characteristics of nursing practice and is reflected in state board definitions.

In general, a profession—whether nursing or another profession, such as medicine, teaching, or law—has certain characteristics (Finkelman, 2016; Huber, 2014; Lindberg, Hunter, & Kruszewski, 1998; Quinn & Smith, 1987; Schein & Kommers, 1972; Bixler & Bixler, 1959):

- A systematic body of knowledge that provides the framework for the profession's practice
- Standardized, formal higher education
- Commitment to providing a service that benefits individuals and the community
- Maintenance of a unique role that recognizes autonomy, responsibility, and accountability

- Control of practice responsibility of the profession through standards and a code of ethics
- Commitment to members of the profession through professional organizations and activities

Does nursing demonstrate these professional characteristics? Nursing has a standardized content, although schools of nursing may configure the content in different ways; there is consistency in content areas such as adult health, maternal–child health, behavioral or mental health, pharmacology, assessment, and so on. The National Council Licensure Examination (NCLEX) covers standardized content areas. This content is based on systematic, recognized knowledge as the profession's knowledge base for practice. The *Nursing Education, Accreditation, and Regulation* chapter discusses nursing education in more detail. It is clear, though, that the focus of nursing is practice—care provided to assist individuals, families, communities, and populations.

Nursing as a profession has a social contract with society, as described in the ANA's *Nursing's Social Policy Statement*, which is now an appendix in the ANA standards, *Nursing: Scope and Standards of Practice*, and *Nursing's* **Code of Ethics** (American Nurses Association [ANA], 2015a, 2015b; Fowler, 2015a, 2015b). The contract between nursing and society is based on professional and regulatory requirements, but also on what society expects from healthcare services and healthcare professionals. As a profession, we have the right to autonomy in our practice, authority to practice based on our education and scope of practice, and self-governance. Society protects a profession through government legislation and regulation (for example, licensure to protect our titles and scope of practice, need to decrease staff safety risk in the workplace, and so on).

Autonomy, **responsibility**, and **accountability** are intertwined with the practice of nursing and are critical components of a profession. Autonomy is the "capacity of a nurse to determine his/her own actions through independent choice, including demonstration of competence, within the full scope

of nursing practice" (ANA, 2015a, p. 85). It is the right to make a decision and take control. Nurses have a distinct body of knowledge and develop competencies in nursing care that should be based on this nursing knowledge. When this is accomplished, nurses can then practice nursing. "Responsibility refers to being entrusted with a particular function" (Ritter-Teitel, 2002, p. 34). "Accountability means being responsible and accountable to self and others for behaviors and outcomes included in one's professional role. A professional nurse is accountable for embracing professional values, maintaining professional values, maintaining competence, and maintenance and improvement of professional practice environments" (Kupperschmidt, 2004, p. 114). A nurse is also accountable for the outcomes of the nursing care that the nurse provides; what nurses do must mean something (Finkelman, 2016). The nurse is answerable for the actions that the nurse takes. Accountability and responsibility do not have the same meaning. A nurse often delegates tasks to other staff members, telling staff what to do and when. The staff member who is assigned a task is *responsible* both for performing that task and for the performance itself. The nurse who delegated the task to the staff person is *accountable* for the decision to delegate the task. Delegation is discussed in more detail in the *Work in Interprofessional Teams* chapter.

Sources of Professional Direction

Professions develop documents or statements about what the members consider is important to guide their practice, to establish control over practice, and to influence the quality of that practice. Some of the important sources of professional direction for nurses follow:

1. *Nursing's Social Policy Statement* (ANA, 2015a) is an important document that describes the profession of nursing and its professional framework and obligations to society. The original 1980 statement has been revised three times—in 1995,

2003, and 2010. The **social policy statement** informs consumers, government officials, other healthcare professionals, and other important stakeholders about nursing and its definition, knowledge base, scope of practice, and regulation. "Nursing is called a helping profession and many of us went into nursing to help others. The social policy statement of our profession is about the multiple ways in which nursing helps others: through direct patient care, and by changing institutions, society, and global health. Nurses can be civic professionals and cosmopolite professionals and be active in any *or* all of these ways of helping between here and nursing's furthest horizon, and to find good colleagues and companions along the way" (Fowler, 2015a, p. xv).

2. *Nursing: Scope and Standards of Practice* (ANA, 2015a) was developed by the ANA and its members; however, these standards as is true for other ANA professional documents apply to all registered nurses. Nursing **standards**, which are "authoritative statements defined and promoted by the profession by which the quality of practice, service, or education can be evaluated" (ANA, 2015a, p. 89), are critical to guiding quality patient care. Standards describe minimal expectations. "We must always remember that as a profession the members are granted the privilege of self-regulation because they purport to use standards to monitor and evaluate the actions of its members to ensure a positive impact on the public it serves" (O'Rourke, 2003, p. 97). Standards also include a **scope of practice** statement that describes the "who, what, where, when, why, and how" of nursing practice. The ANA definition of nursing is the critical foundation. As noted in **Exhibit 1-3**, the definition of nursing evolved and will most likely continue to evolve over time as healthcare needs change and healthcare delivery and practice evolve. Nursing knowledge and the integration of science and art, which

are discussed in more detail in *The Essence of Nursing: Knowledge and Caring* chapter, are part of the scope of practice, along with the definition of the "what and why" of nursing. Nursing care is provided in a variety of settings by the professional registered nurse, who may have an advanced degree and specialty training and expertise. Additional information about the standards, as well as the nurse's roles and functions, is found throughout this text. Part of being a professional is a commitment to the profession—a commitment to lifelong learning, adhering to standards, maintaining membership in professional organizations, publishing, and ensuring that nursing care is of the highest quality possible.

3. *Code of Ethics for Nurses* (ANA, 2015b) describes nursing's central beliefs and assists the profession in controlling its practice. This code "makes explicit the primary obligations, values, and ideals of the profession. In fact, it informs every aspect of the nurse's life" (ANA, 2015a, p. vii). Implementation of this code is an important part of nursing's contract with society. As nurses practice, they need to reflect these values. The *Ethics and Legal Issues* chapter focuses on ethical and legal issues related to nursing practice and describes the code in more detail.

To go full circle and return to the social contract, nursing care must be provided and should include consideration of health, social, cultural, economic, legislative, and ethical factors. Content related to these issues is discussed in other chapters in this text. Nursing is not just about making someone better; it is about providing health education, assisting patients and families in making health decisions, providing direct care and supervising others who provide care, assessing care and applying the best evidence in making care decisions, communicating and working with the interprofessional treatment team, developing a plan of care with the team that includes the patient and family when the patient agrees to family participation, evaluating patient outcomes, advocating for patients, and much more.

The *Apply Quality Improvement* chapter discusses quality care in more detail, but as the student becomes more oriented to nursing education and nursing as a profession, it is important to recognize that establishing and maintaining standards is part of being in a profession. The generic standards and their measurement criteria, which apply to all nurses, are divided into two types of standards: standards of practice and standards of professional performance. The major content areas of the standards follow (ANA, 2015a).

Standards of Practice (competent level of practice based on the nursing process)

1. Assessment
2. Diagnosis
3. Outcomes identification
4. Planning
5. Implementation (coordination of care, health teaching and health promotion, consultation, and prescriptive authority)
6. Evaluation

Standards of Professional Performance (competent level of behavior in the professional role)

1. Ethics
2. Culturally congruent practice
3. Communication
4. Collaboration
5. Leadership
6. Education
7. Evidence-based practice and research
8. Quality of practice
9. Professional practice evaluation
10. Resource utilization
11. Environmental health*

Nursing specialty groups—in some cases, in partnership with the ANA—have developed specialty standards, such as those for cardiovascular nursing, neonatal nursing, and nursing informatics. However, all nurses must meet the generic standards regardless of their specialty.

State boards of nursing also assume an important role in guiding and, in some cases, determining professional direction through legislation. Each state board operates under a state practice act, which allows the state government to meet its responsibility to protect the public—in this case, the health of the public—through nursing licensure requirements. Each nurse must practice, or meet the description of, nursing as identified in the state in which the nurse practices. Regulation is discussed in more detail in the *Nursing Education, Accreditation, and Regulation* chapter.

Professional Nursing Associations

Nurses have a history of involvement in organizations that foster the goals of the profession. The existence of professional associations and organizations is one of the characteristics of a profession. A **professional organization** is a group that has specific goals, objectives, and functions that relate to the mission of a specific profession. Typically, membership is open to members of that profession and requires payment of dues. Some organizations have more specific membership requirements or may be by invitation only. Nursing has many organizations at the local, state, national, and international levels, and some organizations function on all of these levels.

Professional organizations often publish journals and other information related to the profession and offer continuing education opportunities through meetings, conferences, and other formats. As discussed previously, many of the organizations, particularly ANA, have been involved in developing professional standards. Professional education is a key function of many organizations. Some organizations are very active in policy decisions at the government level, taking political action to ensure that the profession's goals are addressed and advocating for health care in general. This activity is generally done through lobbying and advocacy. Some of the organizations are involved in advocacy in the work environment, for example, a union, with the aim of making the workplace environment better for nurses.

Major Nursing Associations

The following description highlights some of the major nursing organizations (keep in mind that many other professional organizations exist). Organizations that focus on nursing specialties have expanded. Other organizations related to nursing education are described in the *Nursing Education, Accreditation, and Regulation* chapter. To give you a perspective of the many organizations representing different aspects of the profession **Exhibit 1-4** lists some of these organizations and their websites.

American Nurses Association. The ANA is the organization that represents all RNs in the United States, but not all RNs belong to the ANA. The ANA also represents nurses who are not members because many in healthcare, government, and business

---

Exhibit 1-4 Specialty Nursing Organizations

Academy of Medical–Surgical Nurses: http://www.medsurgnurse.org

Academy of Neonatal Nursing: http://www.academyonline.org

American Academy of Ambulatory Care Nursing, http://www.aaacn.org

American Academy of Nurse Practitioners: http://www.aanp.org

American Academy of Nursing: http://www.aannet.org

American Assembly for Men in Nursing: http://aamn.org

American Association for the History of Nursing: http://www.aahn.org

American Association of Colleges of Nursing: http://www.aacn.nche.edu

American Association of Critical-Care Nurses: http://www.aacn.org

American Association of Legal Nurse Consultants: http://www.aalnc.org

American Association of Neuroscience Nurses: http://www.aann.org

American Association of Nurse Anesthetists: http://www.aana.com

American Association of Nurse Attorneys: http://www.taana.org

American Association of Occupational Health Nurses: http://www.aaohn.org

American College of Nurse–Midwives: http://www.midwife.org

American College of Nurse Practitioners: http://www.acnpweb.org

American Holistic Nurses' Association: http://www.ahna.org

American Nephrology Nurses' Association: http://www.annanurse.org

American Nurses Association: http://www.nursingworld.org

American Nurses Foundation: http://www.anfonline.org

American Nursing Informatics Association: http://www.ania.org

American Organization of Nurse Executives: http://www.aone.org

American Psychiatric Nurses Association: http://www.apna.org

American Public Health Association–Public Health Nursing: http://www.apha.org

American Society of PeriAnesthesia Nurses: http://www.aspan.org

American Society of Plastic Surgical Nurses: http://www.aspsn.org

(Continues)

Exhibit 1-4 *(continued)*

Association for Nursing Professional Development: http://anpd.org

Association of Camp Nurses: http://www.campnurse.org

Association of Nurses in AIDS Care: http://www.nursesinaidscare.org

Association of Pediatric Hematology/Oncology Nurses: http://www.apon.org

Association of periOperative Registered Nurses: http://www.aorn.org

Association of Rehabilitation Nurses: http://www.rehabnurse.org

Association of Women's Health, Obstetric and Neonatal Nurses: http://www.awhonn.org

Commission on Graduates of Foreign Nursing Schools: http://www.cgfns.org

Council of International Neonatal Nurses: http://www.coinnurses.org

Emergency Nurses Association: http://www.ena.org

Home Healthcare Nurses Association: http://www.hhna.org

Hospice and Palliative Nurses Association: http://www.hpnaadvancingexpertcare.org

Infusion Nurses Society: http://www.ins1.org

International Association of Forensic Nurses: http://www.forensicnurses

International Council of Nurses: http://www.icn.ch

International Home Care Nurses Association: http://ihcno.org

International Society for Psychiatric–Mental Health Nurses: http://www.ispn-psych.org

International Transplant Nurses Society: http://itns.org

National Alaskan Native American Indian Nurses Association: http://www.nanainanurses.org

National Association of Clinical Nurse Specialists: http://www.nacns.org

National Association of Neonatal Nurses: http://www.nann.org

National Association of Orthopaedic Nurses: http://www.orthonurse.org

National Association of Pediatric Nurse Practitioners: http://www.napnap.org

National Association of School Nurses: http://www.nasn.org

National Black Nurses Association: http://www.nbna.org

National Council of State Boards of Nursing: https://www.ncsbn.org

National Gerontological Nursing Association: http://www.ngna.org/

National League for Nursing: http://www.nln.org

National Nursing Staff Development Organization: http://www.nnsdo.org

National Student Nurses Association: http://www.nsna.org

Oncology Nursing Society: http://www.ons.org

Society of Gastroenterology Nurses and Associates: http://www.sgna.org

Society of Pediatric Nurses: http://www.pedsnurses.org

Society of Trauma Nurses: http://www.traumanurses.org

State Nurses Associations: http://www.nursingworld.org/functionalmenucategories/aboutana/whoweare/cma.aspx

The Association for Radiologic & Imaging Nursing: http://www.arinursing.org

Transcultural Nursing Society: http://www.tcns.org

Wound, Ostomy and Continence Nurses Society: http://www.wocn.org

view the ANA as the voice of nursing. When the ANA lobbies for nursing, it is lobbying for *all* nurses, not just its membership. This organization represents more than 3.6 million RNs through its multiple constituent member associations and state and territorial associations, although the actual membership is much less than the total number of RNs (ANA, 2016). This shift in membership must be considered in light of generational issues. New nurses typically do not join organizations, and there is continual unrest regarding the perception by some nurses of the ANA's lack of response to vital nursing issues. In addition to being a professional organization, some state chapters have formed labor unions. Participation in the labor union is optional for members, and each state organization's stance on unions has an impact on membership. The ANA's major publication is *American Nurse Today*. The organization's 2017–2020 strategic plan identifies the three goals (ANA, 2017):

1. Increase the number and engagement of nurses in ANA.
2. Stimulate and disseminate innovation that increases recognition of the value of nursing and drives improvement in health and health care.
3. Leverage the ANA Enterprise to position nurses as integral partners consumers' health and health care journeys.

The ANA has three affiliated organizations: the American Nurses Foundation (ANF), the American Academy of Nursing (AAN), and the American Nurses Credentialing Center (ANCC).

American Nurses Foundation. The ANF is "dedicated to transforming the nation's health through the power of nursing. It is the only philanthropic organization with a mission to improve health care and support the 3.6 million nurses across the United States health through the power of nursing. We help nurses step into leadership roles in their communities and workplaces to ensure that they can play a meaningful role in shaping decisions on the quality and capacity of health care" (American Nurses Foundation [ANF], 2017). As of 2015, more

than 1,000 nursing scholars have received ANF grants representing more than $5 million (ANF, 2015).

American Academy of Nursing. The AAN was established in 1973, and it serves the public and the nursing profession through its activities to advance health policy and practice (American Academy of Nursing [AAN], 2015a). The academy is considered the "think tank" for nursing. Membership as an academy fellow is by invitation; fellows may then list "FAAN" in their credentials. There are approximately 2,100 fellows, representing nursing's leaders in education, management, practice, and research. This is a very prestigious organization, and fellows have demonstrated their leadership in practice, management, and academic nursing. The AAN also publishes the journal *Nursing Outlook*. Examples of some of the AAN's current initiatives follow (AAN, 2015b):

- *Choosing Wisely* is a campaign to ensure that more Americans hear about and understand the need for the right care provided at the right time. ANA fellows are working in partnership with other organizations in this initiative.
- The AAN provides expert panels to address current healthcare concerns.
- The Council for the Advancement of Nursing Science serves as a voice for nurse scientists and supports development of nursing science.
- *Have You Ever Served?* An AAN initiative in collaboration with other organizations and the federal government to improve the health of veterans.
- *Institute for Nursing Leadership* supports nurse appointments and leadership development.

American Nurses Credentialing Center. The ANA established the ANCC in 1973 to develop and implement a program that would provide tangible recognition of professional achievement. Additional programs were added to the work done by the ANCC including (American Nurse Credentialing Center, 2016):

- *Accreditation Program:* The ANCC Accreditation program recognizes the importance of high-quality continuing nursing education (CNE) and skills-based competency programs. Around the world, ANCC-accredited organizations provide nurses with the knowledge and skills to help improve care and patient outcomes.

- *Certification Program:* ANCC's Certification Program enables nurses to demonstrate their specialty expertise and validate their knowledge to employers and patients. Through targeted exams that incorporate the latest nursing practice standards, ANCC certification empowers nurses with pride and professional satisfaction.
- *Pathway:* The Pathway to Excellence Program recognizes a healthcare organization's commitment to creating a positive nursing practice environment. The Pathway to Excellence in Long Term Care program is the first to recognize this type of supportive work setting. Pathway organizations focus on collaboration, career development, and accountable leadership to empower nurses.
- *Magnet Recognition Program®:* ANCC's Magnet Recognition Program is the most prestigious distinction a healthcare organization can receive for nursing excellence and quality patient outcomes. Organizations that achieve Magnet recognition are part of an esteemed group that demonstrates superior nursing practices and outcomes.
- *Nursing Knowledge Center:* The Nursing Knowledge Center provides educational materials and guidance to support nurses and organizations in their quest to achieve success through its credentialing programs.

National League for Nursing.   The NLN is a nursing organization that focuses on excellence in nursing education. Its membership is primarily composed of schools of nursing and nurse educators. The organization began in 1893 as the American Society of Superintendents of Training Schools. It holds a number of educational meetings annually and provides continuing education and certification for nurse educators. This organization has four major goals (National League for Nursing, 2017):

- *Goal I—Leader in Nursing Education:* Enhance the NLN's national and international impact as the recognized leader in nursing education.
- *Goal II—Commitment to Members:* Build a diverse, sustainable, member-led organization with the capacity to deliver the NLN's mission effectively, efficiently, and in accordance with the NLN's values.
- *Goal III—Champion for Nurse Educators:* Be the voice of nurse educators and champion their interests in political, academic, and professional arenas.
- *Goal IV—Advancement of the Science of Nursing Education:* Promote evidence-based nursing education and the scholarship of teaching.

American Association of Colleges of Nursing.   The AACN is the national organization for educational programs at the baccalaureate level and higher. The organization is particularly concerned with development of standards and resources and promotes innovation, research, and practice to advance nursing education. The organization represents more than 780 schools of nursing at the baccalaureate and higher levels (AACN, 2016, 2015b). The dean or director of a school of nursing serves as a representative to the AACN. The organization holds annual meetings for nurse educators that focus on different levels of nursing education. The AACN has been involved in creating and promoting new roles, such as the clinical nurse leader and the DNP, as well as educational programs, which are discussed in other chapters of this text. The major AACN publication is the *Journal of Professional Nursing.* This organization's strategic goals for 2017–2019 are as follows (AACN, 2017):

- *Goal 1*: AACN is the driving force for innovation and excellence in academic nursing.
- *Goal 2*: AACN is a leading partner in advancing improvements in health, health care, and higher education.
- *Goal 3*: AACN is a primary advocate for advancing diversity and inclusivity with academic nursing.

- *Goal 4:* AACN is the authoritative source of knowledge to advance academic nursing through information curation and synthesis.

Organization for Associate Degree Nursing. The Organization for Associate Degree Nursing (OADN) [formerly N-OADN] represents associate degree (AD) nurses, AD nursing programs, and individual member nurse educators. The organization joined the ANA as an organizational affiliate in December 2016 along with 30 other specialty nursing organizations that are ANA affiliates (*The American Nurse*, 2017). The OADN focuses on enhancing the quality of AD nursing education, strengthening the professional role of the AD nurse, and protecting the future of AD nursing in the midst of healthcare changes. Its major goals follow (Organization for Associate Degree Nursing, 2016):

- *Collaboration Goal:* Advance associate degree nursing education through collaboration with a diversity of audiences.
- *Education Goal:* Advance associate degree nursing education.
- *Advocacy Goal:* Advocate for issues and activities that support the organization's mission.

Sigma Theta Tau International.   Sigma Theta Tau International (STTI) is a not-for-profit international organization based in the United States. This nursing honor society was created in 1922 by a small group of nursing students at what is now the Indiana University School of Nursing. Its mission is to provide leadership and scholarship in practice, education, and research to improve the health of all people (Sigma Theta Tau International, 2016). Membership in this organization is by invitation to baccalaureate and graduate nursing students who demonstrate excellence in scholarship and to nurse leaders who demonstrate exceptional achievements in nursing. STTI has more than 135,000 active members, and 85 countries are represented in its membership.

Schools of nursing may form STTI association chapters. The chapters are where most of the work

of the organization takes place. There are about 500 chapters at approximately 695 institutions of higher education, which include schools in Armenia, Australia, Botswana, Brazil, Canada, Colombia, England, Ghana, Hong Kong, Japan, Kenya, Lebanon, Malawi, Mexico, the Netherlands, Pakistan, Portugal, Singapore, South Africa, South Korea, Swaziland, Sweden, Taiwan, Tanzania, Thailand, the United Kingdom, and the United States. Other countries are considering establishing chapters. This is an important organization, and students should learn more about their school's chapter (if the school has one) and aspire to an invitation for induction into STTI. Inductees meet specific academic and leadership standards. The major STTI publications are *Journal of Nursing Scholarship*, *Reflections on Nursing Leadership*, and the newest publication, *Worldviews on Evidence-Based Nursing*. The organization manages the major online library for nursing resources, the Virginia Henderson International Nursing Library, through its website.

International Council of Nurses.   The ICN, founded in 1899, is a federation of 130 national nurses' associations representing approximately 16 million nurses worldwide, representing more than 130 national nurse associations such as the ANA (International Council of Nurses [ICN], 2015). This organization is the international voice of nursing and focuses on activities to better ensure quality care for all and sound health policies globally. Its activities focus on (1) professional nursing practice (for example, specific health issues, International Classification of Nursing Practice), (2) nursing regulation (for example, regulation and credentialing, ethics, standards, continuing education), and (3) socioeconomic welfare for nurses (for example, occupational health and safety, salaries, migration, and other issues). The ICN headquarters is in Geneva, Switzerland.

National Student Nurses Association.   The National Student Nurses Association (2016) has a membership of approximately 60,000 students enrolled in diploma, AD, baccalaureate, and general graduate nursing programs in 50 states, the District of

Columbia, Puerto Rico, and the U.S. Virgin Islands. It is a national organization with chapters within schools of nursing. Its major publication is *Imprint*. Joining the NSNA is a great way to get involved and to begin to develop professional skills needed for the future (such as learning more about being a leader and a follower, critical roles for practicing nurses). The NSNA website provides an overview of the organization and its activities. Attending a national convention is also a great way to find out about nursing in other areas of the country and network with other nursing students. Annual conventions attract more than 3,000 nursing students and are held at different sites each year. This professional networking also affords students opportunities to learn about graduate education, specialty groups, and nursing careers. Active engagement in your school's NSNA chapter and national activities provide you with opportunities to develop leadership competencies. Hopefully, these experiences will provide a springboard to later professional engagement in nursing professional organizations.

Why Belong to a Nursing Professional Organization?

The previous section described many nursing professional organizations, and there is further information in the *Nursing Education, Accreditation, and Regulation* chapter about some of these organizations. Why is it important to belong to a professional organization? Joining a professional organization and becoming active in the organization's activities is a professional obligation. Membership and, it is hoped, active involvement can help nurses develop leadership skills, improve networking, and find mentors. Additionally, membership gives nurses a voice in professional issues and in some cases, health policy issues. It provides a range of opportunities for professional development. Nurses represent the single largest voting bloc in any state. By using this political power through nursing and other professional organizations, nurses can speak in one powerful voice. Yet as nurses, we have often failed to pull together. Membership in a professional organization is one way to develop one strong voice.

Nurses who attend meetings, hold offices, and serve on committees or as delegates to large meetings benefit more from membership than those who do not participate. Submitting abstracts for a presentation or poster at a meeting is excellent experience for nurses and offers even more opportunities for networking with other nurses who might also provide resources and mentoring for professional development. There are some factors that are important to recognize as you consider joining a professional organization. Belonging to a nursing association requires money for membership and commitment to the association, which means it takes time to engage in the organization.

Students can begin to meet this professional obligation by joining local student organizations, which may or may not be directly related to the nursing program but to the campus in general, and developing skills that can be used after graduation when they join professional organizations. Membership offers opportunities to serve as a committee member and even chair a committee. Organization communication methods can be observed, and the student can participate in the processes, developing leadership competencies. Engagement in organizations allows members to participate in making decisions about nursing and health care in general. When new nurses enter the profession today, they find a healthcare system that is struggling to improve its quality and keep up with medical changes, and nurses need to be engaged in the process to improve health care. Organizations also sometimes band together—increasing collaboration to have a greater voice about critical healthcare policy issues such as the need to expand the nursing profession or improve care in a local area.

Nursing Workforce

Nursing is one of the largest healthcare professions, and nurses have many opportunities to serve as leaders in health care. Nurses work in a variety of settings, such as hospitals, clinics, home health care, hospice care, long-term care, rehabilitation, physician offices, school health, employment services, and numerous other service sites. The majority of nurses work in acute care hospital settings, but this is changing as more care moves into the community.

According to the U.S. Bureau of Labor Statistics' (2015) employment projections for 2014–2024, employment opportunities for registered nurses are expected to increase 16%, which is faster than expected for most other occupations. Over this period, another 495,500 nursing workforce replacements may be needed, bringing the total number of job openings for nurses due to growth and replacements to 1.2 million by 2020. We have experienced a number of years of fluctuating nursing shortages. As the number of nurses in practice and nursing school enrollments fluctuate, any nursing shortage, whether this is geographic specific or healthcare organization specific, affects access to care in the years to come—and there can be great variation from one area of the country to another. Because of demographic changes, the older adult population in the United States is increasing rapidly, and from 2010 to early 2017, the ACA extended insurance coverage to more people. Taken together, these developments signal that the demand for nurses and other healthcare professionals will increase. Changes in future federal legislation and their impact on states need to be followed by the nursing profession to determine impact on nursing practice and need for nurses.

The 2014 Health Resources and Services Administration (HRSA) report, *The Future of the Nursing Workforce: National- and State-Level Projections, 2012–2025*, indicates that the United States is on track to meet the projected demand for nursing staff (registered nurses and licensed practical nurses in the next 10 years (HHS, HRSA, & BHW, 2014). The number of new graduates entering the workforce has increased. Many factors impact supply and demand for nursing staff. This report notes some trends and study limitations that might alter this projection; for example:

- While not considered in this study, emerging care delivery models, with a focus on managing health status and preventing acute health issues, will likely contribute to new growth in demand for nurses—for example, nurses taking on new and/or expanded roles in preventive care and care coordination (p. 2).
- Supply and demand will continue to be affected by numerous factors, including population growth and the aging of the nation's population, overall economic conditions, aging of the nursing workforce, and changes in healthcare reimbursement (p. 4).
- While the evidence in this report points toward the United States currently educating slightly more nurses than required to meet future demand, a reduction in people choosing nursing as a career or a combination of factors such as early retirement or increased demand could be sufficient to erase projected surpluses for RNs and LPNs (licensed practical nurses) (p. 14).
- If the growing emphasis on care coordination, preventive services, and chronic disease management in care delivery models leads to a greater need for nurses, this brief may underestimate the projected nurse demand (p. 15).

Nursing is a profession. It meets all the requirements for a profession and serves as a major profession in healthcare delivery and the healthcare workforce. In the early part of its history, nursing was not viewed as a profession, as noted in the review of nursing history described earlier in this chapter, but it is now recognized as a profession built on knowledge that reflects its dual components of science and art with clear roles and responsibilities in the healthcare workforce. The *Essence of Nursing: Knowledge and Caring* chapter explores the art and

Stop and Consider #2

It is easy to see how nursing is a profession.

science of the profession of nursing, expanding on the view of nursing as a profession and an active member of the healthcare workforce.

The Image of Nursing

The image of nursing may appear to be an unusual topic for a nursing text, but it is not. Image is part of any profession. It is the way a person appears to others, or in the case of a profession, the way a profession appears to other professionals and others in the work environment and to the general public—in nursing's case, consumers of health care. Image and the perception of the profession affect recruitment of students; the view of the public; funding for nursing education and research; relationships with healthcare administrators and other healthcare professionals, government agencies, and legislators at all levels of government; and, ultimately, the profession's self-identity. Just as individuals may feel depressed or less effective if others view them negatively, so can professionals experience similar reactions if their image is not positive. Image influences everything the profession does or wishes to do. How nurses view themselves—their professional self-image—has an impact on professional self-esteem (Buresh & Gordon, 2006). How one is viewed has an impact on whether others seek that person out and how they view the effectiveness of what that person might do. Every time a nurse says to family, friends, or members of the public that he or she is a nurse, the nurse is representing the profession. "We cannot expect outsiders to be the guardians of our visibility and access to public media and health policy arenas. We must develop the skills of presenting ourselves in the media and to the media—we have to take the responsibility for moving from silence to voice" (Buresh & Gordon, 2006, p. 15). The professional introduction is an example of critical communication that sets the stage for a nurse–patient relationship, and it is associated with the image of nursing. Saying one's name, first and last, and title and explaining your role is an important step in establishing trust and maintaining accountability—demonstrating professionalism (LeBlanc, Burke, & Henneman, 2016). Most nurses do not even consider the implications of the introduction and quickly move on to a task that must be done. They may not provide their first and last name due to concerns about their privacy, though this does not really protect privacy because it is easy for a patient to find out a nurse's name.

The public's views of nursing and nurses are typically based on personal experiences with nurses, which can lead to a narrow view of a nurse often based on only a brief personal experience. This experience may not provide an accurate picture of all that nurses can and do provide in the healthcare delivery process. In addition, this view may be influenced by the emotional response of a person to the situation and the encounter with a nurse.

But the truth is that most often the nurse is invisible. "Although nurses comprise the majority of healthcare professionals, they are largely invisible. Their competence, skill, knowledge, and judgment are—as the word 'image' suggests—only a reflection, not reality" (E. Sullivan, 2004, p. 45). Consumers (patients, families) may not understand the knowledge and competencies required to be a registered nurse, may not recognize they are interacting with a nurse, or they may think someone is a nurse who is not. When patients go to their doctor's office, they interact with staff, and often these patients think that they are interacting with a registered nurse. Most likely, they are not—the staff person may be a medical assistant of some type or a licensed practical/vocational nurse. When in the hospital, patients interact with many staff members, and there is little to distinguish one from another, so patients may refer to most staff as nurses. Uniforms do not help identify roles because many staff wear scrub clothes and lab coats, and there has been less emphasis placed on professional attire. In the past, hospitals had strict dress codes, with standard uniforms per type of staff. Over time, this approach changed—affecting not only what staff wore, but also appearance such as hair, wearing of jewelry, and so on. Healthcare organizations now find it difficult to change dress codes with staff complaining this is not needed. One organization conducted an extensive study of the issue of dress and image, examining how patients viewed nurses, and noted at the conclusion of the study that standardizing nurse uniforms would have a positive impact on the nurse's professional image and this then would affect the nurse–patient relationship (West et al., 2016).

This does not mean that the public does not value nurses—quite the contrary. When a person tells another that he or she is a nurse, the typical response is positive. However, many people do not know about the education required to become a nurse and to maintain current knowledge or about the great variety of educational entry points into nursing that all lead to the RN qualification. Consumers generally view nurses as good people who care for others. In 2017, nurses continue to rank number one in ethics and honesty in the annual Gallup Poll compared to other occupations (Jimenez, 2016). This high vote of confidence has been a consistent annual result in this poll. What is not mentioned in the poll is the knowledge and competency required to do the job properly—important aspects of the nursing profession.

You might wonder why it is so important for nurses to make themselves more visible. You chose nursing, so you know that it is an important profession. Nevertheless, many students have a narrow view of the profession, much closer to what is portrayed in the media—the nurse who cares for others, albeit with less understanding of the knowledge base required and competency needed to meet the complex needs of patients. There is limited recognition that nursing is a scientific field. The profession needs to be more concerned about visibility because the profession needs to attract qualified students and keep current nurses in practice.

The nurse's voice is typically silent, and this factor has demoralized nursing (Pike, 2001). This is a strong statement and may be a confusing one. What is the nurse's voice? It is the "unique perspectives and contributions that nurses bring to patient care" (Pike, 2001, p. 449). Nurses have all too often been silent about what they do and how they do it, but this has been a choice that nurses have made—to be silent or to be more visible. Both external and internal factors affect the nurse's voice and this silence. The external factors include the following (Pike, 2001):

- Historical role of nurse as handmaiden (not an independent role)
- Hierarchical structure of healthcare organizations (may limit the role of nurses in decision making and leadership)
- Perceived authority and directives of physicians (may limit the independent role of nurses)
- Hospital policy (may limit nursing actions and leadership)
- Threat of disciplinary or legal action or loss of job (may limit a nurse when he or she needs to speak out—advocate)

Nurses who can deal with the internal factors can be more visible and less silent about nursing and better advocate for patients. The internal factors to consider include:

- Role confusion
- Lack of professional confidence
- Timidity
- Fear
- Insecurity
- Sense of inferiority

Nurses' loss of professional pride and self-esteem can also lead to a more serious professional problem: Nurses feel like victims and then act like victims. Victims do not take control, but rather see others as being in control; they abdicate responsibility. They play passive–aggressive games to exert power. This can be seen in the public image of nurses, which is predominantly driven by forces outside the profession. It also affects the nurse's ability to collaborate with others—both other nurses and other healthcare professionals.

It is all too easy for nurses to feel like victims, and this perception has led in many ways to nurses viewing physicians in a negative light, emphasizing that "physicians have done this to us." As a consequence, nurses may have problems saying they are colleagues with other healthcare professionals and acting like colleagues. **Colleagueship** "involves entering into a collaborative relationship that is characterized by mutual trust and response and an understanding of the perspective each partner contributes" (Pike, 2001, p. 449). Colleagues have the following characteristics:

- Control interprofessional and intraprofessional competition and antagonism from the past conflict that may influence the present and the future.
- Integrate work to provide the best care.
- Acknowledge they share a common goal: quality patient care.
- Recognize their interdependence and also independent responsibilities.
- Share responsibility and accountability for patient care outcomes.
- Respond to conflict in a positive manner before it accelerates.

What is unexpected is how nurses' silence may actually have a negative impact on patient care. This factor may influence how a nurse speaks out or advocates for care that a patient needs, how effective a nurse can be on the interprofessional treatment team, and how nurses participate in healthcare program planning and implementation of services. Each nurse has the responsibility and accountability to define himself or herself as a colleague, and empowerment is part of this process.

The role of nursing has experienced many changes, and many more will occur in the future. How has nursing responded to these changes and communicated them to the public and other healthcare professionals? Suzanne Gordon, a journalist who has written extensively about the nursing profession, noted that often the media are accused of representing nursing poorly when, in reality,

the media are simply reflecting the public image of nursing (Buresh & Gordon, 2006). Nurses have not taken the lead in standing up and discussing their own image of nursing—what it is and what it is not. It is not uncommon for a nurse to refuse to talk to the press because the nurse feels no need to do so, may not feel competent to do so, or fears reprisals from his or her employer. When nurses do speak to the press—often when being praised for an action—they say, "Oh, I was just doing my job." This statement undervalues the reality that critical thinking and clinical reasoning and judgment on the part of nurses makes a difference in the health of patients (individuals, families, communities) every day. What is wrong with taking that credit? Because of these types of responses in the media, nursing is not directing the image, but rather accepting how those outside the profession describe nursing.

Gordon and Nelson (2005) comment "nursing needs to move away from the 'virtue script' toward a knowledge-based identity" (p. 62). The "virtue script" continues to be present in current media campaigns that are supported by the profession. For example, a video produced by the NSNA mentions knowledge but not many details; instead, it includes statements such as "[Nursing is a] job where people will love you" (Gordon & Nelson, 2005). How helpful is this approach? Is this view of being loved based on today's nursing reality? Nursing practice involves highly complex care; it can be stressful, demanding, and at times rewarding, but it is certainly not as simple as "everyone will love you." Why do nurses continue to describe themselves in this way? "One reason nurses may rely so heavily on the virtue script is that many believe this is their only legitimate source of status, respect, and self-esteem" (Gordon & Nelson, 2005, p. 67). This, however, is a view that perpetuates the victim mentality.

Stop and Consider #3
The image of nursing is not simple to describe.

CHAPTER HIGHLIGHTS

1. Nursing history provides a framework for understanding how nursing is practiced today.
2. The history of nursing is complex and has been influenced by social, economic, and political factors.
3. Florence Nightingale was instrumental in changing the view of nursing and nursing education to improve care delivery, but she is not the only nurse leader who has led the profession.
4. Nursing meets the critical requirements for a profession.
5. The sources of professional direction include ANA documents that describe the scope of practice, standards, and an ethical code.
6. Professional organizations have a key role in shaping nursing as a profession. Nurses should participate in these organizations to have a voice in the profession.
7. The public, the media, interprofessional colleagues, and nurses have an influence on the image of nursing. Nursing's image as a profession has both positive and negative aspects.

ENGAGING IN THE CONTENT

Discussion Questions

1. How might knowing more about nursing history affect your personal view of nursing?
2. How did the image of nursing in Nightingale's time influence nursing from the 1860s through the 1940s?
3. How would you compare and contrast accountability, autonomy, and responsibility?
4. Based on content in this chapter, how would you define *professionalism* in your own words?
5. Why are standards important to the nursing profession and to healthcare delivery?
6. Review the ANA standards of practice and professional performance. Are you surprised by any of the standards? If so, why?
7. How would you explain to someone who is not in health care the reason that nursing emphasizes its social policy statement?

CRITICAL THINKING ACTIVITIES

1. Describe how the Nightingale Pledge may or may not have relevance today and how it might be altered to be more relevant. Work with a team of students to accomplish this activity and arrive at a consensus statement.
2. Interview two registered nurses, ask them if they think nursing is a profession, and determine the rationale for their viewpoints. How does what they say compare with what you have learned about professionalism in this chapter?
3. Attend an NSNA meeting at your school. What did you learn about the organization? What did you observe in the meeting about leadership and nursing? Do you have any criticisms of the organization and how it might be improved? If your school does not have an NSNA chapter, why is this the case?
4. Complete a mini-survey of six people (non-nurses), asking them to describe their image of nursing and nurses. Try to pick a variety of people. Summarize and analyze

(Continues)

CRITICAL THINKING ACTIVITIES (CONTINUED)

your data to identify any themes and unusual views. How does what you learned relate to the content in this chapter? List the similarities and differences, and then discuss your findings with a group of your classmates and compare with their findings.

5. You are told that the profession of nursing needs to abandon its image of nurses as angels and promote an image of nurses as competent professionals who are both knowledgeable and caring. *Review this article*: Rhodes, M., Morris, A., & Lazenby, R. (2011, May). Nursing at its best: Competent and caring. *OJIN, 16*. Retrieved from http://www.nursingworld.org/MainMenuCategories/ ANAMarketplace/ANAPeriodicals/OJIN /TableofContents/Vol-16-2011/No2-May-2011 /Articles-Previous-Topics/Nursing-at-its-Best. html. Debate this issue in class.

6. Analyze a television program that focuses on a healthcare situation/story line. How are nurses depicted compared with other healthcare professionals? Compose a letter to the program describing your analysis, and document your arguments to support your viewpoint. This could be done with a team of students; watch the same program and then discuss opinions and observations.

ELECTRONIC REFLECTION JOURNAL

You are asked to develop an *Electronic Reflection Journal* that you will use after you complete each chapter. This is the place for you to reflect on some aspect of the chapter's content identified at the end of the chapter. You may also want to keep notes about issues that you want to expand on as you progress through your nursing education. If you are using technology that allows you to make visuals, use drawings and graphics as one method to reflect in your journal.

In your first entry in your *Electronic Reflection Journal*, consider the following questions related to the image of nursing. Connect your responses so that you can better understand the importance of image to the profession and the meaning of profession.

1. Why is the image of nursing important to the profession? To health care in general?
2. What role do you think you might have as a nurse in influencing the image of nursing? Provide specific examples.
3. What is your opinion about nursing uniforms, and how do you think they influence the image of nursing?
4. What stimulated your interest in nursing as a profession? Was the image of nursing in any way related to your decision, and in what way did it affect your decision?

Special assignment for this chapter: Write your own definition of nursing and include it in your *Electronic Reflection Journal*. Work on this definition throughout this course as you learn more about nursing. Save the final draft, and at the end of each semester or quarter, go back to your definition and make any changes you feel are necessary. Keep a draft of each definition so that you can see your changes. When you graduate, review all your definitions, illustrating how you have developed your view of professional nursing. Ideally, you might then review your definition again one-year post graduation.

CASE STUDIES

Case 1

You and your friends in the nursing program are having lunch after a class that covered content found in this chapter. One of your friends says, "I was bored when we got to all that information on professionalism and nursing organizations. What a waste of time. I just want to be a nurse." All of you are struggling to figure out what you have gotten yourself into. You turn to your friends and suggest it might be helpful to have an open discussion on the comment just made. So over lunch, you all talk about the comment. It was clear that the students who had read the chapter were better able to discuss the issue, but everyone had an opinion.

Case Questions

1. What is the purpose of nursing organizations?
2. What role should professional organizations assume to increase nursing status in the healthcare system?
3. What are some of the advantages and disadvantages to joining a professional organization?
4. What do you know about your school's NSNA chapter?
5. Which nursing organization mentioned in this chapter interests you, and why? Compare your response with those of your other classmates.
6. Search on the Internet for a specialty nursing organization and pick one that interests you. What can you find out about the organization?

Case 2

The NSNA chapter in your school wants to help the school develop a campaign to increase enrollment. You have volunteered along with three other members to meet with the associate dean to discuss ideas for the campaign. The associate dean tells you that the school is going to use its standard marketing materials. She shows them to you. The materials focus on the importance of being a caring person to be a "good" nurse. When you ask to see print materials and materials to be posted on the Internet, you are told that the focus is on print, and you see a photo of a nurse holding a patient's hand.

Case Questions

1. How do you respond to this marketing material?
2. What recommendations would you make?
3. How might you get data from fellow students to support your recommendations?

Working Backward to Develop a Case

This type of case is a different format from usual cases. It is a "backward case." Students are provided with several questions and are asked to develop a case scenario that would

CASE STUDIES (CONTINUED)

relate to the questions and chapter content (paragraph or two). After the scenario is written, students answer the questions. A second option is for this to be a team activity. A team of students develops the scenario and then passes it on to another team to answer the questions. Following this, the teams discuss the case. *This description and use of this learning activity will not be repeated in each chapter guide.*

Write a brief paragraph that describes a case related to the following questions and comments.

1. What do we need to do to be more professional as students?
2. I think this topic is not important now as we are students. We deal with it when we get our first job.
3. We now have to wear our uniforms in the simulation lab. What is all this about? So annoying as we have other things to think about.

REFERENCES

American Academy of Nursing. (2015a). *About AAN.* Retrieved from http://www.aannet.org/about-the-academy

American Academy of Nursing. (2015b). *AAN initiatives.* Retrieved from http://www.aannet.org/home

American Assembly for Men in Nursing. (2017). *20 X 20 choose nursing.* Retrieved from http://www.aamn.org/resources/20x20-choose-nursing

American Association of Colleges of Nursing. (2004, September 20). *AACN endorses the Sullivan Commission report on increasing diversity in the health professions* (press release). Washington, DC: Author.

American Association of Colleges of Nursing. (2015a). *Enrollment.* Retrieved from http://www.aacn.nche.edu/news/articles/2015/enrollment

American Association of Colleges of Nursing. (2015b). *Fact sheet: Enhancing diversity in the nursing workforce.* Retrieved from http://www.aacn.nche.edu/media-relations/diversityFS.pdf

American Association of Colleges of Nursing. (2016). *AACN fact sheet.* Retrieved from http://www.aacn.nche.edu/media-relations/fact-sheets/aacn-fact-sheet

American Association of Colleges of Nursing. (2017). *Strategic plan 2017–2019.* Retrieved from http://www.aacn.nche.edu/about-aacn/strategic-plan

American Nurses Association. (2015a). *Nursing: Scope and standards of practice.* Silver Spring, MD: Author.

American Nurses Association. (2015b). *Guide to the code of ethics for nurses. Interpretation and application.* Silver Spring, MD: Nursesbooks.org

American Nurses Association. (2016). *Home page.* Retrieved from http://www.anfonline.org/Homepage-Category/Publications/AnnualReports/2015-Annual-Report.pdf

American Nurses Association. (2017). *ANA strategic plan 2017-2020.* Retrieved from http://www.nursingworld.org/FunctionalMenuCategories/AboutANA/ANAStrategicPlan

American Nurse Credentialing Center. (2016). *About ANCC.* Retrieved from http://www.nursecredentialing.org/FunctionalCategory/AboutANCC

American Nurses Foundation. (2015). *Annual report, 2015.* Retrieved from http://www.anfonline.org/Homepage-Category/Publications/AnnualReports/2015-Annual-Report.pdf

American Nurses Foundation. (2017). *About us.* Retrieved from http://www.anfonline.org/Main/AboutANF

Ashley, J. (1976). *Hospitals, paternalism, and the role of the nurse.* New York, NY: Teachers College Press.

Benner, P., Sutphen, M., Leonard, V., & Day, L. (2010). *Educating nurses: A call for radical transformation.* San Francisco, CA: Jossey-Bass.

Bixler, G., & Bixler, R. (1959). The professional status of nursing. *American Journal of Nursing, 59,* 1142–1147.

Boughn, S. (2001). Why women and men choose nursing. *Nursing and Healthcare Perspectives, 22,* 14–19.

Brooks, J., & Kleine-Kracht, A. (1983). Evolution of a definition of nursing. *Advances in Nursing Science, 5*(4), 51–63.

Bullough, V. (2006). Nursing at the crossroads: Men in nursing. In P. Cowen & S. Moorhead (Eds.), *Current issues in nursing* (7th ed., pp. 559–568). St. Louis, MO: Mosby.

Bullough, V., & Bullough, B. (1978). *The care of the sick: The emergence of modern nursing.* New York, NY: Prodist.

Buresh, B., & Gordon, S. (2006). *From silence to voice: What nurses know and must communicate to the public* (2nd ed.). Toronto, Ontario: Canadian Nurses Association.

Chinn, P. (2001). Feminism and nursing. In J. Dochterman & H. Grace (Eds.), *Current issues in nursing* (6th ed., pp. 441–447). St. Louis, MO: Mosby.

Cohen, S. (2007). The image of nursing. *American Nurse Today, 2*(5), 24–26.

Connolly, C. (2004). Beyond social history: New approaches to understanding the state of and the state in nursing history. *Nursing History Review, 12,* 5–24.

Dietz, D., & Lehozky, A. (1963). *History and modern nursing.* Philadelphia, PA: Davis.

Donahue, M. (1985). *Nursing: The finest art.* St. Louis, MO: Mosby.

Farmer, R. (2015, July 1). Why gender diversity in the workforce matters. *Minority Nurse.* Retrieved from http://minority nurse.com/why-gender-diversity-in-the-workforce -matters/

Finkelman, A. (2016). *Leadership and management for nurses: Competencies for quality care.* (3rd. ed.). Upper Saddle River, NJ: Pearson Education.

Fowler, M. (2015a). *Guide to nursing's social policy statement.* Silver Spring, MD: American Nurses Association.

Fowler, M. (2015b). *Guide to the code of ethics for nurses with interpretive statements.* Silver Spring, MD: American Nurses Association.

Freeman, L. (2007). Commentary. *Nursing History Review, 15,* 167–168.

Gordon, S. (2005). *Nursing against the odds.* Ithaca, NY: Cornell University Press.

Gordon, S., & Nelson, S. (2005). An end to angels. *American Journal of Nursing, 105*(5), 62–69.

Gorenberg, B. (1983). The research tradition of nursing: An emerging issue. *Nursing Research, 32,* 347–349.

Huber, D. (Ed.). (2014). *Leadership and nursing care management* (5th ed.). Philadelphia, PA: Saunders.

International Council of Nurses. (2015). *Our mission.* Retrieved from http://www.icn.ch/who-we-are/our -mission-strategic-intent-core-values-and-priorities/

Institute of Medicine. (2003). *Healthcare education: A bridge to quality.* Washington, DC: The National Academies Press.

Institute of Medicine. (2010). *The future of nursing. Leading change, advancing health.* Washington, DC: The National Academies Press.

Jacobs, M., & Huether, S. (1978). Nursing science: The theory practice linkage. *Advances in Nursing Science, 1,* 63–78.

Jimenez, S. (2016, December 21). *Nurses rank #1 once again in the Gallop Poll for ethics and honesty.* Retrieved from https://www.nurse.com/blog/2016/12/21/nurses-rank -1-once-again-in-gallup-poll-for-ethics-and-honesty/

Kalisch, P., & Kalisch, B. (1986). *The advance of American nursing* (2nd ed.). Boston, MA: Little, Brown and Company.

Kalisch, P., & Kalisch, B. (2005). Perspectives on improving nursing's public image. *Nursing Education Perspectives, 26*(1), 10–17.

Keller, M. (1979). The effect of sexual stereotyping on the development of nursing theory. *American Journal of Nursing, 79,* 1584–1586.

Kidd, P., & Morrison, E. (1988). The progression of knowledge in nursing: A search for meaning. *Image, 20,* 222–224.

Kupperschmidt, B. (2004). Making a case for shared accountability. *Journal of Nursing Administration, 34,* 114–116.

LeBlanc, R., Burke, M., & Henneman, E. (2016). The professional introduction. The key to establishing the relationship between nurse and patient. *AJN, 116*(6), 11.

Lindberg, B., Hunter, M., & Kruszewski, K. (1998). *Introduction to nursing* (3rd ed.). Philadelphia, PA: Lippincott.

Lynaugh, J., & Fagin, C. (1988). Nursing comes of age. *Image, 20,* 184–190.

Masters, K. (2005). *Role development in professional nursing practice.* Burlington, MA: Jones & Bartlett Learning.

National League for Nursing. (2017). *Mission/goals/core values.* Retrieved from http://www.nln.org/aboutnln /ourmission.htm

National Student Nurses Association. (2016). *Who are we?* Retrieved from http://www.nsna.org/AboutUs.aspx

Nightingale, F. (1858a). *Notes on matters affecting the health, efficiency, and hospital administration of the British army.* London, UK: Harrison and Sons.

Nightingale, F. (1858b). *Subsidiary notes as to the introduction of female nursing into military hospitals.* London, UK: Longman, Green, Longman, Roberts, and Green.

Nightingale, F. (1859). *Notes on hospitals.* London, UK: Harrison and Sons.

Nightingale, F. (1992). *Notes on nursing: What it is, and what it is not* (Commemorative ed.). Philadelphia, PA: Lippincott Williams & Wilkins. (Original work published 1860).

Organization for Associate Degree Nursing. (2016). *Mission and goals.* Retrieved from https://www.oadn.org /about-us/about-oadn

O'Rourke, M. (2003). Rebuilding a professional practice model: The return of role-based practice accountability. *Nursing Administrative Quarterly, 27*, 95–105.

Perry, J. (1985). Has the discipline of nursing developed to the stage where nurses do "think nursing"? *Journal of Advanced Nursing, 10*, 31–37.

Pike, A. (2001). Entering collegial relationships. In J. Dochterman & H. Grace (Eds.), *Current issues in nursing* (6th ed., pp. 448–452). St. Louis, MO: Mosby.

Quinn, C., & Smith, M. (1987). *The professional commitment: Issues and ethics in nursing*. Philadelphia, PA: Saunders.

Ritter-Teitel, J. (2002). The impact of restructuring on professional nursing practice. *Journal of Nursing Administration, 32*, 31–41.

Rosen, G. (1958). *A history of public health*. New York, NY: M.D. Publications.

Schein, E., & Kommers, D. (1972). *Professional education*. New York, NY: McGraw-Hill.

Seymer, L. (Ed.). (1954). *Selected writings on Florence Nightingale*. New York, NY: Macmillan.

Shames, K. (1993). *The Nightingale conspiracy: Nursing comes to power in the 21st century*. Montclair, NJ: Enlightenment Press.

Shaw, M. (1993). The discipline of nursing: Historical roots, current perspectives, future directions. *Journal of Advanced Nursing, 18*, 1651–1656.

Sigma Theta Tau International. (2016). *STTI organizational fact sheet*. Retrieved from http://www .nursingsociety.org/connect-engage/about-stti /sigma-theta-tau-international-organizational-fact-sheet

Slater, V. (1994). The educational and philosophical influences on Florence Nightingale, an enlightened conductor. *Nursing History Review, 2*, 137–151.

Sullivan, E. (2002). In a woman's world. *Reflections on Nursing Leadership, 28*(3), 10–17.

Sullivan, E. (2004). *Becoming influential: A guide for nurses*. Upper Saddle River, NJ: Pearson Education.

Sullivan, L. (2004). *Missing persons: Minorities in the health professions*. Battle Creek, MI: W. K. Kellogg Foundation.

The American Nurse. (2017, January). ANA welcomes the national organization for associate degree nursing. Retrieved from http://www.theamericannurse .org/2014/03/03/ana-welcomes-the-national -organization-for-associate-degree-nursing/

U.S. Bureau of Labor Statistics. (2015). *Employment projection*. Retrieved from http://www.bls.gov/opub /mlr/2015/article/occupational-employment -projections-to-2024.htm

U.S. Department of Health and Human Services, Health Resources and Services Administration, & Bureau of Health Professions. (2010). *The registered nurse population: Findings from the March 2008 national sample survey of registered nurses*. Retrieved from http://datawarehouse.hrsa.gov/nursingsurvey .aspx

U.S. Department of Health and Human Services, Health Resources and Services Administration, & Bureau of Health Workforce. (2014, December). *The future of the nursing workforce: National- and state-level projections, 2012-2025*. Retrieved from https://bhw .hrsa.gov/sites/default/files/bhw/nchwa/projections /nursingprojections.pdf

Wall, B. (2003). Science and ritual: The hospital as medical and sacred space, 1865–1920. *Nursing History Review, 11*, 51–68.

West, M., Wantz, D., Campbell, P., Rosler, G., Troutman, D., & Muther, C. (2016). Contributing to a quality patient experience: Applying evidence-based practice to support changes in nursing dress code policies. *OJIN, 21*(1). Retrieved from http://www.nursing world.org/MainMenuCategories/ANAMarketplace /ANAPeriodicals/OJIN/TableofContents/Vol-21-2016 /No1-Jan-2016/Quality-Patient-Experience-Nursing -Dress-Code-Policies.html

Widerquist, J. (1997). Sanitary reform and nursing. *Nursing History Review, 5*, 149–159.

Woodham-Smith, C. (1951). *Florence Nightingale: 1820–1910*. New York, NY: McGraw-Hill.

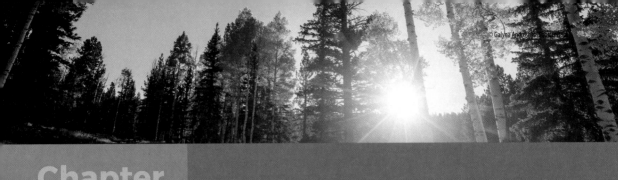

© Galyna Andrushko/Shutterstock

Chapter 2

The Essence of Nursing: Knowledge and Caring

CHAPTER OBJECTIVES

At the conclusion of this chapter, the learner will be able to:

- Discuss issues related to defining nursing.
- Examine nursing knowledge and the knowledge–caring dyad, knowledge workers, and knowledge management.
- Explain the relevance of scholarship to nursing and implications of research.
- Compare and contrast major nursing roles and responsibilities.

CHAPTER OUTLINE

KEY TERMS

Advocate	Dichotomous thinking	Provider of care
Applied or clinical research	Educator	Reality shock
Basic research	Entrepreneur	Reflective thinking
Caring	Groupthink	Research
Change agent	Identity	Researcher
Clinical judgment	Intuition	Role
Clinical reasoning	Knowledge	Role transition
Collaboration	Knowledge management	Scholarship
Competency	Knowledge workers	Sensemaking
Counselor	Leader	Status
Critical thinking	Management	Theory

Introduction

In the fall of 2016, the National Institute of Nursing Research (NINR) celebrated its 30th anniversary with activities to communicate the theme of "Advancing Science, Improving Lives. A Window to the Future" (NINR, 2016). Nursing has developed into a profession that now has greater emphasis on research and application of research. This chapter focuses on knowledge representing the science of nursing and the art and caring of nursing. We must always consider both aspects of the profession. A 2006 publication by Nelson and Gordon, *The complexities of care: Nursing reconsidered*, expanded on this topic. The authors stated, "Because we take caring seriously, we (the authors) are concerned that discussions of nursing care tend to sentimentalize and decomplexify the skill and knowledge involved in nurses' interpersonal or relational work with patients" (p. 3). Nelson and Gordon make a strong case that there is an ongoing problem of nurses devaluing the care they provide, particularly regarding the required knowledge component of nursing care and technical competencies needed to meet patient care needs, although caring is important part of the process—both of these aspects relate to the goal of providing quality care. This chapter explores the knowledge and caring of nursing practice. Both

must be present for quality nursing care. Content includes the effort to define nursing, knowledge and caring, competency, scholarship in nursing, major nursing roles, and leadership.

Nursing: How Do We
Define It?

Defining nursing is relevant to this chapter and requires further exploration. Can nursing be defined, and if so, why is it important to define it? Before this discussion begins, you should review your personal definition of nursing. You may find it strange to spend time on the question of a definition of nursing, but the truth is, there is no universally accepted definition by healthcare professionals and patients. The easy first approach to developing a definition is to describe what nurses do; however, this approach leaves out important aspects and essentially reduces nursing to tasks. Diers noted that even Florence Nightingale's and Virginia Henderson's definitions are not definitions of what nursing *is*, but more of what nurses *do*—more consideration needs to be given to (1) what drives nurses to do what they do or why they do what they do (rationales, evidence-based practice [EBP]) and (2) what is achieved by what they do (outcomes) (2001). Henderson's definition focuses more on a personal concept of nursing rather than a true definition. Henderson herself even said that what she wrote was not the complete definition of nursing (Henderson, 1991). Diers also commented that there really are no complete definitions for most disciplines. Yet nursing is still concerned with a definition. Having a definition serves several purposes that really drive what that definition will look like (Diers, 2001, p. 7):

- Providing an operational definition to guide research
- Acknowledging that changing laws requires a definition that will be politically accepted—for example, in relationship to a nurse practice act
- Convincing legislators about the value of nursing—for example, to gain funds for nursing education
- Explaining what nursing is to consumers/patients (although no definition is totally helpful because patients/consumers respond to a description of the work, not a definition)
- Explaining to others in general what one does as a nurse, which often represents a personal description of nursing

One could also say that a definition is helpful in determining what to include in a nursing curriculum, but nursing has been taught for years without a universally accepted definition. As mentioned in other content in this text, the American Nurses Association (ANA, 2015a) defines *nursing* as "the protection, promotion, and optimization of health and abilities, prevention of illness and injury, alleviation of suffering through the diagnosis and treatment of human response, and advocacy in the care of individuals, families, communities, and populations" (p. 88). Some of the critical terms in this definition include the following; others are discussed in the ANA standards:

- *Promotion of health:* Assisting people to maintain their health within their abilities; supporting families, populations and communities to maintain a healthy lifestyle.

- *Health:* "An experience that is often expressed in terms of wellness and illness, and may occur in the presence or absence of injury" (ANA, 2015a, p. 87).
- *Prevention of illness and injury:* Interventions taken to keep illness or injury from occurring—for example, immunization for tetanus or teaching parents how to use a car seat.
- *Illness:* "The subjective experience of discomfort" (ANA, 2015a, p. 88).
- *Injury:* Harm to the body—for example, a broken arm caused by a fall from a bicycle.
- *Diagnosis:* "A clinical judgment about the patient's response to actual or potential health conditions or needs. The diagnosis provides the basis for determination of a plan to achieve expected outcomes. Registered nurses utilize nursing and medical diagnosis depending upon educational and clinical preparation and legal authority" (ANA, 2015a, p. 86).
- *Treatment:* To give care through interventions—for example, administering medication, teaching a patient how to give him- or herself insulin, wound care, preparing a patient for surgery, and ensuring that the patient is not at risk for an infection.
- *Advocacy:* The act of pleading for or supporting a course of action on behalf of individuals, families, communities, and populations—for example, a nurse who works with the city council to improve health access for a community.

Essential features of professional nursing are identified from definitions of nursing (ANA, 2015a, pp. 7–9):

1. Caring and health are central to the practice of the registered nurse.
2. Nursing practice is individualized.
3. Registered nurses use the nursing process to plan and provide individualized care for healthcare consumers.
4. Nurses coordinate care by establishing relationships.

5. A strong link exits between the professional work environment and the registered nurse's ability to provide quality health care and achieve optimal outcomes.

Knowledge and caring are the critical dyad in any description or definition of nursing, and both relate to nursing scholarship and leadership and are integrated in the above features.

As part of a project to define the work of nursing, the North American Nursing Diagnosis Association (2016) described nursing diagnoses and developed the Nursing Interventions Classification (NIC) (University of Iowa, 2016a) and the Nursing Outcomes Classification (NOC) (University of Iowa, 2016b). Maas (2006) discussed the importance of these initiatives, which she described as the building blocks of nursing practice theory, and noted that "rather than debating the issues of definition, nursing will be better served by focusing those energies on its science and the translation of the science of nursing practice" (p. 8). In summary, there are three conclusions about defining nursing that are important to consider: (1) No universally accepted definition of nursing exists, although several definitions have been developed by nursing leaders and nursing organizations; (2) individual nurses may develop their own personal description of nursing to use in practice; and (3) a more effective focus is the pursuit of nursing knowledge to build nursing scholarship. The first step is to gain a better understanding of knowledge and caring in relationship to nursing practice.

Stop and Consider #1

Your personal definition of nursing is as important as a formal definition of nursing.

Knowledge and Caring

Understanding how knowledge and caring form the critical dyad for nursing is essential to providing effective quality care. **Knowledge** is specific information about something, and **caring** is behavior that demonstrates compassion and respect for another. But these are very simple definitions. The depth of nursing practice goes beyond basic knowledge and the ability to care. Nursing encompasses a distinct body of knowledge coupled with the art of caring. As stated by Butcher (2006), "A unique body of knowledge is a foundation for attaining the respect, recognition, and power granted by society to a fully developed profession and scientific discipline" (p. 116).

Knowledge

Knowledge can be defined and described in a number of ways. There are five ways of knowing that are useful in understanding how one knows something. A nurse might use all or some of these ways of knowing when providing care (Cipriano, 2007):

1. *Empirical knowing* focuses on facts and is related to quantitative explanations—predicting and explaining.
2. *Ethical knowing* focuses on a person's moral values—what should be done.
3. *Personal knowing* focuses on understanding and actualizing a relationship between a nurse and a patient, including knowledge of self (nurse).
4. *Aesthetic knowing* focuses on the nurse's perception of the patient and the patient's needs, emphasizing the uniqueness of each relationship and interaction.
5. *Synthesizing*, or pulling together the knowledge gained from the other types of knowing, allows the nurse to understand the patient better and to provide higher-quality care.

The ANA (2015b) identifies key issues related to the knowledge base for nursing practice, including both theoretical and evidence-based knowledge (pp. 189–190):

- Promotion of health and wellness
- Promotion of safety and quality of care
- Care, self-care processes, and care coordination
- Physical, emotional, and spiritual comfort, discomfort, and pain

- Adaptation to physiologic and pathophysiologic processes
- Emotions related to experiences of birth, growth and development, health, illness, disease, and death
- Meanings ascribed to health and illness and other concepts
- Linguistic and cultural sensitivity
- Health literacy
- Decision making and the ability to make choices
- Relationships, role performance, and change processes within relationships
- Social policies and their effects on health
- Healthcare systems and their relationships to access, cost, and quality of health care
- The environment and the prevention of disease and injury

This is the basic knowledge that every nurse should have to practice. Nurses use this knowledge, but they also must integrate it as they collaborate with patients and the healthcare team to assess, plan, implement, and evaluate care.

Knowledge Management

Knowledge work is a critical component of healthcare delivery today, and nurses are knowledge workers. Forty percent or more of workers in knowledge-intensive businesses, such as a healthcare organization, are **knowledge workers** (Sorrells-Jones & Weaver, 1999). **Knowledge management** includes both routine work (such as taking vital signs, administering medications, and walking a patient) and nonroutine work, which (1) involves exceptions, (2) requires judgment and use of knowledge, and (3) may be confusing or not fully understood. In a knowledge-based environment, a person's title is not as important as the person's expertise, and use of knowledge and learning are important. Knowledge workers actively use the following skills:

- Communication
- Collaboration

- Teamwork
- Coordination
- Analysis
- Critical thinking, clinical reasoning, and judgment
- Evaluation
- Willingness to be flexible

Knowledge workers recognize that change is inevitable and that the best approach is to be ready for change and view it as an opportunity for learning and improvement. Nurses use knowledge daily in their work. They work in an environment that expects healthcare providers to use the best evidence in providing care. "Transitioning to an evidence-based practice requires a different perspective from the traditional role of nurse as 'doer' of treatments and procedures based on institutional policy or personal preference. Rather, the nurse practices as a 'knowledge worker' from an updated and ever-changing knowledge base" (Mooney, 2001, p. 17). The knowledge worker focuses on acquiring, analyzing, synthesizing, and applying evidence to guide practice decisions (Dickenson-Hazard, 2002). The knowledge worker uses synthesis, competencies, multiple intelligences, a mobile skill set, outcome practice, and teamwork, as opposed to the old skills of functional analysis, manual dexterity, fixed skill set, process value, process practice, and unilateral performance (Porter-O'Grady & Malloch, 2007). This nurse is a clinical scholar. The employer and patients should value a nurse for what the nurse knows and how this knowledge is used to meet patient care outcomes—not just for technical expertise and caring, although these aspects of performance are also important (Kerfoot, 2002).

This change in a nurse's work is also reflected in the Carnegie Foundation Report on nursing education, as reported by Patricia Benner and colleagues (2010). Benner suggests that instead of focusing on content, nurse educators should focus on teaching nurses how to access information, use and manipulate data (such as data from patient information systems), and document effectively in the electronic interprofessional format—using knowledge to improve practice and care.

Critical Thinking and Clinical Thinking and Judgment: Impact on Knowledge Development and Application

Critical thinking, reflective thinking, and intuition are different approaches to thinking and can be used in combination. Nurses use all of them to explore, understand, develop new knowledge, and apply knowledge as evidence for best practice and caring in the nursing process. Experts such as Dr. Patricia Benner suggests that we often use the term *critical thinking*, but there is high variability and little consensus on what constitutes critical thinking (Benner, Sutphen, Leonard, & Day, 2010). Clinical reasoning and judgment are also very important and include critical thinking.

Critical thinking is clearly a focus of nursing practice. The ANA standards state that the nursing process is a critical thinking tool, albeit not the only one used in nursing (ANA, 2015a). This skill emphasizes purposeful thinking, rather than sudden decision making that is not based on thought and knowledge. Alfaro-LeFevre (2011) identified four key critical thinking components:

- Critical thinking characteristics (attitudes/behaviors)
- Theoretical and experiential knowledge (intellectual skills/competencies)
- Interpersonal skills/competencies
- Technical skills/competencies

In reviewing each of these components, one can easily identify the presence of knowledge, caring (interpersonal relationships, attitudes), and technical expertise. The nursing process (assessment, diagnosis, planning, implementation, and evaluation) applies all of these components and is discussed in more detail in later content in this text.

Critical thinking requires nurses to generate and examine questions and problems, use intuition, examine feelings, and clarify and evaluate evidence.

It means being aware of change and willing to take some risks. Critical thinking allows the nurse to avoid using **dichotomous thinking**—seeing situations as either good or bad, or Black or White. This limits possibilities and clinical choices for patients (Finkelman, 2001).

Critical thinking skills that are important to develop include affective learning; applied moral reasoning and values (relates to ethics); comprehension; application, analysis, and synthesis; interpretation; knowledge, experience, judgment, and evaluation; learning from mistakes when they happen; and self-awareness (Finkelman, 2001). A person uses four key intellectual traits in critical thinking (Paul, 1995). Each of the traits can be learned and developed.

- *Intellectual humility:* Willingness to admit what one does not know. (This is difficult to do, but it can save lives. A nurse who cannot admit that he or she does not know something and yet proceeds is taking a great risk. It is important for students to be able to use intellectual humility as they learn about nursing.)
- *Intellectual integrity:* Continual evaluation of one's own thinking and willingness to admit when thinking is not adequate. (This type of honesty with self and others can make a critical difference in care.)
- *Intellectual courage:* Ability to face and fairly address ideas, beliefs, and viewpoints for which one may have negative feelings. (Students enter a new world of health care and may experience confusing thoughts about ideas, beliefs, and viewpoints, and sometimes their personal views may need to be put aside in the interest of the patient and quality care.)
- *Intellectual empathy:* Conscious effort to understand others by putting one's own feelings aside and imagining oneself in another person's place.

Critical thinking also helps to reduce the tendency toward dichotomous thinking and groupthink, avoiding focus on just two options. Dichotomous thinking is related to **groupthink**, which occurs when all group or team members think alike. While all of the team members might be working together smoothly, groupthink limits choices, discourages open discussion of possibilities, and diminishes the ability to consider alternatives. Problem solving is not a critical thinking skill, but effective problem solvers use critical thinking.

The following methods will help develop your critical thinking skills (Finkelman, 2001, p. 196):

1. Seek the best information and data possible to allow you to fully understand the issue, situation, or problem. Questioning is critical. Examples of some questions that might be asked are: What is the significance of _____? What is your first impression? What is the relationship between _____ and _____? What impact might _____ have on _____? What can you infer from the information/data?

2. Identify and describe any problems that require analysis and synthesis of information—thoroughly understand the information/data.

3. Develop alternative solutions—more than two is better because this forces you to analyze multiple solutions even when you discard one of them. Be innovative, and avoid proposing only typical or routine solutions.

4. Evaluate the alternative solutions and consider the consequences for each one. Can the solutions really be used? Do you have the resources you need? How much time will it take? How well will the solution be accepted? Identify pros and cons.

5. Make a decision, choosing the best solution, even though there is risk in any decision making.

6. Implement the solution but continue to question.

7. Follow-up and evaluate; plan for evaluation from the very beginning. Self-assessment of critical thinking skills is an important part of using critical thinking. How does one use critical thinking, and is it done effectively?

Reflective thinking needs to become a part of daily learning and practice. Critical reflective thinking requires that the student or nurse examine the underlying assumptions and really question or even doubt the arguments, assertions, or facts of a situation or case (Benner, Hughes, & Sutphen, 2008). This allows the nurse to better grasp the patient's situation. Conway (1998) noted that nurses who use reflective thinking implement care based on the individualized care needs of the patient, whereas nurses who may not use reflective thinking or use it less often tend to provide illness-oriented care. Reflection is seen as a part of the art of nursing, which requires "creativity and conscious self-evaluation over a period of time" (Decker, 2007, p. 76). Reflection helps nurses cope with unique situations.

The skills needed for reflective thinking are the same skills required for critical thinking—the ability to monitor, analyze, predict, and evaluate (Pesut & Herman, 1999) and to take risks, be open, and have imagination (Westberg & Jason, 2001). Guided reflection with faculty who assist students in using reflective thinking during simulated learning experiences can enhance student learning and help students learn reflective learning skills. It is recommended that this process be done with faculty to avoid negative thoughts that a student may experience (Decker, 2007; Johns, 2004). The student should view the learning experience as an opportunity to improve and examine the experience from different perspectives. Some strategies that might be used to develop reflective thinking are keeping a journal (such as the Electronic Reflection Journal and the Working Backward Cases offered as an end-of-chapter activities), engaging in one-to-one dialogue with a faculty facilitator, joining in email dialogues, and participating in structured team/group forums in the classroom or online to help you understand how others examine an issue and learn more about constructive feedback. Reflective thinking strategies are not usually used for grading or evaluation, but rather are intended to help you think about your learning experience in an open manner.

Intuition is part of thinking. Including intuition in critical thinking and clinical reasoning and judgment helps to expand the person's ability to know (Hansten & Washburn, 2000). The most common definition of intuition is having a gut feeling about something. Nurses often have this feeling as they provide care—"I just have this feeling that Mr. Wallace is heading for problems." It is hard to explain what this is, but it happens. The following are examples of thoughts that a person might have related to intuition (Rubenfeld & Scheffer, 2015):

- I felt it in my bones.
- I couldn't put my finger on why, but I thought instinctively I knew.
- My hunch was that . . . .
- I had a premonition/inspiration/impression.
- My natural tendency was to . . . .
- Subconsciously I knew that . . . .
- Without thought I figured it out.
- Automatically I thought that . . . .
- While I couldn't say why, I thought immediately that . . . .
- My sixth sense said I should consider . . . .

Intuition is not science, but sometimes intuition can stimulate research and lead to greater knowledge and questions to explore. Intuition is related to experience. A student would not likely experience intuition about a patient care situation, but over time, as nursing expertise is gained, the student may be better able to use intuition. Benner's (2001) work, *From Novice to Expert*, suggests that intuition for nurses is really the putting together of the whole picture based on scientific knowledge and clinical expertise, not just a hunch, and intuition continues to be an important part of the nursing process (Benner, Hughes, & Sutphen, 2008).

Clinical reasoning and **clinical judgment** require more than recall and understanding of content or selection of the correct answer; they also require the ability to apply, analyze, and synthesize knowledge (Del Bueno, 2005). Nursing clinical judgment is the process, or the "ways in which nurses come to understand the problems, issues or concerns of clients/patients, to attend to salient information, and to respond in concerned and involved ways" (Benner, Tanner, & Chesla, 1996, p. 2). This process includes both deliberate, conscious decision making and intuition. "In the real world, patients do not present the nurse with a written description of their clinical symptoms and a choice of written potential solutions" (Del Bueno, 2005, p. 282). Beginning nursing students, however, are looking for the clear picture of the patient that matches what the student has read about in the text. This patient really does not exist, so critical thinking and clinical reasoning and judgment become more important as the student learns to compare and contrast what might be expected with what is reality (Benner, Sutphen, Leonard, & Day, 2010).

A systematic review of studies published between 1980 and 2012 arrived at a sample of 23 studies to examine the status of knowledge on clinical judgment and reasoning (Cappelletti, Engle, & Prentice, 2014). The following results from the study describe some aspects of clinical judgment (2014, pp. 455–456):

- Clinical judgments are more influenced by what the nurse brings to the situation than the objective data about the situation at hand.
- Sound clinical judgment rests to some degree on knowing the patient and his or her typical pattern of responses, as well as engagement with the patient and his or her concerns.
- Clinical judgments are influenced by the context in which the situation occurs and the culture of the nursing unit.
- Nurses use a variety of reasoning patterns alone or in combinations.
- Reflection on practice is often triggered by breakdown in clinical judgment and is critical for the development of clinical knowledge and improvement in clinical reasoning.

Sensemaking is a term that has been applied to "making sense of a problem." It is part of using critical thinking and clinical reasoning and judgment. You do this all the time in your daily life and then carry it forward into your nursing practice—solving a problem effectively requires understanding the situation. Individuals experience situations; confront gaps better; understand and/or take action; and then, after the experience, evaluate information that was used in the process. This is all done primarily unconsciously (Linderman, Pesut, & Disch, 2015). You use data that you receive through observation, communication, and other methods to make sense of the experience or situation. From this, you move on to other experiences and may or may not reflect on past sensemaking or apply what was learned. We also help others, such as our patients and their families, to get a better sense of what is happening to them. Sensemaking happens on the cognitive level as we use our cognitive tools to understand and formulate a view, physical level when we take actions, and emotional levels as we experience a situation and respond. Nursing leaders should make more use of sense making to build on their experiences and apply these to new experiences.

Caring

There is no universally accepted definition for caring in nursing, but it can be described from four perspectives (Mustard, 2002). The first is the sense of caring, which is probably the most common perspective for students to appreciate. This perspective emphasizes compassion or being concerned about another person. This type of caring may or may not require knowledge and expertise, but in nursing, effective caring requires both knowledge and expertise. The second perspective is doing for other people what they cannot do for themselves. Nurses do this all the time, and it requires knowledge and expertise to be effective. The third perspective is to care for the medical problem; this, too, requires knowledge of the problem, interventions, and so on, as well as expertise to provide the care. Providing wound care

or administering medications is an example of this type of caring. The fourth perspective is "competence in carrying out all the required procedures, personal and technical, with true concern for providing the proper care at the proper time in the proper way" (Mustard, 2002, p. 37). Not all four types of caring must be used at one time to be described as caring. Caring practices have been identified by the American Association of Critical-Care Nurses (2011) in the organization's synergy model for patient care as "nursing activities that create a compassionate, supportive, and therapeutic environment for patients and staff, with the aim of promoting comfort and healing and preventing unnecessary suffering". The model is discussed in other chapters in this text. Caring is an important component of patient-centered care and supports quality care.

Nursing theories often focus on caring. Theories are discussed later in this chapter, but here it is important to note one theory in particular that is known for its focus on caring—Watson's theory on caring. In 1979, Watson defined *nursing* "as the science of caring, in which caring is described as transpersonal attempts to protect, enhance, and preserve life by helping find meaning in illness and suffering, and subsequently gaining control, self-knowledge, and healing," and this continues to be relevant today (Scotto, 2003, p. 289). Patients today need caring. They feel isolated and are often confused by the complex medical system. Many patients have chronic illnesses such as diabetes, arthritis, and cardiac problems that require long-term treatment, and these patients need to learn how to manage their illnesses and be supported in the self-management process. Even many patients with cancer who have longer survival rates today are now described as having a chronic illness.

How do patients view caring? Patients may not see the knowledge and skills that nurses need, but they can appreciate when a nurse is there with them. The nurse–patient relationship can make a difference when the nurse uses caring consciously (Schwein, 2004). Characteristics of the patient-centered relationship are as follows:

- Being physically present with the patient
- Having a dialogue with the patient
- Showing a willingness to share and hear—to use active listening
- Avoiding assumptions
- Maintaining confidentiality
- Showing intuition and flexibility
- Believing in hope

As will be discussed in this text, patient-centered care is now a critical focus of healthcare delivery and nursing. Caring is part of focusing on patients—who should make decisions about their health care and expect respect from healthcare professionals during the care process.

Caring is offering of self. As Scotto (2003) comments, this means "offering the intellectual, psychological, spiritual, and physical aspects one possesses as a human being to attain a goal. In nursing, this goal is to facilitate and enhance patients' ability to do and decide for themselves" (p. 290). To be competent to care there are four aspects that need to be considered (Scotto, 2003, pp. 290–291):

- The *intellectual aspect* of nurses consists of an acquired, specialized body of knowledge, analytical thought, and clinical judgment, which are used to meet human health needs.
- The *psychological aspect* of nurses includes the feelings, emotions, and memories that are part of the human experience.
- The *spiritual aspect* of nurses, as for all human beings, seeks to answer the questions, "Why? What is the meaning of this?"
- The *physical aspect* of nurses is the most obvious. Nurses go to patients' homes, the bedside, and a variety of clinical settings where they apply their strength, abilities, and skills to attain a goal. For this task, nurses first must care for themselves, and then they must be accomplished and skillful in nursing interventions.

For students to be able to care for others, they need to also care for themselves. This is also important for practicing nurses. It takes energy to care for another person, and this effort is draining. Developing positive, healthy behaviors and attitudes can protect a nurse later when more energy is required in the practice of nursing and also have an impact on performance and thus on quality care outcomes, as discussed in other chapters in this text.

As students begin their nursing education program (and indeed throughout the program), the issue of the difference between medicine and nursing often arises. Caring is something that only nurses do, or so nurses say. Nurses are not the only healthcare professionals—for example, physicians would say they have a caring attitude and caring is part of their profession; however, what has happened with nursing (which may not have been so helpful) is that when caring is discussed in relation to nursing, it is described only in emotional terms (Moland, 2006). This view ignores the fact that caring often involves competent assessment of the patient to determine what needs to be done and the ability to subsequently provide that care. For both of these endeavors to be effective, the healthcare provider must have knowledge. The typical description of medicine is curing; for nursing, it is caring. This type of extreme dichotomy is not helpful for either the nursing or medical profession individually and also has implications for the interrelationship between the two professions, adding conflict and creating difficulty in communication in the interprofessional team.

The use of technology in health care has increased steadily since 1960, particularly since the end of the 20th century. Nurses work with technology daily, and more and more care involves some type of technology. This has a positive impact on care; however, some wonder about the negative impact of technology on caring. Does technology create a barrier between the patient and the nurse that interferes with the nurse–patient relationship? Because of this concern, "nurses are placing more emphasis on the 'high touch' aspect of a 'high tech' environment, recognizing that clients (patients) require human interactions, such as warmth, care, acknowledgement of self-worth, and collaborative decision-making" (Kozier, Erb, & Blais, 1997, p. 10). There must be an effort to combine technology and caring because both are critical to positive patient outcomes. This synergistic relationship is referred to as "technological competency as caring" in nursing (Locsin, 2005). Nurses who use technology but ignore the patient as a person are just technologists; they are not nurses who use knowledge, caring, critical thinking, clinical reasoning and judgment, technological skills, and recognition of the patient as a person as integral parts of the caring process. For example, the nurse who focuses on the computer monitor in the room may get the data needed but does not engage the patient or demonstrate caring in an effective manner—and may miss some important observation data.

Competency

Competency is the behavior that a student is expected to demonstrate. The ANA (2015a) standards define competency as "an expected and measurable level of nursing performance that integrates knowledge, skills, abilities, and judgment based on established scientific knowledge and expectations for nursing practice" (p. 86). The ultimate goal of competence is to promote quality care. The report, *The Future of Nursing. Leading Change, Advancing Health*, recommends, that that all nurses to engage in lifelong learning (Institute of Medicine [IOM], 2010). Competency levels change over time as students gain more experience. Development of competencies continues throughout a nurse's career. Nurses in practice have to demonstrate certain competencies to continue practice. Meeting staff development/education requirements assist in improving staff practice at level expected, but it does not ensure it. Students, however, must satisfy competency requirements to progress through the nursing program

and graduate. Competencies include elements of knowledge, caring, and technical skills and affect curricula as discussed in other chapters in this text.

After a number of reports described serious problems with health care, including errors and poor-quality care, an initiative was developed to identify core competencies for all healthcare professions, including nursing, to build a bridge across the quality chasm to improve care (IOM, 2003). It is hoped that these competencies will have an impact on education for, and practice in, health professions. The core competencies are identified here and discussed throughout this text (2003, p. 4).

1. *Provide patient-centered care:* Identify, respect, and care about patients' differences, values, preferences, and expressed needs; relieve pain and suffering; coordinate continuous care; listen to, clearly inform, communicate with, and educate patients; share decision making and management; and continuously advocate disease prevention, wellness, and promotion of healthy lifestyles, including a focus on population health. The description of this core competency relates to content found in definitions of nursing, nursing standards, nursing social policy statement, and nursing theories.

2. *Work in interdisciplinary [interprofessional] teams:* Cooperate, collaborate, communicate, and integrate care in teams to ensure that care is continuous and reliable. There is much knowledge available about teams and how they impact care. Leadership is a critical component of working on teams—both as team leader and as followers or members. Many of the major nursing roles that are discussed in this chapter require working with teams.

3. *Employ evidence-based practice:* Integrate best research with clinical expertise and patient values for optimal care, and participate in learning and research activities to the extent feasible. EBP has been mentioned in this chapter about knowledge and caring as it relates to research.

4. *Apply quality improvement:* Identify errors and hazards in care; understand and implement basic safety design principles, such as standardization and simplification; continually understand and measure quality of care in terms of structure, process, and outcomes in relation to patient and community needs; and design and test interventions to change processes and systems of care, with the objective of improving quality. Understanding how care is provided and which problems in providing care arise often leads to the need for additional knowledge development through research.

5. *Utilize informatics:* Communicate, manage knowledge, mitigate error, and support decision-making using information technology. This chapter focuses on knowledge and caring, both of which require use of informatics to meet patient needs.

Stop and Consider #2

Critical thinking and clinical reasoning and judgment are related but not the same.

Scholarship in Nursing

There is a great need to search for better solutions and knowledge and to disseminate knowledge in health care. This discussion about scholarship in nursing explores the meaning of scholarship, the meaning and impact of theory and research, use of professional literature, and new scholarship modalities.

What Does Scholarship Mean?

The American Association of Colleges of Nursing (AACN, 2005) defines **scholarship** in nursing "as those activities that systematically advance the teaching, research, and practice of nursing through rigorous inquiry that: (1) is significant to the profession, (2) is creative, (3) can be documented, (4) can be replicated or elaborated, and (5) can be peer-reviewed through various methods" (p. 1). The common response when asking which activities might be considered scholarship is "research." Boyer (1990), however, questioned this view of scholarship, suggesting that other activities may also be scholarly:

- *Discovery*, in which new and unique knowledge is generated (research, theory development, philosophical inquiry)
- *Teaching*, in which the teacher creatively builds bridges between his or her own understanding and the students' learning
- *Application*, in which the emphasis is on the use of new knowledge in solving society's problems (practice)
- *Integration*, in which new relationships among disciplines are discovered (publishing, presentations, grant awards, licenses, patents, or products for sale; must involve two or more disciplines, thus advancing knowledge over a broader range)

These four aspects of scholarship are critical components of academic nursing and support the values of a profession committed to both social relevance and scientific advancement.

Some nurses think that the AACN definition of scholarship limits scholarship to educational institutions only. Mason (2006) commented that this is a problem for nursing; science needs to be accessible to practitioners, defining *scholarship* as "an in-depth, careful process of exploring current theory and research with the purpose of either furthering the science or translating its findings into practice or policy" (p. 11). The better approach, then, is to consider scholarship in both the education and practice arenas and still emphasize that nursing is a patient-centered practice profession. Nursing theory and research are described in this chapter—and by Mason—as integral parts of knowledge and caring and scholarship of nursing. If all nurses should demonstrate scholarship and leadership, it is important that nurses understand what they mean and how they affect practice.

Nursing has a long history of scholarship, although some periods seem to have been more active than others in terms of major contributions to nursing scholarship. **Exhibit 2-1** describes some of the milestones that are important in understanding nursing scholarship as the profession developed first in Britain and then in the United States.

Exhibit 2-1 A Brief History of Selected Nursing Scholarship Milestones

1850	Nightingale conducted first nursing research by collecting healthcare data during the Crimean War.
1851	Florence Nightingale, age 32, attended the Institution of Deaconesses at Kaiserswerth to train in nursing. She was interested in care focused on spirituality and healing. This experience had an impact on her later work in nursing and nurses' training (education).
1854–1855	Nightingale created the first standards for care.
1854–1856	Nightingale applied knowledge of statistics and care training. She took charge of lay nurses and the Anglican sisters.
1860	The first training school for nurses was founded in London.
1860	*Notes on Nursing* by Nightingale was published.
	Early in the history of the United States, some steps were taken that later would serve as stepping-stones to a more structured healthcare system and affect the education and roles and responsibilities of nurses. • A lack of organized nursing and care led to the development of Bellevue Hospital, which was founded in 1658 in New York. • In 1731, the Philadelphia Almshouse was started by the Sisters of Charity, spearheaded by Elizabeth Ann Bayley Seton, a physician's daughter who married, was widowed, and then entered religious life and provided nursing care. • Charity Hospital in New Orleans, Louisiana, was founded in 1736 and funded by private endowment.
1860–1865	During the Civil War, Dorothea Dix was Superintendent of Female Nurses for the Union Army. She identified the first qualifications for nurses in the United States.
1860s	Dr. Elizabeth Blackwell, first female U.S. physician, started the Women's Central Association for Relief in New York City, which later became the city's Sanitary Commission. The New England Hospital for Women and Children in Boston, Massachusetts, opened in 1860. During its early years, there was no structured care, such as what we know of care today, in the hospital. Woman's Hospital of Philadelphia opened in 1861, also with no structured care but a place sick people came for general caring. In 1863, the state of Massachusetts established the state first board of nursing, which was the first attempt at regulation of the practice of nursing in the United States.

(continues)

Exhibit 2-1 *(continued)*

1870s	The first U.S. nursing school graduate was Linda Richards in 1873 from the New England Hospital for Women and Children in Boston, Massachusetts. Although Nightingale had made a plea for attention to the hospital environment in Britain, it was not until the 1870s that lights were introduced in hospitals. Written patient reports were instituted during this time, replacing the use of only verbal reports. Hospitals began to examine the causes of mortality among their patient population, representing initial steps toward quality improvement. Mary Mahoney, the first Black nurse, graduated in 1879.
1873	Three nursing schools were founded: Bellevue Training School in New York City; Connecticut Training School in New Haven, Connecticut; and Boston Training School in Boston, Massachusetts.
1882	Clara Barton, a schoolteacher, founded the American Red Cross.
1884	Isabel Hampton Robb wrote *Nursing: Its Principles and Practice for Hospital and Private Use*.
1885	The first nursing text was published: *A Textbook of Nursing for the Use of Training Schools, Families and Private Students*.
1890s	The Visiting Nurses Group started in England.
1893	The American Society of Superintendents of Training Schools was formed. Lillian Wald founded the Henry Street Settlement, a community center in New York City. This was the beginning of community-based care.
1897	The nursing school in Galveston, Texas, moved its undergraduate nursing education into the university setting—the University of Texas at Galveston.
1900–1930s	A shortage of funds put nursing education under the control of doctors and hospitals. This situation resulted from: • Leaders believing that the only way to change was to organize. • The need to provide protection for the public from poorly educated nurses. • A lack of sanitation. • Schools providing cheap services for hospitals.
1900	Columbia Teachers College offered the first graduate nursing degree. As nursing moved from a practice-based discipline to a university program, subjects such as ethics were introduced for the first time. Isabel Hampton Robb, considered the architect of American nursing, wrote *Nursing Ethics*, the first ethics text for nurses. Both textbooks and journals for nurses became available. Among the first of the journals was the *American Journal of Nursing*.
1901	Mary Adelaide Nutting started a 3- to 6-month preparatory course for nurses; by 1911, 86 schools had some form of formalized, structured nurse training.
1907	Mary Adelaide Nutting became the first nursing professor and began the first state nursing association in Maryland. At this time, nursing was moving toward a more formal educational system, similar to that of the discipline of medicine. A professional organization at a state level gave recognition to nursing as a distinct discipline.

Exhibit 2-1 *(continued)*

	As a distinct discipline, nursing needed standards to guide practice and education. Isabel Hampton Robb wrote *Educational Standards for Nurses*.
1908	Other professional organizations grew, including the National Association of Colored Graduate Nurses.
1909	The first baccalaureate degree program in nursing was started at the University of Minnesota.
1911	The development of specialties within nursing began with Bellevue Hospital's midwifery program.
1912	The American Society of Superintendents of Training Schools became the National League for Nursing Education (NLNE). The National Organization for Public Health Nursing was founded. The *Public Health Nursing* journal was started.
1917	The National League for Nursing Education identified its first *Standard Curriculum for Schools of Nursing*, a remedy for the lack of standards in nursing education.
1920	The first master's program in nursing began at Yale School of Nursing.
1922	Sigma Theta Tau International (STTI), the nursing honor society, was formed.
1923	The Goldmark Report called for nursing education to be separate from (and precede) employment; it also advocated nursing licensure and proper training for faculty at nursing institutions.
1925	Mary Breckenridge founded the Frontier Nursing Service in Kentucky. Her intent was to provide rural health care; this organization was the first to employ nurses who could also provide midwifery services. As the status of women increased, nurses were among the first women to lead the women's rights movements in the United States.
1930	A total of 41 (out of 48) states established regulatory state boards of nursing.
1934	New York University and the Teachers College started PhD and EdD in programs in nursing.
1940	The Nursing Council on National Defense, formed after World War I (1917–1918), underwent changes during 1940. As nursing education moved into university settings, nursing research became more important for well-educated nurses to study. The first research studies focused on nursing education.
1948	The Brown Report recommended that nursing education programs be located in universities; this report also formed the basis for evaluating nursing programs.
1950s–1960s	Early nursing theory was developed.
1950	The American Nurses Association published the first edition of the *Code for Nurses*. Graduate nursing education began programs to prepare clinical nurse specialists.

(continues)

Exhibit 2-1 *(continued)*

1952	The NLNE changed its name to the National League for Nursing (NLN). Publication of *Nursing Research* began under the direction of the ANA. Mildred Montag started the first associate degree-nursing program.
1954	The University of Pittsburgh started a PhD program in nursing (academic doctorate).
1955	The American Nurses Foundation was formed to obtain funds for nursing research.
1956	Columbia University granted its first master's degree in nursing.
1960	The doctorate in nursing science (DNS) degree was started at Boston University (professional doctorate).
1960s	Federal monies were made available for doctoral study for nurse educators.
1963	The initial publication of *International Journal of Nursing Studies* became available.
1964	Loretta Ford established the first nurse practitioner program at the University of Colorado.
1965	The first nursing research conference was held. The ANA made the statement that a baccalaureate degree should represent the entry level for nursing practice. As of 2017, this recommendation was still not fully implemented, although there has been significant improvement since the publication of *The Future of Nursing. Leading Change, Advancing Health* (IOM, 2010).
1967	The STTI launched its publication *Image* (Now known as the *Journal of Nursing Scholarship*.)
1969	The American Association of Colleges of Nursing (AACN) formed, with its 121 members serving as representation for baccalaureate degree and higher education nursing programs.
1970s–1990s	This period of development saw the birth of most nursing theories; some of these theories have been tested and expanded upon.
1973	The first nursing diagnosis conference was held. The American Academy of Nursing (AAN) was formed under the aegis of the ANA to recognize nursing leaders. The ANA published the first edition of *Standards of Nursing Practice*.
1978–1979	Several new nursing research journals had their initial publication.
1985	The National Center for Nursing Research was established at the National Institutes of Health, later to become the National Institute of Nursing Research (NINR).
1990s	Evidence-based practice became a major focus.

Exhibit 2-1 *(continued)*

1993	The ANA published its position statement on nursing education.
	The American Association of Colleges of Nursing (AACN) established the Commission on Collegiate Nursing Education (CCNE) to accredit nursing programs, with an emphasis on baccalaureate and master's degree programs.
	The Cochrane Collaborative was formed in Britain to develop and publish systematic reviews, expanding access to evidence-based literature.
1995	The ANA published the first edition of *Nursing's Social Policy Statement*.
1996	The Joanna Briggs Institute for Evidence-Based Practice, which focused on nursing to provide access to this literature, was founded in Adelaide, Australia.
1997	The National League for Nursing Accrediting Commission (NLNAC) became a separate corporation from the NLN. It changed its name to the Accreditation Commission for Education in Nursing (ACEN) in 2013.
1999	The AACN published its position statement on nursing research.
2004	The NLN established Centers for Excellence in Nursing Education to recognize exemplar schools of nursing and later the Academy of Nursing to recognize nurse educators.
	The AACN endorsed the development of and called for pilot schools to create the Clinical Nurse Leader (CNL).
	The AACN issued a statement endorsing the movement of the level of preparation for advanced practice nursing from master's level to doctorate by 2015—date has been revised for some specialty areas.
2010	The landmark nursing education report, *Educating Nurses: A Call for Radical Transformation* (Benner, Sutphen, Leonard, and Day), was published.
	A significant Institute of Medicine report, *The Future of Nursing: Leading Change, Advancing Health*, was published (IOM, 2010). In 2015, a progress report was published indicating need to continue work on the report's recommendations.
	Passage of the Patient Protection and Affordable Care Act (ACA), which had an impact on the number of people with healthcare coverage in the United States (from 2010 to early 2017) and included provisions that affect nursing and nursing education, such as funding. *Status of this legislation may change over time and change these outcomes and provisions.*

Nursing Theory

A simple description of a **theory** is "words or phrases (concepts) joined together in sentences, with an overall theme, to explain, describe, or predict something" (Sullivan, 2006, p. 160). Theories help nurses understand and find meaning in nursing. A number of nursing theories have been developed since Nightingale's contributions to nursing, particularly during the 1960s through 1980s. These theories vary widely in their scope and approach. This surge in development of nursing theories was related to the need to "justify nursing as an academic discipline"—the need to develop and describe nursing knowledge" (Maas, 2006, p. 7). Some of the major theories are described in **Exhibit 2-2** from the perspective of how each description, beginning with Nightingale, consider the concepts of the person, the environment, health, and nursing.

Since the late 1990s, nursing education has placed less emphasis on nursing theory. This change has been controversial. Theories may be used to provide frameworks for research studies and to test their applicability. In addition, practice may be guided by one of the nursing theories. In hospitals and other healthcare organizations, the nursing department may identify a specific theory or a model on which the staff bases its mission. In these organizations, it is usually easy to see how the designated theory is present in the official

Exhibit 2-2 Overview of Major Nursing Theories and Models

Theories and Models	Person	Environment	Health	Nursing
Systematic approach to health care Florence Nightingale	Recipient of nursing care.	External (temperature, bedding, ventilation) and internal (food, water, and medications).	Health is "not only to be well, but to be able to use well every power we have to use" (Nightingale, 1969 [reissue], p. 24).	Alter or manage the environment to implement the natural laws of health.
Theory of caring in nursing Jean Watson	A "unity of mind body spirit/ nature" (Watson, 1996, p. 147).	A "field of connectedness" at all levels (Watson, 1996, p. 147).	Harmony, wholeness, and comfort.	Reciprocal transpersonal relationship in caring moments guided by curative factors.
Science of unitary human beings Martha E. Rogers	An irreducible, irreversible, pandimensional, negentropic energy field identified by pattern; a unitary human being develops through three principles: helicy, resonancy, and integrality (Rogers, 1992).	An irreducible, pandimensional, negentropic energy field, identified by pattern and manifesting characteristics different from those of the parts and encompassing all that is other than any given human field (Rogers, 1992).	Health and illness area a part of a continuum (Rogers, 1970).	Seeks to promote symphonic interaction between human and environmental fields, to strengthen the integrity of the human field, and to direct and redirect patterning of the human and environmental fields for realization of maximum health potential (Rogers, 1970).

Exhibit 2-2 *(continued)*

Self-care deficit nursing theory Dorothea E. Orem	A person under the care of a nurse; a total being with universal, developmental needs, and capable of self-care (patient).	Physical, chemical, biologic, and social contexts with which human beings exist; environmental components include environmental factors, environmental conditions, and developmental environment (Orem, 1985).	"A state characterized by soundness or wholeness of developed human structures and of bodily and mental functioning" (Orem, 1995, p. 101).	Therapeutic self-care designed to supplement self-care requisites. Nursing actions fall into one of three categories: wholly compensatory, partly compensatory, or supportive educative system (Orem, 1985).
Roy adaptation model Callista Roy	"A whole with parts that function as a unity" (Roy & Andrews, 1999, p. 31).	Internal and external stimuli; "the world within and around humans as adaptive systems" (Roy & Andrews, 1999, p. 51).	"A state and process of being and becoming an integrated and whole human being" (Roy & Andrews, 1999, p. 54).	Manipulation of stimuli to foster successful adaptation.
Neuman systems model Betty Neuman	A composite of physiological, psychological, sociocultural, developmental, and spiritual variables in interaction with the internal and external environment; represented by central structure, lines of defense, and lines of resistance.	All internal and external factors of influences surrounding the client system.	A continuum of wellness to illness.	Prevention as intervention; concerned with all potential stressors.

(continues)

Exhibit 2-2 *(continued)*

Systems framework and theory of goal attainment Imogene M. King	A personal system that interacts with interpersonal and social systems (human being).	A context "within which human beings grow, develop, and perform daily activities" (King, 1981, p. 18). "The internal environment of human beings transforms energy to enable them to adjust to continuous external environmental changes" (1981, p. 5).	"Dynamic life experiences of a human being, which implies continuous adjustment to stressors in the internal and external environment through optimum use of one's resources to achieve maximum potential for daily living" (King, 1981, p. 5).	A process of human interaction; the goal of nursing is to help patients achieve their goals.
Behavioral systems model Dorothy Johnson	A biophysical being is a behavioral system with seven subsystems of behavior (human being).	Includes internal and external environment.	Efficient and effective functioning of system; behavioral system balance and stability.	An external regulatory force that acts to preserve the organization and integrity of the patient's behavior at an optimal level under those conditions in which the behavior constitutes a threat to physical or social health or in which illness is found (Johnson, 1980, p. 214).
Theory of human becoming Rosemarie Parse	An open being, more than and different from the sum of parts in mutual simultaneous interchange with the environment, who chooses from options and bears responsibility for choices (Parse, 1987, p. 160).	In mutual process with the person.	Continuously changing process of becoming.	Use of true presence to facilitate the becoming of the participant.

Exhibit 2-2 *(continued)*

Transcultural nursing model Madeleine Leininger	Human beings, family, group, community, or institution.	"Totality of an event, situation, or experience that gives meaning to human expressions, interpretations, and social interactions in physical, ecological, sociopolitical, and/or cultural settings" (Leininger, 1991, p. 46).	"A state of well-being that is culturally defined, valued, and practiced" (Leininger, 1991, p. 46).	Activities directed toward assisting, supporting, or enabling with needs in ways that are congruent with the cultural values, beliefs, and lifeways of the recipient of care (Leininger, 1995).
Interpersonal relations model Hildegard Peplau	"Encompasses the patient (one who has problems for which expert nursing services are needed or sought) and the nurse (a professional with particular expertise)" (Peplau, 1952, p. 14).	Includes culture as important to the development of personality.	"Implies forward movement of personality and other ongoing human processes in the direction of creative, constructive, productive, personal, and community living" (Peplau, 1952, p. 12).	The therapeutic, interpersonal process between the nurse and the patient.

Data from Johnson, D. (1980). The behavioral systems model for nursing. In J. Riehl & C. Roy (Eds.), *Conceptual models for nursing practice* (2nd ed., pp. 207–216). New York, NY: Appleton-Century-Crofts; King, I. M. (1981). *A theory of nursing: Systems, concepts, process.* New York, NY: Wiley; Leininger, M. M. (1991). *Culture care diversity and universality: A theory of nursing.* New York, NY: National League for Nursing; Leininger, M. M. (1995). Transcultural nursing perspectives: Basic concepts, principles, and culture care incidents. In M. M. Leininger (Ed.), *Transcultural nursing: Concepts, theories, research, and practices* (2nd ed., pp. 57–92). New York, NY: McGraw-Hill; Nightingale, F. (1969 [reissue]). *Notes on nursing: What it is and what it is not.* New York, NY: Dover; Orem, D. (1985). *Nursing: Concepts of practice* (3rd ed.). St. Louis, MO: Mosby; Orem, D. (1995). *Nursing: Concepts of practice* (5th ed.). St. Louis, MO: Mosby; Parse, R. R. (1987). *Nursing science: Major paradigms, theories, and critiques.* Philadelphia, PA: Saunders; Peplau, H. (1952). *Interpersonal relations in nursing.* New York, NY: G. P. Putnam's Sons; Rogers, M. E. (1970). *An introduction to the theoretical basis of nursing.* Philadelphia, PA: Davis; Rogers, M. E. (1992). *Nursing science and the space age. Nursing Science Quarterly, 5,* 27–34; Roy, C., & Andrews, H. A. (1999). *The Roy adaptation model.* New York, NY: Appleton-Lange; Watson, J. (1996). Watson's philosophy and theory of human caring in nursing. In J. P. Riehl-Sisca (Ed.), *Conceptual models for nursing practice* (pp. 219–235). Norwalk, CT: Appleton & Lange, as cited in K. Masters (2005), *Role development in professional nursing practice.* Sudbury, MA: Jones & Bartlett Learning.

documents about the department, but it is not always so easy to see how the theory impacts the day-to-day practice of nurses in the organization. It is important to remember that theories do not tell nurses what they must do or how they must do something; rather, they are guides—abstract guides. **Figure 2-1** describes the relationship among theory, research, and practice.

Most of the existing nursing theories were developed from the 1970s through 1990s. What issues might future theories address? In 1992, the following were predicted as possible areas to be included in nursing theories (Meleis, 1992, pp. 112–114):

- The human science underlying the discipline that is predicated on understanding the meanings of daily-lived experiences as they are perceived by the members or the participants of the science
- The increased emphasis on practice orientation, or actual, rather than "ought-to-be," practice
- The mission of nursing to develop theories to empower nurses, the discipline, and clients (patients)
- Acceptance of the fact that women may have different strategies and approaches to knowledge development than men
- Nursing's attempt to understand consumers' experiences for the purpose of empowering

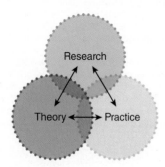

Figure 2-1 Relationship Theory, Research, Practice

Reproduced from Masters, K. (2005). *Role development in professional nursing practice*. Sudbury, MA: Jones & Bartlett Learning.

them to receive optimum care and to maintain optimum health

- The effort to broaden nursing's perspective, which includes efforts to understand the practice of nursing in third world countries

These potential characteristics of nursing are somewhat different from those evidenced in past theories. Consumerism is highlighted through better understanding consumers/patients and empowering them. Empowering nurses is also emphasized. The suggestion that female nurses and male nurses might approach care issues differently has not really been addressed in the past. The effort to broaden nursing's perspective is highly relevant today, given the increase in globalization and the emphasis on culturally appropriate care. Developed and developing countries can share information via the Internet in a matter of seconds. There are fewer boundaries than ever before, such that better communication and information exchange have become possible. A need for nursing to expand its geographic scope certainly exists because globally nursing issues and care problems are often the same or very similar. Indeed, efforts to solve these problems on a worldwide scale are absolutely necessary. Take, for example, issues such as infectious diseases: Because of the ease of travel, they can quickly spread from one part of the world to another in which the disease is relatively unknown. How we understand nursing and the knowledge required to improve performance are critical aspects that may be assisted by greater sharing of experiences globally. In conclusion, theory development is not as active today as it was in the past—it is not really clear what role nursing theories might play and how theories might change in the future.

Nursing Research

Nursing **research** is "systematic inquiry that uses disciplined methods to answer questions and solve problems" (Polit & Beck, 2013, p. 4). The major purpose of doing research is to expand nursing knowledge to improve patient care and outcomes. Research helps to explain and predict care that nurses provide. Two major types of research exist: basic and applied. **Basic research** is conducted to gain knowledge for knowledge sake, and basic research results may then be used in **applied or clinical research**.

Connecting research with practice has improved both in nursing education and practice. There needs to better collaboration between the nurses in practice and the research process. Nursing needs to know more about "whether and how nurses produce knowledge in their practice" (Reed, 2006, p. 36). Nursing—indeed, all health care—needs to be patient-centered (IOM, 2003), and research should also be patient-centered. This does not mean that there is no need for research in administration/management and in education, because there are critical needs in these areas; rather, it means that nursing needs to gain more knowledge about the nursing process with patients as the center. Because of these issues, EBP has become more central in nursing practice, as discussed later in this chapter. The research process is similar to the nursing process in that there is a need to identify a problem using data, determine goals, describe what will be done, and then assess results.

Professional Literature

Professional literature is an important part of nursing scholarship, but it is important to remember that "because of the changing healthcare environment and the proliferation of knowledge in health care and nursing, much of the knowledge acquired in your nursing education program may be out of date 5 years after you graduate" (Zerwekh & Claborn, 2006, p. 197). This literature is found in textbooks and in professional journals. It represents a repository of nursing knowledge that is accessible to nursing students and nurses. It is important that nurses keep up with the literature including research in their specialty areas, given the increased emphasis on EBP. Increased access to journals is now available

through the Internet, and this is a positive change because it makes knowledge more accessible when it is needed along with many other information resources now accessible through the Internet.

Textbooks typically are a few years behind current information because of the length of the publication schedule. Although this gap is improving, it still takes significantly longer to write and publish a textbook than a journal and its articles. It is also more expensive to publish a book, so new editions do not come out annually or, as in the case of many journals, monthly. The content found in textbooks provides the background information and detail on particular topics. A textbook is peer reviewed when content is shared with experts on the topic for feedback to the author(s). Today, many textbook publishers offer companion websites to provide additional material and, in some cases, more updated content or references. More publishers are publishing textbooks in e-book format; some offer both hard copy and e-books, and others offer only e-books. This change might reduce the delay in getting textbooks published and provide a method for updating content quickly.

Content in journals is typically more current than in textbooks and usually focuses on a very specific topic in less depth than a textbook. Higher-quality journals are peer reviewed. This means that several nurses who have expertise in the manuscript's topic review submitted manuscripts. A consensus is then reached with the editor regarding whether to publish the manuscript. Online access to journal articles has made this literature more accessible to nurses. A newer option for publishing in journals today is open access journals—which offer unrestricted access and unrestricted reuse (for example, no copyright fees or permission is required if one uses content from an open access journal). These journals are usually available free online to anyone who wants access. Publishing in these journals can vary, for example, some use peer review and some do not. Authors must pay fees to publish in the journal, and sometimes these fees are high. Authors will typically choose nonopen access journals with more prestige if they can get their manuscripts accepted. This is still a relatively new area and thus it is unknown how this will develop in the future—but the Internet encourages free use of information, and this has had an impact on how we get professional information and the many barriers set up in the past on publishing and sharing information.

Nursing professional organizations often publish journals. Studies published in the last 25 years in scientific nursing journals have primarily focused on adults and psychological factors, with a decrease in theory-based studies and an increase in qualitative studies (Oermann & Jenerette, 2013). Any nurse with expertise in an area can submit an article for publication; however, this does not mean all manuscripts are published. The profession needs more nurses publishing, particularly in journals. Publications are listed on nurse's resumes or curriculum vita as scholarly endeavors and have an impact on career goals and promotion. **Exhibit 2-3** identifies examples of nursing journals.

New Modalities of Scholarship

Scholarship includes publications, copyrights, licenses, patents, or products for sale. Nursing is expanding into a number of new modalities that can be considered scholarship. Many of these modalities relate to web-based learning—including course development and learning activities and products such as case software for simulation experiences—and involve other technology, such as tablets and smartphones. Most of these new modalities relate to teaching and learning in academic programs, although many have expanded into staff development/education and continuing education and even to tools used in practice. In developing these modalities, nurses are creating innovative methods, developing programs and learning outcomes, improving professional development, applying technical skills, and sharing scholarship in a timelier manner with the goal of improving nursing practice. Interprofessional

Exhibit 2-3 Examples of Nursing Journals
American Journal of Nursing (AJN)
American Nurse Today
Archives of Psychiatric Nursing
Home Healthcare Nurse
International Journal of Nursing Knowledge
Journal for Nurses in Professional Development
Journal of Cardiovascular Nursing
Journal of Emergency Nursing
Journal of Nursing Administration
Journal of Nursing Care Quality
Journal of Nursing Informatics
Journal of Nursing Management
Journal of Nursing Scholarship
Journal of Pediatric Nursing
Journal of Perinatal and Neonatal Nursing
Journal of Professional Nursing
Journal of Psychiatric Nursing and Mental Health Nursing
Nurse Leader
Nursing Management
Nursing Outlook
Nursing Research
Nursing 2017
Oncology Nursing
Online Journal of Nursing
World Views of Evidence-Based Nursing

approaches are used more today, and this improves integrative scholarship—something nurses need to be aware of and engage in as improvements are made.

Stop and Consider #3

Because scholarship is a critical aspect of professionalism, you need to demonstrate scholarship as a professional nurse.

Multiple Nursing Roles
and Leadership

Nurses use knowledge and caring as they provide care to patients; however, there are other aspects of nursing that are important. As nurses apply knowledge and caring, they function in multiple roles.

Key Nursing Roles

Before discussing nursing roles, it is important to discuss some terminology related to roles. A role can vary depending on the context. **Role** means the expected and actual behaviors that one would associate with a position such as a nurse, physician, teacher, pharmacist, and so on. Connected to role is **status**, which is a position in a social structure, with rights and obligations—for example, a nurse manager would have more status compared with a staff nurse. As a person assumes a new role, the person experiences **role transition**. Nursing students are in role transition as they gradually learn about nursing roles. All nursing roles are important in patient care, and typically these roles are interconnected in practice. Students learn about the roles and what is necessary to be competent to meet role expectations. **Identity** is also involved: "Identity is foundational to professional nursing practice. Identity in nursing can be defined as the development within nurses of an internal representation of people–environment interactions in the exploration of human responses to actual or potential health problems. Professional identity is foundational to the assumption of various nursing roles" (Cook, Gilmer, & Bess, 2003, p. 311).

Nursing is a complex profession and involves multiple types of consumers of nursing care (for example, individuals, families, specific populations, and communities), multiple types of problems (for example, physical, emotional, sociological, economic, and educational), and multiple settings (for example, hospitals, clinics, communities, schools, the patient's home), and specialties within each of these dimensions. Some roles such as teaching, administration, and research do not focus as much on the teacher, administrator, or researcher providing direct patient care. Different levels of knowledge, caring, and education may be required for different roles. All of the roles require leadership. The key roles found in nursing are discussed in the following sections. Within a position title such as a staff nurse, the nurse may actually have multiple roles such as provider of care, patient educator, and so on.

Provider of Care

The **provider of care** role is probably what students think nursing is all about—this is the role typically seen in the hospital setting and the role that most people think of when they think of a nurse. Caring is attached most to this role, but knowledge is critical to providing quality care. When the nurse is described, it is often caring that is emphasized, with less emphasis on knowledge and expertise required to provide quality care. This perspective is not indicative of what really happens because nurses need to use knowledge and be competent, as discussed earlier in this chapter. Providing care has moved far beyond the hospital, with nurses providing care in clinics, schools, the community, homes, industry, and at many more sites.

Educator

Nurses spend a lot of time teaching—teaching patients, families, communities, and populations. In the **educator** role, nurses focus on health promotion and prevention and helping the patient (individuals, families, communities, and populations) cope with illness and injury and maintain health. Teaching needs to be planned and based on needs, and nurses must know about teaching principles and methods. Some nurses teach other nurses and healthcare providers in healthcare settings—an activity called staff development or staff education or in nursing schools. Nursing education is considered to be a type of nursing specialty/advanced practice.

Counselor

A nurse may act as a **counselor**, providing advice and counseling to patients, families, communities, and populations. This is often done in conjunction with other roles.

Manager

In daily practice, nurses act as managers, even if they do not have a formal management position. **Management** is the process of getting something done efficiently and effectively through and with other people. Nurses might do this by ensuring that a patient's needs are addressed—for example, the nurse might ensure that the patient receives needed laboratory work or a rehabilitation session. The nurse who provides patient care needs to plan the care (interventions, timeline, and who will provide specific care), implements the plan, and evaluates outcomes, making changes as need. Managing care involves critical thinking, clinical reasoning and judgment, planning, decision making, delegating, collaborating, coordinating, communicating, working with interprofessional teams, and leadership. There are also nurses in formal management positions such as a manager of a unit, director of nursing or vice president of nursing, dean of a school of nursing, and so on—all are formal managers.

Researcher

Only a small percentage of nurses are actual nurse **researchers** leading research studies; however, nurses may participate in research in other ways. The most critical means is by using EBP or evidence-based management (EBM), which is one of the five core healthcare professions competencies. Some nurses now hold positions in research studies that may or may not be nursing research studies. These nurses assist in obtaining informed consent, data collection, and may manage research projects.

Collaborator

Every nurse is a collaborator. "**Collaboration** [boldface added] is a cooperative effort that focuses on a win-win strategy. Each individual needs to recognize the perspective of others who are involved and eventually reach a consensus of common goal(s)" (Finkelman, 2016, p. 318). A nurse collaborates with other healthcare providers, members of the community, government agencies, and many other individuals and organizations. Teamwork is a critical component of daily nursing practice.

Change Agent (Intrapreneur)

It is difficult to perform any of the nursing roles without engaging in change. Change may be found in how care is provided, where care is provided and when, to whom care is provided, and why care is provided. Change is normal today in our personal lives. The healthcare delivery system experiences constant change. Nurses deal with change wherever they work, but they may also initiate change for care improvement. When a nurse acts as a **change agent** within the organization where the nurse works, the nurse is an intrapreneur. This requires risk and the ability to see change in a positive light. An example of a nurse acting as a change agent would be a nurse who sees the value in extending visiting hours in the intensive care unit. The nurse reviews the literature on this topic to support EBP interventions and then approaches management with the suggestion about making a change. The nurse then works with the interprofessional team to plan, implement, and evaluate this change to assess the outcomes.

Entrepreneur

This role is not as common as other roles, though it is found more often today. The **entrepreneur** works to make changes in a broader sense. Examples include nurses who are healthcare consultants and legal nurse consultants and nurses who establish businesses related to health care, such as a staffing agency, a business to develop a healthcare product, a healthcare media business, or a collaboration with a healthcare technology venture.

Patient Advocate

Nurses serve as an **advocate** on behalf of the patient (individual, groups, populations, communities) and family. In this role, the nurse acts as a change agent and a risk taker. The nurse speaks for the patient but does not take away the patient's independence. A nurse caring for a patient in the hospital, for example, might advocate with the physician to alter care so as to allow a dying patient to spend more time with his or her family. A nurse might also advocate for better health coverage by writing to the local congressional representative or by attending a meeting about care in the community—influencing health policy.

Leader

In all of these roles, nurses need to act as **leaders**; however, it is important to recognize that being a leader is a role that nurses assume, either formally by taking an administrative position or informally with others recognizing that someone has leadership characteristics. Leadership is discussed throughout this text.

Summary Points: Roles and What Is Required

To meet the demands of these multiple roles, nurses need to be prepared and competent. Prerequisites and the nursing curriculum, through its content, simulation laboratory experiences, and clinical experiences, help students to transition to these roles. The prerequisites provide content and experiences related to biological sciences, English and writing, sociology, government, languages, psychology, mathematics, and statistics. In nursing, course content relates to the care of diverse patients in hospitals, homes, and communities; planning, implementing, and evaluating care; communication and interpersonal relationships; culture; legal and ethical issues; teaching; public/community health; epidemiology; quality improvement; research and EBP and EBM; health policy; and leadership and management. As discussed earlier in this chapter, this content relates to the required knowledge base.

When students transition to the work setting as registered nurses, they should be competent as beginning nurses; even so, the transition is often difficult. **Reality shock** may occur. This reaction may occur when a new nurse is confronted with the realities of the healthcare setting and nursing, which are typically very different from what the nurse experienced in school (Kramer, 1985). Knowledge and competency are important, but new nurses also need to build self-confidence, and they need time to adjust to the differences between the academic world and real-life practice. Some schools of nursing, in collaboration with hospitals, now offer internship/externship and residency programs for new graduates to decrease reality shock, which are discussed in more detail in other chapters. The major nursing roles that you will learn about in your nursing programs are important in practice, but it is also important for you to learn about being an employee, working with and in teams, communicating in real situations, and functioning in complex organizations.

More nurses—particularly new graduates—work in hospitals than in other healthcare settings, although the number of nurses working in hospitals is decreasing. Hospital care has changed, with sicker patients staying in the hospital for shorter periods and with greater use of complex technology. These changes have an impact on what is expected of nurses—namely, in terms of competencies.

Nursing standards, nurse practice acts, professional ethics, and the nursing process influence nursing roles. Health policy also has an impact on roles; for example, legislation and changes in state practice guidelines were required before the advanced practice registered nurse could obtain have prescriptive authority (ability to prescribe medications). This type of role change requires major advocacy efforts from nurses and nursing organizations.

Stop and Consider #4

Though holding one position, a nurse may have multiple roles as part of that position.

CHAPTER HIGHLIGHTS

1. The definition of nursing varies depending on the source.
2. The need to define nursing relates to the ability to describe what nursing is and what nurses do.
3. Effective nursing practice utilizes critical thinking and clinical reasoning and judgment.
4. Caring and knowledge are critical components of the nursing profession.
5. Today, the trend is toward preparing nurses to serve as knowledge workers.
6. Competency is defined by and related to the skills that a nurse needs to function in today's healthcare environment.
7. Nursing scholarship is demonstrated in nursing theory, research, and professional literature.
8. The key roles of the nurse are care provider, educator, manager, advocate, counselor, researcher, collaborator, change agent (intrepreneur), entrepreneur, and leader.

ENGAGING IN THE CONTENT

Discussion Questions

1. Discuss the relationship between knowledge and caring in nursing.
2. How might a definition of nursing impact your practice?
3. What does *knowledge worker* mean?
4. Why is leadership important in nursing?
5. Describe nurses' roles in today's healthcare system.
6. Why are competencies important?
7. Discuss the role of critical thinking in nursing education and explain why there is little agreement about what constitutes critical thinking. What is the importance of clinical reasoning and judgment? Identify examples from your own practice that apply to critical thinking and clinical reasoning and judgment and their application to nursing roles.

CRITICAL THINKING ACTIVITIES

1. Based on what you have learned about critical thinking, assess your own ability to use critical thinking. Make a list of your strengths and limitations regarding your use of critical thinking. Determine several strategies that you might use to improve your critical thinking. Write down these strategies and track your improvement over the semester. Apply the critical thinking skills mentioned in this chapter to guide you in this activity.
2. Review the descriptions of the nursing theories found in **Exhibit 2-2**. Compare and contrast the theories in relationship to their views of person, environment, health, and nursing. Identify two similarities and dissimilarities in the theories. Select a theory that you feel represents your view of nursing at this time. Why did you select this theory?
3. Go to the National Institute of Nursing Research (NINR) website (http://www.ninr.nih.gov/AboutNINR/) and click on "Mission

(Continues)

CRITICAL THINKING ACTIVITIES (CONTINUED)

& Strategic Plan." Explore the Ongoing Research Interests section. What are some of the interests? Do any of them intrigue you? If so, why? What is the NINR's current strategic plan? What can you learn about past and current nursing research? Did you think of these areas of study as part of nursing before this course? Why or why not? What impressed you about the research results? Do you think these results are practice oriented?

4. Do you think nursing scholarship is important? Provide your rationale for your response.

5. Select one of the major nursing roles and describe it. Explain why you would want to function in this role.

6. Develop questions you will use in an interview of a staff nurse, a nurse manager, or an educator to inquire about their definition of nursing. You can do this in a team and then compare answers. Why do you believe there are differences? How do these definitions relate to what you have learned in this chapter?

7. Ask a patient to describe the role of a nurse then compare this description with your view of nursing. Is it similar or different, and why?

ELECTRONIC REFLECTION JOURNAL

What does *caring* mean to you? How does your view of caring compare with what you have learned in this chapter?

CASE STUDIES

Case 1

A nurse who works in a community clinic has a busy day ahead of her. The first half of the day is focused on seeing four patients as follow-up to their appointments last week for high blood pressure (hypertension). The nurse checks each patient's blood pressure, asks about symptoms, weighs each patient, and asks if the patient has any questions. If there are negative changes, the patient sees the physician. The nurse also assists the physician with physical examinations as needed. Two new patients require patient education about their diets. A dietician appointment is scheduled for one patient who needs more intensive assistance. In the afternoon, the nurse leads a group for diabetic patients. At the end of the day, the nurse meets with her nurse manager for her annual performance evaluation, and the nurse manager tells the nurse that she should write a journal article about the group for patients with diabetes. The nurse is getting into her car to go home and thinks to herself, "Now when would I have time to write a journal article!"

CASE STUDIES (CONTINUED)

Case Questions

1. During the day, which ways of knowing did the nurse use in providing care?
2. What makes this nurse a knowledge worker?
3. Identify what the nurse did that was routine and nonroutine (knowledge management).
4. How did change impact this nurse?

Case 2

A Historical Event to Demonstrate the Importance of the Art and Science of Nursing, Nursing Roles, and Leadership

The following case is a summary of a change in healthcare delivery that had an impact on nursing. After reading the case, respond to the questions.

In the 1960s, something significant began to happen in hospital care, and ultimately in the nursing profession. But first, let's go back to the 1950s for some background information. There was increasing interest in coronary care during this time, particularly for acute myocardial infarctions. It is important to remember that changes in health care are influenced by changes in science and technology, but incidents and situations within the country as a whole also drive change and policy decisions. This situation was no exception. Presidents Dwight D. Eisenhower and Lyndon B. Johnson both had acute myocardial infarctions, which received a lot of press coverage. The mortality rate from acute myocardial infarctions was high. There were also significant new advances in care monitoring and interventions: cardiac catheterization, cardiac pacemakers, continuous monitoring of cardiac electrical activity, portable cardiac defibrillators, and external pacemakers. This really was an incredible list to come onto the scene at the same time.

Now, what was happening with nursing in the 1950s regarding the care of cardiac patients? Even with advances, nurses were providing traditional care, and the boundaries between physicians and nurses were very clear.

Physicians
- Examined the patient
- Administered the electrocardiogram
- Drew blood for laboratory work
- Diagnosed cardiac arrhythmias
- Determined interventions

Nurses
- Made the patient comfortable
- Took care of the patient's belongings
- Answered the family's questions
- Assessed vital signs (blood pressure, pulse, and respirations)
- Made observations and documented them
- Administered medications
- Provided the diet ordered and ensured patient rest

CASE STUDIES (CONTINUED)

In the 1960s, change began to happen. Dr. Hughes Day, a physician at Bethany Hospital in Kansas City, had an interest in cardiac care. The hospital redesigned its units, moving away from open wards to private and semiprivate rooms. This was nice for the patients, but it made it difficult for nurses to observe patients. (This is a good example of how environment and space influence care.) Dr. Day established a Code Blue to communicate the need for urgent response to patients having critical cardiac episodes (Day, 1972). This was a great idea, but the response often came too late for many patients who were not observed early enough. Dr. Day then instituted monitoring of patients with cardiac problems who were unstable. Another good idea, but if there was a problem, what would happen? Who would intervene, and how? Dr. Day would often be called during the day and when he was at home at night, but in such a critical situation, how could he get to the hospital in time? Nurses had no training or experience with the monitoring equipment or in recognizing arrhythmias or knowledge about what to do if there were problems. Dr. Day was beginning to see that his ideas needed revision.

At the same time that Dr. Day was exploring cardiac care, Dr. L. Meltzer was involved in similar activity at Presbyterian Hospital in Philadelphia. These physicians did not know of the work that the other was doing. Dr. Meltzer went about the problem a little differently. He knew that a separate unit was needed for cardiac patients, but he was less sure about how to design it and how it would function. Dr. Meltzer approached the Division of Nursing, U.S. Public Health Services, for a grant to study the problem. He wanted to establish a two-bed cardiac care unit (CCU). His research question was: *Will nurse monitoring and intervention reduce the high incidence of arrhythmic deaths from acute myocardial infarctions*? At this time (and a development that was good for nursing), Faye Abdella, PhD, RN, was leading the Division of Nursing. She really liked the study proposal, but she felt that something important was missing. To receive the grant, Dr. Meltzer needed to have a nurse lead the project. Dr. Meltzer proceeded to look for that nurse. He turned to the University of Pennsylvania and asked the dean of nursing for a recommendation. Rose Pinneo, MSN, RN, a nurse who had just completed her master's degree and had experience in cardiac care, was selected. Dr. Meltzer and Pinneo became a team. Pinneo liked research and wanted to do this kind of work, and by chance, she had her opportunity. What she did not know was this study and its results would have a major long-term impact on cardiac care and the nursing profession.

Dr. Zoll, who worked with Dr. Meltzer, recognized the major barrier to success in changing patient outcomes: Nurses had no training in what would be required of them in the CCU. The proposed change represented a major shift in what nurses usually did. They needed to examine the role of the nurse and it needed to be changed, and so a study was conducted. Notably, Dr. Meltzer, a physician not a nurse, then proposed a new role for nurses in the CCU:

- The nurse has specific skills in monitoring patients using the new equipment.
- Registered nurses (RNs) would provide all the direct care. Up until this time, the typical care organization consisted of a team of licensed practical nurses and aides, who provided most of the direct care, led by an RN (team nursing). This led to changes in CCU staffing and increased the need for more qualified RNs in CCU.
- RNs would interpret heart rhythms using continuous-monitoring electrocardiogram data.

CASE STUDIES (CONTINUED)

- RNs would initiate emergency interventions when needed.
- RNs, not physicians, would be central in providing care in CCU 24 hours a day, 7 days a week, but they must practice with the physicians.

There were questions as to whether RNs could be trained for this new role, but Dr. Meltzer had no doubt that they could be.

Based on Dr. Meltzer's plan and the new nursing role, Pinneo needed to find the nurses for the units. She wanted nurses who were ready for a challenge and who were willing to learn the new knowledge and skills needed to collect data. Collecting data would be time consuming, plus the nurses had to provide care in a very new role. The first step after finding the nurses was training. This, too, was unique. An interprofessional approach was taken, and it took place in the clinical setting, the CCU. Once the unit opened, clinical conferences were held to discuss the patients and their care.

The nurses found that they were providing care for highly complex problems. They were assessing and diagnosing, intervening, and helping patients with their psychological patients with their psychological responses to having had an acute myocardial infarction. Clearly, knowledge and caring were important, but added to this was curing. With the interventions that nurses initiated, they were helping to save lives. Dr. Meltzer developed standing orders telling CCU nurses what to do in certain situations based on clinical data they collected. House staff—physicians in training—began to turn to the nurses to learn more about cardiac care because the CCU nurses had experience with these patients. Dr. Meltzer called his approach the scientific team approach. In 1972, he wrote, "Until World War II even the recording of blood pressure was considered outside the nursing sphere and was the responsibility of a physician. As late as 1962, when coronary care was introduced, most hospitals did not permit their nursing staff to perform venipunctures or to start intravenous infusions. That nurses could interpret the electrocardiograms and defibrillate patients indeed represented a radical change for all concerned" (Meltzer, Pinneo, & Kitchell, 1972, p. 8).

What were the results of this study? Nurses could learn what was necessary to function in the new role. Nurses who worked in CCU gained autonomy, but now the boundaries between physicians and nurses were less clear. This began to spill over into other areas of nursing. There is no doubt that nursing began to change. CCUs opened across the country. They also had an impact on other types of intensive care and then nursing in general.

Case Questions

If you do not know any terms in this case, look them up in a medical dictionary.

1. Based on this case, discuss the implications of the art and science of nursing.
2. What were the differences in how Dr. Day and Dr. Meltzer handled their interests in changing cardiac care?
3. Who led this initiative? Why is this significant?
4. Compare and contrast the changes in nursing roles before the Meltzer and Day studies. What was the new role supported by their work?
5. What is unique and unexpected about this case?
6. What does this case tell you about the value of research?

Sources: Day, H. (1972). History of coronary care units. *American Journal of Cardiology, 30,* 405; Meltzer, L., Pinneo, R., & Kitchell, J. (1972). *Intensive coronary care: A manual for nurses.* Philadelphia, PA: Charles Press.

CASE STUDIES (CONTINUED)

Working Backward to Develop a Case

Write a brief paragraph that describes a case related to the following questions and comments.

1. A nurse says, "I think to get our message across we need to look at who we are and how we have changed as a profession."
2. What do we mean when we say "we all care about patients"?
3. A nurse says, "Our patients and families do not know what we really do."

REFERENCES

Alfaro-LeFevre, R. (2011). *Applying nursing process: A tool for critical thinking.* Philadelphia, PA: Lippincott Williams & Wilkins.

American Association of Colleges of Nursing. (2005). *Position statement on defining scholarship for the discipline of nursing.* Washington, DC: Author.

American Association of Critical-Care Nurses. (2011). The AACCN synergy model for patient care. Retrieved from http://www.aacn.org:88/wd/certifications/content/synmodel.pcms?pid=1&&menu=

American Nurses Association. (2015a). *Nursing scope and standards of practice.* Silver Spring, MD: Author.

American Nurses Association. (20105b). *Nursing's social policy statement.* Silver Spring, MD: Author. Published as an appendix in *Nursing scope and standards of practice (ANA, 2015).*

Benner, P. (2001). *From novice to expert: Excellence and power in clinical nursing practice* (commemorative ed.). Upper Saddle River, NJ: Prentice Hall.

Benner, P., Hughes, R., & Sutphen, M. (2008). Clinical reasoning, decision-making, and action: Thinking critically and clinically. In R. Hughes (Ed.), *Patient safety and quality: An evidence-based handbook for nurses* (pp. 103–125). Rockville, MD: Agency for Health Research and Quality, AHRQ Publication #08-0043.

Benner, P., Tanner, C., & Chesla, C. (1996). *Expertise in nursing practice: Caring, clinical judgment and ethics.* New York, NY: Springer.

Benner, P., Sutphen, M., Leonard, V., & Day, L. (2010). *Educating nurses: A call for radical transformation.* San Francisco, CA: Jossey-Bass.

Boyer, E. (1990). *Scholarship reconsidered: Priorities for the professionate.* Princeton, NJ: Carnegie Foundation for the Advancement of Teaching.

Butcher, H. (2006). Integrating nursing theory, nursing research, and nursing practice. In J. Cowen & S. Moorehead (Eds.), *Current issues in nursing* (7th ed., pp. 112–122). St. Louis, MO: Mosby.

Cappelletti, A., Engel, J., & Prentice, D. (2014). Systematic review of clinical judgment and reasoning in nursing. *Journal of Nursing Education, 53*(8), 453–458.

Cipriano, P. (2007). Celebrating the art and science of nursing. *American Nurse Today, 2*(5), 8.

Conway, J. (1998). Evolution of the species "expert nurse": An examination of practical knowledge held by expert nurses. *Journal of Clinical Nursing, 7*(1), 75–82.

Cook, T., Gilmer, M., & Bess, C. (2003). Beginning students' definitions of nursing: An inductive framework of professional identity. *Journal of Nursing Education, 42*(7), 311–317.

Decker, S. (2007). Integrating guided reflection into simulated learning. In P. Jeffries (Ed.), *Simulation in nursing education* (pp. 73–85). New York, NY: National League for Nursing.

Del Bueno, D. (2005). A crisis in critical thinking. *Nursing Education Perspectives, 26,* 278–282.

Dickenson-Hazard, N. (2002). Evidence-based practice: "The right approach." *Reflections in Nursing Leadership, 28*(2), 6.

Diers, D. (2001). What is nursing? In J. Dochterman & H. Grace (Eds.), *Current issues in nursing* (pp. 5–13). St. Louis, MO: Mosby.

Finkelman, A. (2001, December). Problem-solving, decision-making, and critical thinking: How do they mix and why bother? *Home Care Provider*, 194–199.

Finkelman, A. (2016). *Leadership and management for nurses: Core competencies for quality care* (3rd. ed.). Upper Saddle River, NJ: Pearson Education.

Hansten, R., & Washburn, M. (2000). Intuition in professional practice: Executive and staff perceptions. *Journal of Nursing Administration, 30*(4), 185–189.

Henderson, V. (1991). *The nature of nursing: Reflections after 25 years.* Geneva, Switzerland: International Council of Nurses.

Institute of Medicine. (2003). *Health professions education: A bridge to quality.* Washington, DC: The National Academies Press.

Institute of Medicine. (2010). *The future of nursing: Leading change, advancing health.* Washington, DC: The National Academies Press.

Johns, C. (2004). *Becoming a reflective practitioner* (2nd ed.). Malden, MA: Blackwell.

Kerfoot, K. (2002). The leader as chief knowledge officer. *Nursing Economics, 20*(1), 40–41, 43.

Kozier, B., Erb, G., & Blais, K. (1997). *Professional nursing practice: Concepts and perspectives.* Menlo Park, CA: Addison Wesley Longman.

Kramer, M. (1985). Why does reality shock continue? In J. McCloskey & H. Grace (Eds.), *Current issues in nursing* (pp. 891–903). Boston, MA: Blackwell Scientific.

Linderman, A., Pesut, D., & Disch, J. (2015). Sense making and knowledge transfer: Capturing the knowledge and wisdom of leaders. *Journal of Professional Nursing, 31*(4), 290–297.

Locsin, R. (2005). *Technological competency as caring in nursing: A model for practice.* Indianapolis, IN: Sigma Theta Tau International.

Maas, M. (2006). What is nursing, and why do we ask? In P. Cowen & S. Moorhead (Eds.), *Current issues in nursing* (7th ed., pp. 5–10). St. Louis, MO: Mosby.

Mason, D. (2006). Scholarly? AJN is redefining a crusty old term. *American Journal of Nursing, 106*(1), 11.

Meleis, A. (1992). Directions for nursing theory development in the 21st century. *Nursing Science Quarterly, 5*, 112–117.

Moland, L. (2006). Moral integrity and regret in nursing. In S. Nelson & S. Gordon (Eds.), *The complexities of care: Nursing reconsidered* (pp. 50–68). Ithaca, NY: Cornell University Press.

Mooney, K. (2001). Advocating for quality cancer care: Making evidence-based practice a reality. *Oncology Nursing Forum, 28*(suppl 2), 17–21.

Mustard, L. (2002). Caring and competency. *JONA's Healthcare Law, Ethics, and Regulation, 4*(2), 36–43.

National Institute of Nursing Research. (2016). *30th anniversary: Advancing science, improving lives. A window to the future.* Retrieved from https://www.ninr.nih.gov/newsandinformation/30years

Nelson, S., & Gordon, S. (Eds.). (2006). *The complexities of care: Nursing reconsidered.* Ithaca, NY: Cornell University Press.

North American Nursing Diagnosis Association. (2016). *Nursing diagnoses: Definitions and classification.* Retrieved from http://www.nanda.org/Diagnosis Development/DiagnosisSubmission/PreparingYour Submission/GlossaryofTerms.aspx

Oermann, M., & Jenerette, C. (2013). Scientific nursing journals over 25 years: Most studies continue to focus on adults and psychological variables, with a decline in theory-testing–based studies and an increase in quali- tative studies. *Evidence-Based Nursing, 16*(4), 117–118.

Paul, R. (1995). *Critical thinking: How to prepare students for a rapidly changing world.* Santa Rosa, CA: Midwest.

Pesut, D., & Herman, J. (1999). *Clinical reasoning: The art and science of critical and creative thinking.* Albany, NY: Delmar.

Polit, D., & Beck, C. (2013). *Essentials of nursing research.* Philadelphia, PA: Lippincott Williams & Wilkins.

Porter-O'Grady, T., & Malloch, K. (2007). *Quantum leader- ship: A resource for health care innovation* (2nd ed.). Burlington, MA: Jones & Bartlett Learning.

Reed, P. (2006). The practitioner in nursing epistemology. *Nursing Science Quality, 19*(1), 36–38.

Rubenfeld, M., & Scheffer, B. (2015). *Critical thinking tactics for nurses* (3rd ed.). Sudbury, MA: Jones and Bartlett.

Schwein, J. (2004). The timeless caring connection. *Nursing Administration Quarterly, 28*(4), 265–270.

Scotto, C. (2003). A new view of caring. *Journal of Nursing Education, 42*, 289–291.

Sullivan, A. (2006). Nursing theory. In J. Zerwekh & J. Claborn (Eds.), *Nursing today* (pp. 159–178). St. Louis, MO: Elsevier.

Sorrells-Jones, J., & Weaver, D. (1999). Knowledge work- ers and knowledge-intense organizations, Part 1: A promising framework for nursing and health care. *JONA, 29*(7/8), 12–18.

University of Iowa, College of Nursing. (2016a). *CNC. Overview: Nursing interventions classification.* Retrieved from https://nursing.uiowa.edu/cncce /nursing-interventions-classification-overview

University of Iowa, College of Nursing. (2016b). *CNC. Overview: Nursing outcomes classification.* Re- trieved from https://nursing.uiowa.edu/cncce /nursing-outcomes-classification-overview

Watson, J. (1979). *Nursing: The philosophy and science of caring.* Boston, MA: Little, Brown.

Westberg, J., & Jason, H. (2001). *Fostering reflection and providing feedback.* New York, NY: Springer.

Zerwekh, J., & Claborn, J. (2006). *Nursing today: Transition and trends.* St. Louis, MO: Saunders.

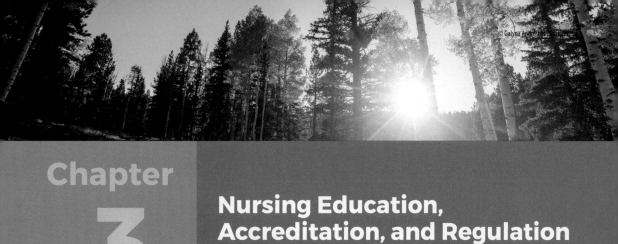

© Galyna Andrushko/Shutterstock

Chapter 3

Nursing Education, Accreditation, and Regulation

CHAPTER OBJECTIVES

At the conclusion of this chapter, the learner will be able to:

- Discuss the differences between nursing education and other types of education.
- Compare the types of nursing programs and degrees.
- Examine the roles of major nursing organizations that affect nursing education.
- Critique examples of methods used to better ensure quality and excellence in nursing education.

- Discuss critical problems in nursing education.
- Examine the need to transform nursing education and possible methods to do so.
- Examine the implications of interprofessional healthcare education.
- Discuss the importance of regulation and critical issues related to the nursing profession.

CHAPTER OUTLINE

- Introduction
- Nursing Education
  - A Brief History of Nursing Education
  - Major Nursing Reports: Improving Nursing Education
  - Entry into Practice: A Long Debate
  - Differentiated Nursing Practice
- Types of Nursing Education Programs
  - Diploma Schools of Nursing
  - Associate Degree in Nursing
  - Baccalaureate Degree in Nursing
  - Master's Degree in Nursing
  - Research-Based Doctoral Degree in Nursing
  - Doctor of Nursing Practice

- Nursing Education Associations
  - National League for Nursing
  - American Association of Colleges of Nursing
  - Organization for Associate Degree Nursing
- Quality and Excellence in Nursing Education
  - Nursing Education Standards
  - NLN Excellence in Nursing Education
  - Focus on Competencies
  - Curriculum
    - Didactic or Theory Content
    - Practicum or Clinical Experience
    - Distance Education

- Accreditation of Nursing Education Programs
- Critical Nursing Education Problems
  - Faculty Shortage
  - Access to Clinical Experiences
  - A Response and Innovation: Laboratory Experiences and Clinical Simulation
  - Transforming Nursing Education
  - Interprofessional Healthcare Education
- Regulation
  - Nurse Practice Acts
  - State Boards of Nursing
  - National Council of State Boards of Nursing
  - Licensure Requirements
  - National Council Licensure Examination
- Critical Current and Future Regulation Issues
  - Nurse Licensure Compact
  - Mandatory Overtime
  - Foreign Nursing Graduates: Entrance to Practice in the United States
  - Global Health Regulatory Issues
- Chapter Highlights
- Engaging in the Content
- Discussion Questions
- Critical Thinking Activities
- Electronic Reflection Journal
- Case Studies
- Working Backward to Develop a Case
- References

KEY TERMS

Academic health center
Academic nursing
Accelerated program
Accreditation
Advanced practice registered nurse
Apprenticeship
Articulation agreement
Associate degree in nursing
Baccalaureate degree in nursing

Clinical experiences
Continuing education
Curriculum
Differentiated practice
Diploma schools of nursing
Direct entry program
Distance education
Doctor of nursing practice
Education
Master's degree in nursing
Nurse licensure compact

Nurse migration
Nurse practice act
Practicum
Preceptor
Prescriptive authority
Regulation
RN-BSN
Research-based doctorate
Self-directed learning
Standard
Training

Introduction

This chapter focuses on three critical concerns in the nursing profession: (1) nursing education, (2) quality of nursing education, and (3) regulatory issues such as licensure. These concerns are interrelated because they change, are dependent on each other (for example, graduating from an accredited program is required for licensure), and require regular input from the nursing profession.

Even after graduation, nurses should be aware of educational issues, such as appropriate and reasonable accreditation of nursing programs and ensuring that regulatory issues support the critical needs of the public for quality health care and the needs of the profession. The Tri-Council for Nursing—an alliance of four nursing organizations (American Association of Colleges of Nursing [AACN], American Nurses Association [ANA], American Organization of Nurse Executives [AONE], and National League for Nursing [NLN])—issued a consensus policy statement in 2010 following Congress's passage of the Patient Protection and Affordable Care Act (ACA). This demonstrates the engagement of the nursing professional in health policy and its collaborative efforts with other healthcare professionals. In part, this policy statement reads as follows: "Current healthcare reform initiatives call for a nursing workforce that integrates evidence-based clinical knowledge and research with effective communication and leadership skills. These competencies require increased education at all levels. At this tipping point for the nursing profession, action is needed now to put in place strategies to build a stronger nursing workforce. Without a more educated nursing workforce, the nation's health will be further at risk" (Tri-Council for Nursing, 2010, p. 1). This statement is in line with the Institute of Medicine (IOM, 2003) recommendations for healthcare professions education. **Figure 3-1** highlights the components of the education-to-practice process.

Nursing Education

A nursing student might wonder why a nursing text has a chapter that includes content about nursing education. By the time, students are reading this text, they have selected a nursing program and enrolled. This content is not included here to help someone decide whether to enter the profession or which nursing program to attend. Rather, it is essential because education is a critical component of the nursing profession. Nurses need to understand the structure and process of the profession's education, education quality issues, and current issues and trends.

Data from 2014 indicate that nursing students represent more than half of all healthcare professionals (American Association of Colleges of Nursing [AACN], 2015a). The number of students enrolling in all levels of nursing programs increased

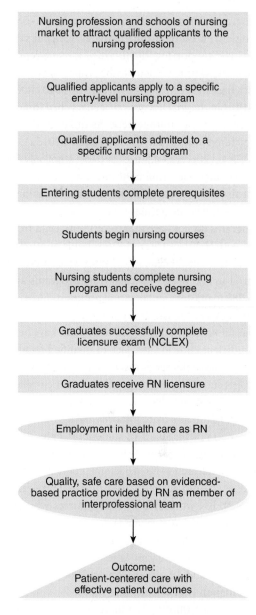

Figure 3-1 From Education to Practice

in 2014: 4.2% increase in entry-level baccalaureate programs (BSN); 10.4% increase in RN-BSN programs (degree completion programs); 6.6% increase in master's programs; 3.2% in research-focused (PhD); and 26.2% practice-focused (DNP) doctoral programs. There was also an increase in RN-BSN program enrollment and graduates, which is very positive, supporting *The future of nursing* report recommendation to increase the proportion of RNs with baccalaureate degrees to 80% by 2010 (IOM, 2010), but the goal has not yet been reached though there has been improvement. As of 2014, 55% of registered nurses held a BSN (AACN, 2015a).

A key concern for nurse educators is not only the need to increase enrollment and completion rates, but also the need to reduce the number of qualified applicants who are not able to enroll because nursing programs do not have places for them. Data from the AACN 2014 survey of 816 schools of nursing indicate that 68,936 qualified applicants could not enroll in entry-level baccalaureate programs and 15,288 to master's and doctoral programs (AACN, 2015a). Over the past few years, the common reasons for programs turning away students have been insufficient clinical sites, lack of qualified faculty, limited classroom space, insufficient preceptors, and budget cuts. The percentage of minorities enrolling in such programs has increased (AACN, 2015a). Nursing students from minority backgrounds increased in 2014: 30.1% of students in entry-level baccalaureate programs, 31.9% in master's programs, 29.7% in research-focused doctoral programs (PhD), and 28.7% in practice-focused doctoral programs (DNP). RN workforce diversity, nurses who are working (2014 AACN data), however, continues to be a problem, though it is slowly improving: 73% White, 11% African American, 9% Asian, 7% Hispanic, and 1% other (Robert Wood Johnson Foundation [RWJF], 2016).

This snapshot of data indicates that there has been improvement in the number of applicants to the various nursing degree programs, in enrollment rates, and in student diversity, but much work remains to reach the desired levels so as to meet the needs of the healthcare delivery system for qualified nurses. Reported data are typically behind the current year, and the AACN website periodically provides updated data as does the NLN.

A Brief History of Nursing Education

It is impossible to discuss the history of nursing education without reflecting on the history of the profession and the history of health care, as discussed in other chapters—all three are interconnected.

A key historical nursing leader was Florence Nightingale. She changed not only the practice of nursing, but also nurses' **training**, which eventually came to be called education rather than training. Training focuses on fixed habits and skills; uses repetition, authority, and coercion; and emphasizes dependency, and **education** focuses more on self-discipline, responsibility, accountability, and self-mastery (Donahue, 1983). Up until the time that Nightingale became involved in nursing, there was little, if any, training for the role. **Apprenticeship** was used to introduce new recruits to nursing, and often it was not done effectively. As nursing changed, so did the need for more knowledge and skills, leading to increasingly structured educational experiences. This did not occur without debate and disagreement regarding the best approach. What did happen, and how does it impact nursing education today?

In 1860, Nightingale established the first school of nursing, St. Thomas, in London, England. She was able to do this because she had received a very good education in the areas of math and science, which was highly unusual for women of her era. With her experience in the Crimean War, Nightingale recognized that many soldiers were dying not just because of their wounds, but also because of infection and failure to place them in the best situation for healing. To improve care, she devoted her energies to upgrading nursing education, placing less focus on on-the-job training and more focus on a structured educational program of study, creating a nurse training school. This training school and those that quickly followed also became a source of cheap labor for hospitals. Students were provided with some formal nursing education, but they also worked long hours in the hospitals and were the largest staff source. The apprenticeship model continued, but it became more structured and included a more formal educational component. This educational component was far from ideal, but over time, it expanded and improved. During the same era, similar programs opened in the United States. These programs were called diploma or hospital schools of nursing.

Hospitals across the United States began to open schools as they realized that students could be used as staff in the hospitals. The quality of these schools varied widely because there were no standards aside from what the individual hospital wanted to do. A few schools recognized early on the need for more content and improved teaching. Over time, some of these schools were creative and formed partnerships with universities so that students could receive some content through an academic institution. Despite these small efforts to improve, the schools continued to be very different from one another, and there were concerns about the lack of standardized quality nursing education.

Major Nursing Reports: Improving Nursing Education

In 1918, an important step was taken through an initiative supported by the Rockefeller Foundation to address the issue of the diploma schools. This initiative culminated in the Goldmark Report (*Nursing and nursing education in the United States*), the first of several major reports about U.S. nursing education. This report included the following key points, which provide a view of some of the common concerns about nursing education in the early 1900s (Goldmark, 1923):

- Hospitals controlled the total education hours, offering minimal content and, in some cases, no content even when that content was needed.

- Inexperienced instructors with few teaching resources often taught science, theory, and practice of nursing.
- Graduate nurses had limited experience and time to assist the students in their learning supervised students.
- Classroom experiences frequently occurred after the students had worked long hours, even during the night.
- Students typically were able to only get the experiences that their hospital provided, with all clinical practice experiences located in one hospital. As a consequence, students might not get experiences in specialties such as obstetrics, pediatrics, and psychiatric–mental health.

The Goldmark Report had an impact, particularly through its key recommendations: (1) separate university schools of nursing from hospitals (this represented only a minority of the schools of nursing); (2) change the control of hospital-based programs to schools of nursing; and (3) require a high school diploma for entry into any school of nursing. These recommendations represented suggestions for major improvements in nursing education. New schools opened based on the Goldmark recommendations, such as Yale University (New Haven, Connecticut) and Case Western Reserve University (Cleveland, Ohio).

In 1948, the Brown report was also critical of the quality of nursing education (Brown, 1948). This led to the implementation of an accreditation program for nursing schools, which was conducted by the NLN. **Accreditation** is a process of reviewing what a school is doing and its curriculum based on established standards. Movement toward the university setting and away from hospital-based schools of nursing and establishment of standards with an accreditation process were major changes for the nursing profession. The ANA and the NLN continue to establish standards for practice and education and to support implementation of those standards. In addition, the AACN developed a nursing education accreditation process, as discussed later in this chapter. Changes were made, but slowly. The NLN started developing and implementing standards for schools, but it took more than 20 years to accomplish this mission.

The third report on the assessment of nursing education was published in 2010, *Educating nurses: A call for radical transformation* (Benner, Sutphen, Leonard, & Day, 2010). This report addressed the need to better prepare nurses to practice in a rapidly changing healthcare system in order to ensure quality care. The conclusion of this qualitative study of nursing education was that there is need for great improvement. Students should be engaged in the learning process. There needs to be more connection between classroom experience and clinical experience, with a greater emphasis on practice throughout the nursing curriculum. Students should be better prepared to use clinical reasoning and judgment and understand the trajectory of illness. To meet the recommendations of this landmark report, nursing education must make major changes and improvements. **Exhibit 3-1** describes the report's recommendations.

The most recent report on the nursing profession, published by the IOM (2010), *The future of nursing: Leading change, advancing health*, delineates several key messages for nurses and nursing education. Nurses should practice to the fullest extent possible based on their level of education. There should be mechanisms for nurses to advance their education easily, act as full partners in healthcare delivery, and be involved in policy making especially as it relates to the healthcare workforce. This report, along with the report by Benner and colleagues (2010), is transforming nursing's role in health care and calling for radical changes in nursing education. In late 2015, a progress report was published to assess the current status of *The future of nursing* recommendations (National Academy of Medicine, 2015). This report is discussed further in other chapters; however, it is important to note in this discussion about nursing education, accreditation,

and regulation that many of the recommendations require more work. For example, the recommendation to double the number of doctoral degrees by 2020 was not progressing as of 2015 in a manner expected to reach this objective.

Entry into Practice: A Long Debate

The challenges in making changes in the entry into practice debate were great when one considers that a very large number of hospitals in communities across the country had diploma schools based on the old model, and these schools were part of, and funded by, their communities. It was not easy to change these schools or to close them without major nursing and community debate and conflict. These schools constituted the major type of nursing education in the United States through the 1960s, and some schools still exist today. The number of diploma schools has decreased primarily because of the critical debate over what type of education nurses need for entry into practice. The drive to move nursing education into college and university settings was great, but there was also great support to continue with the diploma schools of nursing.

In 1965, the NLN and the ANA made strong statements endorsing college-based nursing education as the entry point into the profession. In 1965, the ANA stated that "minimum preparation for beginning technical (bedside) nursing practice at the present time should be associate degree education in nursing" (p. 107). The situation was very tense. The two largest nursing organizations at the time—one primarily focused on education (NLN) and the other more on practice (ANA)—clearly took a stand. From the 1960s through the 1980s, these organizations tried to alter accreditation, advocated for the closing of diploma programs, and lobbied all levels of government (Leighow, 1996). It was an emotional issue, and even today it continues to be a tense topic because it has not been fully resolved, although stronger statements were made

Exhibit 3-1 Recommendations from *Educating Nurses: A Call for Radical Transformation*

Entry and Pathways

- Come to agreement about a set of clinically relevant prerequisites.
- Require the BSN for entry to practice.
- Develop local articulation programs to ensure a smooth, timely transition from ADN to BSN programs.
- Develop more ADN-to-MSN programs.

Student Population

- Recruit a more diverse faculty and student body.
- Provide more financial aid, whether from public or private sources, for all students, at all levels.

The Student Experience

- Introduce pre-nursing students to nursing early in their education.
- Broaden the clinical experience.
- Preserve post-clinical conferences and small patient-care assignments.
- Develop pedagogies that keep students focused on the patient's experience.
- Vary the means of assessing student performance.
- Promote and support learning the skills of inquiry and research.
- Redesign the ethics curricula.
- Support students in becoming agents of change.

Teaching

- Fully support ongoing faculty development for all who educate student nurses.
- Include teacher education courses in master's and doctoral programs.
- Foster opportunities for educators to learn how to teach students to reflect on their practice.
- Support faculty in learning how to coach students.
- Support educators in learning how to use narrative pedagogies.
- Provide faculty with resources to stay clinically current.
- Improve the work environment for staff nurses, and support them in learning to teach.
- Address the faculty shortage.

Entry to Practice

- Develop clinical residencies for all graduates.
- Change the requirements for licensure.

National Oversight

- Require performance assessments for licensure.
- Cooperate on accreditation.

Data from Benner, P., Sutphen, M., Leonard, V., & Day, L. (2010). *Educating nurses. A call for radical transformation.* San Francisco, CA: Jossey-Bass.

in 2010 to change to a baccalaureate entry level (Benner, Sutphen, Leonard, & Day, 2010; IOM, 2010). Since 1965, however, there have been many changes in the educational preparation of nurses:

- The number of diploma schools have gradually decreased, but they still exist.

- The number of associate degree in nursing (ADN) programs has increased. However, there was, and continues to be, concern over the potential development of a two-level nursing system—ADN and baccalaureate degree in nursing (BSN)—with one viewed as technical and the other as professional. In fact, this did not happen. ADN programs continue to increase, and there has been no change in licensure for any of the nursing programs—graduates of all RN pre-licensure programs continue to take the same exam and receive the same license.

- BSN programs continue to grow but still have not outpaced ADN programs, though there has been some decrease in ADN programs.

Differentiated Nursing Practice

Another issue related to entry into practice is differentiated nursing practice. **Differentiated practice** is not a new idea; it has been discussed in the literature since the 1990s. It is described as a "philosophy that structures the roles and functions of nurses according to their education, experience, and competence," or "matching the varying needs of clients [patients] with the varying abilities of nursing practitioners" (AONE, 1990, as cited in Hutchins, 1994, p. 52).

How does this actually work in practice? Does a clinical setting distinguish among RNs who have a diploma, associate degree, and BSN degree? Does this affect role function and responsibilities? Does the organization even acknowledge degrees on name badges? Most healthcare organizations do note differences when it comes to RNs with graduate degrees, and many do not necessarily note other degrees such as the BSN. This approach does not recognize that there are differences in the educational programs that award each degree or diploma. The ongoing debate remains difficult to resolve because all RNs, regardless of the type and length of their basic nursing education program, take the same licensing exam. Patients and other healthcare providers rarely understand the differences or even know that differences exist. A difference in salaries due to degrees is the highest level of recognition, and this is done in some healthcare organizations.

In 1995, a joint report was published by the AACN in collaboration with the American Organization of Nurse Executives and the National Organization (AONE) and the National Organization for Associate Degree Nursing (now known as the Organization for Associate Degree Nursing or OADN). This document described the two roles of the BSN and the ADN graduate (p. 28):

- The BSN graduate is a licensed RN who provides direct care that is based on the nursing process and focused on patients/clients with complex interactions of nursing diagnoses. Patients/clients include individuals, families, groups, aggregates, and communities in structured and unstructured healthcare settings. The unstructured setting is a geographical or a situational environment that may not have established policies, procedures, and protocols and has the potential for variations requiring independent nursing decisions.

- The ADN graduate is a licensed RN who provides direct care that is based on the nursing process and focused on individual patients/clients who have common, well-defined nursing diagnoses. Consideration is given to the patient's/client's relationship within the family. The ADN functions in a structured healthcare setting, which is a geographical or situational environment where the policies, procedures, and protocols for provision of health care are established. In the structured setting, there is recourse to assistance and support from the full scope of nursing expertise.

Despite increased support, such as from AONE, for making the BSN the entry-level educational requirement, this question continues to be one of the most frustrating issues in the profession and has not been clearly resolved (AACN, 2005a). The AACN believes that "education has a direct impact on the skills and competencies of a nurse clinician. Nurses with a baccalaureate degree are well-prepared to meet the demand placed on today's nurse across a variety of settings and are prized for their critical thinking, leadership, case management, and health promotion skills" (AACN, 2005a, p. 1).

Since 2001, there has been an increase in the number of students enrolling in entry-level BSN programs, and the number of RNs returning to school for their BSN also continues to increase. The result has been nine years of steady growth in the number of RNs with baccalaureate degrees (ANA, 2011). A study by Aiken, Clarke, Cheung, Sloane, and Silber (2003) indicates that there is a "substantial survival advantage" for patients in hospitals with a higher percentage of BSN RNs. Other studies (Estabrooks, Midodzi, Cummings, Ricker, & Giovannetti, 2005) support these outcomes. McHugh and Lake (2010) examined how nurses rate their level of expertise as a beginner, competent, proficient, advanced, and expert and how often they were selected as a preceptor or consulted by other nurses for their clinical judgment. The survey, which was done in 1999 and then the data used in this 2010 study, included 8,611 nurses. More highly educated nurses rated themselves as having more expertise than less educated nurses, and this correlated with how frequently they were asked to be preceptors or consulted by other nurses. The long-term impact of these types of studies on the entry into practice is unknown, but there is more evidence now to support the decision made in 1965 along with recommendations from major reports (Benner, Sutphen, Leonard, & Day, 2010; IOM, 2010).

Aiken and colleagues published a study in 2014 addressing nurse staffing and hospital mortality in nine European countries. This study received major recognition by healthcare organizations and the media. The sample included discharge data for 422,730 patients aged 50 years or older who had common surgeries in the nine countries. The survey included 26,516 nurses in the study hospitals. The findings indicate that increasing a nurse's workload by one patient increased the likelihood of a patient dying within 30 days of admission by 7%; in contrast, every 10% increase in the number of nurses with baccalaureate degrees was associated with a 7% decrease in the likelihood of a patient dying within 30 days of admission. These associations imply that patients receiving care in hospitals in which 60% of nurses had baccalaureate degrees and nurses cared for an average of six patients would have almost a 30% lower mortality than patients in hospitals in which only 30% of nurses had baccalaureate degrees and nurses cared for an average of eight patients. The results indicate there is value in using BSN-prepared nurses in these hospitals, whereas reducing nursing staff may have a negative impact on patient outcomes.

In the last few years, many more hospitals have implemented initiatives to hire only RNs with BSN degrees and to encourage staff members without a BSN degree to return to school. Studies such as the ones mentioned here have had an impact on increasing hospital support for RNs with BSN degrees. This decision by hospitals, however, is highly dependent on the availability of RNs with the BSN degree in the local area and has also been influenced by the Magnet Recognition Program®, which supports the BSN degree as a requirement for initial practice, though it does make this a requirement to receive Magnet recognition.

Stop and Consider #1

The nursing degree required for entry into practice continues to be a problem.

Types of Nursing
Education Programs

Nursing is a profession with a complex education pattern: It has many different entry-level pathways to the same license to practice and many different graduate programs. The following content provides descriptions of the major nursing education programs. Because several types of entry-level nursing programs exist, this complicates the issue and raises concerns about the best way to provide education for nursing students.

Diploma Schools of Nursing

Diploma schools of nursing still exist, now representing less than 10% of all entry-level nursing programs. Many of these programs have transitioned to other types of degree programs—for example, by forming partnerships with colleges or universities where students might take some of their courses. Many of these schools have closed—some have been converted into associate degree and baccalaureate programs, and some have partnered with ADN and BSN programs. These programs still interest some employers when they are short of staff and degree programs are not meeting these needs. The Association of Diploma Schools of Professional Nursing represents these schools. Diploma schools are accredited by the NLN. Graduates take the same licensing exam as graduates from all the other types of nursing programs. The nursing curriculum is similar; the graduates need the same nursing content for the licensing exam. The students, however, typically have fewer prerequisites, particularly in liberal arts and sciences, though they do have some science content. Curricula requirements may vary in these schools because some schools allow students to take some of their required courses in local colleges.

Associate Degree in Nursing

Programs awarding an **associate degree in nursing** (AD/ADN) began when Mildred Montag published a book on the need for a different type of nursing program—a 2-year program that would be established in community colleges (Montag, 1959). The first programs opened in 1958. At the time Montag created her proposal, the United States was experiencing a shortage of nurses. For students, ADN programs are less expensive and shorter. The percentages of ADN and BSN programs vary from state to state—for example, in California, 61% of RNs completed a BSN or higher degree; however, more than half the students entering nursing are

still doing so in ADN programs (RWJF, 2015). The big difference is the increase in RN-BSN programs pushing the number of nurses with a BSN up. In 2014, there were 67 diploma programs and 1,092 ADN programs identified in the NLN Survey of Schools of Nursing (NLN, 2014). From 2005 to 2014, the NLN data indicate there was a slight fluctuation in the data for these two programs. Associate degree programs are accredited by the NLN's accrediting services. The ADN curriculum includes some liberal art and science courses at the community college level and focuses more on technical nursing. Graduates take the same licensing exam as graduates from all other pre-licensure nursing programs.

Recently, a variety of models and opportunities for ADN students and graduates have been introduced. Montag envisioned the ADN as a terminal degree, but this perception has since changed, with the degree now typically viewed as part of a career mobility path. The **RN-BSN** or BSN completion programs are a way for ADN graduates to complete the requirements for a BSN. There are also LPN-ADN and LPN-BSN programs to assist staff in their career paths. Typically, in all of these programs, nurses work for a time and then go back to school, often on a part-time basis, to complete a BSN in a university-level program. Some prerequisite courses must be taken before these students enter most BSN programs. Examples of additional nursing courses these students may take in the RN-BSN program are health assessment, public/community health with clinical practice, leadership and management, research/evidence-based practice, and health policy. Until recently, these students rarely took additional clinical courses, as this is not the major focus of the RN-BSN programs; however, all programs accredited by AACN must now include **clinical experiences** or a **practicum**. The Commission on Collegiate Nursing Education (CCNE, 2013), accrediting body for the AACN, defines *clinical practice experiences* as "planned learning activities in nursing practice that allow students to understand, perform, and refine professional competencies at the appropriate program level" (p. 21). The content typically included for the clinical experience is public/community health, focusing on what these students typically do not cover in an ADN program. Today, many of the RN-BSN programs offer courses online. The type of clinical experiences can vary greatly; however, not having any clinical experiences in a RN-BSN program may be a problem for students who want to continue on to a graduate degree.

Greater efforts are now made to facilitate the transition from the ADN program to the BSN program. The overall goal is to guide all ADN graduates back to school for a BSN, though this has not yet been accomplished. These graduates do not have to take the licensure exam because they are already RNs, but to participate in a RN-BSN program, they are expected to maintain an active registered nurse license. ADN and BSN programs have increased their efforts to partner with each other to provide a seamless transition from one program to the other. Establishing an **articulation agreement** describing the responsibilities of the partners, benefits to the students, and how the students will meet the expected BSN outcomes or competencies clarifies these partnerships. "Articulation agreements are important mechanisms that enhance access to baccalaureate level nursing education. These agreements support education mobility and facilitate the seamless transfer of academic credit between associate degree (ADN) and baccalaureate (BSN) nursing programs" (AACN, 2005c, p. 1). Academic progression supports "life long learning through the attainment of academic credentials" (Organization for Associate Degree Nursing & American Nurses Association, 2015, p. 5). State law may mandate these agreements, which may be partnerships between individual schools or may be part of statewide articulation plans to facilitate more efficient transfer of credits. Typically, in these partnerships, students spend their first 2 years in the ADN program and then complete the last 2 years of the BSN degree in the partner BSN program.

In these types of programs, both the participating ADN and BSN programs collaborate on the curriculum and determine how to best transition the students. One benefit of this model is for the first 2 years students pay the community college fees, which are less costly than the university fees. Another advantage is if there is no BSN program in a community students have the option of staying within their own community while they pursue a nursing degree and then transition to a more distant BSN program or complete the BSN online.

Baccalaureate Degree in Nursing

The idea for the **BSN**, an entry-level degree, was introduced in the Goldmark Report (Goldmark, 1923), although it took many years for this recommendation to have an impact on nursing education. The original programs took 5 years to complete, with the first 2 years focused on liberal arts and sciences courses, followed by 3 years in nursing courses. Most BSN programs have changed to a 4-year model, with various configurations of liberal arts and sciences and then 2 years in nursing courses. Some schools introduce students to nursing content during the first 2 years, but typically the amount of nursing content is limited during this period. In many colleges of nursing, students are not formally admitted to the school/college of nursing until they complete the first 2 years, although the students are in the same university. These programs may be accredited by the NLN or through the AACN, both of which have accrediting services. (More information about accreditation appears later in the chapter.) The licensure exam is taken after successful completion of the BSN program. A BSN is required for admission to a nursing graduate program, and this has influenced more nurses to return to school to get a BSN degree.

The movement of many nursing schools into the university setting was not all positive. Nursing programs lost their strong connection with hospitals. Rather than establish different educational models with hospitals, the nursing education community sought to get away from the control of hospitals and move to an academic setting; however, now nursing educators and students are visitors in hospitals with little feeling of partnership and connection. This has an impact on clinical experiences, in some cases limiting effective clinical learning.

Master's Degree in Nursing

Graduate education and the evolution of the **master's degree in nursing (MSN)** have a long history. Early in the development of graduate-level nursing, it was called postgraduate education, and the typical focus areas were public health, teaching, supervision, and a few clinical specialties. The first formal graduate program was established in 1899 at Columbia University Teachers College (Donahue, 1983). The NLN supported the establishment of graduate nursing programs, and these programs were developed in great numbers and developed new models. For example, some of the early programs, such as Yale School of Nursing, admitted students without a BSN who had a baccalaureate degree in another major. Today, this is very similar to the **accelerated programs** or **direct entry programs** in which students with other degrees are admitted to a BSN program that is shorter, covering the same basic entry-level nursing content but with an accelerated approach. These students are typically categorized as graduate students because of their previous degree even though the degree is not in nursing. Even so, they must complete pre-licensure BSN requirements, including successful completion of the licensure exam before they can take nursing graduate clinical courses, and in some cases, they are not admitted to the nursing graduate program automatically until completion of a direct entry program. They must apply to the program in same manner as any student who wants to attend a graduate program in nursing.

The master's programs in nursing have evolved since the 1950s. The typical length for a master's program is 2 years, and students may attend full-time or part-time. The following are examples of master's degree programs:

- *Advanced practice registered nurse (APRN):* This master's degree can be offered in any clinical area, but typical areas are adult health, pediatrics, family health, women's health, neonatal health, and psychiatric–mental health. Graduates take APRN certification exams in their specialty area and must then meet specific state requirements, such as for **prescriptive authority**, which gives them limited ability to prescribe medications. These nurses usually work in independent roles. The American Nurses Credentialing Center (ANCC) provides national certification exams for **advanced practice registered nurses** in a variety of areas.
- *Clinical nurse specialist (CNS):* This master's degree can be offered in any clinical area. Specialty exams may also be taken. These nurses usually work in hospital settings. The ANCC provides national certification for CNSs in a variety of areas, as discussed later in this chapter.
- *Certified registered nurse anesthetists (CRNA):* This has been a master's degree and is not offered at all colleges of nursing. This is a highly competitive graduate program. The Council on Accreditation of Nurse Anesthesia Educational Program, as part of the American Association of Nurse Anesthetists, focuses on accreditation of these programs and certification. This educational program is now moving to the level of **doctor of nursing practice** (DNP). All master's-level programs must transition to entry-level DNP programs by 2022, and thereafter, all new programs must be entry-level DNP programs. The data indicate that the programs are rapidly moving in this direction. As of December 2016, 53 programs have been approved for

entry-level doctoral degrees; 27 programs offer post-master's doctoral degree completion programs for CRNAs; and 63 programs remain to be approved for entry-level doctoral degrees by the deadline of January 1, 2022 (Council on Accreditation, 2017).

- *Certified nurse–midwife:* This master's degree focuses on midwifery—pregnancy and delivery—as well as gynecologic care of women and family planning. These programs are accredited by the American College of Nurse–Midwives.

- *Clinical nurse leader (CNL):* This is one of the newer master's degrees, which prepares nurses for leadership positions that have a direct impact on patient care. The CNL is a provider and a manager of care at the point of care to individuals and cohorts. The CNL serves as a nurse leader and designs, implements, and evaluates patient care by coordinating, delegating, and supervising the care provided by the healthcare team, including licensed nurses, technicians, and other health professionals, and advocates for patients (AACN, 2013). Certification is available for CNLs.

- *Master's degree in a functional area:* This type of master's degree focuses on the functional areas of administration or education. It was more popular in the past, but with the growing need for nursing faculty, there has been a resurgence of master's programs in nursing education. In some cases, colleges of nursing are offering certificate programs in nursing education. In these programs, a nurse with a nursing master's degree may take a certain number of credits that focus on nursing education; then, if the nurse successfully completes the NLN certification exam, the nurse is then a certified nurse educator. This provides the nurse with additional background and experience in nursing education.

Research-Based Doctoral Degree in Nursing

The doctoral degree (doctor of philosophy—PhD) (**research-based doctorate**) in nursing has had a complicated development history. The doctorate of nursing science (DNSc) was first offered in 1960, but this degree program has since transitioned to other types of doctoral programs. There were PhD programs in nursing education as early as 1924, and New York University started the first PhD program in nursing in 1953. Today, not enough students are entering these programs, and this has an impact on nursing faculty because schools of nursing want faculty with doctoral degrees. Someone with a PhD is not always required to teach but is encouraged to do so. Nurses with PhDs usually are involved in research, although a nurse at any level can be involved in research and may or may not teach. Study for a PhD typically takes place after receiving a master's degree in nursing and includes coursework and a research-focused dissertation. This process can take 4 to 5 years to complete, and much depends on completion of the dissertation. Nurses with PhDs may be called "doctor"; this is not the same as the "medical doctor" title, but rather a designation or title indicating completion of academic doctoral work in the same way that an English professor with a doctorate is called "doctor."

Some schools of nursing now offer BSN-PhD or BSN-DNP options. This means the student does not have to obtain a master's degree prior to entering the program, and the students typically enter the process as BSN students and complete with a PhD or DNP degree. The goal is to increase the number of nurses with doctoral degrees (terminal degree) by encouraging nursing students to make this career decision early.

Doctor of Nursing Practice

The DNP is the newest nursing degree. The DNP is not a traditional PhD program, although nurses with a DNP degree are also called "doctor." However, this does not represent the same title as someone with a PhD or a doctor or medicine. The DNP is a practice-focused doctoral degree program. This position has been controversial within nursing and within health care, particularly among physicians. The ANCC defines *advanced nursing practice* as "any form of nursing intervention that influences outcomes for individuals or populations, including the direct care of individual patients, management of care for individuals and populations, administration of nursing and health organizations, and the development and implementation of health policy" (AACN, 2015b, p. 11). This description is important due to transition of the requirement of master's programs for APRNs to the DNP degree. APRN refers to the nursing role for a nurse who meets certain qualifications; some refer to this also as advanced practice nurse.

Practice-focused doctoral nursing programs prepare leaders for nursing practice. The long-term goal is to make the DNP the terminal practice degree for APRN preparation, including clinical nurse specialists, certified registered nurse anesthetists, certified nurse–midwifes, and nurse practitioners. This means that by 2015—a date identified by the AACN—and by 2022—a date identified by the American Association of Nurse Anesthetists—APRNs would be required to have a DNP degree or an entry-level DNP for advanced practice nursing. As of 2017 much more needs to be done to meet this goal.

Some of the reasons that the DNP degree was developed relate to the process for obtaining an APRN master's degree, which requires a large number of credits and clinical hours. It was recognized that students should be getting more credit for their coursework and effort. Going on to a DNP program allows them to apply some of this credit toward a doctoral degree. As of April 2016, there are 289 DNP programs, with 128 in the planning stages; 62 are post-baccalaureate and 66 are post-master's programs (AACN, 2016a). Our healthcare system and healthcare service needs demand the highest

level of scientific knowledge and expertise for quality care. The change is based on "the rapid expansion of knowledge underlying practice; increased complexity of patient care; national concerns about the quality of care and patient safety; shortages of nursing personnel which demands a higher level of preparation for leaders who can design and assess care; shortages of doctoral-prepared nursing faculty; and increasing educational expectations for the preparation of other members of the healthcare team" (AACN, 2016a, p. 1).

Because the DNP is a relatively new degree and has led to the development of new roles, it is not clear at this time what its long-term impact will be on nursing and on healthcare delivery. Some have questioned the decision to confer such a degree in light of the need for a greater number of APRNs for primary care (Cronenwett et al., 2011); others have questioned it because there is need for nurses with research-focused degrees (PhDs). There is concern that nurses who might have once considered pursuing a PhD would instead seek a DNP; indeed, data indicate that there is now greater enrollment in DNP programs, so this prediction has proven correct.

Stop and Consider #2

We have confusion when it comes to our pre-licensure degree programs.

Nursing Education
Associations

There are three major nursing education organizations, each with a different program focus. These organizations are the NLN, the AACN, and the OADN.

National League for Nursing

The NLN is an older organization than the AACN. It "promotes excellence in nursing education to build a strong and diverse nursing workforce to advance the health of our nation and the global community," and the NLN's goals are as follows (NLN, 2017a):

- *Leader in nursing education:* Enhance the NLN's national and international impact as the recognized leader in nursing education.
- *Commitment to members:* Engage a diverse, sustainable, member-led organization with the capacity to deliver our mission effectively, efficiently, and in accordance with our values.
- *Champion for nurse educators:* Be the voice of nurse educators and champion their interests in political, academic, and professional arenas.
- *Advancement of the science of nursing education:* Promote research that generates evidence about nursing education and the scholarship of teaching.

The NLN represents several types of registered nurse programs (diploma, ADN, BSN, master's) and vocational/practical nurse programs. Accreditation of nursing education programs is discussed in a later section of this chapter. The NLN offers educational opportunities for its members (individual membership and school of nursing membership) and addresses policy and standards issues related to nursing education.

American Association of Colleges of Nursing

The AACN is the national organization that represents baccalaureate and graduate programs in nursing, including doctoral programs. It has approximately 725 members (schools/colleges of nursing). Its activities include educational research, government advocacy, data collection, publishing, and initiatives to establish standards for baccalaureate and graduate degree nursing programs, including implementation of the standards. Its goals for 2017–2019 are as follows: (1) The AACN is the driving force for innovation and excellence in academic nursing; (2) the AACN is a leading partner in advancing

improvements in health, health care, and higher education; (3) the AACN is a primary advocate for advancing diversity and inclusivity within academic nursing; and (4) the AACN is the authoritative source of knowledge to advance academic nursing through information (AACN, 2017). The organization also offers accreditation of baccalaureate and master's degree nursing programs as described in another section in this chapter.

Organization for Associate Degree Nursing

The Organization for Associate Degree Nursing (OADN) began in 1984 after Mildred Montag proposed the ADN degree in 1952. The OADN, formerly known as N-OADN, is the organization that advocates for associate degree nursing education and practice. Its major goals are as follows (OADN, 2017):

- *Education:* Advance associate degree nursing education.
- *Leadership:* Develop leadership within associate degree nursing to create meaningful change.
- *Inclusivity:* Foster an environment in associate degree nursing that advances inclusivity.
- *Collaboration:* Further associate degree nursing education through collaboration with a diverse group of stakeholders.
- *Advocacy:* Advocate for associate degree nursing as it relates to the delivery of quality health care.

The organization supports academic progression of its graduates so that they can reach their potential. The organization does not offer accreditation services. Accreditation of ADN programs is done through the NLN accrediting organization (CNEA).

Stop and Consider #3

We have three nursing education organizations; maybe due to the confusion over our degree programs.

Quality and Excellence in
Nursing Education

There is greater emphasis today on quality health care, as discussed in this text, but also, for us to have quality care, we need to have healthcare providers who meet standards for quality performance. This requires us to consider the quality of our nursing education programs.

Nursing Education Standards

Nursing education standards are developed by the major nursing professional organizations that focus on education: NLN, AACN, and OADN. The accrediting bodies of the NLN and the AACN also set nursing education standards. State boards of nursing are involved as well. In addition, colleges and universities must meet certain standards for non-nursing accreditation at the overall college or university level. **Standards** guide decisions, organizational structure, process, policies and procedures, budgetary decisions, admissions and progress of students, evaluation/assessment (program, faculty, and student), curriculum, and other academic issues. Critical standard documents published by the AACN are *The Essentials* covering baccalaureate, master's, and DNP degrees (AACN, 2006, 2008, 2011). The baccalaureate *Essentials* emphasizes the three roles of the baccalaureate generalist nurse: provider of care; designer/manager/coordinator of care; and member of a profession, which includes advocating for the patient and profession by applying the *Essential* standards. These standards include student learning outcomes expected for nursing pre-licensure graduates related to the following topical areas and associated percentage of the outcomes: 25% nursing across the lifespan, 25% professional identity/communication, 25% leadership, 13% population health, and 12% evidence-based practice/quality improvement (Godfrey & Martin, 2016). These authors also note, "in today's healthcare environment, nurses must be able to not only deliver care but also intentionally design care, assign care, and supervise others who provide care. To achieve desired patient outcomes, nurses must be proficient in understanding how to establish and maintain healthy work environments; use research-based knowledge to adjust their standards of practice; collect, interpret, and recommend changes to care on the use of established quality improvement" (2016, p. 396). In addition, as noted in the outcome categories, there is need for community understanding and focus and inclusion of systems at all levels and professional input through professional organizations.

NLN Excellence in Nursing Education

The NLN Hallmarks of Excellence© identifies 30 hallmarks or indicators, which are posed as questions focusing on students, faculty, continuous quality improvement, curriculum, teaching/learning evaluation strategies, resources, innovation, educational research, environment, and leadership (NLN, 2017c). These indicators are applied in two of its programs that recognize excellence.

The NLN Center of Excellence in Nursing Education identifies schools of nursing that demonstrate "sustained, evidence-based, and substantive innovation in the selected area; conduct ongoing research to document the effectiveness of such innovation; set high standards for themselves; and are committed to continuous quality improvement" (NLN, 2017d). These schools make a commitment to pursue excellence in (1) student learning and professional development, (2) development of faculty expertise in pedagogy, and/or (3) advancing the science of nursing education. The award is given to a school or college of nursing—not a program within a school—and remains in effect for 3 years. After this period, the school must be reviewed again to retain the Center of Excellence recognition. This NLN initiative is an excellent example of efforts to improve nursing education.

Another NLN initiative to recognize excellence is the Academy of Nursing Education. The purpose of the Academy of Nursing Education is to "foster excellence in nursing education by recognizing and capitalizing on the wisdom of outstanding individuals in and outside the profession who have contributed to nursing education in sustained and significant ways" (NLN, 2017d). It selects nurse educator fellows that demonstrate significant contributions to nursing education in one or more areas (teaching/learning innovations, faculty development, research in nursing education, leadership in nursing education, public policy related to nursing education, or collaborative education/practice/community partnerships) and continue to provide visionary leadership in nursing education and in the academy (NLN, 2017d, 2017e). It inducted its first nurse education fellows in 2007, and continues to do so annually.

Focus on Competencies

In 2003, the IOM published the *Health Professions Education* report to address the need for education in all major health professions describing critical common competencies. The development of this report was motivated by grave concerns about the quality of care in the United States and the need for healthcare education programs to prepare professionals who provide quality care. "Education for health professions is in need of a major overhaul. Clinical education [for all healthcare professions] simply has not kept pace with or been responsive enough to shifting patient demographics and desires, changing health system expectations, evolving practice requirements and staffing arrangements, new information, a focus on improving quality, or new technologies" (IOM, 2001, as cited in IOM, 2003, p. 1). The core competencies are also emphasized in the *Essentials of Baccalaureate Education* (AACN, 2008); however, schools of nursing need to make changes to include the competencies and, in some cases, add new content to meet these needs.

The nursing curriculum should identify the competencies expected of students throughout the nursing program. There is greater emphasis today on implementing healthcare professions competencies, particularly the core competencies for all healthcare professions: (1) provide patient-centered care, (2) work in interdisciplinary/interprofessional teams, (3) employ evidence-based practice, (4) apply quality improvement, and (5) utilize informatics (IOM, 2003). This does not mean that profession-specific competencies are not relevant, such as the Quality and Safety Education for Nurses (QSEN, 2017) competencies, but rather recognizes the existence of basic competencies that all healthcare professions should demonstrate. See **Table 3-1** comparing the core competencies and QSEN competencies.

You need to know what the expected competencies are so that you can be an active participant in your own learning to reach these competencies. The competencies are used in evaluation and to identify the level of learning or performance expected of the student. Nursing is a profession—a practice profession—so performance is a critical factor. Competency is "the application of knowledge and the interpersonal, decision-making, and psychomotor skills expected for the nurse's practice role, within the context of public health, welfare, and safety" (National Council of State Boards of Nursing [NCSBN], 2005, p. 1). The ANA (2015) defines *competency* as "an expected and measurable level of nursing performance that integrates knowledge, skills, abilities, and judgment, based on established scientific knowledge and expectations for nursing practice" (p. 86). Competencies should clearly state the expected parameters related to the behavior or performance. The curriculum should support the development of competencies by providing necessary prerequisite knowledge and learning opportunities to meet the competency. The ultimate goal is a competent RN who can provide quality care.

Curriculum

A nursing program's **curriculum** is the plan that describes the program's philosophy, levels, student

Table 3-1 Comparing the Five Healthcare Professions Core Competencies and the QSEN Competencies for Nurses

Healthcare Professions Core Competencies*	QSEN Competencies for Nurses**
Provide patient-centered care.	Patient-centered care: knowledge, skills, attitudes
Work on interdisciplinary [interprofessional] teams.	Teamwork and collaboration: knowledge, skills, attitudes
Employ evidence-based practice.	Evidence-based practice: knowledge, attitudes, skills
Apply quality improvement.	Quality improvement: knowledge, skills, attitudes
Utilize informatics.	Safety: knowledge, skills, attitudes
	Informatics: knowledge, skills, attitudes

Data from *Institute of Medicine (IOM). (2003). *Health Professions Education. A Bridge to Quality*. Washington, DC: The National Academies Press;

**QSEN Institute (2015). *Pre-licensure competencies*. Retrieved from http://qsen.org/competencies/pre-licensure-ksas/ and graduate level competencies retrieved from http://qsen.org/competencies/graduate-ksas/

terminal competencies (outcomes or what students are expected to accomplish by the end of the program), and course content (described in course syllabi). Also specified are the sequence of courses and a designation of course credits and learning experiences, such as didactic courses (typically offered in a lecture/classroom, seminar setting or both venues; in some cases in online format) and clinical or practicum experiences. In addition, simulation laboratory experiences are included either at the beginning of the curriculum or throughout the curriculum. The nursing curriculum is very important. It informs potential students what they should expect in a nursing program and may influence a student's choice of programs, particularly at the graduate level. It helps orient new students and is important in the accreditation of nursing programs. State boards of nursing also review the curricula of schools of nursing in their state. To keep current, faculty need to review the curriculum regularly, in a manner that allows changes to be made as easily and quickly as possible and includes student input. Standards for nursing education accreditation also

have an impact on the curriculum; for example, *The essentials of baccalaureate education for professional nursing practice* provides guidelines for baccalaureate curricula (AACN, 2008).

Didactic or Theory Content

Nursing curricula may vary as to titles of courses, course descriptions and objectives/learning outcomes, sequence, number of hours of didactic content, and clinical experiences, but there are some constants even within these differences. To ensure consistency in the practice of nursing and to prepare for the licensure exam nursing content needs to include the following broad topical areas:

- Professional issues and trends
- Health assessment
- Pharmacology
- Adult health or medical–surgical nursing
- Psychiatric/mental health nursing
- Pediatrics
- Maternal–child nursing (obstetrics, women's health, neonatal care)
- Public/community health

- Gerontology
- Leadership and management
- Palliative care and care of the dying patient
- Communication, collaboration, and coordination
- Teamwork
- Evidence-based practice
- Research
- Health policy
- Legal and ethical issues
- Quality improvement

Many schools offer courses focused on other topics, such as informatics and genetics. Quality improvement content is often weak, even though it is now considered critical knowledge that every practicing nurse needs to have if care is to be improved.

Nursing content may be provided in clearly defined courses that focus on only one overall topical area, or it may be integrated with multiple topics. Clinical experience/practicum may be blended with related didactic content—for example, pediatric content and pediatric clinical experience—such that they are considered one course; alternatively, the clinical/practicum and didactic content may be offered as two separate courses, typically in the same semester. Faculty who teach didactic content may or may not teach in the clinical setting.

Practicum or Clinical Experience

Clinical experience or practicum is a critical component of a nursing curriculum. These experiences must be planned; correlate with the curriculum; require intensive faculty supervision to facilitate effective learning; and focus on active student engagement in the experiences, requiring extensive time and effort.

Extensive faculty effort and coordination with clinical sites is required for effective planning, implementing, and evaluating of student clinical experiences. A critical issue today for many schools is access to clinical sites. This has led to various methods to alleviate the problem to ensure effective clinical experiences for students—some have

been more successful than others. The hours for the practicum or clinical experiences can be highly variable within one school and from school to school (for example, the number of hours per week and sequence of days, such as practicum on Tuesdays and Thursdays from 8 a.m. to 3 p.m.). Many schools are now offering 12-hour clinical sessions. There is greater acknowledgment that 12-hour work shifts may lead to staff fatigue and an increased number of errors, but this has not stopped some schools from offering this time schedule for student practica. Some schools offer clinical experiences in the evenings, at night, and on weekends. It is important for students to understand the time commitment and scheduling related to clinical experience requirements, which have a great impact on students' personal lives, time with family, and social relationships. If a student is employed while going to school, scheduling will be complex. In addition, these clinical experiences require preparation time. The types of clinical settings are highly variable and depend on the objectives and the available sites. Typical types of settings are acute care hospitals (all clinical areas); mental health/psychiatric hospitals; pediatric hospitals; women's health (may include obstetrics) clinics; public/community health clinics and other health agencies; home health agencies; hospice centers, including freestanding sites, hospital-based centers, and patients' homes; schools; camps; health-oriented consumer organizations such as the American Diabetes Association; health mobile clinics; homeless shelters; doctors' offices; clinics of all types; ambulatory surgical centers; emergency centers; Red Cross centers; businesses with occupational health services; and many more. In some of these settings—for example, in acute care—faculty remain with the students for the entire rotation time. In other settings, particularly public/community healthcare settings, faculty visit students at the site because, typically, only 1 to 4 students are in each site, and the clinical group might include as many as 10 students at different sites—which is different from acute care, when a group (8 to 10 students) is usually assigned to a faculty member in on clinical area for hospital experiences. The ratio of students to faculty in clinical settings may vary depending on the state board of nursing requirements. The number of hours per week in clinical experiences increases each year in the program, with the most hours assigned at the end of the program.

During some part of a nursing program, schools of nursing use preceptors in the clinical settings, in both undergraduate and graduate programs. In entry-level programs, preceptor experiences are typically used toward the end of the program, but some schools use preceptors throughout the program for certain courses such as in master's programs. A **preceptor** is an experienced and competent staff member (for example, an RN for undergraduate students; APRN graduate or medical doctor for APRN students; certified registered nurse anesthetist or a certified nurse–midwife for graduate nursing students in these specialties). Preceptors should have formal training to function in this role. The preceptor serves as a role model and a resource for the nursing student and guides learning. The student is assigned to work alongside the preceptor. Faculty provide overall guidance to the preceptor regarding the nature of, and objectives for, the student's learning experiences; monitor the student's progress by meeting with the student and the preceptor; and are on call for communication with the student and preceptor as needed. The preceptor participates in evaluations of the student's progress, along with the student, but the faculty member has the ultimate student evaluation responsibility. The state board of nursing may dictate how many total hours may be assigned to preceptor experiences for undergraduate students. At the graduate level, the number of preceptor hours is much higher.

Distance Education

Distance education, which is often offered online, has become quite common in nursing education, although not all schools offer courses in this manner.

The AACN describes *distance education* as "a set of teaching and/or learning strategies to meet the learning needs of students separate from the traditional classroom and sometimes from traditional roles of faculty" (AACN, 2005b; Reinert & Fryback, 1997). This definition is still applicable today. Distance education technologies have expanded over the past few years as technology developed. Some of the common distance education technologies that are used are email, audiotaped instruction, conference by telephone or via Internet, desktop videoconference, and Internet-based programming or online format. There is no doubt that these methods will continue to expand as new ones are added and some discarded as not effective or efficient. The most common and increasingly more widely adopted education approach is online courses. Distance education can be configured in several ways, including the following:

- Self-study or independent study
- Hybrid model—distance education combined with traditional classroom delivery (the most common configuration; an example is the flipped classroom)
- Faculty-facilitated online learning with no classroom activities (the approach that is growing most rapidly)

Distance education courses must require students to meet the same course competencies or outcomes as described in the program curriculum. Students who participate in distance education typically have certain characteristics that lead to success in this type of educational program. Most notably, they need to be responsible for their own learning, with faculty facilitating their learning. Computer competencies are critical for completing coursework and reducing student stress. Nursing programs must be clear about required hardware and software needed to complete course work. Students who are organized and able to develop and meet a schedule will be able to handle the course requirements. If students are assertive, ask questions, and request help when they need it they will be more successful. Effective online learning also requires active, engaged competent faculty.

Self-directed learning is important for all nursing students because it leads to greater ability to achieve lifelong learning as a professional. There are a variety of definitions of self-directed learning, most of which are based on Knowles's (1975, p. 18, as cited in O'Shea, 2003, p. 62) definition: "a process in which individuals take the initiative, with or without the help of others, in diagnosing their learning needs, formulating learning goals, identifying human and material resources for learning, choosing and implementing appropriate learning strategies and evaluating learning outcomes." Student-centered learning approaches assist effective student learning by helping students apply learning—for example, problem-based learning or team-based learning. This type of approach means that the faculty must also change how they teach. Faculty members assume the role of a facilitator of learning, which requires establishing a more collaborative relationship between faculty and students. Faculty work with students to develop active participation and goal setting: help students in setting goals, make plans with clear strategies to meet the goals, and encourage self-assessment. The flipped classroom approach is also used, for example, with content provided online, in textbooks, and so on and the expectation that students come to class prepared so that they can actively participate in learning activities in the classroom rather than listening to lectures. Compared to the traditional classroom approach, distance education typically emphasizes adult teaching and learning principles more, and approaches such as the flipped classroom also focus more on these principles. Knowles (1984) originally described principles that emphasized how learners engage with this type of educational program:

- Accept responsibility for collaborating in the planning of their learning experiences
- Set goals
- Actively participate

- Pace their own learning
- Participate in monitoring their own progress; perform self-assessment

As noted in the report on nursing education (Benner, Sutphen, Leonard, & Day, 2010), there is need for greater student engagement in the classroom, which emphasizes adult principles of learning.

The quality of distance education is as important as the quality of traditional classroom courses. Syllabi that provide the course description, credits, objectives or learning outcomes, and other information about the course should ensure that the same general structure and expectations are followed whether a course is taught using a traditional approach or through distance education—ensuring this is part of a school's evaluation process. Student evaluation must be built into a distance education course just as it is in traditional courses; however, more details are typically provided in distance education course materials and teaching–learning practices may be different. Students and faculty also need access to timely technology support. Schools should ensure that students provide anonymous evaluations of the course and faculty, as required for traditional course format.

Accreditation of Nursing
Education Programs

Accreditation is important in assessing and maintaining standards to better ensure effective programs for students that meet practice requirements. Potential nursing students may not be as aware of accreditation of the schools they are considering, but they should be. **Accreditation** is a process in which an organization is assessed regarding how it meets established standards. The focus here is on education accreditation; in other chapters, accreditation of healthcare organizations is discussed. The accrediting organization identifies minimum standards that guide the process, and nursing schools incorporate these standards into their programs. The accrediting organization then reviews the school and its programs. This is supposedly a voluntary process, but in reality, it is not; to be effective, a school of nursing must be accredited—to attract faculty, students, funding for education programs and research grants, and so that their graduates can attend other nursing programs such as graduate programs. Attending a nursing program that is not accredited can lead to complications in licensure, employment, and opportunities to continue on to higher degree programs. Currently, two organizations offer accreditation of nursing programs: NLN and AACN through their accrediting services CNEA and CCNE.

What is accreditation? The process is complex and takes time. Schools of nursing must pay for the review. Schools may or may not receive initial accreditation, and when they do, programs may be required to make changes. During the time period in which they are accredited, the accrediting body may determine that a school is not in compliance with the expected standards; therefore, the school may lose accreditation or additional reviews may be required. Accreditation is not a legal requirement, but state boards of nursing require this type of accreditation from the NLN or AACN to maintain state board of nursing accreditation. Some specialty organizations accredit specific graduate programs within a school, such as the American College of Nurse Midwifery and the American Association of Nurse Anesthetists. A school may choose which organization (CNEA or CCNE) accredits its school unless mandated by state agency or law; however, schools with diploma and associate degree programs can be accredited only by the CNEA (NLN, 2017b). The state board of nursing in each state is involved in this requirement and in its own state accreditation process.

During the accreditation process, the review team assesses the schools of nursing for the following, based on the accrediting organization's standards:

- Mission and vision
- Structure and governance
- Resources and physical facilities, including budget

- Faculty and faculty outcomes
- Curriculum and implementation
- Student support services
- Admissions process and other academic processes
- Policies and procedures
- Ongoing assessment process (continuous quality improvement, student and program outcomes)

The standards are periodically reviewed and revised; for example, in 2016, the CNEA revised its standards (NLN, 2016). The NLN accrediting standards support diversity in schools' missions, curricula, students, and faculty as well as support continuous quality improvement in education; in doing so, the NLN has an impact on a caring and competent nursing workforce (NLN, 2017b).

After the school of nursing completes a self-study based on the accreditation standards established by the accrediting organization, the written self-study results are submitted to the accrediting organization. The next step in the accreditation process is the onsite survey at the school. Surveyors visit the school: They observe classes and clinical experience/practicum, meet with staff at clinical sites, review documents (for example, curriculum, completed student assignments, budget, faculty organization, grants, and so on), and meet with school administrative staff. If the school of nursing is part of a university, they also meet with university administrative staff. In addition, surveyors meet with faculty, students, and alumni. They typically remain at the school for several days. Students have an obligation to participate in accreditation surveys and provide feedback. The goal is maintenance of minimum standards to ensure an effective learning environment that supports student learning and meets the needs of the profession. Schools must undergo reviews after they receive initial accreditation to continue their accreditation status, typically at a designated time period, but such reviews may occur if changes in the school or problems arise.

Stop and Consider #4
Continuous improvement is not only needed in healthcare delivery, but also in nursing education.

Critical Nursing
Education Problems

Today, two critical problems that concern participants in nursing education programs are the growing faculty shortage and the need to find clinical experiences for students, particularly as efforts are made to increase enrollment. These complex problems require more than one solution, and they have a great impact on the quality of nursing education and student outcomes.

Faculty Shortage

The faculty shortage has an impact on the availability of graduates to practice because it means that fewer new nurses can enter the profession. As noted earlier in this chapter, one of the reasons that potential qualified students cannot enroll in a nursing program is the shortage of qualified faculty. A school's faculty should reflect a balance of expert clinicians who can teach, expert researchers and grant writers who can teach and meet research obligations, and expert teachers who are pedagogical scholars (NLN, 2016). Today, schools of nursing, regardless of the type of program, are struggling to meet the demand for greater enrollment of students because of the limited number of faculty. They have problems recruiting experienced faculty, and thus many faculty are new to teaching. Some of the same factors that affect the fluctuating nursing shortage have an impact on the faculty shortage, such as faculty retirement (for example, 2013–2014 data indicate average ages of doctoral-prepared faculty range from 61.6 to 51.4 years; master's prepared range is 57.1 50 51.2 years [AACN, 2015a]). This challenge will only increase in the future because a large number of nursing faculty members are approaching retirement

age. It is also difficult to attract nurses to teaching because the pay is lower than for nursing practice; for this reason, nurses with graduate degrees often opt to stay in active practice. Attracting nurses to attend graduate school is an issue, particularly at the doctoral level. The DNP degree has attracted more nurses to these advanced degree programs, but these nurses may not be interested in teaching—and the DNP program was not intended to prepare faculty but rather to prepare practitioners. However, even if more students apply to DNP programs, they may be denied admission due to the lack of sufficient faculty to teach in the programs. The ACA offers some opportunities to expand nursing faculty through provisions supporting funding for education so that nurses can prepare for the faculty role, and this has improved the situation. Changes in the law may impact these provisions.

Access to Clinical Experiences

Aside from having a limited number of faculty, nursing programs struggle to provide space for clinical laboratories and to secure a sufficient number of clinical sites at healthcare facilities—all of this requires a certain number of faculty to meet standards for quality education and faculty–student ratios. With the drive to increase student enrollment, securing enough clinical sites to meet course objectives is a challenge for schools of nursing. If a number of nursing schools are located in the same area, there is also competition for clinical slots. This is particularly a problem in healthcare specialties that may have fewer patient services in a location, which translates into tight demand for clinical slots—such as pediatrics, obstetrics, and mental health. Schools of nursing need to be more innovative and recognize that every student may not get the same clinical experiences. For example, there is increasing use of non–acute care pediatric settings. Some communities do not have pediatric hospitals and may have limited beds assigned to pediatric care in other hospitals. Other sites that might be used are pediatrician offices, pediatric clinics, schools, daycare centers, and camps. For obstetrics, possible clinical sites are birthing centers, obstetrician offices, and midwifery practices. Mental health clinical experiences may take place in clinics, homeless shelters, mental health emergency and crisis centers, and may even use a mental health association or other type of community organization focused on health needs.

This difficulty in getting sites has forced some schools to move away from the traditional clinical hours offered—Monday through Friday during the day. Some schools are recognizing that operating on a 9-month basis with a long summer break affects the availability of clinical experiences. To accommodate the needs of all schools of nursing and the need to increase student enrollment, community-area healthcare providers often collaborate with schools to determine how all these needs can be met effectively.

A Response and Innovation: Laboratory Experiences and Clinical Simulation

Laboratory and simulation experiences have become important teaching–learning settings for developing competencies, partly because of problems in accessing clinical experiences, but also as a result of the recognition that they provide effective learning experiences for students with no risk of harm to patients. A new simulation dictionary developed and published by the Agency for Healthcare Research and Quality (AHRQ) defines *healthcare simulation* as: "A technique that creates a situation or environment to allow persons to experience a representation of a real healthcare event for the purpose of practice, learning, evaluation, testing, or to gain understanding of systems or human actions; the application of a simulation activity to training, assessment, research, or systems integration toward patient safety" (Lopreiato, 2016, p. 15). Simulation helps students develop confidence in their skills

in a safe setting before they begin caring for real patients and can help students to develop teamwork competencies. This is supported by the NCSBN study on the role and outcomes of simulation in pre-licensure programs, which indicates that, "up to 50 percent of traditional clinical experiences under conditions comparable to those described in the study" may be used instead of clinical experiences (NLN, 2015, p. 2; Hayden, Smiley, Alexander, Kardong-Edgren, & Jeffires, 2014). The simulated environment provides opportunities for teams of nurses, or ideally, interprofessional students to work together to respond to simulated clinical situations. Student evaluation and real-time feedback can be done in a simulated structured learning situation. Simulated experiences should be as close to real life as possible—although they are not, of course, totally real. This does not, however, mean that these learning situations are not very helpful for student learning. Clinical training laboratories that are not as high-tech as simulation centers may be used to learn basic skills. Most schools do not have their own full simulation laboratories due to the expense of setting up and running such labs. The simulation laboratory may be established through a partnership of multiple health practice education programs and/or hospitals to reduce the financial burden on each institution and offer simulation to a variety of students, often as an interprofessional student and/or staff experience.

A simulation laboratory is expensive to develop and maintain. Students need to respect the equipment and supplies and follow procedures so that costs can be managed. Faculty supervision in the simulation laboratory may be based on a higher ratio of students to faculty than the required ratio for clinical experiences, providing more cost-effective teaching and learning. With the development of more sophisticated technology, computer simulation can even be incorporated into distance education. State boards of nursing may have requirements as to the number of simulation hours that can be substituted for clinical hours.

Stop and Consider #5
The critical problems in nursing education are interrelated.

Transforming Nursing
Education

Recent reports on quality in healthcare delivery indicate an urgent need to institute changes in nursing education. In fact, the most recent major nursing education report identified preparation of nurses to meet these quality demands as a critical topic (Benner, Sutphen, Leonard, & Day, 2010). Thus, quality improvement relies, in part, on improvement of nursing education. Nursing students need to be included in the evaluation of nursing education and changes. As a student, you can help meet this need by providing course feedback and participating in curriculum committees when requested. Nursing education leaders should always review content and improve curriculum, but they must have methods to do this in a timely, effective manner. When accreditation surveyors come to schools of nursing, they talk to students to get their feedback, as there is recognition that students need to be engaged in the transformation of nursing education.

One aspect of transforming health care related to nursing education was addressed in a recent report sponsored by the AACN focusing on academic health centers (AHCs) and nursing education (academic nursing) and practice—noting that nurses are the primary care givers and advocates for patients (Manatt Health Project Team, 2016). The report clarifies two key terms. An **AHC** is a center of multiple health profession schools, accredited, and connected to a teaching healthcare organization, such as a hospital or health system. **Academic nursing** is the integration of practice, education, and research associated with baccalaureate and graduate schools of nursing—academic nursing faculty demonstrate "a commitment to inquiry, generate new knowledge for the discipline, connect practice with education, and lead scholarly pursuits that improve health and health care" (Manatt Health Project Team, 2016, p.5). The findings from the report indicate that academic nursing is not currently positioned as a real partner in healthcare transformation—for example, nursing has limited participation in governance and faculty leadership roles in the AHCs. This needs to change, though resources will be needed to increase this participation and collaboration. An example that was given as a barrier is lack of nursing faculty practices that bring in income and the over-reliance on tuition for academic nursing budgets. The AACN (2016b)report's recommendations are to "embrace a new vision for academic nursing, enhance the clinical practice of academic nursing, partner in preparing the nurses of the future, partner in the implementation of accountable care, invest in nursing research programs and better integrate research into clinical practice, and implement the advocacy agenda in support of a new era for academic nursing" (p. 1).

Stop and Consider #6
Transforming nursing education is connected to nursing practice.

Interprofessional
Healthcare Education

One of the healthcare professions core competencies is focused on interprofessional teams; an important competency for nursing education and has impact on patient care (IOM, 2003). Emphasis on this competency has stimulated collaboration toward better understanding of interprofessonal collaborative practice. The interprofessional education collaborative (IPEC) established key competencies in 2009 and published updates in 2011 and 2016. Initially, IPEC identified four topical areas or domains as values and ethics, roles and responsibilities, interprofessional communication, and teams and teamwork; however, a fifth domain has been added as the central domain: interprofessional collaboration supported by four competencies (IPEC, 2016, p. 11):

- Work with individuals of other professions to maintain a climate of mutual respect and shared values (values and ethics domain).
- Use the knowledge of one's own role and those of other professions to assess and address the healthcare needs of the patients and populations served (roles and responsibility domain).
- Communicate with patients, families, communities, and other health professionals in a responsive and responsible manner that supports a team approach to health maintenance and the treatment of disease (interprofessional communication domain).
- Teams and teamwork: Apply relationship-building values and the principles of team dynamics to perform effectively in different team roles to plan and deliver patient-/population-centered care that is safe, timely, efficient, effective, and equitable (teams and teamwork domain).

Figure 3-2 describes a model for interprofessional collaboration and its associated domains.

These efforts strongly support the need for "safe, high-quality, accessible, patient-centered care" for all and interprofessional collaboration is required to accomplish this" (IPEC, 2016, p. 4). Not only are healthcare profession education programs including more on interprofessional content and experiences with interprofessional teams, but also there is more faculty development on the topic. This emphasis on interprofessional teams is also now included in accreditation of education programs. Interprofessional education occurs, "when students from two or more professions learn about, from and with each other to enable effective collaboration and improve health outcomes" (World Health Organization, 2010). To meet these needs,

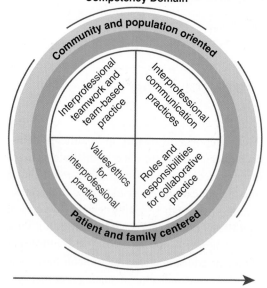

Interprofessional Collaborative Competency Domain

Figure 3-2 The Learning Continuum Pre-Licensure through Practice Trajectory

Reproduced with permission from Interprofessional Education Collaborative. (2016). Core competencies for interprofessional collaborative practice: 2016 update. Washington, DC: Interprofessional Education Collaborative. p. 9. Retrieved from https://ipecollaborative.org/uploads/IPEC-2016-Updated-Core-Competencies-Report__final_release_.PDF

nursing education must work to provide effective learning experiences for nursing students so that they are prepared to work on interprofessional teams. Nursing students, pre-licensure and graduate, also have responsibilities, such as to actively engage in the learning activities planned by faculty and to seek out learning situations that support interprofessional competencies. Students might do this by observing work teams in clinical, asking to join an interprofessional activity in clinical, and working to increase communication with and respect of other healthcare professionals.

Stop and Consider #7

Interprofessional education is critical for effective interprofessional teams.

Regulation

How are professional regulation and nursing regulation for practice licensure related? **Regulation** for practice or licensure is clear, though problematic in some cases. This type of regulation is based on state laws and regulations and leads to licensure. However, this is different from the professional regulation, in which the profession itself regulates its practice. State boards of nursing are not nursing professional organizations, but rather state government agencies. This distinction can make it difficult to make changes in a state's practice of nursing, which requires state legislative changes. Professional organizations do have an impact on practice through the standards they propose and other elements of support and data that they provide. "For effective nursing workforce planning to occur and be sustained, [state] boards of nursing must collaborate with nursing education and practice to support the safe and effective evolution of nursing practice" (Damgaard, VanderWoude, & Hegge, 1999, as cited in Loquist, 2002, p. 34).

"In 1950, nursing became the first profession for which the same licensure exam, the State Board Test Pool (now called NCLEX), was used throughout the nation to license nurses. This increased mobility for the registered nurse and resulted in a significant advantage for the relatively new profession of nursing" (Lundy, 2005, pp. 21–22). The major purpose of regulation is to protect the public, and it is based on the Tenth Amendment of the U.S. Constitution, the states' rights amendment. Each state has the right to regulate professional practice, such as nursing practice, within its own state.

In general, the regulatory approach selected should be sufficient to ensure public protection. The following criteria are still relevant today in providing a framework for professional licensure (NCSBN, 1996, pp. 8–9):

- *Risk of harm for the consumer:* The evaluation of a profession to determine whether unregulated practice endangers the public should focus on recognizable harm. That harm could result from the practices inherent in the nature of the profession, the characteristics of the clients/patients, the settings, or supervisory requirements, or a combination of these factors. Licensure is applied to a profession when the incompetent or unethical practice of that profession could cause greater risk of harm to the public unless there is a high level of accountability; at the other extreme, registration is appropriate for professions where such a high level of accountability is not needed.
- *Skill and training needed:* The more highly specialized the services of the professional, the greater the need for an approach that actively inquires about the education and competence of the professional.
- *Level of autonomy:* Licensure is indicated when the professional uses independent judgment and practices independently with little or no supervision. Registration is appropriate for individuals who do not use independent judgment and practice with supervision.
- *Scope of practice:* Unless there is a well-demarcated scope of practice for the profession that is distinguishable from other professions and definable in enforceable legal terms, there is neither basis nor need for licensure. This scope may overlap other professions in specific duties, functions, or therapeutic modalities.
- *Consumer expectation:* Consumers expect that those professions that have a potentially high impact on the consumer or on their physical, mental, or economic well-being will be subject to regulatory oversight. The costs of operating regulatory agencies and the restriction of practitioners who do not meet the minimum requirements are justified to protect the public from harm.
- *Alternative to regulation:* There are no alternatives to the selected regulatory approach

that would adequately protect the public. It should also be the case that when it is determined that regulation of the profession is required; the least restrictive level of regulation consistent with public protection is implemented.

Influenced by the above, today eight guiding principles apply to nursing regulation: (1) protection of the public, (2) competence of all practitioners regulated by the board of nursing, (3) due process and ethical decision making, (4) shared accountability, (5) strategic collaboration, (6) evidence-based regulation, (7) response to the marketplace and healthcare environment, and (8) globalization of nursing (NCSBN, 2007).

Nurse Practice Acts

Each state has a **nurse practice act** that determines the nature of nursing practice within the state. The nurse practice act is a state law passed by the state legislative body. Nurse practice acts for each state can be found on state government websites. Every licensed nurse should be knowledgeable about the nurse practice act that governs practice in the state where the nurse practices under his or her RN license, and nursing students should be aware of the nurse practice act in the state in which they are enrolled as a student. Typically, nurse practice acts do the following for their state (Masters, 2005, p. 166):

- Define the authority of the board of nursing, its composition, and its powers.
- Define nursing and boundaries of the scope of practice.
- Identify types of licenses and titles.
- State the requirements for licensure.
- Protect titles.
- Identify the grounds for disciplinary action.

The most important function of the nurse practice act is to define the scope of practice, boundaries of practice, for nurses in the state to protect public safety.

State Boards of Nursing

State boards of nursing implement the state's nurse practice act and recommend state regulations and changes to this act when appropriate. This board is part of state government, although how it fits into a state's governmental organization varies from state to state. RNs serve on state boards of nursing, and the governor typically selects board members who serve for a specific term of office. Licensed vocational/practical nurses (LVN/LPNs) and laypersons or consumers (non-nurses) may also have representation on the board. The primary purpose of the state board of nursing is to protect the health and safety of the public (citizens of the state). A board of nursing has an executive director who runs the business of the board, along with staff who work for the state board—all are state employees. The size of the state has an impact on the size of the board of nursing and its staff. Boards are not only involved in setting standards and licensure of nurses (RNs and LVN/LPNs), but also are responsible for monitoring nursing education (RN and LPN) programs in the state. The board serves a regulatory function; as part of this function, it can issue administrative rules or regulations consistent with state law to facilitate the enforcement of the nurse practice act.

The board of nursing in each state also reviews problems with individual licensure and is the agency that administers disciplinary actions. If a nurse fails to meet certain standards, participates in unacceptable practice, or has problems that interfere with safe practice and if any of these violations are reported to the board, the board can conduct an investigation and review and determine actions that might need to be taken. Examples of these issues are assault or causing harm to a patient; having a problem with illegal drugs or with alcohol (substance abuse); conviction of, or pleading guilty to, a felony (examples of felonies are murder, robbery, rape, and sexual battery); and having a psychiatric illness that is not managed effectively and interferes with safe functioning. A nurse may be reprimanded by the board or denied a license, may be subject to suspended or revoked licensure, or may face licensure restriction with stipulations (for example, the nurse must attend an alcohol treatment program to retain licensure).

The board must follow strict procedures when taking any disciplinary action, which must first begin with an official complaint to the board. Anyone can make a complaint to the board—another nurse, another healthcare professional, a healthcare organization, or a consumer. The state nursing practice act identifies the possible reasons for disciplinary action. Boards of nursing publish their disciplinary action decisions because they are part of the public record. When nurses obtain a license in another state, they are asked to report any disciplinary actions that have been taken by another state's board of nursing. Not reporting disciplinary board actions has serious consequences for obtaining (and losing) licensure. A key point is that licensure is a privilege, not a legal right. It is important to consider this point as a student because the same rules apply when getting the first license—even if a student graduates from a nursing program, this does not mean he or she has a right to take the NCLEX exam or to be given a license.

National Council of State Boards of Nursing

The NCSBN is a not-for-profit organization that represents all of the boards of nursing in the 50 states, the District of Columbia, and 4 U.S. territories (American Samoa, Guam, Northern Mariana Islands, and Virgin Islands). Through this organization, all state boards of nursing work together on issues related to the regulation of nursing practice that affect public health, safety, and welfare, including the development of registered nurse licensing examinations. Although the NCSBN cannot dictate change to individual state boards of nursing, it can make recommendations, which often carry significant weight. Individual state boards of nursing, unlike the NCSBN, are part of, and report to, state government. The NCSBN performs the following functions (NCSBN, 2013):

- Develops the NCLEX-RN, NCLEX-PN, NNAAP, and MACE examinations.
- Monitors trends in public policy, nursing practice, and education.
- Promotes uniformity in relationship to the regulation of nursing practice.
- Disseminates data related to the licensure of nurses.
- Conducts research on nursing practice issues.
- Serves as a forum for information exchange for members (individual state boards of nursing).
- Provides opportunities for collaboration among its members and other nursing and healthcare organizations by maintaining the Nursys database, which coordinates national publicly available nurse licensure information.

Licensure Requirements

Each state's board of nursing determines its state's licensure requirements based on state law; however, all states require passage of the NCLEX-RN, which is a national exam. Other requirements include criminal background checks for initial licensure and continuing education (CE) for renewal, though the latter requirement varies from state to state. Many nurses hold licenses in several states, which is obtained through endorsement, or may be on inactive status in some states. An RN should always maintain one license, even if not practicing, to make it easier to return to practice. Fees are paid for the initial license and for license renewal. States in which a nurse is licensed notify the nurse when the license is up for renewal. It is the nurse's responsibility to complete the required forms and submit payment, and many states now do this electronically. Examples of initial licensure and renewal requirements, which vary from state to state, include the following:

- Fee (always required, though the amount varies and depends on whether the nurse has active or inactive licensure status)
- Passage of NCLEX (required for first licensure but no further testing required for renewals or change of license from one state to another)
- For renewal, **CE** contact hours within a specified time period (number of contact hours varies from state to state, and some states do not require any CE for licensure renewal)
- Criminal background check (required typically for initial licensure in a state; also asked if any felonies when renewing license or getting a license in a different state may require background check)
- For renewal or new state, active employment for a specific number of hours within a specified time period (varies from state to state)
- For renewal or new state, number of hours of professional nursing activities (varies from state to state)

Ultimately, each RN is responsible for maintaining competency for safe practice. Any person who practices nursing without a valid license commits a minor misdemeanor. If licensed in one state, the nurse can typically do the following in another state in which the nurse is not licensed: consult, teach as guest lecturer, and conduct evaluation of care as part of an accreditation process.

National Council Licensure Examination

The NCLEX is the national nursing exam that is developed and administered through the NCSBN (2017a). There are two forms of the exam: NCLEX-RN for RN licensure and NCLEX-PN for practical nurse licensure. In each jurisdiction (state) in the United States and its territories, licensing authorities regulate entry into practice of nursing. To ensure public protection, each jurisdiction requires a candidate for licensure to pass an examination that measures the competencies needed to perform safely and effectively as a newly licensed, entry-level RN (or LPN/LVN). RN content relates to the following patient/client needs categories: safe effective care environment (management of care, safety, and infection control), health promotion and maintenance, psychosocial integrity, and physiological integrity (basic care and comfort, pharmacologic and parenteral therapies, reduction of risk potential, physiological adaptation).

The examination is offered online. Most of the questions are written at the cognitive level of application or higher, requiring the candidate to use problem-solving skills to select the best answer. The exam is a computerized adaptive test. In this type of exam, the computer adjusts questions to the individual candidate so that the exam is then highly individualized, offering challenging questions that are neither too easy nor too difficult. The exam ends when the computer determines with 95% certainty that the person's ability is either below or above the passing standard. The exam can also end when the time runs out or there are no more questions. Because of these factors, all candidates do not receive the same number of questions. The exam includes a variety of types of questions such as multiple-response, fill-in-the-blank, and hot spot items using a picture or graphic.

If a candidate does not pass the NCLEX, he or she may retake the exam. Most schools of nursing provide some type of preparation (for example, throughout the nursing program or near the end); some may recommend that students complete a prep course on their own. These prep courses require a fee and are of varying length. Many publications are also available to assist with NCLEX preparation. In reality, exam preparation takes place every day in nursing programs—in courses and clinical experiences as students learn and practice receiving faculty feedback.

Students are asked by their school to complete an application for NCLEX in the final semester before graduation. This application is sent to the state board of nursing in the state where the student is seeking licensure. After a student completes the nursing program, the school must verify that the student has graduated. At this point, the student becomes an official NCLEX candidate. The student receives an authorization to test and exam instructions and information about scheduling the exam. The authorization to test is the nursing graduate's pass to take the exam, so it is important to keep it. Students then schedule their own exam within the given time frame.

Testing sites are available in every state, and a candidate may take the exam in any state. Licensure, however, is awarded by the state in which the candidate has applied for licensure. On the scheduled date, the student goes to the designated testing site to take the computerized exam. Candidates are fingerprinted and photographed to ensure security for the exam and are provided an orientation and a brief practice session prior to taking the exam. An exam session lasts several hours, but because of the computerized adaptive test method, the amount of time that an individual candidate takes on the exam varies; that time is not an indicator of passing or failing.

Passing scores are the same for every state and are set by the NCSBN; they can vary from year to year. Candidates are usually informed of their results within 4 weeks; the result is pass or fail, with no specific score provided. Schools of nursing receive composites of student results. Data on individual school pass rates are available on state board of nursing websites and are open to the public. Results from the NCLEX are an important element in a school of nursing's evaluation/assessment process. The first-time pass rate is reviewed routinely and must be reported to the school's accreditation organization; in addition, the state board monitors these results. Schools of nursing can be put on probation by their state boards of nursing if pass rates are a problem. This leads to further evaluation of the program and monitoring of outcomes. The state boards of nursing protect students and potential students in ensuring that the education provided will prepare them at the level expected.

Critical Current and Future Regulation Issues

Nursing regulation covers many issues related to legal requirements about nursing practice. Most of the focus and responsibility for nursing regulation falls on the state boards of nursing and their respective legislative bodies; however, the National Council for State Boards of Nursing offers advise to state boards of nursing. Nursing professional organizations also offer their advice but cannot formally regulate practice. There have been some regulatory efforts at the federal level, though this is not common but if done more routinely would lead to more consistency across states.

Nurse Licensure Compact

There has been a growing need to design licensure methods that address the following situations: a nurse lives in one state but works in an adjacent state, a nurse works for a healthcare company in several states, and a nurse works in telehealth with care provided via technology in more than one state. To address these types of issues, the NCSBN created a new model for license portability called mutual recognition or **nurse licensure compact** (NLC) (Wallis, 2015). Each state in a mutual recognition compact must enact legislation or regulation authorizing the NLC and also adopting administrative rules and regulations to implement the compact. Each compact state must also appoint an NLC administrator to facilitate the exchange of information between the states that relates to compact nurse licensure and regulation. Twenty-five states have adopted this model (NCSBN, 2017a). Other states have decided that this model is unconstitutional in their states because it delegates authority for licensure decisions to other states. A list of current states offering this multistate licensure is available from the NCSBN website. There have been suggestions that what is needed is national licensure, but it is not likely to occur at this time (Wallis, 2015).

The same type of licensure questions applies to APRNs. In 2002, the NCSBN Delegate Assembly approved the adoption of model language for a licensure compact for APRNs. Only those states that have adopted the RN and LPN/LVN licensure compact may implement a compact for APRNs. Many states are now working on implementation regulations, which must be put into effect prior to implementation of the compact. The APRN compact offers states the mechanism for mutually recognizing APRN licenses and authority to practice.

Mandatory Overtime

A critical concern in practice today is requiring nurses to work overtime. Employers make this decision, and it is called mandatory overtime. This policy impacts the quality of care and has affected staff satisfaction and burnout. Some state boards of nursing have become involved in state legislative efforts related to mandatory overtime.

Although legislative and regulatory responses have provided nurses with additional support for creating safer work environments, each of these legislative responses has a significant effect on the numbers and types of nursing personnel that will be required for care delivery systems in the future as well as the cost of care. Clearly, there is concern at the state and national levels regarding the impact that fewer staff will have on the health and safety of patients (Loquist, 2002, p. 37).

As students and new graduates interview for their first positions, they should ask about mandatory overtime if they are not in a state that has a law to protect them from it. Research has been done regarding sleep deprivation and its connection to the rising number of medical errors (Girard, 2003; Manfredini, Boari, & Manfredini, 2006; Montgomery, 2007; Sigurdson & Ayas, 2007). This area of research is fairly new, and researchers will need to continue to provide concrete evidence of the links among sleep deprivation, long work hours, and medical errors. Other work areas and professions have examined this problem and taken steps to reduce hours, for example, the aviation industry has cut back the number of hours that flight crews can work without sleep; the number of hours that medical residents can work consecutively has been decreased because of concern about fatigue and errors.

Foreign Nursing Graduates: Entrance to Practice in the United States

The number of nurses from other countries coming to the United States to work and/or study has increased. Some nurses want to work here only temporarily; others want to stay permanently. This movement of nurses internationally typically increases during a shortage, and today there is a worldwide shortage and a lot of nursing migration (International Centre on Nurse Migration, 2017). **Nurse migration** is a complex area—affecting the country of origin, which may then experience a shortage and the need to effectively integrate foreign nurses in the United States who may not have had a the type of nursing education we expect (Jacobson, 2015). The International Centre for Nurse Migration provides resources for nurses who are moving from one country to another and information about this critical topic to increase the profession's understanding of this issue.

The NCSBN notes that each state board of nursing is responsible for RN licensure for its state. States may vary in requirements, but all internationally educated nurses must pass the NCLEX exam; comply with standards of approved or comparable education, hold a verified valid and unencumbered state license, and be proficient in their written and spoken English language skills (NCSBN, 2017b).

What do these nurses have to do to meet practice requirements in the United States? The Commission on Graduates of Foreign Nursing Schools (2017) is an organization that assists these nurses in evaluating their credentials and verifies their education, registration, and licensure. This is an internationally recognized, immigration-neutral, nonprofit organization that protects the public by ensuring that these nurses are eligible and qualified to meet U.S. licensure and immigration requirements. These nurses must also take the English as a Foreign Language Exam to ensure that their English language ability is at an acceptable level. This requirement also applies to students who want to enter U.S. nursing education programs. A nurse who is licensed in another country must successfully complete the NCLEX and meet the state licensure requirements where the nurse will practice. If the nurse wants to enter a graduate nursing program, the nurse needs to get a U.S. RN license for clinical work that is required in the educational program. Licensure is not required to enter a pre-licensure program (BSN) in nursing, but it is required for a graduate nursing program.

Global Health Regulatory Issues

With the development of the Internet, telehealth and global migration have forced nursing to confront the need to examine changes related to interstate nursing practice and possible responses. Globalization has had a similar impact on migration (Fernandez & Hebert, 2004). This migration phenomenon supports the need for an international credentialing of immigrant nurses to ensure public safety as defined by the International Council of Nurses (Schaefer, 1990). "New models for practice will continue to emerge to manage change, care, and plan for the future. Electronic technologies provide an opportunity to develop a new identity for nursing practice. New regulatory requirements will emerge to meet the need of practitioners to ensure public safety. As a new paradigm for ensuring competencies and self-regulation in a global market evolves, the need to explore global licensure will emerge. The future belongs to those who will accept the challenge to make a difference in a global marketplace and take the necessary risks to make things happen" (Fernandez & Hebert, 2004, p. 132).

The Global Alliance for Leadership in Nursing Education (GANES, 2017) is a nursing organization that focuses on getting nurse educators from around the world to work together to develop and facilitate nursing education and professional development for nurses worldwide in order to improve care globally. These efforts recognize the need for international standards in nursing education. Nursing has moved from a focus on individual hospitals, to the state level, to the national level, and now to a global level.

Stop and Consider #8
Regulation protects patients.

CHAPTER HIGHLIGHTS

1. The evolution of nursing education influences how nursing is taught.
2. Nursing has multiple types of programs and degrees: diploma, associate degree, baccalaureate, master's, and doctoral levels.
3. Nursing organizations, such as AACN and NLN, guide nursing education, provide resources, and accreditation.
4. There is a need to improve nursing education to better meet patient care needs—for example, use of standards, competencies, recognition of excellence, and accreditation.
5. Licensure and regulation of nursing practice set standards and rules for nursing education.

   Different levels of nursing pre-licensure education have different competencies and expectations, yet nurses at all levels take the same licensure examination.
6. Nursing education is undergoing changes to improve and meet needs.
7. Interprofessional education is now an important consideration in nursing education.
8. Examples of critical concerns related to education, regulation, and practice are compact licensure, mandatory overtime, and global migration of nurses.

ENGAGING IN THE CONTENT

Discussion Questions

1. Why do you think it is important that nursing now emphasize education over training? Consider Donahue's definitions for education and training found in the chapter. How has apprenticeship been adapted to current nursing education needs?

2. Compare and contrast the types of entry programs in nursing: diploma, ADN, BSN, and accelerated or direct entry programs.

3. Select one of the following graduate nursing programs (master's—any type; DNP or PhD) and find, through the Internet, two different universities that offer the program. Compare and contrast admission requirements and the curricula.

4. Visit the NCLEX website (https://www.ncsbn .org/nclex.htm). Review and describe the exam process and what happens on exam day. Go to https://www.ncsbn.org/1287 .htm and review the current NCLEX-RN detailed test plan for candidates. Which type of information is included in the plan? How might this information help you, both now and closer to the time when you take the NCLEX?

5. Does your state participate in the NLC? Visit https://www.ncsbn.org/158.htm to find out. Why might this be important to you if you choose to be licensed in your state after graduation?

CRITICAL THINKING ACTIVITIES

1. Conduct a debate in class with another classmate. Take the side of diploma, associate degree, or both levels of entry into practice, with the other classmate supporting the BSN as the entry into practice level. The class should then vote on the side that presents the best support for one of the perspectives. You will need to research your issue and present a substantiated rationale for your side of the issue.

2. Conduct a debate in class with another classmate. Take the side supporting the PhD in nursing, with the other classmate supporting the DNP. The class should then vote on the side that presents the best support for one of the perspectives. You will need to research your issue and present a substantiated rationale for your side of the issue.

3. Consider your nursing education program. What aspects do you think are effective for you as a student, and why? What are problems you identify, and what ideas do you have for solutions?

ELECTRONIC REFLECTION JOURNAL

Assess your current nursing program—you may not be in the program long, but consider your admission process, orientation, any courses you have taken (non-nursing and nursing), communication with faculty, relationships with other students and the culture of the school, and any clinical or lab experiences you have had. How might you use your reflection to improve your nursing education experiences?

CASE STUDIES

Case 1

The executive committee of your school's Student Nurses' Association chapter is meeting to plan a program for the membership. A lively discussion is going on to select the topic. One board member mentions the need to have a program about nursing education accreditation because the school will have an accreditation survey visit next semester. The SNA chapter president speaks up and says, "Many of us are getting ready to take NCLEX, and we have many questions about licensure." Both of these topics are important topics. Consider the questions that follow.

Case Questions

1. Which topic would you choose, and why?
2. If someone said to you, "Accreditation is the business of the faculty," what would you say?
3. Which type of content might you include in the content for a program on accreditation and a program on licensure for your membership?

Case 2

Nursing education and the profession in general have experienced a very long disagreement about the appropriate entry-level degree for nursing. This debate first emerged in 1965, as noted in this chapter. In addition, authors such as Kutney-Lee, Sloane, and Aiken have conducted studies that have concluded the BSN should be the entry-level degree (2013). Cynthia Maskey, PhD, RN, CNE, in the March 2013 issue of *Health Affairs*, responded to this study. Dr. Maskey is an OADN board member. Review the study and Dr. Maskey's response:

- Article: Kutney-Lee, A., Sloane, D., & Aiken, L. (2013). An increase in the number of nurses with baccalaureate degrees is linked to lower rates of postsurgery mortality. *Health Affairs, 32*, 3579–3586.
- At the link for this study see response by C. Maskey, The study focuses on problems, not solutions. Retrieved from http://content.healthaffairs.org/content/32/3/579 /reply#healthaff_el_476350

Case Questions

After reading this article and visiting the website with Maskey's response, consider the following questions.

1. What is the study that is highlighted? Why is it important?
2. What is your view of the entry-level disagreement?
3. Does it surprise you that this issue is cause for disagreement? If so, why does it surprise you?
4. What is your opinion of the response from the ADN perspective?
5. What are the possible negative results from such a disagreement in the profession?

CASE STUDIES (CONTINUED)

Working Backward to Develop a Case

Write a brief paragraph that describes a case related to the following questions.

1. What is the purpose of nursing education accreditation?
2. Why do we as students need to be involved?
3. What do we want to share about our school?

REFERENCES

Aiken, L., Clarke, S., Cheung, R., Sloane, D., & Silber, J. (2003). Educational levels of hospital nurses and surgical patient mortality. *Journal of the American Medical Association, 290,* 1617–1623.

Aiken, L. et al. for the RN4CAST consortium. (2014, February 15). Nurse staffing and education and hospital mortality in nine European countries: A retrospective observational study. *Lancet.* doi: 10.1016/S0140-6736(13)62631-8

American Association of Colleges of Nursing. (2005a, May 6). *AACN applauds decision of the AONE board to move registered nurse education to the baccalaureate level* (press release). Washington, DC: Author.

American Association of Colleges of Nursing. (2005b). *Alliance for Nursing Accreditation statement on distance education policies.* Retrieved from http://www.aacn.nche.edu/education/disstate.htm

American Association of Colleges of Nursing. (2005c). *Fact sheet: Articulation agreements among nursing education programs.* Washington, DC: Author.

American Association of Colleges of Nursing. (2006). *The essentials of doctoral education for advanced nursing practice.* Washington, DC: Author. Retrieved from http://www.aacn.nche.edu/dnp/Essentials.pdf

American Association of Colleges of Nursing. (2008). *The essentials of baccalaureate education for professional nursing practice.* Washington, DC: Author. Retrieved from http://www.aacn.nche.edu/Education/pdf/BaccEssentials98.pdf

American Association of Colleges of Nursing. (2011). *The Essentials of masters education for nursing.* Washington, DC: Author. Retrieved from http://www.aacn.nche.edu/education-resources/MasEssentials96.pdf

American Association of Colleges of Nursing. (2013). *Competencies and curricular expectations for clinical nurse leader education and practice.* Washington, DC: Author.

American Association of Colleges of Nursing. (2015a). *New AACN data confirm enrollment surge in schools of nursing.* Retrieved from http://www.aacn.nche.edu/news/articles/2015/enrollment

American Association of Colleges of Nursing. (2015b). *The doctor of nursing practice: Current issues and clarifying recommendations.* Retrieved from http://www.aacn.nche.edu/aacn-publications/white-papers/DNP-Implementation-TF-Report-8-15.pdf

American Association of Colleges of Nursing. (2016a). *DNP fact sheet.* Retrieved from http://www.aacn.nche.edu/media-relations/fact-sheets/dnp

American Association of Colleges of Nursing. (2016b). *About AACN.* Retrieved from http://www.aacn.nche.edu/about-aacn

American Association of Colleges of Nursing. (2017). *AACN strategic plan 2017–2019.* Retrieved from http://www.aacn.nche.edu/about-aacn/strategic-plan

American Association of Colleges of Nursing, American Organization of Nurse Executives, & National Organization for Associate Degree Nursing. (1995). *A model for differentiated nursing practice.* Washington, DC: Author.

American Nurses Association. (1965). Education for nursing. *American Journal of Nursing, 65*(12), 107–108.

American Nurses Association. (2011). *ANA fact sheet.* Retrieved from http://nursingworld.org/NursingbytheNumbersFactSheet.aspx

American Nurses Association. (2015). *Nursing scope and standards of practice*. Silver Spring, MD: Author.

American Organization of Nurse Executives. (1990). *Current issues and perspectives of differentiated practice*. Chicago, IL: American Hospital Association.

Benner, P., Sutphen, M., Leonard, V., & Day, L. (2010). *Educating nurses: A call for radical transformation*. San Francisco, CA: Jossey-Bass.

Brown, E. (1948). *Nursing for the future: A report prepared for the National Nursing Council*. New York, NY: Russell Sage Foundation.

Commission on Collegiate Nursing Education. (2013). *Standards for accreditation of baccalaureate and graduate nursing programs*. Retrieved from http://www.aacn.nche.edu/ccne-accreditation/Standards-Amended-2013.pdf

Commission on Graduates of Foreign Nursing Schools. (2017). *CGFNS website*. Retrieved from http://www.cgfns.org/about/

Council on Accreditation. (2017, January). *Transition nurse anesthesia programs to doctoral degree*. Retrieved from http://home.coa.us.com/Pages/default.aspx

Cronenwett, L., Dracup, K., Grey, M., McDauley, L., Meleis, A., & Salmon, M. (2011). The doctor of nursing practice: A national workforce perspective. *Nursing Outlook, 59*(1), 9–17.

Damgaard, G., VanderWoude, D., & Hegge, M. (1999). Perspectives from the prairie: The relationship between nursing regulation and South Dakota nursing workforce development. *Journal of Nursing Administration, 29*(11), 7–9, 14.

Donahue, M. (1983). Isabel Maitland Stewart's philosophy of education. *Nursing Research, 32*, 140–146.

Estabrooks, C., Midodzi, W., Cummings, G., Ricker, K., & Giovannetti, P. (2005). The impact of hospital nursing characteristics on 30-day mortality. *Nursing Research, 54*(2), 74–84.

Fernandez, R., & Hebert, G. (2004). Global licensure. New modalities of treatment and care require the development of new structures and systems to access care. *Nursing Administration Quarterly, 28*, 129–132.

Girard, N. J. (2003). Lack of sleep another safety risk factor (editorial—medical errors). *AORN Journal, 78*, 553–556.

Global Alliance for Leadership in Nursing Education. (2017). *GANES about*. Retrieved from http://ganes.info/About.php

Godfrey, N., & Martin, D. (2016). Breakthrough thinking in nursing education. The Baccalaureate big 5. *Journal of Nursing Administration, 46*(7/8), 393–399.

Goldmark, J. (1923). *Nursing and nursing education in the United States*. New York, NY: Macmillan.

Hayden, J., Smiley, R., Alexander, M., Kardong-Edgen, S., & Jeffries, P. (2014). Supplement: The NCSBN national simulation study: A longitudinal, randomized, controlled study replacing clinical hours with simulation in pre-licensure nursing education. *Journal of Nursing Regulation, 5*(2), C1–S64.

Hutchins, G. (1994). Differentiated interdisciplinary practice. *Journal of Nursing Administration, 24*(6), 52–58.

Institute of Medicine. (2001). *Crossing the quality chasm: A new health system for the 21st century*. Washington, DC: The National Academies Press.

Institute of Medicine. (2003). *Health professions education: A bridge to quality*. Washington, DC: The National Academies Press.

Institute of Medicine. (2010). *The future of nursing: Leading change, advancing health*. Washington, DC: The National Academies Press.

International Centre on Nurse Migration. (2017). *ICNM website*. Retrieved from http://www.intlnursemigration.org/

Interprofessional Education Collaborative. (2016). *Core competencies for interprofessional collaborative practice: 2016 update*. Washington, DC: Author. Retrieved from https://ipecollaborative.org/uploads/IPEC-2016-Updated-Core-Competencies-Report__final_release_.PDF

Jacobson, J. (2015). The complexities of nurse migration. *AJN, 115*(12), pp. 22–23.

Knowles, M. (1975). *Self-directed learning: A guide for learners and teachers*. Chicago, IL: Follett.

Knowles, M. (1984). *Andragogy in action*. San Francisco, CA: Jossey-Bass.

Kutney-Lee, A., Sloane, D., & Aiken, L. (2013). An increase in the number of nurses with baccalaureate degrees is linking to lower rates to post surgery mortality. *Health Affairs 30*(3), 579–586.

Leighow, S. (1996). Backrubs vs. Bach: Nursing and the entry-into-practice debate: 1946–1986. *Nursing History Review, 4*, 3–17.

Lopreiato, J. (2016, October). *Healthcare simulation dictionary*. Rockville, MD: Agency for Healthcare Research and Quality, AHRQ Publication No. 16(17)-0043.

Loquist, R. (2002). State boards of nursing respond to the nurse shortage. *Nursing Administration Quarterly, 26*(4), 33–39.

Lundy, K. (2005). A history of health care and nursing. In K. Masters (Ed.), *Role development in professional nursing practice* (Ch. 1). Burlington, MA: Jones & Bartlett Learning.

Manatt Health Project Team. (2016). *Advancing healthcare transformation. A new era for academic nursing*. Washington, DC: American Association of Colleges of Nursing. Retrieved from http://www.aacn.nche.edu/AACN-Manatt-Report.pdf

Manfredini, R., Boari, B., & Manfredini, F. (2006). Adverse events secondary to mistakes, excessive work hours, and sleep deprivation. *Archives of Internal Medicine*, *166*, 1422–1433.

Masters, K. (2005). *Role development in professional nursing practice*. Burlington, MA: Jones & Bartlett Learning.

McHugh, M., & Lake, E. (2010). Nurse education, experience, and the hospital context. *Research in Nursing & Health, 33*, 276–287.

Montag, M. (1959). *Community college education for nursing: An experiment in technical education for nursing*. New York, NY: McGraw-Hill.

Montgomery, V. (2007). Effect of fatigue, workload, and environment on patient safety in the pediatric intensive care unit. *Pediatric Critical Care Medicine, 8*(suppl. 2), S11–S16.

National Academy of Medicine. (2015). *Assessing progress on the Institute of Medicine report The Future of Nursing*. Washington, DC: The National Academies Press.

National Council of State Boards of Nursing. (1996). *Why regulation paper: Public protection or professional self-preservation?* Retrieved from https://www.ncsbn.org/why_regulation_paper.pdf

National Council of State Boards of Nursing. (2005). *Position paper: Clinical instruction in pre-licensure nursing programs*. Retrieved from http://www.ncsbn.org/pdfs/Final_Clinical_Instr_Pre_Nsg_programs.pdf

National Council of State Boards of Nursing. (2007). *Guiding principles of nursing regulation*. Retrieved from https://www.ncsbn.org/Guiding_Principles.pdf

National Council of State Boards of Nursing. (2013). *About NCSBN*. Retrieved from https://www .ncsbn.org/about.htm

National Council of State Boards of Nursing. (2017a). *Nurse license compact*. Retrieved from https://www.ncsbn.org/nurse-licensure-compact.htm

National Council of State Boards of Nursing. (2017b). *U.S. nursing licensure for internationally educated nurses*. Retrieved from https://www.ncsbn.org/171.htm

National League for Nursing. (2014). *NLN Biannual survey of schools of nursing, 2014*. Retrieved from http://www.nln.org/docs/default-source/newsroom/nursing-education-statistics/number-of-basic-rn-programs-total-and-by-program-type-2005-to-2014.pdf?sfvrsn=0

National League for Nursing. (2015). *A vision for teaching with simulation*. Retrieved from http://www.nln.org/docs/default-source/about/nln-vision-series-(position-statements)/vision-statement-a-vision-for-teaching-with-simulation.pdf?sfvrsn=2

National League for Nursing. (2016, February). Commission for Nursing Education Accreditation. *Accreditation standards for nursing education programs*. Retrieved from http://www.nln.org/docs/default-source/accreditation-services/cnea-standards-final-february-201613f2bf5c78366c709642ff00005f0421.pdf?sfvrsn=4

National League for Nursing. (2017a). *Mission and goals*. Retrieved from http://www.nln.org/about/mission-goals

National League for Nursing. (2017b). *National league for nursing commission for nursing education accreditation (CNEA)*. Retrieved from http://www.nln.org/accreditation-services/overview

National League for Nursing. (2017c). *Hallmarks of excellence*. Retrieved from http://www.nln.org/professional-development-programs/teaching-resources/hallmarks-of-excellence

National League for Nursing. (2017d). *Academy of nursing education*. Retrieved from http://www.nln.org/recognition-programs/academy-of-nursing-education

National League for Nursing. (2017e). *Eligibility criteria*. Academy of Nursing Education. Retrieved from http://www.nln.org/recognition-programs/academy-of-nursing-education/eligibility-requirements

Organization for Associate Degree Nursing , & American Nurses Association. (2015). *Organization for Associate Degree Nursing and the American Nurses Association joint position statement on academic progression to meet the needs of the registered nurse, the healthcare consumer, and the U.S. health care system*. Retrieved from http://www.nursingworld.org/MainMenuCategories/Policy-Advocacy/Positions-and-Resolutions/ANAPositionStatements/Position-Statements-Alphabetically/Academic-Progression-to-Meet-Needs-of-RN.html

Organization for Associate Degree Nursing. (2017). *About OADN*. Retrieved from https://www.oadn.org/about-us/about-oadn

O'Shea, E. (2003). Self-directed learning in nurse education: A review of the literature. *Journal of Advanced Nursing, 43*(1), 62–70.

Quality and Safety Education for Nurses. (2017). *QSEN*. Retrieved from http://qsen.org/

Reinert, B., & Fryback, P. (1997). Distance learning and nursing education. *Journal of Nursing Education, 36*(9), 421.

Robert Wood Johnson Foundation. (2015, September 9). *In historic shift, more nurses graduate with bachelor's degrees*. Retrieved from http://www.rwjf.org/en/library/articles-and-news/2015/09/more-nurses-with-bachelors-degrees.html

Robert Wood Johnson Foundation. (2016, January). Changing face of nursing: Creating a workforce for an increasingly diverse nation. *Charting Nursing's Future, 27*, p. 1. Retrieved from http://www.rwjf.org/content/dam/farm/reports/issue_briefs/2016/rwjf425988

Schaefer, B. (1990). International credentials review: Crucial and complex. *Nursing Healthcare, 11,* 431–432.

Sigurdson, K., & Ayas, N.T. (2007). The public health and safety consequences of sleep disorders. *Canadian Journal of Physiology and Pharmacology, 85,* 179–183.

Tri-Council for Nursing. (2010). *Tri-Council for Nursing issues new consensus policy statement on the educational advancement of registered nurses.* Retrieved from http://www.tricouncilfornursing.org/

Wallis, L. (2015). The case for license portability. *AJN, 115*(9), 18–19.

World Health Organization. (2010). *Framework for action on interprofessional education and collaborative practice.* Geneva, Switzerland. Retrieved from http://apps.who.int/iris/bitstream/10665/70185/1/WHO_HRH_HPN_10.3_eng.pdf

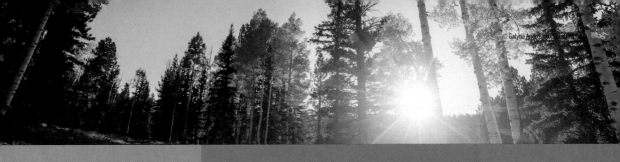

Chapter 4

Success in Your Nursing Education Program

© Galyna Andrushko/Shutterstock

CHAPTER OBJECTIVES

At the conclusion of this chapter, the learner will be able to:

- Examine how you can make the most of your nursing education experiences.
- Describe the roles of the nursing student and faculty.
- Assess your learning style.
- Apply tools for success in a nursing education program.
- Explain the use of clinical learning in nursing education.
- Compare various methods to expand graduate competency, such as cooperative learning, internships, and residencies.
- Explain the importance of lifelong learning.
- Compare certification and credentialing.
- Examine the need for care of self and methods to support oneself as a student and as a nurse.

CHAPTER OUTLINE

- Introduction
- Your Pursuit of a Profession: Making the Most of Your Educational Experience to Reach Graduation and Licensure
- Roles of the Student and the Faculty
- Student Learning Styles
- Tools for Success
  - Time Management
  - Study Skills
    - Preparation
    - Reading
- Using Class Time Effectively
  - Using the Internet
  - Preparing Written Assignments and Team Projects
  - Preparing to Take Quizzes and Exams
- Participating in Team Discussions in the Classroom and Online
- Networking and Mentoring
- Clinical Learning Experiences
- Clinical Lab and Simulation
- Clinical Experiences or Practicums

- Additional Learning Experiences to Expand Graduate Competency
  - Cooperative Experiences
  - Nurse Internships/Externships
  - Nurse Residency Programs
- Lifelong Learning for the Professional
- Certification and Credentialing
- Caring for Self

- Chapter Highlights
- Engaging in the Content
- Discussion Questions
- Critical Thinking Activities
- Electronic Reflection Journal
- Case Studies
- Working Backward to Develop a Case
- References

KEY TERMS

Burnout	Debriefing	Nurse residency
Certification	Internship/externship	Professional socialization
Clinical experiences/	Learning style	Reality shock
practicum	Lifelong learning	Simulation
Compassion fatigue	Mentor	Stress
Continuing education	Mentoring	Stress management
Credentialing	Networking	Time management

Introduction

There is much work to do to become a professional nurse. The history of nursing indicates that the development of the profession and its education has been a long process. As you strive to reach your goal, you will find that the program of study is rigorous and not like other learning experiences you have had. This chapter focuses on each student and the experience of a nursing student—what it is and what you need to understand and do to be successful. Nursing education differs from other types of education programs and requires extensive experiences in labs, simulation, and clinical settings. Students are encouraged to assess their learning styles and methods used to successfully meet the education outcomes. Long-term education is an important part of any profession, but especially for nursing. Caring for self is important both as a student and as a practicing nurse as you prepare to be a nurse and then when you practice.

Your Pursuit of a Profession:
Making the Most of Your Educational Experience to Reach Graduation and Licensure

Beginning a nursing program is a serious decision. It means that you have chosen to become a professional registered nurse (RN). This text introduces you to the profession and provides an orientation to a variety of important material that will be covered in more depth in your future courses. One topic that needs to be addressed in the initial stages of your nursing education is how to make the most of the experience to reach your goal of graduation and licensure to practice as an RN and provide quality care. The following content discusses the roles of the student and faculty, tools for success, different teaching and learning practices used in nursing education, opportunities to expand your experiences, and caring for self. This is all critical content—it may not be something you will be tested on, but the content provides some guidance to help you navigate through the nursing education process effectively.

This Is Not an English Lit Course! Nursing education is different—different from other educational programs and courses. Students who enter a college- or university-based nursing program complete many courses in liberal arts and sciences as prerequisites to entering the full nursing curriculum. When they enter a nursing program, they arrive with certain expectations that are derived from their previous experiences. Students expect a didactic course similar to other courses they have taken, such as an English literature course. That is, they expect to go to the class, sit at their desk and listen, and then periodically turn in assignments and take exams. Recently, in some cases, students have taken some of these courses online and now may even expect that nursing courses are online.

Whether you take courses in a face-to-face venue or online, nursing courses demand more. Much of the content relies on knowledge gained in previous courses and builds to subsequent courses. The expectation is that students will apply content from their previous courses to their current courses and to their clinical experiences. Learning becomes more of a continuum, as opposed to neat packages of content that can be filed away when a course ends. Understanding is more important than memorizing (though some memorization is required), and application of information becomes more important on exams and in practice. As this chapter makes clear, nursing education is definitely not English lit! Nursing education is demanding and complex—but how did it get this way, and why is it this way?

Professional socialization is part of nursing education. It is described as follows: "[T]ransition into professional practice is characterized by the acquisition of the skills, knowledge, and behaviors needed to successfully function as a professional nurse. This process involves the new nurse's internalization of the values, attitudes, and goals that comprise his

or her occupational identity" (Young, Stuenkel, & Bawel-Brinkley, 2008, p. 105). This process takes time and is integrated throughout your nursing education experiences and continues through the first few years of your professional life as an RN.

Stop and Consider #1

You can gain control of your nursing education experience.

Roles of the Student
and the Faculty

Throughout your nursing education, you need to assume a very active role in the learning process and take responsibility for your own learning; this is not passive learning. Students who ask questions, read and critique, apply information even if it is risky, and are interested in working with others—not just patients and their families, but also fellow students and faculty—will be more successful. Students who wait to be told what to do and when to do it will not be as successful.

Nursing faculty facilitate student learning. This is done by developing course content and by using teaching–learning practices to assist the student in learning the required content and developing the required competencies. Faculty enhance learning situations in the simulation laboratory and in clinical settings by guiding students to practice and become competent in areas of care delivery. The best learning takes place when faculty and students work together and communicate about needs and expectations. Faculty members not only plan for a group of students, but also assess the learning needs of individual students and work with them to meet the course and program objectives or outcomes. A critical key to success with faculty is communication: Ask questions, ask for explanation if confused, meet course requirements when due, and use the faculty as a resource to enhance learning.

Becoming an RN involves more than just graduating from a nursing program. New graduates must pass the NCLEX, an examination that is not offered by the school of nursing but rather through the National Council of State Boards of Nursing (NCSBN) and state boards of nursing as discussed in other content in this text. Throughout the nursing program, students may be offered opportunities to complete practice exams and receive feedback. In addition, course exam questions are typically written in the formats found in the NCLEX, such as application of knowledge questions rather than questions relating to memorized content. Becoming comfortable with this format is often difficult for new nursing students because they are accustomed to taking exams in non-nursing courses that focus less on application and do not build on knowledge gained from course to course. For example, in nursing you complete the anatomy and physiology course, and then you are expected to apply this information later when you take exams on clinical content. You learn about blood flow through the heart, and then, in conjunction with adult health content, you are expected to understand this content and apply it when providing care to a patient with a myocardial infarction (heart attack). Months or even a year or more may elapse between when you complete the anatomy and physiology course and when you take an adult health course or care for a patient with a myocardial infarction.

Stop and Consider #2

Both faculty and students have responsibilities in the nursing education process.

Student Learning Styles

As you enter nursing courses, it is helpful for you to consider your own preferred learning style and to determine how your style might or might not be effective. If it is not effective, you may need to consider changes.

What does learning style mean? **Learning style** is a student's preferences for different types of learning and instructional activities. There are a variety of views of these styles. In doing a personal learning style self-assessment, you might apply Kolb's (1984) learning style inventory, which was further developed by Honey and Mumford (1986, 1992). Kolb described a continuum of four learning styles: (1) concrete experiences, (2) reflective observation, (3) abstract conceptualization, and (4) active experimentation. No person can be placed in only one style category, but most people have a predominant style (Kolb, 1984, as cited in Rassool & Rawaf, 2007, pp. 36–37):

- *Divergers:* Sensitive, imaginative, and people oriented; often enter professions such as nursing; excel in brainstorming sessions.
- *Assimilators:* Less focused on people and more interested in ideas and abstract concepts. Excel in organizing and presenting information; prefer formal education formats; prefer reading, lectures, exploring analytical models, and having time to think things through.
- *Convergers:* Solve problems and prefer technical tasks; less concerned with people and interpersonal aspects; often choose careers in technology; excel in getting things done.
- *Accommodators:* People-oriented, active learners; excel in concrete experience and active experimentation; prefer to take a practical or experimental approach; attracted to new challenges and experiences.

Adapting Kolb's proposed styles, the following has been described by Rassool and Rawaf (2007):

- *Activists:* Having an experience. Focus on immediate experience; interested in here and now; like to initiate new challenges and be the center of attention.
- *Reflectors:* Reviewing the experience.
- *Observers:* Prefer to analyze experiences before taking action; good listeners; cautious; tend to adopt a low profile.

- *Theorists:* Concluding from experience. Adopt a logical and rational approach to problem solving but need some structure with a clear purpose or goal; learning is weakest when they do not understand the purpose, when activities are less structured, and when feelings are emphasized.
- *Pragmatists:* Planning the next steps. Prefer to try out new ideas and techniques to see if they work in practice; are practical and down to earth; like solving problems and making decisions.

Understanding your style can help you when you approach new content, read assignments, and participate in other learning activities. It can affect how easy or difficult the content and assignments may be for you. You may need to stretch—that is, to try to learn or do something that is challenging for you—and you may need to adapt your learning style.

Stop and Consider #3

Your past learning styles may or may not effective for you in the nursing program.

Tools for Success

Organization and time management are very important tools for success in a nursing program. In the past, you may have gone to class for a few hours a day, but in nursing programs, some courses meet once or several times a week for several hours. Some courses may be taught online but require some attendance in a classroom setting—but maybe none. In addition,

the clinical component of the program has a major impact on your schedule. You need to prepare for the clinical component and work this activity into your schedule to meet course requirements. Study skills and test-taking skills are critical. This educational experience will not be without some stress; thus, if you develop stress management skills to help you cope, you will find that the experience can be handled better. **Exhibit 4-1** provides some links to websites with tools for student success.

Time Management

Time management is not difficult to define, but it is difficult to achieve. Learning how to manage time and requirements is also very important to effective nursing practice. Time management skills in school are not different from what is required for clinical practicums and after graduation in practice. **Figure 4-1** describes how to get started with time management.

There never is enough time, it seems, and no one can make more time, so it is best to figure out how to make the most of your available time. Everyone has felt unproductive or been guilty of squandering time. In simple terms, productivity is the ratio of inputs to outputs. What does a person put into a task or activity (resources such as time, energy, money, give up doing something else, and so forth) that then leads to outcomes or results? For example, one student studies 12 hours for an exam and then gives up going to a film with friends; another student studies 5 hours and goes to the same film. These two students put different levels of resources into exam

Exhibit 4-1 Links for Student Success

Study tips: https://www.studytips.org/
Controlling procrastination: http://www.how-to-study.com/study-skills-articles/procrastination.asp
Test-taking strategies: http://www.d.umn.edu/kmc/student/loon/acad/strat/test_take.html
Test-taking checklist: http://www.d.umn.edu/kmc/student/loon/acad/strat/testcheck.html

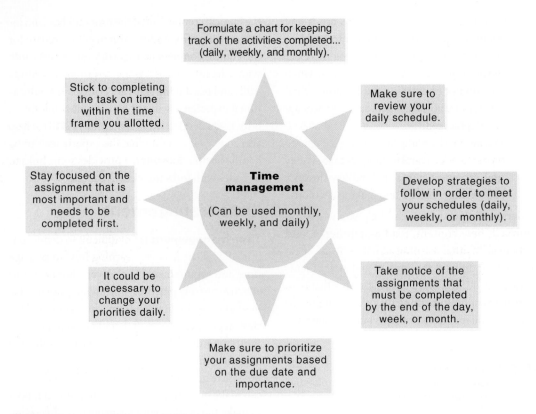

Figure 4-1 Getting Started with Time Management

Reproduced from Wilfong, D., Szolis, C., & Haus, C. (2007). *Nursing school success: Tools for constructing your future.* Sudbury, MA: Jones & Bartlett Learning.

preparation, and they get different results—the first student makes an A on the exam and the second a B. The second student then has to decide if it was worth it. Should more time be spent on studying for exams and the personal schedule arranged to allow for some fun, but after exams? Or is the B grade acceptable? The student with the A grade may decide too much time was spent on studying, was not productive, and could have been organized better to reduce study time. This more global perspective is certainly one aspect of time management, but time management also gets into the details of how one uses time to be efficient and effective, such as what the student with the A grade considered. You need to know yourself and what works for you.

Time analysis is used to assess how one uses time. You might keep a log for a week and record all of your activities, including time spent on each activity and interruptions. If you commit to doing this, you need to be honest so that the data truly reflect your activities. After the data are collected, you then need to analyze the data using these questions:

- Did you set any priorities, and did you adhere to them?
- What were your activities, and how long did each take?
- Do you see a difference on certain days as to activities and time?
- What did you complete, and what did you not complete? Can you identify reasons for not completing a task or project?
- Which types of interruptions did you have? How many interruptions were really important, and why?

- Did you procrastinate? Are there certain activities that you put off more than others? Why?
- Did you jump from one task to another, and why?
- Look at your telephone calls, e-mails, texting, and so on. How did they affect your time management?
- Did you spend time getting ready to do a task, to communicate with others, and so on? Was some of this required, or could it have been done more effectively?
- Did you take breaks? (Breaks are important.) How many breaks did you take, how long were they, and what did you do? Did it refresh you?
- Did you consult your calendar and use it as a guide?
- Are there times during the day when you are more productive? Knowing when you tend to be more productive provides you with opportunity to capitalize on this and be more productive.

You need to work on time management and planning as a student because nurses need to be able to plan their day's work and still be flexible as changes occur. Ideally, nurses set priorities and follow through, evaluate how they use their time, and cut down on wasted time so that care can be delivered effectively and in a timely manner. They use communication effectively and prepare for procedures and other care delivery activities in an organized manner so that they are not running back and forth to get supplies and so on. They handle interruptions by determining what is important and what can wait. Your success in meeting these demands relates to your need to assess your own time management and learn time management skills.

Technology has made life easier and more organized in some respects, especially the use of computers, smartphones, and tablets, as well as emails, text messaging, and other communication methods. However, these new devices and methods can also interfere with time management. For example, you may stop what you are doing to answer an email or a text message that just arrived, or you may spend so much time syncing all this technology that the work does not get done. Managing time today means managing personal technology, too.

Many people struggle with the same time management problems. Consider these examples and how they might apply to you:

- No planning—not using a calendar effectively or not using one
- Not setting goals and priorities, or having unclear goals and priorities
- Allowing too many interruptions
- Getting started without preparing
- Inability to say, "No," often leading to over-commitment (the most common problem for many people)
- Inability to concentrate
- Insufficient rest, sleep, exercise, and unhealthy diet, making one feel perpetually tired
- High stress level
- Too much socializing when work needs to be done—not knowing how to find the right balance
- Ineffective use of communication tools, including overuse of email, computer and Internet, cell phone, and so on
- Too much crisis management—waiting too long to act so that it is then a crisis to get the work done
- Inability to break down large projects into smaller projects or steps
- Wasting time—little tasks, procrastination

Other, more serious problems can have a major impact on time management. These difficulties arise when the student does not feel competent or does not know what is expected. Students often experience these problems, although they may not recognize them or want to admit them. Nevertheless, these feelings can lead to problems with time management as students struggle to feel better and/or try to figure out what they are supposed to do. If you experience one or both of these feelings, you need to talk to your faculty openly about your concerns. You are not expected to be perfect. The educational process is focused on helping you gradually build your competence. In some cases, perfectionism actually becomes a barrier to completing a task; you may fear that the task will not be completed perfectly, so you avoid the task or work on it longer than needed.

Benner (2001) described the experience of moving from novice to expert in nursing, which is a practice profession. Beginners or novices have no experience as nurses, and therefore, must gain clinical knowledge and expertise (competence) over time. A beginning student may enter a nursing program with some nursing care experience, such as nursing aide experience. That student may then be at a different novice level but still a novice. A graduate will not be an expert; this comes with time and experience. This change in status can be difficult for students who may have felt that they were competent in understanding the content after a course such as American history or introduction to sociology. Nursing competency, however, is developed over time. Each course and its content are relevant to subsequent courses. There is no neat packaging that allows one to say, "I have mastered all there is to know about nursing" or this topic. Health care is ever changing. The profession must adapt to changes, new knowledge and technology, identification of new health problems, and so on.

Another component of time management is setting clear goals and priorities. This helps to organize your time and focus your activities. You need to consider what is needed now and what is needed later. This is not always advice that is easy to follow; sometimes a student might prefer to work on a task that is not due for a while, avoiding work that needs to be done sooner. Sometimes writing down goals and priorities and putting this information where it can be seen to focus more on a time management plan. Delegation plays a major role in health care and is related to time management. One of the key issues when prioritizing is determining who should complete the task. Perhaps someone else is a better choice to complete the task; in this case, the task may be delegated, a topic discussed in this text.

Tasks and activities can be dissected. Consider what the needs of the task are; when it is due; how long it will take; how critical it is; what impact it will have; and what the consequences will be if it is postponed or not completed. Plan how the work will be done to meet the due date. Large projects are best broken into smaller parts or steps. For example, the preparation of a major paper should be broken into a series of tasks, such as identifying the topic or problem, working with a team (if writing the paper is a team assignment), completing the research for the paper, writing the paper (which should begin with an outline), reviewing and editing, and polishing the final draft. Building in deadlines for the steps will help ensure that the final due date is met. Many large papers or projects in nursing courses cannot be completed overnight. They may require active learning, such as interviews, assessments, and other types of activities. A presentation may need to be developed after the paper is written or a poster designed. Often, this type of work is done with a team of students, which is important because nurses work in teams. Group efforts take more time because team members have to learn to work together, develop a teamwork plan, and meet if necessary. Some team assignments are now done "virtually," through online activities in which students never physically meet. Getting prepared for the clinical experience/practicum is also a larger task that will be described later in this chapter. All of this takes organization.

Some strategies for improving time management that you might consider include the following:

- Use a calendar or electronic method for a calendar; update it as needed.
- Develop a daily time management plan (see **Figure 4-2**).
- Decrease socializing at certain times to improve production.

DAILY TIME MANAGEMENT WORKSHEET

Primary Task	Projected Start Time	Projected Finish Time	Actual Time Taken to Complete Task

Secondary Task

Figure 4-2 Daily Time Management Worksheet

Reproduced from Wilfong, D., Szolis, C., & Haus, C. (2007). *Nursing school success: Tools for constructing your future.* Sudbury, MA: Jones & Bartlett Learning.

- Limit use of your cell phone, text messaging, and email during key times.
- Identify typical interruptions and control them.
- Anticipate—flexibility is necessary because something can happen that will disturb the plan.
- Determine the best time to read, study, prepare for an exam, write papers, and so on. Some people do better in early morning; others are more effective late at night. Know what works best for you.
- Work in blocks of time, minimizing interruptions.
- Develop methods for note taking and organizing learning materials to decrease the need to hunt for these materials.
- Conquer procrastination. Try dividing tasks into smaller parts to get a project done.
- Come prepared to class, clinical laboratory, and clinical settings. Preparation means that less time will be spent figuring out what needs to be done when you need to be doing it.

- Do not use electronic communication during class for non-class-related interaction or during clinical experiences.
- Do the right thing right, working effectively and efficiently.
- Remember that time management is not a static process, but rather a dynamic one; your time management needs will change.
- Organize your electronic course files so that they are easy to use.

Study Skills

Study skills are developed over time; however, this does not mean that these skills cannot always be improved. You may also find you need to use different study skills for nursing courses and clinical experiences. This is the time to review your study skills and determine what can be done to improve them. Typical components of study skills are reading, using class time effectively, preparing written assignments and team projects, and preparing for discussions and other in class learning activities, quizzes, and exams. In nursing, clinical preparation, which is new for students entering nursing programs, is also a key area.

Preparation

Students need to prepare for class, whether it is a face-to-face class, a seminar, or an online course. The first issue is what to prepare. The guide for this is the focus of the experience and its objectives/learning outcomes. Use the course syllabus and other course materials as a guide to the course and the expectations of students. The format influences preparation—for example, use of a class session with 60 students versus a seminar with 10 students. The latter is an experience in which the student will undoubtedly be expected to respond to questions and discuss issues. The larger class may vary; it could be a straight lecture, with little participation expected, or it could include participation requiring preparation—in class team discussion. You need to be clear about the course expectations. If the course syllabus or other course materials do not provide clear explanations, you are responsible for asking about expectations or seeking clarification of confusing expectations. You then need to complete any work such as reading or research a topic that is expected prior to the class or the learning experience to improve your learning. Class time often emphasizes application of information.

Reading

There is much reading to do in a nursing program, ranging from textbooks and published articles to Internet resources and handout materials that faculty may provide. It is very easy to become overwhelmed by these materials. Explore the textbook(s) for the course from front to back. Sometimes students do not realize that a textbook has a valuable glossary, appendix, and index that could help them. Review the table of contents to become familiar with the text content. Some faculty may assign specific pages

rather than entire chapters, so making note of the details of a reading assignment is critical. Review a chapter to become familiar with its structure. Typically, there are objectives or outcomes, chapter outline, and key terms; content divided into sections; additional elements, such as exhibits, figures, and boxed information; and finally the summary, learning activities, and references. An increasing number of textbooks have an affiliated website that offer additional information and learning activities and, in some cases, quiz-style questions.

Many textbooks are now published as e-books, as an option or offered in both e-book and hard copy. E-books are often highly interactive (for example, you can highlight material, take notes, and search for content in the text) and can be downloaded to computers and tablets, smartphones, and so on. These trends are likely to continue.

Yes, this is all overwhelming, and where does one begin? How do you make the best use of your reading time? Reading should focus on four goals:

1. Learning information for recall is memorizing. This is important for some content, but if it is the only focus of reading, you will not be able to apply the information and build on learning.

2. Comprehension of general principles, facts, and examples is an important component of effective reading.

3. Critical evaluation of the content should be part of your reading process. Ask yourself questions and challenge the content. Does it make sense?

4. Application of content is critical in nursing because nursing is a practice-oriented profession. For example, at some point you will take a course that focuses on maternal–child content; later, you will be expected to apply that content in a clinical pediatric unit. How you read and understand the content will make a difference on your ability to apply the content to a case in the classroom, a simulation experience, or in a clinical setting.

As noted in the previous section on time management, time is precious. The student who is trying to develop more effective reading skills should not waste time reading ineffectively, but rather should accomplish specific goals in a timely manner. The following are some tips to use in tackling a chapter:

- Take a quick look at the chapter elements—objectives, terms, and major headers—and compare them with the course content expectations. Pay particular attention to the chapter outline, if there is one, and to the summary, conclusions, and/or key points at the end of the chapter.
- Read through the chapter not for details, but to get a general idea of the content.
- Go back and use a marker to highlight key concepts, terms, and ideas. If this is done first, it can lead to over-marking. Using different colors for different levels of content may be useful for some students. You will need to go back and study the content; just highlighting content is not studying. The goal is to find a system that works for you. If using an e-book, understand and use its features.

- Note exhibits, figures, and boxes. (This is when it is important to check the reading assignment. Does it specify pages or content to read or ignore?)
- Some students make notes in the margins, highlight key points, and so on.

Figures 4-3 and **4-4** illustrate two different formats for organizing notes from readings (if notes are taken). The format in Figure 4-3 can also be used to take notes in class.

Using Class Time Effectively

Attending a class session can be a positive or negative learning experience. Preparation is important. In addition, how you approach the course and an individual course session is important. If you have trouble concentrating, sitting in the back of the room may not be the best approach. Sitting with friends can be helpful, but if it means you cannot concentrate, alternatives need to be considered. It is often difficult to disconnect from other issues and problems, but class time is not the place to focus

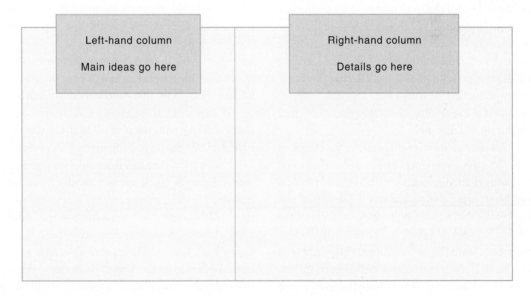

Figure 4-3 Taking Two-Column Notes

Reproduced from Wilfong, D., Szolis, C., & Haus, C. (2007). *Nursing school success: Tools for constructing your future.* Sudbury, MA: Jones & Bartlett Learning.

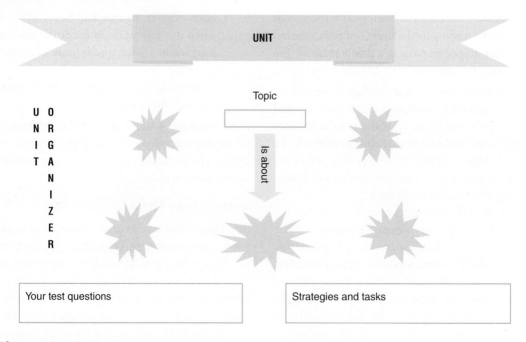

Figure 4-4 Unit Organizer

Reproduced from Wilfong, D., Szolis, C., & Haus, C. (2007). *Nursing school success: Tools for constructing your future.* Sudbury, MA: Jones & Bartlett Learning.

on them. One of the most common issues in class involves students who use class time to prepare for another class—working on assignments, studying for an exam, and so on. In the end, the learning experience on both ends is less effective. Students waste their time if they come to class without completing the reading, analyzing the content, or preparing assignments.

Another element of preparation for class and other learning experiences involves identifying and accessing needed resources, such as the textbook, a notebook, assignments, and so on. Some students use laptops and tablets, so planning for access if the battery runs out is important. Learning will be compromised if a student uses electronic equipment such as a laptop, tablet, or smartphone for purposes that do not involve course content. Today, tablets are used more frequently in the classroom and for studying. Student options with tablets have expanded with the development of apps and pens for tablet writing and

access to e-books. If you choose to use these options, research carefully what is available and how it might provide support for your learning. Make sure you know how to use the new options prior to using them in a course. The Internet includes a lot of information and reviews of apps that may be used by students.

If a course has face-to-face sessions, taking notes is important. Figures 4-3 and 4-4 illustrate two methods for organizing notes. It is critical to find a note-taking strategy that works for you. Some students may be visual learners, in which case they may draw figures, charts, concept maps, and so on to help them remember something—for example, using a tablet with a stylus pen to make sketch figures. Going back and reviewing notes soon after a class session will help you remember items that may need to be added and to recall information over the long term. As notes are taken in class, include comments from faculty that begin with "This is important," "You might want to remember this," and similar indicators of the material's importance. Questions that faculty ask should be noted.

It is easy to get addicted to PowerPoint slide presentations and think that if you have these available in a handout or in electronic form learning has taken place. In reality, this presentation content is only part of the content that nursing students are expected to learn—and just having them does not mean you understand the material. The faculty may make additional comments related to the content on the slides. Students need to pay attention to content found in reading assignments, research, written assignments, and clinical experiences. Online courses also may include PowerPoint slide presentations, and some may have audio components.

Using the Internet

The Internet has become a critical tool in the world today. As students increasingly turn to the Internet to get information, it is important that reputable websites are used. Government sites are always appropriate sources, and professional organization sites also have valuable and appropriate information. Identify who sponsors the site. Bias is always a concern; for example, the site for a pharmaceutical company will inevitably praise that company's own products. Wikipedia is not considered a scholarly resource for references. When using a site, check when it was last updated. Sites that are not updated regularly have a greater chance of including outdated information.

In addition, the Internet is now used frequently for literature searches, usually through university libraries that offer online access to publications. Students need to learn about the resources available to them through their school libraries and learn how to use them effectively. Often, libraries offer short workshops to assist you (face-to-face and online) and also orientation materials on the library website. It is important to properly attribute the source for content taken from the Internet for an assignment, using the correct citation format required by your school of nursing.

Preparing Written Assignments and Team Projects

The critical first step for any written assignment is to understand the assignment—what is expected. Read directions for assignments carefully and ask questions if unsure of expectations. What are the evaluation rubrics? You then complete the assignment based on these expectations. If the assignment describes specific areas to cover in a paper, this should be an important part of the outline for the paper—and these areas may even be used as key headers in the paper. Faculty will look for the content based on the assignment outline. If you have questions about the assignment as you work on the assignment, ask prior to submission.

For some assignments, students select their topics. If possible, selecting a topic similar to one used for a different assignment might save some time, but this does not mean that the student may submit an assignment that was done for another course. Plagiarism and submitting the same paper or assignment for more than one course are not acceptable. You need to be aware of and apply your school's honor code. This includes cheating on exams or quizzes, which demonstrates a lack of professional ethics.

Correct grammar, spelling, writing style, and citation format are critical for every written assignment. Nurses need to know how to communicate both orally and in written form. Use your school's required method for citations. Editing your work and checking is your responsibility before you submit it.

Some assignments will require that you work with a team or group of students. Some students do not like this type of project, but these experiences provide great opportunities to learn about working on teams, which is important in nursing. Teamwork requires clear communication among members and an understanding of the expectations for the work that the team needs to do. Effective teams spend time organizing their work and determining how they will communicate with one another. To complete team projects successfully, teams must decide how to complete the assignment, which might involve analysis of a case; writing a paper; developing a poster, presentation, or educational program; or another type of activity. Having a clear plan of what needs to be done, by whom, and when will help guide the work and decrease conflict. Everyone is busy, and preventing conflicts and miscommunication decreases the amount of time needed to do the work. If serious problems arise with communication or equality in workload that the team cannot resolve, faculty should be consulted for guidance. Conflicts may occur, and these conflicts need to be dealt with before they get worse. If the team must document its work and evaluate peer members, this should be done honestly, with appropriate feedback and comments about the work. Such evaluations are not easy to do. Additional information on teams is provided in other chapters in this text and apply to work you may do with a student team to complete a team project.

Preparing to Take Quizzes and Exams

Quizzes and exams are inevitable parts of nursing education. Students who routinely prepare for them will experience less pressure at quiz or exam time—but this takes discipline. Building reviews into your study time, even if a review lasts for only a short period, does make a difference.

As is true for any aspect of a learning experience, knowing what is expected comes first during quiz and exam preparation. What content will be covered in a specific quiz or exam? What is the timeframe for the quiz or the exam? What types of questions are expected, and how many? Exams in nursing typically use multiple-choice, true or false, essay, and some fill-in-the-blank questions, although the most common format is multiple-choice questions. The first quiz or exam is always the hardest, as students get to know the faculty and the style of questions. Some faculty may provide a review guide, which should always be used.

Before a major exam, getting enough rest is an important aspect of preparation. Fatigue and sleep deprivation interfere with functioning—reading, thinking, managing time during the exam, clinical practice, and so on. Eating is also important. Students usually know how they respond if they eat too little or too much before an exam.

One aspect of nursing exams that seems to create problems for new students is the use of application questions. Preparing for a nursing exam by just memorizing facts will not lead to a positive result. You do need to know factual information, but you must also know how to use that information in examples.

Another common exam-taking problem is the inability to understand a multiple-choice question and its possible responses/answers. Students may skip over words and think something is included in the question that is not. They may not be able to define all the words in the question and may not identify the key words. Reading the question and the response options carefully will make a difference. You should identify the key words and define them. If you do not know the answer to a question, you should narrow the choices by eliminating responses that you do understand or think might be wrong. Then, you should look for qualifiers such as "always," "all," "never," "every," and "none" because these may indicate that the answer is not correct. **Figure 4-5** describes a system for preparing for multiple-choice exams.

Essay questions require different preparation and skills. You need to have a greater in-depth understanding of the content to respond to an essay question. Some questions may ask for opinions. In all cases, it is important that your answer is clear and concise, provides rationales, includes content relevant to the question and to the material covered in the course, and presents the response in an organized manner. This requires you to read the question carefully and make sure you understand it. Sometimes the exam directions may provide guidelines as to the length of response expected, but in many cases, this must

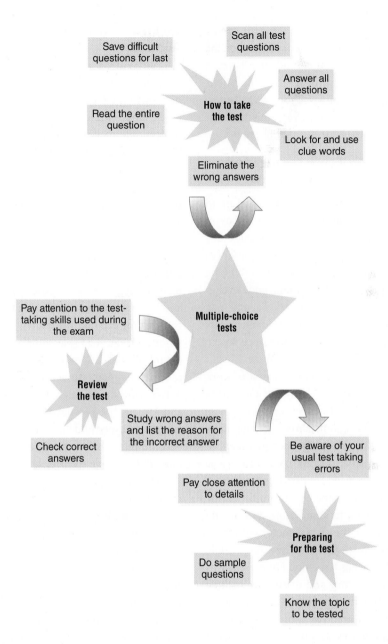

Figure 4-5 Multiple-Choice Exams

Reproduced from Wilfong, D., Szolis, C., & Haus, C. (2007). *Nursing school success: Tools for constructing your future.* Sudbury, MA: Jones & Bartlett Learning.

be judged according to what is required to answer the question. The amount of space provided on the exam may be a good indication, but may not be. Grammar, spelling, and writing style are also important. Jotting down a quick outline will help in focusing your response and manage your time during the exam. It is important for you to review the essay response to make sure the question (or questions) has been answered. As is true for all types of exams, you must pace yourself based on the allotted time for essay questions and other types of exam questions. Spending a lot of time on questions that may be difficult is unwise. You can return to difficult questions and should keep this tactic in mind when managing time during the exam.

Participating in Team Discussions in the Classroom and Online

Nursing courses often include team discussion in the classroom and/or online. You need to focus on the assignment requirements such as the questions to consider. These are critical learning experiences that allow you to apply content, use critical thinking and clinical reasoning and judgment, and develop your communication and teamwork. Faculty may assign students to small teams to analyze and discuss cases in the classroom or work on projects in the classroom and outside the classroom. You may work with the same team throughout the course or work with a team for a specific assignment; sometimes multiple teams may work together. Why is this not called *group* discussion? Nurses are members of *teams* in healthcare settings, not members of groups. Students need to think of themselves as team members. You need to start thinking about teams and teamwork in the classroom, in online learning experiences, in simulation, and during clinical experiences. The critical factor with these experiences is each student must feel responsible for the work that needs to be done in these learning activities, which may and often does include preparation prior to the experience such as reading assignments or research for more information. During the experiences all students on the team should be actively engaged.

Networking and Mentoring

Professional nurses use networking and mentoring to develop themselves and to help peers. Consequently, you need to understand what these concepts are

and begin to work toward using networking and mentoring.

Networking is a strategy that involves using any contact that might be helpful to you. Applying networking effectively is a skill that takes time to develop. Nurses typically use networking at professional meetings. You can begin to network in student organization activities, whether local, statewide, or national. Networking allows a person to meet and communicate with a wide variety of people, exchange ideas, explore new approaches, and obtain information that might be useful. Some networking skills are knowing how to meet new people, approaching an admired person, learning how to start a conversation and keep it going, remembering names, asking for contact information, and sharing because networking works both ways. Networking can take place anywhere: in school, in a work setting, at a professional meeting or during organizational activities, and in social situations. It can even happen online through the use of social networking media such as LinkedIn, Facebook, and Twitter, but you have to be careful with what is communicated and how—today information can become public very quickly and once public it is difficult to change it or delete it.

Mentoring is a career development tool. A mentor–mentee relationship cannot be assigned or forced. A **mentor** is a role model and a career advisor. The mentor should not have a formal relationship, such as a supervisory or managerial relationship, with the mentee. Such a linkage could cause stress and not allow the mentor and mentee to communicate openly without concern about possible repercussions; however, there may come a time when a past supervisor becomes a mentor to a former employee.

The mentee needs to feel comfortable with the mentor and usually chooses the mentor. The mentor, of course, must agree to be part of this relationship. A mentorship can be short term or long term. It does take some time to develop the mentor–mentee relationship. Today, such a relationship could occur virtually.

When entering a nursing education program, you might think about acquiring a mentor, yet not know when a possible mentor might be met. Keep your eye out for possible future mentors. The mentor may be a nurse who works in an area where a student has clinical experience/practicum. New graduates can benefit from a mentorship relationship to help guide them in early career decisions. Mentors can give them constructive feedback about their strengths and limitations and suggest improvement strategies. The mentor does not make decisions for the mentee, but rather serves as a sounding board to discuss options and allow the mentee to benefit from the mentor's expertise. In this way, the mentor acts as a guide and a teacher. An effective mentor has the following characteristics:

- Expert in an area related to the mentee's needs and interests
- Honest and trustworthy
- Professional
- Supportive
- Effective communicator
- Teacher and motivator
- Respected and influential
- Accessible

Stop and Consider #4
Trying out different tools for success in learning may lead you to greater success.

Clinical Learning
Experiences

As a new student begins a nursing program, it usually quickly becomes clear that nursing programs are different from past learning experiences. Students need to develop competencies to provide quality care to patients, families, communities, and populations. Nursing education not only uses traditional didactic learning experiences, which may be offered through face-to-face classes offering didactic/theory- or content-focused experiences, but also clinical experiences in clinical lab or simulation labs and in clinical experiences in healthcare settings (practicum). What does this mean to you as a student?

Clinical Lab and Simulation

Schools of nursing use a variety of methods for developing student clinical competencies. A competency is an expected behavior that you must demonstrate. Two methods of developing clinical competencies that have become common in nursing education are the clinical laboratory (lab) and **simulation** learning, which is often combined with the lab experience. The simulation lab is a learning environment that is configured to look like a hospital or other type of clinical setting and provides structured learning experiences. The lab may take the form of a hospital room, a room with multiple beds, or a specialty room such as a procedure room or operating room. It contains the same equipment and supplies that are used in a healthcare setting, typically a hospital. Some schools have a simulation area that looks like a patient's home so that students can practice home care prior to an actual home care visit or a clinic. The clinical lab is typically not configured to replicate a clinical setting in the same way as simulation lab; although it will have some of the same equipment, it typically does not use the high-level equipment. Some schools have only one type of lab—that is, a lab for developing basic nursing skills—with less opportunity for more complex learning in a simulated environment.

Students are assigned specific times in the lab as part of a course. Some didactic content might be delivered prior to the lab experience. Students are expected to come to the lab prepared (for example, having completed a reading assignment, viewed a video, or completed online learning activities). Preparation makes the lab time more effective, and well-prepared students will be able to practice applying what they have learned. To succeed in this setting, students need to be motivated and self-directed learners. (This is true for any learning experience in the nursing program.) Schools have different guidelines about dress and behavior in the lab. In some schools, the lab is treated as if it were an actual clinical setting/agency with certain dress and behavior expectations, such as wearing the school uniform or a lab coat and meeting all other uniform requirements related to appearance and professional behavior in the clinical setting.

Simulation is an effective method to develop clinical competency and is used as part of the educational experiences of nursing students at all levels—pre-licensure and graduate (Hovancsek, 2007). Practice is important, but guided practice is even more important, and ideally this should be risk free. Practicing on a real patient always carries a risk. It is not realistic to expect that a student will be able to provide care without some degree of harm potential the first time such care is given. For this reason, practicing in a setting without a real patient allows students to develop competence and gain self-confidence. What does the student learn in the lab? Most procedures and related competencies can be taught in a lab, such as health assessment, wound care, catheterization, medication administration, enema, general hygiene, and much more. Complex care may also be practiced in the simulation lab setting using teams of students.

Simulation is a method that provides students with as near-to-life experience as possible in which no patient is at risk. Levels of simulations vary, ranging from low fidelity to high fidelity. The difference between levels lies in how close the simulated scenario comes to reality (Jeffries & Rogers, 2007). Simulation also can involve task trainers for learning skills such as IV insertion. Some simulation labs provide experiences for students in which they interact with standardized patients (actors) who role play for the student, following a script and scenario.

Simulation also allows faculty to design learning experiences that meet a variety of learning styles—visual, auditory, tactile, or kinesthetic—and give students time to incorporate their learning. Time is devoted to discussing the care provided without concern for additional care that needs to be provided, as would occur in a clinical setting. This kind of **debriefing** is an important component of the simulation experience. During a simulation, students may work alone, with faculty, and with other nursing students, as well as with other healthcare professions students in an interprofessional team. Faculty can better control the types of experiences in which students engage, whereas in the clinical setting it is not always easy to find a patient who needs a specific procedure or has certain complex care needs at one time. Simulation is an active learning method, which helps the student improve critical thinking/clinical reasoning and judgment (Billings & Halstead, 2005). Some schools are developing interprofessional simulation experiences that involve medical, pharmacy, respiratory therapy, and other healthcare professions students. These can be very important experiences that improve interprofessional teamwork over the long term.

Clinical Experiences or Practicums

Clinical experience or practicum is part of every nursing program. This experience occurs when students, with faculty supervision, provide care to patients. Such care may be provided to individual patients or to their families or significant others (for example, providing care to a patient after surgery and teaching the family how to provide care after discharge), to communities (for example, working with a school nurse in a community), or to specific populations (for example, developing a self-management education program for a group of patients with diabetes). Some nursing programs begin this experience early in the program and others later, but all include it as part of the nursing curriculum. In addition, many nursing courses include a clinical or practicum component, or they may have no didactic component and only a clinical focus. A student might think that these courses are equivalent to a chemistry lab, but this is not a fair comparison. A nursing clinical experience/practicum usually covers several hours per session and, in some cases, can require 8 to 12 hours several days each week. Students must prepare for these experiences and work these hours as students. Faculty are available to guide student learning, and in some situations, students are assigned to *preceptors*, who are nurses working in the healthcare organization. Students do their clinical work in a variety of clinical settings, such as hospitals, clinics, homes, and community settings. Such experiences are not equivalent to taking a 2-hour chemistry lab once a week.

Typically, these practicums are conducted in blocks of time—for example, students are in clinical practice 2 days a week for 6 hours each day. Faculty may be present the entire time or may be available at the site or by telephone. The amount of supervision depends on the level and competency of the student, the type of setting, and the objectives of the experience. The clinical setting may also dictate the student–faculty ratio and supervision. Settings are highly variable in their requirements—a hospital, clinic, physician's office, school, community health service, patient home, rehabilitation center, long-term care facility, senior center, child daycare center, or mental health center, among others. Some experiences require that you are with a group of students; in others, you may be alone. In the latter case, for example, you may be assigned to work with a school nurse or with a preceptor in the intensive care unit.

Participating in clinical experiences (practicums) requires preparation. For many assigned experiences, you may need to go to the site of the clinical practicum before the clinical day begins (sometimes the day before) to obtain information about your patient(s) and plan the care for the assigned time. This is done so that you are ready to provide care. You need to understand the patient's history and problems, laboratory work, medications,

procedures, and critical care issues, and plan care effectively. Often, the student develops a written plan—perhaps in the form of a nursing care plan or a concept map—that is evaluated by faculty. Students who arrive at clinical care settings unprepared will likely be unable to meet the requirements for that day.

Typically, the clinical day begins with a short pre-conference where faculty may highlight particular goals for the experience and students may introduce their assigned patients by sharing information, and then the day ends with an in-depth post-conference to discuss the day's experiences and outcomes.

Sometimes students are assigned an observation experience. In this case, the student does not participate in the care provided but observes. The observation should be planned. If the student knows ahead of time, the student should prepare by reviewing relevant information. During the observation, the student should note factors such as what was done, team member roles and communication, quality care, and so on. Time should be provided to discuss the observation, or other methods should be used to report on the observation such as a written summary. These are important learning activities allowing the students and faculty to reflect on content and application in practice.

Another important aspect of clinical experiences relates to professional responsibilities and appearance. When a nursing student is providing care, the student is representing the profession—a point pertinent to content in this text about the image of nursing. The student needs to meet the school's uniform requirement for the assigned experience, be clean, and meet safety requirements (such as appearance of hair) to decrease infection risk—for example, washing hands as required. Students who go to their clinical experience site and do not meet these requirements may be sent home. Making up clinical experiences is very difficult, and in some cases impossible, because it requires reserving a clinical site again and securing faculty time, student time, and so on. Minimizing absences is critical; however, if the student is sick, the student should not care for patients. Schools have specific requirements related to illness and clinical experiences that should be followed. You should show up for every clinical experience dressed appropriately, prepared, and with any required equipment, such as a stethoscope. In addition, you need to be on time—set your alarm to allow plenty of preparation time and plan for delays in traffic. All this relates to the practicing nurse: Employers expect nurses to come to work dressed as required, prepared, and on time.

Students need to recognize that when they are in clinical, they should practice at the level expected for their education level and to respond in a professional manner. Faculty expect this as do staff. Family view students as part of the healthcare team and also expect that faculty and staff supervise students. Each student must ask for help when the situation is something the student does not feel comfortable doing. A critical factor with students is communication at times of transition or handoffs. Students are responsible for sharing information with staff just as staff are responsible for providing the information the students need to care for patients.

Stop and Consider #5
Your preparation for clinical experiences makes a difference in your learning.

Additional Learning
Experiences to Expand Graduate Competency

When students approach their first nursing job after graduation, many experience **reality shock**. This is a shock reaction that occurs when an individual who has been educated in a nursing education system with one view of nursing encounters a different view of nursing in the practice setting (Kramer, 1985). New graduates do not have to experience reality shock, but many do. One measure that can prevent reality shock is developing better stress management techniques during the nursing education experience. This will not make the difference between your clinical experience and the real world of work completely disappear, but it will help the new graduate cope with this change in roles and views of what is happening in the healthcare delivery system. Another method that helps with adjustment later after graduation is to discuss situations with faculty that seem out of sync with what should be done in practice. Faculty should be used as resources to openly discuss your concerns and to learn from these experiences. To try to reduce the postgraduate stress as one transitions to practice and professional nursing has led to an increasing number of healthcare organizations creating externship/internship and residency programs to guide new graduates through the first year of transition to graduate nursing status. Some schools of nursing have also developed cooperative learning experiences for their students. Nursing, unlike medicine, pushes its "young" out of the nest without the safety net of a residency period (Goode, 2004, 2007). Some of these newer methods may assist with this problem.

Cooperative Experiences

Some schools of nursing offer cooperative (co-op) experiences during the nursing program. These experiences are not common and vary in their design. Such a program might allow students (or even require students) to take a break from courses and work in healthcare settings. Students receive guidance in job searches, résumé development, interviews, and selecting the best experience. Some schools maintain lists of healthcare organizations that students often use. A co-op experience typically means the student is hired by the healthcare organization for several months and functions in an aide or assistant position supervised by RNs.

Nurse Internships/Externships

Students frequently want more clinical experiences in the summer, when many schools of nursing do not offer courses, and they also want to be employed. The nurse **internship/externship** is a program that offers this kind of opportunity for students. Students are often concerned about their first job as well; they wonder if they are ready, and this type of experience can help students later as they adjust to their first positions. Nurse internships/externships are available in some communities as opportunities sponsored by hospitals (Beecroft, Kunzman, & Krozek, 2001). These programs are not usually associated with a school of nursing. They are short programs, such as 10 weeks, usually offered in the summer for students who will enter their senior year in the fall. There is variation in the length of these programs, in what is offered to the student in the program, and in how much support the student receives in the program. The student is employed by the hospital and provided with orientation to the hospital, some content experiences, and preceptored and/or mentored experiences. Students need to investigate these programs and find out what each program offers and whether it meets their needs. This type of program is particularly helpful if students want more time in an organization to determine if they might want to work there after graduation.

Nurse Residency Programs

Because of concern about nursing staff turnover, replacing nurses who leave, and other job-related issues, such as staff burnout and concern about the level of new graduates' preparation and retention, some hospitals have developed **nurse residency** programs (Bowles & Candela, 2005; Casey, Fink, Krugman, & Propst, 2004; Halfer & Graf, 2006a, 2006b). After the nurse passes the licensure exam, the residency program offers the new graduate a structured transition to professional nursing practice.

The American Association of Colleges of Nursing (AACN) conducted a pilot program to examine the use of a national accreditation program based on standards it developed for nurse residency programs. The National Council of State Boards of Nursing (NCSBN, 2017a) has also worked on a pilot residency program known as Transition to Practice (TTP) in combination with its Taxonomy of Error, Root Cause Analysis, Practice-Responsibility (TERCAP) initiative. TTP and TERCAP are based on the five healthcare professions core competencies and quality care definitions identified by the Institute of Medicine (Institute of Medicine [IOM], 2003; NCSBN, 2011; IOM, 2003). **Figure 4-6** describes the transition to practice model. Both *The Future of Nursing* report (IOM, 2010) and the recent nursing education report (Benner, Sutphen, Leonard, & Day, 2010) recommend residency programs as a standard part of nursing education, although at this time they are not required. The progress report for *The Future of Nursing* report also supports the need for more residency programs in acute care and also in public/community care (National Academy of Medicine, 2015).

A residency program requires that a healthcare organization assign staff to manage the program; develop content and learning activities, precepted experiences, and mentoring; and support gradual adjustment to higher levels of responsibility. These are paid positions, and typically the nurse resident must commit to working for the institution for a period of time after the residency. Such programs are proving to be helpful to new nurses and are decreasing new graduate turnover and improving staff retention. However, not all hospitals have residencies, and admission to these programs is competitive.

Some residency programs partner with schools of nursing—a relationship recommended by the AACN residency standards. Residencies focus on leadership, patient safety outcomes, and professional development (American Association of Colleges of Nursing [AACN], 2016a). In the first 6 years of the implementation of the AACN's residency program, the organization established 62 sites in 30 states, and more have been added (AACN, 2016b). Students

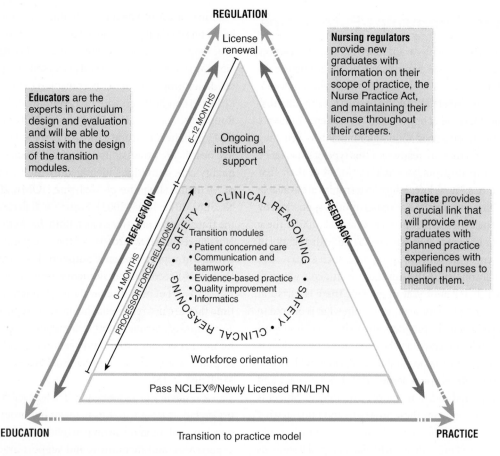

REGULATION

License renewal

Nursing regulators provide new graduates with information on their scope of practice, the Nurse Practice Act, and maintaining their license throughout their careers.

Educators are the experts in curriculum design and evaluation and will be able to assist with the design of the transition modules.

6–12 MONTHS

Ongoing institutional support

CLINICAL REASONING

SAFETY

REFLECTION

0–4 MONTHS

PROCESSOR FORCE RELATIONS

Transition modules
• Patient concerned care
• Communication and teamwork
• Evidence-based practice
• Quality improvement
• Informatics

CLINICAL REASONING

SAFETY

FEEDBACK

Practice provides a crucial link that will provide new graduates with planned practice experiences with qualified nurses to mentor them.

Workforce orientation

Pass NCLEX®/Newly Licensed RN/LPN

EDUCATION

Transition to practice model

PRACTICE

Figure 4-6 Transition to Practice Model

Reproduced from National Council State Boards of Nursing. (2017) *Transition to practice model.* Retrieved from https://www.ncsbn.org/transition-to-practice.htm

who are interested in a residency experience need to investigate these opportunities early in their senior year. Only BSN graduates can participate in residency programs that follow the AACN residency model, but some other residency programs do not require a BSN and are open to ADN graduates. These programs usually encourage new ADN graduates to consider completing a BSN degree.

Stop and Consider #6

Nurse residency programs might be a good choice for you.

Lifelong Learning
for the Professional

Lifelong learning is one of the major characteristics of a professional. This model of learning includes three major components:

- *Academic education:* The courses students take for academic credit—undergraduate and graduate—in an institution of higher learning that typically lead to a degree or completion of a certificate program. Nurses who return to school are pursuing lifelong learning goals.

- *Staff development education:* The systematic process of assessing and developing oneself to enhance performance or professional development—continued competence. Included in staff development are orientation (the process of introducing nursing staff to the organization and position), training required to do a job, and professional development.
- *Continuing education:* Systematic professional learning designed to augment knowledge, skills, and attitudes.

In 2010, the American Nurses Association (ANA) published a revised version of *Nursing professional development: scope and standards of practice.* The following is a summary description of the standards (American Nurses Association & National Nursing Staff Development Organization, 2010).

- Assessment of educational needs
- Identification of issues and trends that might require further education
- Outcomes identification for learning activities
- Planning of learning activities
- Implementation of learning activities including coordination of the activities, the learning and practice environment, and consultation with others to enhance the learning
- Evaluation of the learning activities
- Quality of nursing professional development practice
- Education of the professional development specialist
- Professional practice evaluation of the professional development specialist
- Collegiality to ensure partnerships to enhance learning activities
- Collaboration to facilitate learning
- Ethics
- Advocacy
- Research findings integrated into learning activities
- Resource utilization to most effectively provide learning activities
- Leadership

As a student, you may wonder why lifelong learning is important to you when you are just now entering nursing education. In fact, lifelong learning—particularly the need to recognize its importance for individual nurses, the profession, healthcare organizations, and patient outcomes—begins when you enter a nursing education program. Students often have opportunities to participate in a variety of these learning activities even as students. Such activities are excellent opportunities to gain further knowledge and to better understand the importance of lifelong learning. You also need to know the requirements for **continuing education** (CE) in the state(s) where you wish to apply for licensure. Lifelong learning must be driven by personal responsibility to improve, even in regard to required practice components. Although professional organizations, regulatory agencies, and employers influence whether nurses participate in lifelong learning, successful lifelong learning is ultimately in the hands of the learner—that is, the nurse. The major report on nursing from the IOM (2010) includes the recommendation that the profession ensure that nurses engage in lifelong learning. In addition, a major report focused on collaboration between nursing and medicine examined the need for a clearer vision for lifelong learning for nurses and physicians (American Association of Colleges of Nursing & American Association of Medical Colleges, 2010). The report's recommendations focus on four areas: CE methods (for example, meetings, rounds, conferences, and so on), interprofessional education, lifelong learning, and workplace learning. Interprofessional education is mentioned in other content about academic nursing education; however, it is also relevant to lifelong learning. If different professions can continue to learn together after completion of academic programs, this can be supportive of interprofessional collaboration and understanding of the roles and responsibilities of other professions. This report also discusses an issue that is not often addressed for CE—regulation. There is great variation among professions, and even within a profession, as to requirements for CE and accreditation of CE. This needs to be improved.

The natural assumption is that all nurses would want to get more education and stay current, but this is not necessarily the case. Required CE is a great motivator. Many states require CE if nurses are to maintain their licensure after initial licensure is received. In these states, the state board of nursing designates the number of CE credits required for licensure renewal. States vary in terms of what is considered CE—short, structured CE programs; academic courses; attending conferences where educational content is presented; publishing; and so on. Nurses must follow their state's requirements. Another reason for obtaining CE is to meet certification requirements. The certification body determines the amount and type of required CE. If a nurse is licensed in more than one state, then the nurse must meet the CE requirements for all states in which he or she is licensed.

Sources for CE contact hours are highly variable. Credit can be obtained, for example, by attending a 1-hour or full-day educational offering, attending part or all of conference, reading an article in a professional journal and then taking an assessment quiz, or participating in an online program. Typically, a fee is charged unless the costs for the program are covered, such as by a grant to the sponsoring organization. Nurses do need to be careful and make sure that the program's credit is accepted by the organization requiring the CE, so it is best that the organizations offering CE be accredited programs. The American Nurses Credentialing Center (ANCC) accredits these programs, and some state boards of nursing may offer an accrediting process. Obtaining accreditation is voluntary, but the reality is that to get nurses to participate, accreditation is critical. When a CE program is accredited through an organization such as ANCC, the consumer is assured that national standards of quality education have been applied (American Nurses Credentialing Center [ANCC], 2007). It is assumed that CE has an impact on patient outcomes and quality care, but this relationship is not easy to prove in a consistent manner. When nurses select learning programs to attend or complete, they should evaluate the following factors:

- Accreditation of the program
- Acceptance of the CE by the required body, such as state board of nursing for licensure or organization sponsoring certification
- Number of CE credits and related time commitment
- Schedule and location, including travel issues
- Cost (registration fee, parking and travel, housing, and meals)
- Qualifications of faculty
- Whether the program is based on adult learning principles (Is the program designed for the adult learner?)
- Identification of needs (What does the nurse need to gain? What are the personal or professional objectives? Does the course offer content to meet these objectives?)
- The program's learner objectives (Do they correlate with personal professional objectives?)
- Whether the program is based on current and relevant content
- Teaching methods
- Past experiences with the provider of the educational program (Quality programs attract nurses who return for other programs.)
- Receipt of documentation of completion with title of program, sponsoring organization, date, and hours noted

Nurses are responsible for maintaining their own CE activity records. In states where CE is required for licensure renewal, nurses may be required to produce documentation of these activities. In addition, nurses need to update their résumés to ensure that learning activities are included. In some cases, employers require documentation of CE activities. Nurses are usually required to document learning activities on an annual or biannual basis.

A current issue in CE is the need for greater emphasis on interprofessional CE to increase support for more interprofessional teamwork. The issue is addressed in a major report, which recommends that a national system be developed to support interprofessional CE: "The current system of continuing education for health professionals is not working. Continuing education for the professional health workforce needs to be reconsidered if the workforce is to provide high quality health care. A more comprehensive system of CE is needed, and CPD (Continuing Professional Development) provides a promising approach to improve the quality of learning. An independent public–private Continuing Professional Development Institute will be key to ensuring that the entire health care workforce is prepared to provide high quality, safe care" (IOM, 2010, p. 3). As a follow-up to these proposals, in 2013, CE accreditor organizations for nursing, pharmacy, medicine, and other healthcare professions met together to discuss interprofessional continuing education (Accreditation Council for Continuing Medical Education, 2013). Participants in this meeting identified goals, including creating standardized terminology and exploring a shared set of expectations and measures for interprofessional education in support of collaborative practice.

Stop and Consider #7

Even after you get your nursing degree and license, you need to continue learning.

Certification and
Credentialing

Certification and credentialing are recognition systems that identify whether nurses meet certain requirements or standards. These recognitions may be required or voluntary, depending on the circumstances. Credentialing is typically required, whereas certification may be voluntary. To obtain certification or meet credentialing requirements, nurses must first be licensed as RNs.

Credentialing is a process that ensures practitioners such as RNs are qualified to perform as demonstrated by having licensure. Typically, it is used by healthcare organizations to check for licensure of healthcare professionals (such as nurses) and to monitor continued licensure. Nurses are required to show their current license to their employer, and the employer may then keep a copy of the license. Every state provides access to online checks of licensure status. Education, certification, and maintenance of malpractice insurance may also be reviewed, although this practice varies from one healthcare organization to another. The goal is to protect the public by ensuring that specific state requirements are met.

Certification is "a process by which a nongovernmental agency validates, based upon predetermined standards, an individual nurse's qualification and knowledge for practice in a defined functional or clinical area of nursing" (American Association of Critical-Care Nurses, 2014, p. 4). It is a method of recognizing expertise through successful completion of an exam focused on the certification specialty, recognition of completed education, and the description of clinical experience in a designated specialty area covered by the certification. Certification of nurse practitioners in the areas of adult, family, and adult–gerontology primary care is managed through the American Academy of Nurse Practitioners Certification Program (AANPCP). Other specialty nurse practitioner certifications are managed through different organizations. Pursuing this type of recognition is voluntary in that nurses are not required to have certification, although many employers acknowledge its importance, and some may require certification for certain positions—for example, for APRNs. This recognition is now available in most specialty areas. For example, the ANCC offers certification in multiple nursing specialties. After the nurse receives the initial certification, recertification is accomplished through demonstrating ongoing practice and through CE. Nurses may be certified in multiple areas as long as they meet the requirements for each area. Professional certification in nursing is a measure of distinctive nursing practice, and the benefits of certification are widely accepted. The value of certification is not just significant for nursing practice—focus on professional certification is also essential to meet multiple standards within the ANCC's Magnet Recognition Program® for excellence in nursing services (ANCC, 2004, as cited in Shirey, 2005, p. 245).

Certification may also be given by a healthcare organization for accomplishing a specific goal, such as learning to perform cardiopulmonary resuscitation, but this is not the same type of certification that is awarded after meeting specific professional standards described above.

The nursing profession has proposed a consensus model for regulation that includes licensure, accreditation, certification, and education to ensure greater consistency and clarity for APRN practice (NCSBN, 2008, 2017b). This model reflects ongoing concern about the need for uniformity in educational requirements for and regulations related to APRNs. The consensus model was fully implemented in 2015 (ANCC, 2017; NCSBN, 2013).

Stop and Consider #8
Certification recognizes specialty nursing.

Caring for Self

Caring for others is clearly the focus of nursing, but the process of caring for others can be a drain on the nurse. Students quickly discover that they are very tired after a long day in their clinical sessions. The number of hours worked and the pace of clinical experiences affect staff fatigue, but stress also has an impact. When you graduate and practice, you may find that the stress does not disappear; indeed, in some cases, it may increase, particularly during early years of practice. Nurses often feel that they must be perfect. They may feel guilty when they cannot do everything they think they should be doing, both

at work with patients and in their personal lives. There is still much to learn about nursing, working with others, pacing oneself, and figuring out the best way to mesh a career with a personal life—finding a balance and accepting that nursing is not a career of perfection. All nurses need to be aware of the potential for **burnout**, which is a "syndrome manifested by emotional exhaustion, depersonalization, and reduced personal accomplishments; it commonly occurs in professions like nursing" (Garrett & McDaniel, 2001, p. 92). You need to be aware of your work–life balance, which is "a state where the needs and requirements of work are weighed together to create an equitable share of time that allows for work to be completed and a professional's private life to get attention" (Heckerson & Laser, 2006, p. 27).

Learning how you routinely respond to **stress** and developing coping skills to manage stress can have a major impact and, it is hoped, prevent burnout later. Symptoms such as headaches, abdominal complaints, anxiety, irritability, anger, isolation, and depression can indicate a high level of stress. A review of anatomy and physiology explains how stress affects the body. When you experience stress, two hormones—adrenaline and cortisol—trigger the body to react and put the nervous, endocrine, cardiovascular, and immune systems on a state of alert. This physiological process actually is helpful because it helps you to cope with the stress. The problem may expand when these stress responses happen frequently and over a period of months or years. Stress can be felt from a real or imagined threat, and the stressed person feels powerless. Exposure to constant or frequent stress can lead to chronic stress, which can have an overall impact on a person's health.

The National Institute of Occupational Safety and Health (NIOSH) provides support for employees, including nurses, to ensure a safe and healthy work experience. Stress is a topic of concern for NIOSH. **Figure 4-7** describes a model of job stress. Six factors generally impact job stress in a variety of settings and influence this model (U.S. Department of Health and Human Services [HHS], Centers for Disease

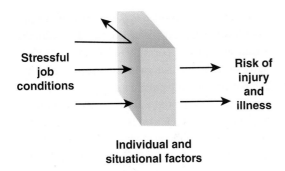

Figure 4-7 Model of Job Stress

Reproduced from U.S. Department of Health and Human Services. Centers for Disease Control and Prevention. National Institute of Occupational Safety and Health. (2014). STRESS...at work. Retrieved from http://www.cdc.gov/niosh/docs/99-101/default.html

Control and Prevention [CDC], & National Institute of Occupational Safety and Health [NIOSH]):

- *Design of tasks:* Aspects to consider are work hours, heavy workload, frequency of breaks, shift work, lack of routine and increased hectic work environment, feeling of loss of control when required to do tasks, and so on
- *Management style:* Lack of staff input into decisions, poor communication, lack of clear policies, and so on

- *Interpersonal relationships:* Poor social environment and communication, lack of support, and so on
- *Career concerns:* Job insecurity, lack of advancement, changes in staff and management, and son on
- *Environmental concerns:* Risky work environment, high levels of noise, air pollution, ergonomic risk, and so on

Nurses are at risk when there is work overload, time pressure, lack of social support, staff incivility, exposure to infections diseases, risk of needlestick injuries, exposure to work-related violence or threats, sleep deprivation, role ambiguity and conflict, understaffing, career development issues, and dealing with difficult or seriously ill patients (HHS, CDC, NIOSH, 2008).

The best time to begin **stress management** is now, while you are still a student. Strategies for coping with stress can be found in a great variety of resources. **Exhibit 4-2** identifies some websites that provide general information about stress. The following are some guidelines that can prevent and/or reduce stress:

- Set some goals to achieve a work–life balance.
- Use effective time management techniques and set priorities.

Exhibit 4-2　Links to Help You Cope with Stress

Understanding and dealing with stress: http://www.mtstcil.org/skills/stress-intro.html

Understanding stress: Signs, symptoms, causes, and effects: http://helpguide.org/mental/stress_signs.htm

Eight immediate stress-busters: http://www.medicinenet.com/script/main/art.asp?articlekey=59875

Psych central: Stress busters: http://psychcentral.com/blog/archives/2009/03/18/10-stress-busters/

Tips to manage anxiety and stress: https://www.adaa.org/tips-manage-anxiety-and-stress

Stress management for nursing students: http://www.ahna.org/Resources/Stress-Management/For-Nursing-Students

How to cope with stress on the job: http://nursingworld.org/Content/Resources/How-to-Cope-with-Stress-on-the-Job.html

- Prepare ahead of time for assignments, quizzes, and exams.
- Ask questions when confused and ask for help—do not view this as a sign of weakness, but rather as strength.
- Take a break—a few minutes of rest can do wonders.
- Get an appropriate amount of exercise, sleep, and a healthy diet. (Watch excessive use of caffeine.)
- Practice self-assertion.
- When you worry, focus on what is happening rather than what might happen.
- When you approach a problem, view it as an opportunity.
- Use humor.
- Set aside some quiet time to just think—even a short period can be productive.
- Care for self.

Two experiences that many nurses have after they practice for a while are burnout and compassion fatigue. These are the costs of caring, and they are similar but have some major differences. *Burnout* occurs when assertiveness–goal achievement intentions are not met, and **compassion fatigue** occurs when rescue-caretaking strategies are not successful (Boyle, 2011). Both lead to physical and emotional responses and affect quality of care and staff retention. Burnout is often discussed as part of an unhealthy work environment that is stressful and may be characterized by disruptive or uncivil staff behavior and lack of staff wellbeing. The nurse may reach the point of not wanting to go to work and have difficulty completing work and difficulty working with others. In a systematic review of 27 studies that measured staff well-being and patient safety, and it was noted that in 16 of the studies there was a significant correlation between poor well-being and patient safety (Hall, Johnson, Watt, Tsipa, & O'Connor, 2016). This is important information because it demonstrates that staff status (burnout, well-being, stress levels, and so on) affects performance, which also affects patient outcomes such as safety and, ultimately,

quality of care. We need to make efforts as individual providers, a healthcare profession, and also healthcare organizations to support staff well-being and reduce burnout. This will have an impact on retaining staff and patient care improvement.

Compassion fatigue is the feeling of emotion that ensues when a person is moved by the distress or suffering of another (Boyle, 2011; Hooper, Craig, Janvrin, Wetsel, & Reimels, 2010; Schantz, 2007). Compassion is necessary for effective caring, but long-term coping with exposure to the distress (both physical and emotional) of others can lead to compassion fatigue or a state of psychic exhaustion. It is the interpersonal connection with patients and families that nursing provides its best care, but this context carries risks for the nurse over time. Burnout is often also a reaction response to work stressors such as staffing, workload, managerial style, staff behavior, and so on, and occurs gradually; in contrast, compassion fatigue is relational, related to caring for others, and has a sudden onset (Boyle, 2011). This topic is included here because it relates to stress management, a set of skills that students need to develop while in school and continue to use throughout their career.

Interventions for burnout and compassion fatigue fall into three categories (Boyle, 2011). First, maintaining a healthy work–life balance is critical, nurturing self when you can. Second, you need to understand the sources of burnout and compassion fatigue. For example, compassion fatigue is often associated with basic communication skills—how do you effectively communicate with patients and families under stress without experiencing fatigue yourself? Third, work-setting interventions are often helpful. For example, onsite counseling, support groups for staff, debriefing, onsite exercise and yoga, space to take a break, stress management techniques, nutritious food and snack offerings, and so on, are important in preventing and reducing burnout and compassion fatigue.

Stop and Consider #9
Self-care is important to every nurse.

CHAPTER HIGHLIGHTS

- The educational experience in nursing differs in important ways from educational experiences in other areas.
- Students and faculty have active roles in the education process, whether in the classroom setting, online, or in lab/simulation/clinical experiences.
- Students need to understand their own learning styles and then use this information to improve their learning methods.
- Tools for success—such as reading methods, taking quizzes and exams, preparing written assignments, and so on—can make a difference in student performance.
- Students use cooperative experiences to expand their learning experiences during their education program. Internships/externships may also be part of a student's education program, but they are more formalized summer programs. Residencies are formal programs, used after completion of a nursing program and obtaining licensure, to provide a gradual integration into nursing.
- Nurses need to be lifelong learners.
- Certification and credentialing are methods used to assess competency, but they do not ensure competency.
- Taking care of self is critical both as a student and a practicing nurse.

ENGAGING IN THE CONTENT

Discussion Questions

1. Why is stress management important to you as a student nurse and to practicing nurses?
2. What is the purpose of a nurse residency program? Search the Internet for information about specific nurse residency programs.
   How do they differ from one another? How are they similar?
3. Participate in a team discussion in class and share tools for success. You might discover some new tools to help you be more successful in your studies.

CRITICAL THINKING ACTIVITIES

1. Consider the learning styles described in this chapter. Where do you fit in? Why do you think the style(s) applies to you? What impact do you think the style(s) you identified will have on your own learning in the nursing program? Are there changes you need to work on?
2. Develop a study plan for yourself that incorporates information about tools for success. Include an assessment of how you use your time.
3. Review your school's philosophy and curriculum. What are the key themes in this information? Do you think that the themes and content are relevant to nursing practice, and if so, why? Do you think anything important is missing, and if so, what is it? As a student, is your responsibility in relation to the curriculum?

ELECTRONIC REFLECTION JOURNAL

During your clinical experiences, observe how nurses use their time. Describe what you observe: Is the nurse effective? Which methods does the nurse use? How might you learn from this observation? Keep track of your time management when in clinical sessions and periodically comment on it in your Electronic Reflection Journal.

CASE STUDIES

Case 1

Bowers, Lauring, and Jacobson (2001) conducted a study to better understand how nurses manage their time in long-term care settings. Their data indicated that the nurses attempted to "create new time" when time was short. As a student, you will be confronted with issues of time when you begin your clinical experience and then throughout your career as a nurse. As you review this study and answer the questions consider the following information this study that discusses the factors of longevity, working faster, changing sequence of tasks, communicating inaccessibility, converting wasted time, and negotiating "wasted time."

Case Questions

1. Consider your own schedule for a week. How would these strategies apply to your own personal methods for handling your time? How would they affect your time management, both positively and negatively?

2. Keep this list, and during your clinical experiences, consider whether you are using these strategies to create more time. Can time really be created? How might you solve this problem?

Source: Bowers, B., Lauring, C., & Jacobson, N. (2001). How nurses manage time and work in long-term care. *Journal of Advanced Nursing, 33*(4), 484–491.

Case 2

A nursing student is completing his first year and meets with his advisor. The discussion is a difficult one. His advisor tells the student that he is passing, but in several courses he is just barely passing. The student is defensive and says that no one said he had to make all A's. The advisor agrees with him that this is not the expectation; however, some of the student's grades are borderline, and more importantly, his performance in clinical sessions has been weak. The advisor tells the student that he needs to improve. The student leaves the meeting discouraged and not sure what to do.

CASE STUDIES (CONTINUED)

Case Questions

1. What more could the advisor have done in this meeting?
2. What does the student need to do? Describe steps the student might take (consider the content in this chapter).

Working Backward to Develop a Case

Write a brief paragraph that describes a case related to the following questions.

1. A staff member asks: What is going on with quality data?
2. How might time management be a factor?
3. Another staff member asks: What is wrong with the staff schedule recently?

REFERENCES

Accreditation Council for Continuing Medical Education. (2013). *CE accreditors meeting focuses on interprofessional education.* Retrieved from http://www.accme.org/news-publications/highlights/ce-accreditors-meeting-focuses-interprofessional-education

American Association of Colleges of Nursing, & American Association of Medical Colleges. (2010). *Life long learning in medicine and nursing.* Washington, DC: Authors.

American Association of Colleges of Nursing. (2016a). *Nurse residency.* Retrieved from http://www.aacn.nche.edu/education-resources/nurse-residency-program

American Association of Colleges of Nursing. (2016b). *Nurse residency locations.* Retrieved from http://www.aacn.nche.edu/education-resources/NRP-Participants-by-State.pdf

American Association of Critical-Care Nurses. (2014). *Certification exam policy handbook.* Retrieved from http://www.aacn.org/wd/certifications/docs/cert-policy-hndbk.pdf

American Nurses Association, & National Nursing Staff Development Organization. (2010). *Nursing professional development: Scope and standards of practice.* Silver Spring, MD: Authors.

American Nurses Credentialing Center. (2004). *Magnet recognition program recognizing excellence in nursing service: Application manual 2005.* Washington, DC: Author.

American Nurses Credentialing Center. (2007). *ANCC Credentialing Center: Primary accreditation.* Retrieved http://www.nursecredentialing.org/Accreditation/Primary-Accreditation.aspx

American Nurses Credentialing Center. (2017). *APRN consensus model.* Retrieved from http://nursecredentialing.org/Certification/APRNCorner

Beecroft, P., Kunzman, L., & Krozek, C. (2001). RN internship: Outcomes of a one-year pilot program. *Journal of Nursing Administration, 31*(12), 575–582.

Benner, P. (2001). *From novice to expert* (commemorative edition). Upper Saddle River, NJ: Prentice Hall Health.

Benner, P., Sutphen, P., Leonard, V., & Day, L. (2010). *Educating nurses: A call for radical transformation.* San Francisco, CA: Jossey-Bass.

Billings, D., & Halstead, J. (2005). *Teaching in nursing: A guide for faculty* (2nd ed.). Philadelphia, PA: Saunders.

Bowers, B., Lauring, C., & Jacobson, N. (2001). How nurses manage time and work in long-term care. *Journal of Advanced Nursing, 33*(4) 484–491.

Bowles, C., & Candela, L. (2005). First job experiences of recent RN graduates. *Journal of Nursing Administration, 35*(3), 130–137.

Boyle, D. (2011, January). Countering compassion fatigue: A requisite nursing agenda. *OJIN, 16.* Retrieved from http://www.nursingworld.org/MainMenuCategories /ANAMarketplace/ANAPeriodicals/OJIN/Table ofContents/Vol-16-2011/ No1-Jan-2011/Countering -Compassion-Fatigue.html

Casey, K., Fink, R., Krugman, M., & Propst, J. (2004). The graduate nurse experience. *Journal of Nursing Administration, 34*(6), 303–311.

Garrett, D., & McDaniel, A. (2001). A new look at nurse burnout. *Journal of Nursing Administration, 31,* 91–96.

Goode, C. (2007, July). Report given at the American Academy of Nursing Workforce Commission Committee on Preparation of the Nursing Workforce, Chicago, IL.

Goode, C., & Williams, C. (2004). Post-baccalaureate nurse residency program. *Journal of Nursing Administration, 34*(2), 71–77.

Halfer, D., & Graf, E. (2006a). Graduate nurse experience. *Journal of Nursing Administration, 34*(6), 303–311.

Halfer, D., & Graf, E. (2006b). Graduate nurse perceptions of the work experience. *Nursing Economics, 24*(2), 150–155.

Hall, L., Johnson, J., Watt, I., Tsipa, A., & O'Connor, D. (2016, July 8). Healthcare staff wellbeing, burnout, and patient safety: A systematic review. *PLOS One, 11*(7). DOI:10.1371 /journal.pone.0159015

Heckerson, E., & Laser, C. (2006). Just breathe! The critical importance of maintaining a work–life balance. *Nurse Leader, 4*(12), 26–28.

Honey, P., & Mumford, A. (1986). *The manual of learning styles.* Maidenhead, UK: Peter Honey.

Honey, P., & Mumford, A. (1992). *The manual of learning styles* (3rd ed.). Maidenhead, UK: Peter Honey.

Hooper, C., Craig, J., Janvrin, D., Wetsel, M., & Reimels, E. (2010). Compassion satisfaction, burnout and compassion fatigue among emergency room nurses compared with nurses in other selected inpatient specialties. *Journal of Emergency Nursing, 36*(5), 420–427.

Hovancsek, M. (2007). Using simulation in nursing education. In P. Jeffries (Ed.), *Simulation in nursing education* (pp. 1–9). New York, NY: National League for Nursing.

Institute of Medicine. (2010a). *Redesigning continuing education in the health professions.* Washington, DC: The National Academies Press.

Institute of Medicine. (2010b). *The future of nursing: Leading change, advancing health.* Washington, DC: The National Academies Press.

Jeffries, P., & Rogers, K. (2007). Evaluating simulations. In P. Jeffries (Ed.), *Simulation in nursing education* (pp. 87–103). New York, NY: National League for Nursing.

Kolb, D. (1984). *Experiential learning: Experience as the source of learning and development.* Toronto, ON: Prentice Hall.

Kramer, M. (1985). Why does reality shock continue? In J. McCloskey & H. Grace (Eds.), *Current issues in nursing* (pp. 891–903). Boston, MA: Blackwell Scientific.

National Academy of Medicine. (2015). *Assessing progress on the IOM report the future of nursing.* Washington, DC: The National Academies Press.

National Council of State Boards of Nursing. (2008). *Consensus model for APRN regulation.* Retrieved from https://www.ncsbn.org/Consensus_Model_for_APRN _Regulation_July_2008.pdf

National Council of State Boards of Nursing. (2011). *TERCAP.* Retrieved from https://www.ncsbn.org /441.htm

National Council of State Boards of Nursing. (2013). *Campaign for consensus.* APRN Retrieved from https:// www .ncsbn.org/2567.htm

National Council of State Boards of Nursing. (2017a). *Transition to practice.* Retrieved from https://www .ncsbn.org/transition-to-practice.htm

National Council of State Boards of Nursing. (2017b). *APRN consensus model.* Retrieved from https://www .ncsbn.org/736.htm

Rassool, G., & Rawaf, S. (2007). Learning style preference of undergraduate nursing students. *Nursing Standard, 32*(21), 35–41.

Schantz, M. (2007). Compassion: A concept analysis. *Nursing Forum, 42*(2), 48–55.

Shirey, M. (2005). Celebrating certification in nursing. Forces of magnetism in action. *Nursing Administration Quarterly, 29,* 245–253.

U.S. Department of Health and Human Services, Centers for Disease Control and Prevention, & National Institute of Occupational Safety and Health. (2008). *Exposure to stress: Occupational hazards in hospitals.* HHS (NIOSH) Publication No. 2008-136. Retrieved from https://www.cdc.gov/niosh /docs/2008-136/pdfs/20080136.pdf

U.S. Department of Health and Human Services, Centers for Disease Control and Prevention, & National Institute of Occupational Safety and Health. (2014). Stress at work. Retrieved from http://www.cdc.gov/niosh/docs /99-101/default.html

Young, M., Stuenkel, D., & Bawel-Brinkley, K. (2008). Strategies for easing the role transition of graduate nurses. *Journal for Nurses in Staff Development, 24*(3), 105–110.

Section 2

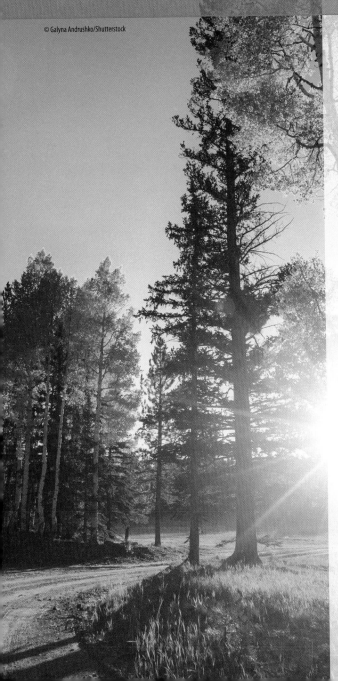

The Healthcare Context

Section II sets the stage for the student by introducing the complex healthcare environment the student now enters. The Health Policy and Political Action *chapter introduces these topics and considers how they relate to the nursing profession. The* Ethics and Legal Issues *chapter discusses these related topics affect on practice. With this background, the* Health Promotion, Disease Prevention, and Illness: A Community Perspective *chapter describes the importance of the public/ community focus on healthcare delivery. The last chapter in this section, The* Healthcare Delivery System: Focus on Acute Care, *examines one type of healthcare organization, the acute care hospital, in depth as an exemplar of how a healthcare organization functions and nurses involvement in these organizations.*

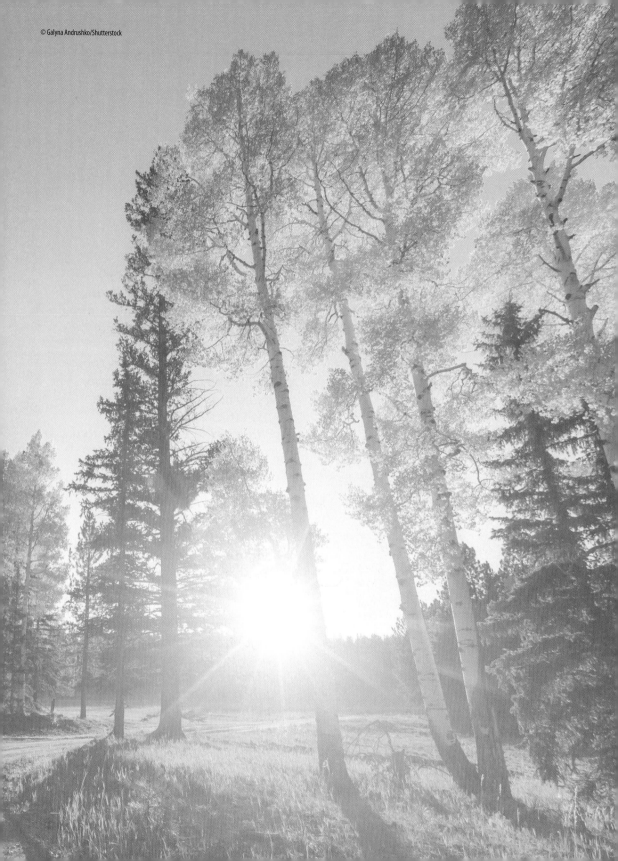

© Galyna Andrushko/Shutterstock

Chapter 5

Health Policy and Political Action

CHAPTER OBJECTIVES

At the conclusion of this chapter, the learner will be able to:

- Discuss the importance of health policy and political action.
- Examine critical health policy issues and their impact on nurses and nursing.
- Critique the policy-making process.

- Discuss the role of the nurse in the political process and its importance to the profession as a whole.
- Analyze the impact of the Patient Protection and Affordable Care Act of 2010.

CHAPTER OUTLINE

- Introduction
- Importance of Health Policy and Political Action
  - Definitions
  - Policy: Relevance to the Nation's Health and to Nursing
  - General Descriptors of U.S. Health Policy
- Examples of Critical Healthcare Policy Issues
  - Cost of Health Care
  - Healthcare Quality
  - Disparities in Health Care
  - Consumers
  - Commercialization of Health Care
  - Reimbursement for Nursing Care
  - Immigration and the Nursing Workforce
- Nursing Agenda: Addressing Health Policy Issues

- The Policy-Making Process
- The Political Process
  - Nurses' Role in the Political Process: Impact on Healthcare Policy
  - Getting into the Political System and Making It Work for Nursing
- Patient Protection and Affordable Care Act of 2010
- Chapter Highlights
- Engaging in the Content
- Discussion Questions
- Critical Thinking Activities
- Electronic Reflection Journal
- Case Studies
- Working Backward to Develop a Case
- References

KEY TERMS

Advocacy
Executive branch
Judicial branch
Legislative branch
Lobbying

Lobbyist
Policy
Political action committee
Political competence
Politics

Private policy
Public Health Act of 1944
Public policy
Social Security Act of 1935

Introduction

This chapter introduces content about health policy and the political process. Both have a major impact on individual nurses, nursing care, the nursing profession, and healthcare delivery. When nurses participate in the policy process, they are acting as advocates for patients, as Abood explained: "Nurses are well aware that today's healthcare system is in trouble and in need of change. The experiences of many nurses practicing in the real world of healthcare are motivating them to take on some form of an advocacy role in order to influence change in policies, laws, or regulations that govern the larger healthcare system. This type of advocacy necessitates stepping beyond their own practice setting and into the less familiar world of policy and politics, a world in which many nurses do not feel prepared to participate effectively" (Abood, 2007, p. 3).

Importance of Health
Policy and Political Action

Understanding healthcare policy requires the nurse to step back and see the broader picture of healthcare needs and delivery while understanding how such policy influences individual care. Political action is part of recognizing the need for health policy; developing policy and implementing policy, including financing policy decisions; and evaluating outcomes. Nurses offer the following resources to health policy making:

- Expertise
- Understanding of consumer (patient, family, community) needs
- Experience in assisting patients in making healthcare decisions
- Understanding of the healthcare system
- Understanding of interprofessional care
- A link to other healthcare professionals and organizations

Nurses may assume roles in policy making at the local, state, and federal levels of government. Within these roles, they demonstrate leadership, expertise, advocacy, and the ability to collaborate with others to meet identified outcomes. Sometimes nurses are successful in getting the policy that they feel is needed for patients and for nursing, and sometimes they are not. The key to policy making is to learn from past experiences and try again.

Definitions

A **policy** is a course of action that affects a large number of people and is inspired by a specific need to achieve certain outcomes. The best approach to understanding health policy is to describe the difference between public policy and private policy. **Public policy** is "policy made at the legislative, executive, and judicial branches of federal, state, and local levels of government that affects individual and institutional behaviors under the government's respective jurisdiction. Public policy includes all policies that come from government at all levels" (Block, 2008, p. 7). Developing and implementing policy is a method for finding solutions to problems, but not all solutions are policies. Many solutions have nothing to do with government. There are two main types of public policies: (1) regulatory policies (for example, registered nurse [RN] licensure that regulates practice) and (2) allocative policies, which involve money distribution. Allocative policies provide benefits for some at the expense of others to ensure that certain public objectives are met. Often the allocative decision relates to funding of certain healthcare programs but not others. Health policy is policy that focuses on health and health-related issues, and it may be a public or private policy. Examples of public policies that have had national impact on health are those prohibiting smoking in public places (initiated through the **legislative branch**, which makes laws) and abortion rulings made by the U.S. Supreme Court (initiated through the **judicial branch**). **Private policy** is made by nongovernmental organizations, such as professional organizations, about a profession and healthcare organizations (for example, hospital, clinic). The second type of private policy, healthcare organization policies, is discussed in later chapters along with procedures that are usually associated with this type of policy.

This chapter focuses on public policy related to health. A general description of these policies includes the following (Block, 2008, p. 6):

- Health-related decisions made by legislators that then become laws
- Rules and regulations designed to implement legislation and laws or are used to operate government and its health-related programs
- Judicial decisions related to health that have an impact on how health care is delivered, reimbursed, and so on

Policy: Relevance to the Nation's Health and to Nursing

Policy has an impact on all aspects of health and healthcare delivery, such as how care is delivered, who receives care, which types of services are received, how reimbursement is doled out, and which types of providers and organizations provide health care. Because nursing is a major part of healthcare delivery policy, nurses need to be involved in policy making and be aware of policy changes.

Each of the areas in **Figure 5-1** relates to individual nurses and to the profession. Roles and standards are found in state laws and rules/regulations. Boards of nursing and each state's nurse practice act set professional expectations and identify the scope of practice for nurses in the state. Federal laws and rules/regulations related to Medicare and Medicaid address issues such as reimbursement for advanced practice registered nurses (APRNs). How nursing care is provided and which care is provided are influenced by Medicare, Medicaid, nurse practice acts, and other laws and rules and regulations made by federal, state, and local governments. Health is influenced by federal policy decisions related to Medicare reimbursement for preventive services, the U.S. Department of Health and Human Services (HHS), and its agencies' rules and regulations. An agency for which rules and regulations are very

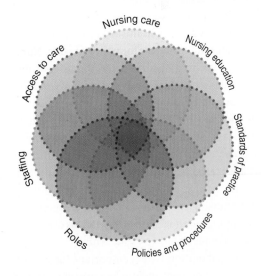

Figure 5-1 Healthcare Policy: Impact on Health Care and Nursing

important is the Food and Drug Administration (FDA), which manages the drug approval process in the United States. State laws, such as those passed in California and other states limiting or eliminating mandatory overtime, may determine staffing levels. Access to care is often influenced by policy, particularly when related to reimbursement policy and limits set on which services can be provided and by whom. This is particularly relevant to Medicare, Medicaid, and state employee health insurance. Individual organizations have their own policies and procedures, and often these are influenced by public policy. Public policy also has an impact on nursing education through laws and rules and regulations—for example, through funding for faculty and scholarships, funding to develop or expand schools of nursing and their programs, evaluation standards through state boards of nursing, funding for new nursing education programs, and much more. Nursing research is also influenced by policy; funding for research primarily comes through government sources, and legislation designates funding for government research (for example, funding for the National Institute of Nursing Research).

Nurses are experts in health care, and in that role they can make valuable contributions to the healthcare policy-making process. Nurses' expertise and knowledge about health and healthcare delivery are important resources for policy makers. Nurses also have a long history of serving as consumer advocates for their patients and patients' families. **Advocacy** means to speak for or be persuasive for another's needs. This does not mean that the nurse takes over for the patient. When nurses are involved in policy development, for example, they are acting as advocates. Nurses may get involved in policy making both as individuals and as representatives of the nursing profession, such as by representing a nursing organization. Each of these forms of advocacy is an example of nursing leadership.

Collaboration is very important for effective policy development and implementation. The goal of health policy should be the provision of better health care for citizens. When nurses advocate for professional issues such as pay, work schedules, the need for more nurses, and so forth, they also influence healthcare delivery. If there is not enough nurses because pay is low, then care is compromised. If there is not enough nurses because few are entering the profession or because schools do not have the funds to increase enrollment or not enough qualified faculty, this compromises care. In other cases, nurses advocate directly for healthcare delivery issues, such as by calling for reimbursement for hospice care or by supporting mental health parity legislation to improve access to care for people with serious mental illness.

General Descriptors of U.S. Health Policy

U.S. health policy can be described by the following long-standing characteristics, which have an impact on the types of policies that are enacted and the effectiveness of the policies (Shi & Singh, 2015). First, whereas most other countries have national, government-run healthcare systems, the United States does not. Instead, the private insurance sector is the dominant player in the U.S. system, which is primarily employer-based insurance. The issue of a universal right to health care has been a contentious one for some time. Government does have an important role in the U.S. healthcare system, but it does not have the only major role. This stance reflects Americans' view that the government's role should be limited.

The second characteristic is the approach taken to achieve healthcare policy, which has been, and continues to be, often fragmented and incremental. This approach does not look at the whole system and how its components work or do not work together effectively; parts are not connected to constitute a whole. Coordination between state and federal policies, and even between the branches of the government, is also limited. The system is further complicated by the wide array of reimbursement sources.

The third characteristic is the role of the states. States have a significant role in policy in the United States, and consequently health policies may vary from state to state. Local government within states also are involved in making policy and supporting or not supporting state-level policy. In some cases, there is a shared role with the state and federal governments—for example, with the Medicaid program.

The last important characteristic is the role of the president (head of the **executive branch** of government), which can be significant. How does the president influence healthcare policy? Consider President Clinton and his initiative to review the quality of health care in the United States. Clinton established a commission to start this process. Although this commission was short term, which is the case for most commissions of this type, it set the direction for extensive reviews and recommendations that have been identified by the Institute of Medicine (IOM). Clinton also pushed to get the Health Insurance Portability and Accountability Act (HIPAA) and the State Children's Health Insurance Program (S-CHIP) passed. Both laws, which are examples of policies, resulted from the work of this healthcare commission. The work of this commission was supposed to be part of a major healthcare reform initiative that did not succeed at the time of the Clinton administration. Its initial goal was to make major changes in healthcare reimbursement, but this did not happen. Some significant policies did emerge from these efforts, such as the two previously mentioned laws and the IOM initiative to further examine the quality of U.S. healthcare delivery. The issue of healthcare reform was not seriously addressed again until the Obama administration, which developed and pushed for passage of the Patient Protection and Affordable Care Act of 2010 (ACA). The Trump administration may initiate changes regarding the ACA; however, if this is done, it will take some time.

Some legislative efforts are diluted over time, canceled as they run out of designated implementation time period (expiring), or they are not renewed. The most recent example is S-CHIP. In 2007, Congress tried to expand this program, but President George W. Bush vetoed the bill. S-CHIP was established to provide states with matching funds from the federal government that would enable states to extend health insurance for children from families with incomes too high to meet Medicaid criteria but not high enough to purchase health insurance. Matching funds is one method used by the government to fund programs. With this method, the federal government pays for half, and the states pay for the other half (or some other configuration of sharing costs). Medicaid is funded with matching funds, whereas only the federal government funds Medicare. The issue of S-CHIP came up again when the legislation was expiring, which opened it up for cancellation or renewal with or without changes. S-CHIP has been an effective program; it has provided reimbursement for needed care for many children, improved access to care and preventive care, and improved the health status of children. Congress and the administration disagreed over expansion and funding of this program, and this dispute reached a stalemate during the Bush administration. When President Obama took office, the first bill he signed was one that continued the expansion of this program, blocking its expiration. This is an example of how legislation can be passed by one administration, vetoed by another administration, not extended, or taken up again by yet another administration.

Stop and Consider #1

Health policy has an impact on healthcare professionals, healthcare organizations, reimbursement, and all aspects of health care from local, state, and national perspectives.

Examples of Critical
Healthcare Policy Issues

Many healthcare policy issues are of concern to local communities, states, and the federal government. **Exhibit 5-1** highlights some of these issues, which

---

Exhibit 5-1 Potential Healthcare Policy Issues

- Access to care
- Acute and chronic illness
- Advanced practice nursing
- Aging
- Changing physician practice patterns
- Healthcare costs
- Healthcare reimbursement
- Disparities in health care
- Diversity in healthcare workforce
- Health promotion and prevention
- Healthcare commercialization and the healthcare industrial complex
- Healthcare consumerism
- Healthcare staff role changes
- Healthcare staffing
- Workforce issues

- Immigration: Impact on care and on providers
- Global health issues
- Mental health parity
- Minority health
- Move from acute care to increased use of ambulatory care
- Nursing education
- Poverty and health
- Public/community health
- Quality care
- Reimbursement
- Rural health care
- Urban health care
- Uninsured and underinsured
- Opioid epidemic

---

are often of particular concern to nurses, nursing, other healthcare professionals, and healthcare delivery in general. How policy is developed or whether policy related to each of these issues is developed at all may vary. Examining some of these issues in more depth provides a better understanding of the complexity of health policy issues. The examples of policy issues related to nursing covered in this section are not the only healthcare policy issues, but they illustrate the types that can be considered health policy issues.

Cost of Health Care

The cost of health care in the United States has risen steadily. There is no doubt that better drugs, treatment, and technology are available today to improve health and meet treatment needs for many problems; unfortunately, these new preventive and treatment interventions typically have increased costs. *Defensive medicine*, in which the physician and other healthcare providers order tests and procedures to protect themselves from lawsuits, also increases

costs. Insurance coverage has expanded, and beneficiaries or enrollees expect to get care when they feel they need it. Insurance costs money—premiums and other payment required of enrollees, cost to employers and to government, insurer costs, and so on. In turn, cost containment and cost-effectiveness have become increasingly important. Health policy often focuses on reimbursement, control of costs, and greater control of provider decisions to reduce costs. The last of these measures has not proved popular with consumers/patients.

For a long time, a critical issue has been whether the United States should move to a universal (national) healthcare system. Coffey (2001) discussed universal health coverage and identified five reasons it should be of interest to nurses, and these reasons still apply today:

- Insuring everyone with one national health program would spread the insurance risk over the entire population.
- The cost of prescription drugs would decrease.
- Billions of dollars in administrative costs would be saved.

- Competition could focus on quality, safety, and patient satisfaction.
- Resources would be redirected toward patients.

The ACA does not establish universal healthcare coverage in the United States, though it does provide insurance coverage through Medicaid for more people who cannot afford insurance and provides other methods for people to enroll in healthcare insurance. It also establishes requirements for health insurance for the U.S. population as a whole. However, it is not clear if future changes in the ACA or new legislation will alter the approach to healthcare reimbursement.

Healthcare Quality

Healthcare quality is a critical topic in health care today, recognizing we need to effectively monitor healthcare delivery and improve outcomes. Following President Clinton's establishment of the Advisory Commission on Consumer Protection and Quality in Healthcare (1996–1998), a whole area of policy development opened up. How can healthcare quality be improved? What needs to be done to accomplish this? This focus led to the federal government's request for the Institute of Medicine, which as of 2015 is known as the National Academy of Sciences, National Academy of Medicine (NAM), to further assess health care in the United States. This resulted in the publication of major reports with recommendations related to quality and patient and staff safety, which are components of quality care. Quality health care is discussed in several chapters in this text. The National Quality Strategy (NQS) is a new addition to the healthcare quality resources for the nation; it is included in this text's discussion about quality (U.S. Department of Health and Human Services [HHS] & Agency for Healthcare Research and Quality [AHRQ], 2017a). The mandate to establish the NQS is included in the ACA of 2010.

Disparities in Health Care

The IOM reports on diversity in health care and disparities and the Sullivan report on healthcare workforce diversity drew attention to a critical policy concern—namely, inequality in access to and services received in the U.S. healthcare system (Institute of Medicine [IOM], 2002, 2004; Sullivan, 2004). Nurses need more knowledge about culture and health needs, health literacy, the ways in which different groups respond to care, and healthcare disparities. How does this impact health policy? Does it mean that certain groups may not get the same services (disparities)? If so, what needs to change? We need regular monitoring of healthcare disparities, and we now do this annually when we monitor healthcare quality (National Healthcare Quality and Disparities Report, QDR) (HHS & AHRQ, 2017b). There is additional content on this critical topic in several chapters in this text, particularly content related to patient-centered care.

Consumers

There is increasing interest in the role of consumers in health care. Today, consumers are more informed about health and healthcare services than members of previous generations. An example of a law that focuses on health and the consumer is the Health Insurance Portability and Accountability Act of 1996 (HIPAA). The major focus of this law addresses the issue of transferring health insurance from one employer to another, but it also includes expectations regarding privacy of patient information, which is now a critical factor considered by healthcare providers in daily practice. With the increased emphasis on patient-centered care and then addition of family-centered care, consumers have gained a stronger voice in their health care.

Commercialization of Health Care

The organization of healthcare delivery systems has been changing into a series of multipronged systems, though not all healthcare organizations are this type. These organizations generally form a corporate model. Such corporations may exist in a local community, statewide, or even nationally. In fact, some of the large healthcare corporations also have hospitals in other countries. This change has had an impact on policies related to financing health care and quality concerns. Over time, commercialization of health care has led to more business practices in healthcare delivery such as marketing, control of budgets, and so on; not all of it is positive.

Reimbursement for Nursing Care

Reimbursement for nursing care must be viewed from two perspectives. The first view considers reimbursement methods for nursing care services, particularly inpatient or hospital services. There has not been much progress in this area. Hospitals still do not clearly identify the specific costs of nursing care in a manner that directly affects reimbursement. The second view involves reimbursement for specific individual provider services instead of reimbursement for an organization provider, such as a hospital. Physicians are reimbursed for their services. There have been major changes in how APRNs are reimbursed; thus, this situation is improving though more needs to be done. For example, if an APRN provides care in a clinic or a private practice, the question arises: How are the APRN services reimbursed? Will the patient's health insurance pay for these services? Some services are covered by federal government plans, but there is great variation in reimbursement from nongovernment plans. The ACA and other initiatives such as those identified in the report, *The future of nursing: leading change, advancing health* (IOM, 2010), have supported greater use of APRNs. To make this work, reimbursement practices will also need to support use of APRNs. There has been, however, more movement to improve APRN reimbursement then there has been clarification of reimbursement for nursing services in hospitals and other types of healthcare organizations.

Immigration and the Nursing Workforce

Immigration of nurses to the United States has an impact on international and U.S. healthcare delivery. This is an important international policy issue, but one that is not yet resolved. Important considerations in this area include regulations (visas to enter the United States and work; nursing licensure), level of language expertise, quality of education, orientation and training needs, and potential limits on immigration of RNs. Some of the issues need to be addressed by laws, rules and regulations, and state boards of nursing and greater global collaboration. Other chapters discuss issues related to this policy concern.

Stop and Consider #2

Multiple healthcare policy issues are influencing us today.

Nursing Agenda:
Addressing Health Policy Issues

The American Nurses Association (ANA) has long advocated for a variety of healthcare issues through its membership and political action. The ANA identifies key issues that it will focus on during each congressional session. The issues vary depending upon need; for example, the ANA advocated for the passage of the ACA and spoke about changes that have been recommended by some experts and politicians. Examples of issues identified on the ANA website for early 2017 include safe staffing, safe patient handling and mobility, home health, nurse workforce development, health reform, APRNs and veterans, RN nursing home staffing, and APRNs and prescribing use of durable medical equipment (DME) (American Nurses Association [ANA], 2017). The latter issue has been successful in that former President Obama signed into law the Medicare Access and CHIP Reauthorization Act of 2015. This law provides better options for merit-based incentive payment and also allows APRNs to order DME for patients and meet documentation requirements for DME (ANA, 2015). This action opens up greater access for patients to easily get DME services with assistance from APRNs rather than just physicians.

Access to care means that care should be affordable for, available to, and acceptable to a great variety of patients. Quality of care remains a problem in the United States. The ANA supports the recommendations of the IOM *Quality Chasm* report series supporting care that is safe, timely effective, efficient, equitable, and patient centered. "The ANA believes that the development and implementation of health policies that reflect these aims, and are based on effectiveness and outcomes research, will ultimately save money" (ANA, 2005, p. 7). The organization's agendas have long addressed the critical nature of the nursing workforce and the need for an "adequate supply of well-educated, well-distributed, and well utilized registered nurses" (ANA, 2005, p. 10).

The ANA agenda is an example of how a professional organization speaks for the profession, delineates issues that need to be addressed through policies, commits to collaborating with others to accomplish the agenda, and advocates for patients through such statements and lobbying efforts. Individual nurses and nursing students should participate in this process. Other nursing professional organizations such as specialty organizations and the major nursing education organizations (the National League for Nursing and the American Association of Colleges of Nursing) are also engaged in policy as it pertains to their members and their organization goals.

Stop and Consider #3

The nursing agenda may have an impact on healthcare policy.

The Policy-Making Process

Health policy is developed at the local, state, and federal levels of government, but the two most common levels are state and federal. At the state level, the typical broad focus areas are public health and safety (for example, immunization, air quality, water safety, and so forth); care for those who cannot afford it; purchasing care through state insurance, such as for state employees; regulation (for example, RN licensure); and resource allocation (for example, funding for care services, research grants, funding for nursing education). At the federal level, there are many different needs and policy makers. The focus areas are much the same as at the state level but apply to the nation as a whole and usually are more complex because they require more collaborative efforts to ensure national acceptance.

Federal legislation is an important source of health policy. Prior to the healthcare reform legislation of 2010, the two laws that had the greatest impact on U.S. health care were the **Social Security Act of 1935** and the **Public Health Act of 1944**. The Social Security Act established the Medicare and Medicaid programs, the two major government-run healthcare reimbursement programs. The Public Health Act consolidated all existing public health legislation into one law, and it, too, has been amended over the years. Some of the programs and issues addressed in this law are health services for migratory workers, establishment of the National Institutes of Health, nurse training funding, prevention and primary care services, rural health clinics, communicable disease control, and family planning services. These laws also provided funding for nursing education through subsequent amendments to the law. An amendment to this law established *Healthy People* in 1990 and its subsequent extensions (its current iteration is *Healthy People 2020*).

The policy-making process is described in **Figure 5-2**. The first step is to recognize that an issue might require a policy. The suggestion of the

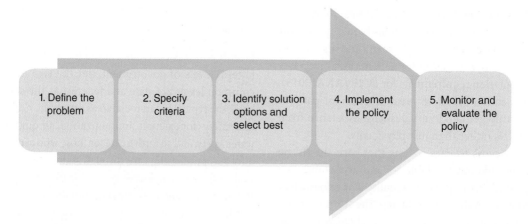

Figure 5-2 The Policy-Making Process

need for a policy can come from a variety of sources, including professional organizations, consumers/citizens, government agencies, and lawmakers.

The second step is not to develop a policy, but rather to learn more about the issue. This investigation may reveal that there is no need for a policy. There may be, and often is, disagreement about the need, and there may also be disagreement about how to resolve it if the need exists. Information and data are collected to get a clearer perspective on the issue from sources such as experts, consumers, professionals, relevant literature (such as professional literature), and research.

Using this information, policy makers then identify possible solutions. They should not consider just one solution because only under rare circumstances is a single solution possible. During this process, policy makers consider the costs and benefits of each potential solution. Costs are more than financial—a cost might be that some people will not receive a service, whereas others will. What impact will this have on both groups? After the cost–benefit analysis is done, a solution is selected, and the policy is developed. It must then go through the approval process, a process that is greatly influenced by politics.

It is at this time that implementation begins, although how a policy might be implemented must

be considered as the solution is selected and policy developed. Perhaps implementation is very complex, which in turn will affect the policy. For example, if a policy decision states that all U.S. citizens should receive healthcare insurance, the policy statement is very simple; however, when implementation is considered, this policy would be very complicated to implement. How would this be done? Who would administer it? Which funds would be used to pay for this system? What would happen to current employer coverage? Would all services be provided? How much decision-making power would the consumer have? How would providers be paid, and which providers would be paid? Many more questions could be asked. Policy development must include an implementation plan. Social, economic, legal, and ethical forces influence policy implementation. The best policy can fail if the implementation plan is not reasonable and feasible. As will be discussed in the next section on the political process, the policy often is legislation (law).

Coalition building is important in gaining support for a new policy and important in the legislative process. As will be discussed in the next section on the political process, gaining support is especially important in getting laws passed. Regarding a healthcare issue, some groups that might be included in coalition building are healthcare providers (for example, physicians, nurses, pharmacists); healthcare organizations, particularly hospitals; professional organizations (for example, the ANA, the American Medical Association, the American Hospital Association, The Joint Commission, the American Association of Colleges of Nursing, the National League for Nursing); state government and other organizations; elected officials; business leaders; third-party payers; and pharmaceutical industry representatives. Members of a coalition that support a policy may offer funding to support the effort, act as expert witnesses, develop written information in support of the policy, and work to get others to support the policy; some, such as lawmakers, may be in a position to actually vote on the legislation.

After a policy is approved and implemented, it should be monitored and its outcomes evaluated. Congress may require routine reports to ensure it is informed of the status. This type of monitoring would also apply to the state legislative process that leads to state policies. This all may lead to future changes or to the determination that a policy is not effective or may not be needed. The process may then begin again.

Stop and Consider #4

To develop effective healthcare policy, the policy-making process should be followed.

The Political Process

The preceding description of the policy-making process may seem to be a clear step-by-step process, but it is not. It is greatly influenced by politics and stakeholders who are either invested in the policy or do not want the policy. **Politics** is "the process of influencing the authoritative allocation of scarce resources" (Kalisch & Kalisch, 1982, p. 31). Typically, nurses participate in the policy-making process by using or participating in the political process. Public policy should meet the needs of the public, but in

reality, it is more complex than this. Politics influences policy development and implementation, and sometimes politics interferes with the effectiveness of policy development and implementation. Political feasibility must be considered because this aspect can mean the difference between a successful policy and an unsuccessful policy. Political support, usually from multiple groups, is critical.

As discussed, most major healthcare policy changes or new policies are made through the legislative process, though some may be made or influenced by executive or judicial components of government. Steps 1–4 of the policy-making process depicted in Figure 5-2 are similar to the legislative process steps. Once the policy is developed in the form of a proposed law, the legislative process merges with the policy-making process. The legislative process varies from state to state, but all states have a legislative process that is similar to the federal process. When a federal bill is written and then introduced in Congress, in addition to its title, it is given an identifier that includes either H.R. (House of Representatives) or S. (Senate), based on which house initiates the bill, plus a number—for example, H.R. 102. The bill is then assigned to a committee or subcommittee by the leadership of the Senate or House, depending on where the bill begins its long process to determine approval through a final vote. In the committee, the bill may figuratively die, meaning that nothing is done with it. Conversely, if there is some support for the bill, the committee or the subcommittee will assess the content. This might include holding hearings on the bill for extensive discussion, often with witnesses. Amendments may be added. If the bill began in a subcommittee, it may be sent on to a full committee, and then progress to the full House or Senate for vote. If the bill began in a committee, it might be sent directly to the full House or Senate.

When the bill gets to the full House, it first goes to the rules committee. There, decisions are made about debate on the bill, such as the length of debate. These decisions can have an impact on the successful passage of the bill. The Senate does not have a rules committee, and senators can add amendments and filibuster or delay a vote on the bill. There is more flexibility in the Senate than in the House. The leader in the Senate (majority leader) and the House leader have a great deal of power over the legislative process. A bill cannot be passed only in the House or only in the Senate and become law; rather, *both* the House and the Senate must pass the bill. Sometimes a bill is introduced at the same time in both the House and the Senate, allowing the approval process to proceed in both simultaneously. Decisions may then need to be made to reconcile differences in the two bills. If this is the case, a conference committee composed of both representatives and senators work to make those decisions. The altered bill must then go back for votes in both the House and the Senate. Funding allocation is a critical aspect of legislation and associated regulations. If both houses of Congress pass the bill, then the bill goes to the president for signature. At this time, the bill moves from the legislative branch of government to the executive branch. **Figure 5-3** identifies the branches of government.

The president has 10 days to decide whether to sign the bill into law. If the president waits longer than 10 days or Congress is no longer in session, the bill automatically becomes law just as if the president had signed it. In some cases, it is made public, either before the bill comes to the president or soon after, that the president is vetoing a bill.

This decision typically is an important political dialogue. In such a case, Congress may decide not to pursue the bill any further or Congress may decide to bring the bill back for another vote to try to override the president's veto. This effort may or may not be successful, but it often is a highly politicized situation. Depending on the number of votes, at this point the bill could either become law or die.

If the president signs the bill or if Congress overrides a presidential veto, the bill goes to the regulatory agency that would have jurisdiction over that particular law. For example, a health law would typically go to the HHS. If the law relates to Medicare, it would go to the Centers for Medicare and Medicaid Services (CMS), an agency within the HHS. It is at this point that a very important step in the process occurs: Rules or regulations are written for the law that state specifically how the law will be implemented, and their content and implementation make a significant difference in the effectiveness of the law. At specific steps in the regulatory development process, the public, including healthcare professionals such as nurses, can participate by providing input. It is important that this input be given. Once the final rules are approved, the law is implemented. There may be a date that the law ends, or "sunsets." If so, the law may expire, or it may be reintroduced into the legislative process.

Not all interested parties accept a policy, and efforts may be made to defeat a policy. Because of the various viewpoints on the same issue, there are often competing interests (Abood, 2007). In addition, partisan issues—that is, Democrat versus Republican—may affect the policy development process. "Decision-makers rely mainly on the political process as a way to find a course of action that is acceptable to the various individuals with conflicting proposals, demands, and values. . . . Throughout our daily lives, politics determines who gets what, when, and how" (Abood, 2007, p. 3).

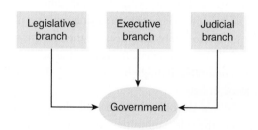

Figure 5-3 The Branches of the U.S. Federal Government

Nurses' Role in the Political Process: Impact on Healthcare Policy

As healthcare professionals, nurses bring a unique perspective to healthcare policy development because of their education, clinical expertise, professional values and ethics, advocacy skills, experience with the interprofessional healthcare team, and understanding of health and healthcare delivery. Significant progress has occurred over the years toward advancing nursing's presence, role, and influence in the development of healthcare policy. However, more nurses need to learn how to identify issues strategically; work with decision makers; understand who holds the power in the workplace, communities, and state- and federal-level organizations and government; and understand who controls the resources for healthcare services (Ferguson, 2001). Many schools of nursing offer courses on health policy particularly graduate courses, or health policy content is integrated in courses such as a course that uses this text. Nursing publications, textbooks, and journals also focus on health policy. These courses or content help to prepare all nurses to better understand policy and how they might be involved in health policy at multiple levels.

Although the nursing profession has gained political power, it is still weaker than it should be. Put simply, given the large number of nurses in the United States, the profession should have more influential power. Each nurse is a potential voter and, therefore, has potential influence over who will be elected and which legislative decisions are made. However, nursing as a profession has struggled with organizing, and this weakness has diluted the political power of nurses in the United States. At the most basic level, nurses have experienced serious problems defining the profession. The use of multiple entry levels, licensure issues, and multiple titles confuse the public and other healthcare professionals. Policy makers may not understand the various nursing roles and titles, which in turn makes it difficult for nurses to speak with one voice for nursing.

Nurses need to develop political competence. **Political competence** involves the ability to use opportunities, including networking, highlighting nursing expertise, using powerful persuasion, demonstrating a commitment to working with others, thinking strategically, and persevering. It means being aware of the rules of the game and recognizing that the other side needs something. Sometimes giving up or modifying one viewpoint or action may lead to more effective results. Collective strength can be powerful, so finding partners makes a difference. Nurses can network to find those partners. Sometimes partners may be found in the least likely groups.

A policy is a tool for change, and nurses are very adept at working with change—something they do in practice on a daily basis. This capability should help nurses develop political competence. "Successful advocacy depends on having the power, the will, the time, and the energy, along with the political skills needed to 'play the game' in the legislative area" (Abood, 2007, p. 3). How can nurses have an impact on healthcare policy? This is what needs to be emphasized.

Getting into the Political System and Making It Work for Nursing

Lobbying is a critical part of the U.S. political process, and nurses are involved in lobbying. A **lobbyist** is a person who represents a specific interest or interest group that tries to influence policy making. The First Amendment to the U.S. Constitution gives citizens the right to lobby—to assemble and to petition the government for redress of grievances. Lobbyists try to influence legislators—the decision makers—as well as public opinion. They often collaborate via coalitions and work with other interest groups to gain more support for a specific interest. Lobbyists particularly want to make contact with legislative staff. The legislative staff assume a major role in getting data about an issue; formulating solutions that may become bills, writing bills, and, if those bills are passed, become laws; and communicating with elected representatives, their bosses, to accept a particular approach or solution. Nurses who visit state and federal representatives typically meet with legislative staff. This is a form of lobbying.

Professional organizations hire staff to be lobbyists at both state and federal levels. The ANA, the National League for Nursing (NLN), the American Association of Colleges of Nursing (AACN), and other nursing organizations, for example, have lobbyists in Washington, DC. Lobbyists may be nurses or persons who are informed about nursing and work with nurses to provide the best information to move an issue forward that supports nursing. **Exhibit 5-2** identifies the federal government agencies monitored by the ANA so that the organization is aware of legislative and regulatory activities and can impact policy.

At both the state and federal levels of government, the legislative branches are highly dependent on committees. Legislative work occurs mainly within committees. If legislation (a bill) gets "stuck" in a committee, this can be the critical barrier to passage of the bill. An example is a recent bill that addresses registered nurse staffing (S.1132), from the 114th Congress (2015–2016) (Congress.gov, 2017). This bill was sent to the Committee on Finance and has not moved forward. The bill focuses on requiring hospital-wide staffing plans to meet needs of patients and delivery of quality care. This bill, at this time, will not pass and is dead. This type of result indicates an inability to gain support for a bill; reasons may vary, such as the bill's policy issue, content of the bill, other bills that may conflict or be more important, disagreement among stakeholders, and more. There are committees on both sides of the federal legislative body, the House and the Senate. Some of the healthcare-related committees in the U.S. Congress are identified in **Exhibit 5-3**.

Within the House and the Senate, committees have representatives from both major parties, Democrat and Republican. The party with the majority in the House and in the Senate decides who will chair committees and who will serve on each committee. To effectively influence legislation, it is important to understand which committee will be involved in the legislation and who is on the committee. What are the chair's and the committee members' views on the issue? How can they be persuaded? Knowing

---

Exhibit 5-2   Important Federal Government Departments and Agencies

U.S. Department of Health and Human Services (HHS): http://www.hhs.gov

Agency for Healthcare Research and Quality (AHRQ): http://www.ahrq.gov

Centers for Medicare and Medicaid Services (CMS): http://www.cms.hhs.gov

Centers for Disease Control and Prevention (CDC): http://www.cdc.gov

U.S. Consumer Product Safety Commission (CPSC): http://www.cpsc.gov

U.S. Food and Drug Administration (FDA): http://www.fda.gov

National Institute for Occupational Safety and Health (NIOSH): http://www.cdc.gov/NIOSH

National Institutes of Health (NIH): http://www.nih.gov

Occupational Safety and Health Administration (OSHA): http://www.osha.gov

Department of Veterans Affairs (VA): http://www.va.gov

Exhibit 5-3 U.S. Congressional Committees with Jurisdiction over Health Matters

U.S. House of Representatives

- House Appropriations Committee
- House Commerce Committee
- House Commerce Committee Subcommittee on Health and Environment
- House Ways and Means Committee
- House Ways and Means Committee Subcommittee on Health

U.S. Senate

- Senate Appropriations Committee
- Health, Education, Labor and Pensions Committee
- Health, Education, Labor and Pensions Committee Subcommittee on Public Health
- Senate Finance Committee
- Senate Finance Committee Subcommittee on Health Care

this information can help develop a more effective strategy to influence the policy content and chance of success, maybe identifying approaches to gain more support from stakeholders. There may need to be some compromises and negotiating.

Political action committees (PACs) are very important in the political process. A PAC is a private group, whose size can vary, that works to get someone elected or defeated. PACs represent a specific issue or group. The Federal Election Campaign Act of 1971 covers PACs and how organizations may use them. The law defines a PAC as an organization that receives contributions or makes expenditures of at least $1,000 for the purpose of influencing an election. Other rules about PAC operations are also identified. PACs do not force organization members to vote on certain candidates—this is always an individual choice even if a PAC supports a candidate.

Why would nurses need to know about PACs? The nursing profession has its own PACs, such as the ANA PAC. The ANA considers political action to be a core mission activity, and its PAC is critical to its success on Capitol Hill (ANA, 2016). The PAC is a form of political advocacy that focuses on supporting candidates who support nursing issues. This organization endorses candidates, makes minimal campaign donations based on legal requirements, and campaigns for candidates. The decision to support a candidate is not based on the candidate's party,

but rather on whether the candidate supports issues important to nursing. In the end, this empowers the PAC members—in this case, nurses. The ANA PAC's overall goal is to improve the healthcare system in the United States. Any nurse can join this PAC by making a contribution to support the PAC's candidate choice and participate in determining who will be supported.

Nurses need to work to get their message across using grassroots advocacy. Many nurses communicate directly with legislators about specific issues of concern. One method of doing so is through written communication. In the past, this was primarily done through letter writing, but now it is easier, and preferred by legislators, to use email for this purpose. Email is more efficient, and it allows nurses to respond quickly to a request to communicate their views. This request may come from a nursing organization, as a result of a personal recognition that something is going on that affects health care and nursing, or from a colleague.

In written communication to legislators, even if through electronic means, it is important to state what the issue is, provide the bill number (if the correspondence is related to a pending bill), succinctly state one's position, and provide a brief rationale. The communication should include one's full name, credentials, employment location, contact information, and voting district. To be more effective, the best contact is the nurse's elected representatives. Another method of communication is to call elected representatives' offices. Before making the call, the nurse should prepare a brief statement that addresses the specific issue. A third method of communication is to visit elected representatives' offices. This could be an elected official's local office, office in the state capital, or in Washington, DC. The nurse probably will meet with the legislative staff, preferably staff responsible for health issues. This is not a step down because staff members play a major role in the process. Make an appointment if possible and be on time. The meeting may be short or long. Be engaging, and let the staff or representative/senator know what you do as a nurse, where you work, and relevant nursing and healthcare concerns. Be prepared to discuss both the topic and the activities of the representative—legislation and other interests. Provide specific information and stories that support facts, avoid generalities, and information should be useful. Present your information concisely—staff and legislators are busy. Students who visit legislators or their staff, for example, might discuss the need for scholarships and financial aid monies, providing examples of how this support helps students to meet career goals and provides more nurses. Follow-up is important; send a thank-you note with a reminder of the discussion.

All these examples related to policy demonstrate leadership by nurses who participate in these efforts to advocate for health care. **Exhibit 5-4** summarizes some tips for making such grassroots efforts more effective.

Exhibit 5-4 Grassroots Tips

Letter or E-Mail Communication with Legislators or Staff

- Make sure your topic is clear.
- Do not assume anything.
- Get the facts and share them as need.
- Be brief and concise.
- Find a local focus—what is important to your city, county, state and so on.
- Make it personal.
- Identify that you are a nurse and include your credentials—for example, "I am a registered nurse who works at Hospital Y in Middletown, Missouri."
- Include your contact information.

Contact with Legislators or Staff

- State: Call the state legislative body, get a directory, or visit your state government's website.
- Federal: Visit senator or representative websites (For federal representatives: http://www.house.gov; http://www.senate.gov).
- Prepare what you will say before you make contact; consider the comments made earlier about written communication.

- Be sure to communicate up front the focus of your contact—why you are contacting the legislator.

Visiting Members of Congress or State Legislature

- You can visit when a representative is in the home district, state capitol office if state legislator, or in Washington, DC.
- You should make an appointment.
- Follow all guides mentioned for other methods of contact. Time will be short, so you need to be on time, prepared, and also be prepared to wait.
- Do not be disappointed if you meet with a staff person. Staff members are very important and give the representative or senator information to make decisions and, in some cases, are very involved in the decision making.
- Be ready to answer questions; prepare for this possibility.
- Dress professionally.
- Enjoy yourself and be proud that you are a professional nurse and an expert.

Nursing organizations are involved in policy development through lobbying, members and officers serving as expert witnesses to government groups and agencies, and publishing information about issues in both professional and nonprofessional literature. Radio and television journalists may interview nurses. These activities place nurses directly in the policy-making process and also improve nurses' public image as experts and consumer advocates.

The AACN holds student policy summits to inform students, such as graduate students, about involvement in Capitol Hill visits and policy work. Student participants then make visits to Capitol Hill with school of nursing deans and directors. Information is provided for all who make these visits so that they are prepared with the facts. The AACN faculty and dean conferences in Washington, DC, typically include visits to Congress and/or conduct sessions in which representatives and senators are invited to speak with attendees about nursing education and the profession in general and implications for healthcare delivery.

There are numerous opportunities for nurses to gain some experience in the area of government practice. For example, fellowships—many of which are short term—at the federal and state levels provide opportunities for nurses to learn more about politics and the legislative process and interact with people who work in government. This is a great way to learn more about health policy and potential government job opportunities. Graduate programs that focus on health policy provide formal academic experiences that can lead to a career in the health policy field.

Some nurses seek election to government positions at local, state, and federal levels. Others serve as staff in health-related government agencies. Nurses who serve in government positions use their nursing expertise, and this provides many opportunities for nurses to be more visible at all levels of the government—legislative, administrative, and judicial. However, there needs to be greater representation of nurses in these positions. Running for office at any level requires political support, finances, and guidance from those experienced in the world of politics and campaigning. If you choose to pursue this path, be aware that it takes time to build up support for a campaign.

There are also government staff who may be nurses in many levels of government. These positions provide great opportunities for nurses to use their expertise and to participate in health policy development and implementation. Nurses have served in high-level government positions. For example, in 2013, Marilyn Tavenner, MHA, BSN, RN, was confirmed as the administrator of the Centers for Medicare and Medicaid Services, which is part of the HHS. This is a very important position providing oversight for the federal government's (and the nation's) largest entitlement program. In 2015, she left this government position and assumed a high level position at the American Health Insurance Plans (AHIP) (Matthews, 2015).

Stop and Consider #5

You can participate in the political process to advocate for health care and for the nursing profession.

Patient Protection and
the Affordable Care Act of 2010

Over the years, there have been many attempts to reform the U.S. healthcare delivery system. Most of these efforts have failed. Political issues have typically limited progress in this area—healthcare delivery is a critical political issue because it affects taxes and is a very expensive business. The 2008 presidential election brought healthcare reform to the forefront again. As was true with other efforts, nursing organizations got involved and spoke out about proposed changes. It was very important that nursing do this because healthcare reform would definitely have an impact on nursing, and it has proven to have an impact during its implementation.

In 2010, Congress passed significant legislation, known as the Patient Protection and Affordable Care Act (ACA); it was signed into law by President Obama. The purpose of the law was to reform some aspects of healthcare insurance coverage in the United States. Although universal healthcare coverage was not included in the final bill owing to a lack of political support, more people in the United States obtained health insurance coverage under this law. It did not change the traditional employer-based approach to U.S. health insurance.

The healthcare delivery system has experienced changes as a result of the various reform efforts. Nurses are assuming new roles and changing old ones—for example, APRNs, nurse managers, clinical nurse leaders, and clinical nurse specialists. Their roles may vary, and more opportunities are opening up. In some cases, nurses with these advanced degrees are eligible for admitting privileges, meaning that they can admit their patients to the hospital from private practice or clinics. This is not the norm, but it does occur. Healthcare reform and other critical sources such as the report, *The future of nursing* emphasize the need to expand use of APRNs in primary care (IOM, 2010). The United States is experiencing a lack of primary care providers, and with the changes in healthcare reform increasing the number of people who have health insurance coverage, there is even greater demand for these providers.

The large number of patients who cannot pay for services and have no insurance coverage causes major financial problems for hospitals. In some situations, this may lead to the closing of units and fewer beds (decreasing the size of the hospital); termination of staff; and, in extreme cases, the closing of hospitals. Patient access to care has become a major problem in some

communities. Access is more than just the ability to get an appointment; it involves the availability of services at times convenient for the patient (time of day and day of week); transportation to and from the care facility; reimbursement for care; and receipt of the right type of care, such as from a specialist. An increase in U.S. citizens with insurance coverage, such as what occurred with the ACA, has an impact on these services and the ability to cover costs.

Healthcare reform continues to have an impact on nursing education, nursing practice, regulation of nursing, and professional roles. There are provisions in the ACA that relate to issues other than reimbursement, such as quality care, funding for healthcare provider education, workforce issues, and more. The provisions did not all go into effect at one time, which means the final results will not be determined for some time, and now with potential changes due to the new administration, this may have an effect, too.

Since the passage of the ACA, there have been efforts made through the court system to diminish the effects of the ACA, and part of the ACA has been declared unconstitutional, so the long-term impact of the 2010 healthcare reform remains unknown due to court issues and to a new administration—changes in the ACA or repeal of the law and a new law. It is important for nurses to engage in the process that might bring changes to this law and be informed of the changes because they will not only affect the number of persons insured, but as noted, there are ACA provisions that focus on quality care and also nursing education, particularly funding. In the future, these provisions could be deleted or changed.

Stop and Consider #6

The Patient Protection and Affordable Care Act of 2010 is a law that is changing.

CHAPTER HIGHLIGHTS

1. Healthcare policy directly affects nurses and nursing.
2. Nurses participate in policy making by sharing their expertise, serving on policy-making committees, working with consumers to get their needs known, and serving in elected offices.
3. A policy is a course of action that affects a large number of people inspired by a specific need to achieve certain outcomes.
4. Policies are associated with roles and standards; specific laws and related programs, such as Medicare and Medicaid; delineation of reimbursement requirements for services; staffing levels; access to care; policies and procedures; and nursing education.
5. Examples of critical healthcare policy issues relevant to nursing are variable nursing shortage and staffing, the cost of health care, healthcare quality and disparities, consumer issues, commercialization of health care, reimbursement for nursing care, and immigration and the nursing workforce.
6. The policy-making process and the political process are connected, and it is important that nurses understand these processes in their advocacy efforts on behalf of consumers and for better health care.
7. Methods that nurses use when involved in the policy-making and political processes are lobbying, interacting with legislative committees, serving on PACs, participating in grassroots advocacy, working with elected officials who are nurses, and serving as elected officials.
8. In 2010, the U.S. Congress passed, and President Obama signed, significant healthcare legislation that has led to increasing the number of citizens with health insurance, but the final result is still not full universal healthcare coverage. This reform (Affordable Care Act of 2010 or ACA) has an impact nursing education, practice, regulation, and roles nurses assume.

ENGAGING IN THE CONTENT

Discussion Questions

1. Why is policy important to nursing?
2. Describe the relationship between the policy-making process and the political process.
3. Discuss the roles of nurses in the policy-making process.
4. Why is advocacy a critical part of policy making?
5. Discuss the methods nurses use to get involved in the policy-making process and the political process.

CRITICAL THINKING ACTIVITIES

1. Select one of the following topics and search the Internet to learn more about the issue. Why would this issue be of interest to nursing? Why would this be a healthcare policy issue for a state or nationally, or both? Has anything been done recently to initiate legislation on this issue? Teams of students can work on an issue and then share their work.

   a. Rural health care
   b. Mental health parity
   c. Aging and long-term care
   d. Healthcare unions
   e. Home care
   f. Emergency room diversions

2. Visit the ANA's *Health Care Reform Headquarters* webpage (http://www.rnaction .org/site/PageServer?pagename=nstat_take _action_healthcare_reform) and review the content provided on healthcare reform and other policy issues. Look at the list of resources and select one to review. What does this resource provide nurses? Look at the Toolkit. Here you will find a list of current legislative/policy. What are they? Select one and examine the issue. Discuss your findings with your classmates.

3. Form a debate team to address the following questions: How would you support or not support universal health care in the United States? How does the ACA affect this problem? The team should base its viewpoint on facts and relevant resources. Present the debate in class or online. Viewers (students who are not on the debate team) should vote for the viewpoint that they think is most persuasive.

4. The AHRQ provides several modules and a toolkit on informed consent. The toolkit on informed consent can be viewed at https:// www.ahrq.gov/funding/policies/informed consent/index.html and the modules at https://www.ahrq.gov/professionals/systems /hospital/informedchoice/index.html. Review the information, and identify three facts you did not know about informed consent.

ELECTRONIC REFLECTION JOURNAL

Describe your personal view of nurses getting involved in politics. Would you get involved? Why or why not?

CASE STUDIES

Case 1

A nurse works in community health in a very large urban neighborhood of mostly African Americans and Hispanics. The socioeconomic level of the area is low, with most people eligible for or covered by Medicaid and Medicare. The nurse is concerned about the level of care that community members' children receive. Clinic services are inadequate, and the

CASE STUDIES (CONTINUED)

hours of the clinics that are available often make it difficult for working parents to access services for their children and for themselves. The teens in the area are involved in a lot of drug activity and have little to do after school. The neighborhood has one high school, one middle school, and one elementary school. There are two small daycare centers for preschoolers run by the city. The nurse is motivated to tackle some of these problems, but she is not sure how to go about it.

Case Questions

1. Identify critical problems the nurse might identify.
2. Do these problems have health policy relevance? Why or why not?
3. What steps do you think the nurse should take in light of what you have learned about health policy in this chapter? Be specific regarding stakeholders, strategies, and political issues to consider.

Case 2

You have joined a nursing specialty organization. After you join, you decide you want to be active by volunteering for the Legislative Committee. At the first meeting you attend, the major topic is the upcoming state elections.

Case Questions

1. How should the committee prepare for the elections?
2. If you are going to visit a candidate, what might you do to prepare, and what type of questions might you ask?
3. What types of election activities might the committee recommend to the organization membership?

Working Backward to Develop a Case

Write a brief paragraph that describes a case related to the following questions.

1. A nurse comments, "Why should we get involved?"
2. The discussion leads to a question, "What is important to us?"
3. How might we use our elected officials?

REFERENCES

Abood, S. (2007). Influencing healthcare in the legislative arena. *Online Journal of Issues in Nursing, 12*(1), 3.

American Nurses Association. (2005). *ANA's health care agenda—2005.* Silver Spring, MD: Author.

American Nurses Association. (2015). *APRNs and DME.* Retrieved from http://www.rnaction.org/site /PageServer?pagename=nstat_take_action_dme.html

American Nurses Association. (2016). *ANA political action committee.* Retrieved from http://www.rnaction.org/site/PageNavigator/NSTAT/nstat_ana_pac

American Nurses Association. (2017). *Take action.* Retrieved from http://www.rnaction.org/site/PageServer?pagename=nstat_issues

Block, L. (2008). Health policy: What it is and how it works. In C. Harrington & C. Estes (Eds.), *Health policy* (5th ed., pp. 4–14). Burlington, MA: Jones & Bartlett Learning.

Coffey, J. (2001). Universal health coverage. *American Journal of Nursing, 101*(2), 11.

Congress.gov. (2017). *S.1132 Registered Nurse Safe Staffing Act of 2015.* Retrieved from https://www.congress.gov/bill/114th-congress/senate-bill/1132

Ferguson, S. (2001). An activist looks at nursing's role in health policy development. *Journal of Obstetric, Gynecologic, and Neonatal Nursing, 30,* 546–551.

Institute of Medicine. (2002). *Unequal treatment: Confronting racial and ethnic disparities in health care.* Washington, DC: The National Academies Press.

Institute of Medicine. (2004). *Health literacy: A prescription to end confusion.* Washington, DC: The National Academies Press.

Institute of Medicine. (2010). *The future of nursing: Leading change, advancing health.* Washington, DC: The National Academies Press.

Kalisch, B., & Kalisch, P. (1982). *Politics of nursing.* Philadelphia, PA: Lippincott.

Matthews, M. (2015, July 17). *Tavenner is the perfect fit for AHIP as big insurers become public utilities.* Retrieved from http://www.forbes.com/sites/merrillmatthews/2015/07/17/tavenner-is-the-perfect-pick-for-ahip-as-big-insurers-become-public-utilities/#47e27e29419b

Shi, L., & Singh, D. (2015). *Delivering health care in America* (6th ed.). Gaithersburg, MD: Aspen.

Sullivan, L. (2004). *Missing persons: Minorities in the health professions.* A report of the Sullivan Commission on diversity in the healthcare workforce. Retrieved from http://www.aacn.nche.edu/Media/pdf/SullivanReport.pdf

U.S. Department of Health and Human Services, & Agency for Healthcare Research and Quality. (2017a). *About the national quality strategy.* Retrieved from https://www.ahrq.gov/workingforquality/about.htm

U.S. Department of Health and Human Services, & Agency for Healthcare Research and Quality. (2017b). *National healthcare quality and disparities report.* Retrieved from https://www.ahrq.gov/research/findings/nhqrdr/index.html

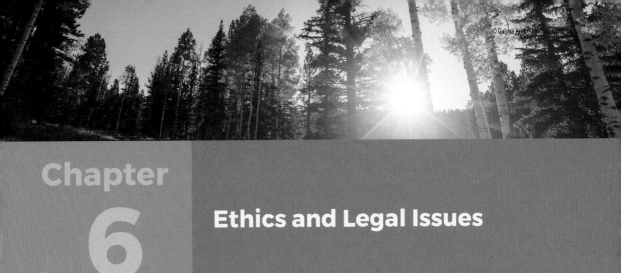

Chapter 6

Ethics and Legal Issues

© Galyna Andrushko/Shutterstock

CHAPTER OBJECTIVES

At the conclusion of this chapter, the learner will be able to:

- Apply ethical principles to decision making with consideration of the importance of ethics to the nursing profession.
- Examine the implications of healthcare fraud and abuse, research ethics, and organizational ethics.
- Discuss the relevance of legal issues such as malpractice to nursing practice.
- Discuss examples of ethical and legal issues in healthcare delivery.

CHAPTER OUTLINE

- Introduction
- Ethics and Ethical Principles
  - Definitions
  - Ethical Principles
  - Ethical Decision Making
  - Professional Ethics and Nursing Practice
  - American Nurses Association Code of Ethics
  - Reporting Incompetent, Unethical, or Illegal Practices
- Critical Ethical Issues in Healthcare Delivery
  - Healthcare Fraud and Abuse
  - Ethics and Research
    - Research: Informed Consent
    - Research: Risk of Physical Harm
    - Research: Risk of Psychological Harm
    - Research: Risk of Social and Economic Harm
  - Organizational Ethics
- Legal Issues: An Overview
  - Critical Terminology
  - Malpractice: Why Should This Concern You?
- Examples of Issues with Ethical and Legal Implications
  - Privacy, Confidentiality, and Informed Consent
  - Rationing Care: Who Can Access Care when Needed
  - Advance Directives, Living Wills, Medical Powers of Attorney, and Do-Not-Resuscitate Orders
  - Organ Transplantation

- Assisted Suicide
- Social Media and Ethical and Legal Issues: A New Concern
- Chapter Highlights
- Engaging in the Content
  - Discussion Questions
- Critical Thinking Activities
- Electronic Reflection Journal
- Case Studies
- Working Backward to Develop a Case
- References

KEY TERMS

Advance directives
Breach of confidentiality
Breach of duty
Confidentiality
Ethical decision making
Ethical dilemma
Ethical principles

Ethics
Fraud
Informed consent
Invasion of privacy
Living will
Malpractice
Medical power of attorney

Moral disengagement
Morals
Negligence
Organizational ethics
Professional ethics
Whistleblowing

Introduction

The content in this chapter addresses ethics and legal issues in nursing. As a profession, nursing has ethical responsibilities, which in some cases are connected to legal issues and in others are not related. In the practice of nursing, ethical and legal issues often arise, and the nurse must understand them and take appropriate steps to address them. These issues involve professionalism, practice concerns, health policy, reimbursement issues, and the organizations that provide health care.

Ethics and Ethical
Principles

All healthcare professionals consider ethics in their practice whether they recognize it or not. Nurses need to understand ethics and the ethical principles that drive healthcare decisions and the nursing profession as a whole.

Definitions

The first question that could be asked in this type of content is *what is ethics*? It is easy to confuse ethics with morals. **Morals** refer to an individual's code of acceptable behavior, and they shape one's values that are influenced by cultural factors and experiences. **Ethics** refers to a standardized code or guide to behaviors. Morals are learned through growth and development, whereas application of ethics typically is learned through a more organized system, such as a standardized ethics code developed by a professional group. Ethics deals with the rightness and wrongness of behavior. Bioethics relates to decisions and behavior related to life-and-death issues. The latter sometimes comes in conflict with a patient's morals, values, and ethics and a nurse's personal morals, values, and ethics. There may also be conflict between a nurse's and an organization's approach to morals, values, and ethics. Health policy also involves ethical decision making, particularly when cost–benefit analysis is used.

Ethical Principles

Four **ethical principles** are used in nursing and healthcare delivery; they are highlighted in **Figure 6-1**. Ethics is a difficult area, and these principles help guide nurses when confronted with ethical issues. Throughout this chapter, the term *patient* will be used, but in the case of a minor or a person who is under legal guardianship or power of attorney, *patient* refers to the family or the guardian, who makes the decisions in such cases. The four principles are autonomy, beneficence, justice, and veracity:

- *Autonomy* focuses on the patient's right to make decisions about matters that affect the patient. This means that if the patient wants to be involved in treatment decisions, the patient makes the final decisions about treatment. To do so, patients need complete and open information or informed consent. The nurse's role is to provide information to better ensure that others, such as the physician,

inform the patient, and then to support the patient's decision. Supporting the patient's decision is not always easy because the nurse may think that the patient is making the wrong decision. It is not the role of the nurse to argue with the patient, but rather to act as the patient's advocate, respecting the patient's choice. The nurse can discuss the decision with the patient and ensure that the patient recognizes the potential consequences of decisions. This principle is directly related to patient-centered care.

- *Beneficence* relates to doing something good and caring for the patient. This principle encompasses more than just physical care—it involves awareness of the patient's situation and needs. In the case of nurses, this also means doing no harm and safeguarding the patient, or non-maleficence.
- *Justice* is about treating people fairly—for example, when deciding which patients receive treatment and which patients do not. There are more concerns about justice in health care today because of problems with disparity (for example, some people are not getting care when they need it). Lack of justice can lead to disparities in health care, and then it can also have an impact on quality care.
- *Veracity* means truth. For example, which information is the patient given during the informed consent process? Trust plays a major role in this principle. Veracity can be a difficult principle to apply because, sometimes, a family member may request that the patient not be fully informed. Such a request is in direct conflict with ethical practices and patient-centered care. Some believe that if another principle is involved, it might be considered first, before veracity comes into play. For example, if it is believed that the truth would cause more harm, does beneficence outweigh veracity? In any ethical dilemma, it is important to remember that

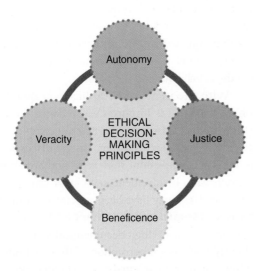

Figure 6-1 Ethical Decision-Making Principles

no two situations are the same. Trust is also related to the requirements for informed consent and patient privacy and confidentiality.

Other principles have been suggested that are applicable in today's healthcare delivery system—for instance, advocacy, caring, stewardship (management of finite resources), respect, honesty, and confidentiality (Koloroutis & Thorstenson, 1999).

Ethical Decision Making

Ethical decision making is about ethical dilemmas. An **ethical dilemma** occurs when a person is forced to choose between two or more alternatives, none of which is ideal. Typically, strong emotions are tied to the issue and the alternative solutions, and it is not possible to say that one is better than the other. If an ethical dilemma arises and the nurse is involved in the care, the nurse should participate in the decision making. If the nurse is not involved in the issue, then the nurse should not step in unless the situation is critical.

Once the ethical dilemma is recognized, the next step is assessment to get facts. What are the medical facts, including information about treatment? What are the psychosocial facts? What does the patient want? Which values are involved, and what is the conflict? Getting this information requires talking to others, including the patient and—if the patient approves—the family, significant others, and other healthcare providers. Neither the nurse nor the physician makes the decision about sharing information with family or significant others, nor do they make the final decision about treatment unless the patient is in an emergency situation and cannot speak for himself or herself. The treatment team provides recommendations to the patient. Sometimes it may be the nurse who thinks that the treatment team does not recognize the presence of an ethical dilemma; in this case, the nurse discusses this observation with the team. After the assessment is concluded, the information is used to develop a plan to address the dilemma. This requires looking at the choices, goals, and parties involved. Options need to be prioritized.

Key to all of this is patient involvement, if the patient is able and willing to participate in the decision-making process. The decision must be one that the patient accepts. During implementation, the nurse must be the patient's advocate, even if the nurse does not agree with the patient's final decision.

Professional Ethics and Nursing Practice

Ethics is a part of any profession, and in nursing, **professional ethics** is part of daily practice. Benner, Sutphen, Leonard, and Day (2010) emphasize that nursing education needs to focus more on ethical conduct. Students need to develop skills to respond ethically when making ethical decisions, which may involve responding to situations in which errors occurred. "Nurses need the skill of ethical reflection to discern moral dilemmas and injustices created by inept or incompetent health care, by an inequitable healthcare delivery system, or by the competing claims of family members or other members of the healthcare team" (Benner et al., 2010, p. 28). It is not easy to find the "right" perspective on ethics in professional roles and in the care provided. Each nurse works to find this perspective and determine how it meshes with the nurse's personal views. This is the potential dilemma between the nurse's view of ethical behavior and the patient's.

With the increased emphasis on quality improvement it is important to recognize that ethical and legal issues are related to quality care, particularly when errors occur. There is discussion in other chapters about staff stress and how this impacts care. Involvement in an error can cause stress or stress may have been a factor in causing the error. **Moral disengagement** is "the process that involves justifying one's unethical actions by altering one's moral perception of those actions" (Hyatt, 2016, p. 15, as cited from Bandura, 1999). A common response is displacement of responsibility or shifting of blame—it was not my responsibility; it was someone else's. Why does this happen to staff? One reason may be the work environment is not healthy and staff members withdraw from taking responsibility. Another reason may be the staff wants to do what is expected (an ethical action), but there are barriers in the organization to achieving this, such as rules, time issues, and so on. This leads to moral distress, which can lead to anger, hopelessness, depression, and compassion fatigue. This works in a cyclic fashion in that moral distress may result in more moral distress for the organization, resulting in a hostile work environment, staff and management passive-aggressive behavior, increased problems with errors, working around the system (discussed in more detail in content about quality improvement), and retention of staff (Hyatt, 2016). It is important that nurses and healthcare organizations support a healthy work environment to prevent or reduce these problems that negatively affect care improvement.

American Nurses Association Code of Ethics

Professional organizations such as the American Nurses Association (ANA) developed a code of ethics with interpretative statements to help nurses understand the intent of the guiding principles. The *Guide to the code of ethics for nurses: Interpretation and application* (ANA, 2015) is the primary source or guide for nurses when ethical issues are encountered. A nursing code of ethics was first discussed in the United States in 1896. Several editions of this code have been issued to ensure that the content and expectations stay current with practice and healthcare issues and analysis of the code (Fowler, 2015). The *Code of Ethics* may change over time, but it also has consistent elements that have been retained.

Obtaining a registered nurse (RN) license and entering the profession requires that nurses meet the professional roles and responsibilities identified by nursing. Ethics is a part of professionalism.

Self-reflection, or the ability to look at a variety of possibilities and consider pros and cons, is also important. It is part of critical thinking and is particularly important when there does not seem to be one right answer, which is the case when an ethical dilemma is experienced. The ANA *Code of Ethics* provisions are described in **Exhibit 6-1**.

Reporting Incompetent, Unethical, or Illegal Practices

Every nurse, regardless of degree preparation or position, has a responsibility to report incompetent, unethical, or illegal practices to the nurse's state board of nursing (ANA, 2015; Burman & Dunphy, 2011; National Council of State Boards of Nursing [NCSBN], 2011), there is, however, variation from state to state as to requirements for reporting. Others can also report nurses, such as employers, consumers, and family members. Each state's nurse practice act (law) serves as the guide for the nurses in the state. This law should be familiar to all licensed nurses. Nurse practice acts vary from state to state because each act is considered part of a state's laws and is not administered at the federal level.

State boards of nursing have specific processes and procedures that must be followed regarding making and handling complaints. The source of a complaint remains private. This confidentiality is intended to protect the person who reports the complaint as well as to eliminate fear of reprisal that would limit reporting of complaints. Among the common complaints brought to a state board of nursing are using illicit drugs or alcohol while practicing, stealing drugs from a healthcare organization, committing a serious error that might demonstrate incompetence, and falsifying records. It is important to remember that a complaint or an initiative by the board to investigate a nurse does not mean that the nurse is guilty. The legal process that must be followed by the state board provides rights for the nurse, rights that can be used to defend one self.

Exhibit 6-1 American Nurses Association Code of Ethics for Nurses

Provision 1

The nurse practices compassion and respect for the inherent dignity, worth, and unique attributes of every person.

Provision 2

The nurse's primary commitment is to the patient, whether an individual, family, group, community, or population.

Provision 3

The nurse promotes, advocates for, and protects and rights, health, and safety of the patient.

Provision 4

The nurse has authority, accountability, and responsibility for nursing practice; makes decisions; and takes action consistent with the obligation to promote health and to provide optimal care.

Provision 5

The nurse owes the same duties to self as to others, including the responsibility to promote health and safety, preserve wholeness of character and integrity, maintain competence, and continue personal and professional growth.

Provision 6

The nurse, through individual and collective effort, establishes, maintains, and improves the ethical environment of the work setting and conditions of employment that are conducive to safe, quality health care.

Provision 7

The nurse, in all roles and settings, advances the profession through research and scholarly inquiry, professional standards development, and the generation of both nursing and health policy.

Provision 8

The nurse collaborates with other health professionals and the public to protect human rights, promote health diplomacy, and reduce health disparities.

Provision 9

The profession of nursing, collectively through its professional organizations, must articulate nursing values, maintain the integrity of the profession, and integrate principles of social justice into nursing and health policy.

Any nurse who is informed of a board of nursing complaint or recognizes that such a complaint might be filed should consult with an attorney. This legal advisor should not be the same attorney who represents the nurse's employer; rather, the nurse should retain the services of a personal attorney.

Dealing with disciplinary actions is a major responsibility of boards of nursing. The media, legislators, and policy makers are interested in disciplinary actions that the boards take. A board of nursing has to find a balance between protecting the public and protecting the individual nurse's right to practice and the nurse's right to due process.

In some situations, such as when a nurse is accused of drug abuse, the state board of nursing may offer the option of entering an alternative program. These programs are not treatment programs, but rather monitoring programs. However, they do give nurses who meet specified criteria the opportunity to maintain their licensure and to practice. The nurse must agree to enter a nondisciplinary program that provides identification and treatment support; agree to monitoring upon return to practice; and often agree to submit to regular drug testing. The risk of public knowledge about a drug problem may compel a nurse to accept the alternative program. Compliance with treatment and aftercare recommendations is also required. Return to practice or continuation of practice is not guaranteed, and the nurse is carefully monitored to ensure public safety.

Stop and Consider #1

RNs are required to report incompetent, unethical, or illegal practice.

Critical Ethical Issues
in Healthcare Delivery

Critical ethical issues change over time due to current issues in healthcare delivery. Three issues that are important today are healthcare fraud and abuse, research ethics, and organizational ethics.

Healthcare Fraud and Abuse

Healthcare fraud and abuse are especially common. **Fraud** is a legal term that means a person deliberately deceived another for personal gain. Fraud also has a non-legal definition, but the focus here is on fraud that involves breaking the law. In health care, it usually involves money and reimbursement. For example, a patient may be charged for care that the patient did not receive or may be charged more than the usual fee. In 2009, the U.S. Department of Health and Human Services (HHS) and the U.S. Department of Justice (DOJ) established the Healthcare Fraud Prevention and Enforcement Action Team (HEAT). Its mission is to prevent and reduce healthcare fraud. Since 2007, more than 2,300 defendants have been charged with Medicare fraud. In 2011, HEAT initiated an effort to attack federal healthcare fraud, which involved $530 million in billing fraud (HHS, 2016).

In 2014, the federal government recovered more than $5.7 billion from fraud-associated federal healthcare programs, representing an increase of $1.9 billion from 2013 (Pawderly, 2015). In 2016, the Department of Justice brought charges against 301 individuals for false billing totaling approximately $900 million (DOJ, 2016). Both of these cases of fraud involve large sums of money that could have been used to provide health care. Recovering the funds is a positive step; however, the magnitude of the collections makes a sad statement about the level of healthcare fraud in the United States. Such actions have led to many legal cases and convictions, all of which are expensive to conduct.

Because of this ongoing major loss of monies, the Affordable Care Act of 2010 (ACA) includes provisions to increase monitoring and enforcement of laws to prevent fraud (U.S. Department of Health and Human Services & Office of the Inspector General, 2011). In March 2011, the Centers for Medicare and Medicaid Services (CMS) began an ambitious project to revalidate all 1.5 million Medicare-enrolled providers and suppliers under the new screening requirements. As of September 2013, more than 535,000 providers were subject to the new screening requirements, and more than 225,000 lost the ability to bill Medicare due to the new requirements and other proactive initiatives. This screening continues to ensure that providers meet Medicare practice requirements to receive reimbursement from CMS. Since the passage of the ACA, the CMS has also revoked 14,663 providers' and suppliers' ability to bill the Medicare program. These providers were removed from the program because they had felony convictions, were not operational at the address CMS had on file, and were not in compliance with CMS rules (HHS, 2014).

Fraud may be committed by physicians, pharmacists, nurses, and other healthcare providers; medical equipment companies; and healthcare organizations. **Exhibit 6-2** identifies examples of Medicaid fraud schemes, which continue to be used. Areas of health care in which fraud is most prevalent include psychiatric care, home care, long-term care, and large corporate healthcare organizations.

Exhibit 6-2 Examples of Medicaid Fraud Schemes

- Billing for "phantom patients"
- Billing for medical goods or services that were not provided
- Billing for more hours than there are in a day
- Paying a "kickback" in exchange for a referral for medical goods or services
- Concealing ownership in a related company
- Using false credentials
- Double-billing for healthcare goods or services not provided

Modified from Department of Health and Human Services, Centers for Medicare and Medicaid Services. (2015). *About fraud.* Retrieved from http://www.stopmedicarefraud.gov/aboutfraud/index.html

Ethics and Research

Research is an area in which complex concerns about ethical and legal issues arise. Research has a history of ethical problems. Some key examples of situations in which research participants were abused include the Nazi medical experiments in World War II; the Tuskegee Syphilis Study, in which African American men with syphilis were not treated so that researchers could observe the course of the disease (1932–1972); and the Willowbrook Study, in which residents of an institution for mentally retarded children were deliberately infected with hepatitis (mid-1950s to the early 1970s). In the late 1970s, recognition of these major abuses led to reforms and the creation of legal guidelines that now must be followed by all healthcare researchers. The Belmont Report (National Commission for the Protection of Human Subjects of Biomedical and Behavioral Research, 1978) identified the key concerns and the need for greater attention to ethical principles in conducting and reporting research. **Exhibit 6-3** contains an excerpt from the Belmont Report's introduction.

Research: Informed Consent

Participation in research must include **informed consent**, and there are rules regarding how this consent must be obtained. The National Institutes of Health (NIH) is a key resource for information about consent. Some of the information that must be revealed includes the nature and purpose of a research intervention; potential risks, discomforts, and benefits to the patient; alternative treatments; compensation if injury occurs; compensation for participating in a study (if offered by the study); and a clear statement how the participant may withdraw at any time without any negative impact on the patient.

The institutional review board (IRB) is an organization's committee or department that ensures that the research process meets ethical and legal requirements in protecting participants in biomedical or behavioral research. Hospitals, universities, and other organizations that conduct research have IRBs. The following passage describes the differences between patient care and research, which can sometimes be confused: "While recognizing that the distinction between research and therapy is often blurred, practice is described as interventions that are designed solely to enhance the well-being of an individual patient or client and that have a reasonable expectation of success. The purpose of medical or behavioral practice is to provide diagnosis, preventive treatment, or therapy to particular individuals. The Commission distinguishes research as designating an activity designed to test a hypothesis, permit conclusions to be drawn, and thereby to develop or contribute to generalizable knowledge (expressed, for example, in theories, principles, and statements of relationships). Research is usually described in

Exhibit 6-3 The Belmont Report

On September 30, 1978, the National Commission for the Protection of Human Subjects of Biomedical and Behavioral Research submitted its report entitled "The Belmont Report: Ethical Principles and Guidelines for the Protection of Human Subjects of Research." The Report, named after the Belmont Conference Center at the Smithsonian Institution where the discussions that resulted in its formulation were begun, sets forth the basic ethical principles underlying the acceptable conduct of research involving human subjects. Those principles—respect for persons, beneficence, and justice—are now accepted as the three quintessential requirements for the ethical conduct of research involving human subjects.

- Respect for persons involves recognition of the personal dignity and autonomy of individuals, and special protection of those persons with diminished autonomy.

- Beneficence entails an obligation to protect persons from harm by maximizing anticipated benefits and minimizing possible risks of harm.
- Justice requires that the benefits and burdens of research be distributed fairly.

The Report also describes how these principles apply to the conduct of research. Specifically, the principle of respect for persons underlies the need to obtain informed consent; the principle of beneficence underlies the need to engage in a risk–benefit analysis and to minimize risks; and the principle of justice requires that subjects be fairly selected. As was mandated by the congressional charge to the Commission, the Report also provides a distinction between "practice" and "research." The text of the Belmont Report is thus divided into two sections: (1) boundaries between practice and research, and (2) basic ethical principles.

Reproduced from U.S. Department of Health and Human Services. (1979). *The Belmont report.* Retrieved from https://www.hhs.gov/ohrp/regulations-and-policy/belmont-report/

a formal protocol that sets forth an objective and a set of procedures designed to reach that objective. The report recognizes that 'experimental' procedures do not necessarily constitute research, and that research and practice may occur simultaneously. It suggests that the safety and effectiveness of such 'experimental' procedures should be investigated early, and that institutional oversight mechanisms, such as medical practice committees, can ensure that this need is met by requiring that 'major innovation[s] be incorporated into a formal research project'" (HHS, 1993).

In healthcare research, participants or subjects may be exposed to multiple risks, typically classified as physical, psychological, social, and economic risks (HHS, 1993). In 2016, new federal regulations were approved focusing on the procedural needs for submitting research sample registration and summary study results information, including adverse event information, from clinical trials of drug products and device products (U.S. Department of Health and Human Services & National Institutes of Health, 2016). These regulations were effective January 2017. This initiative is directed at protecting patients in trials and to ensure rapid, accurate sharing of information about studies, improving public access to information. The regulations are complicated and require institutions and researchers to be more vigilant about sharing information. If this is not done, there will be penalty fees, and organizations and researchers may lose research funding.

Research: Risk of Physical Harm

Some medical research is designed only to measure more carefully the effects of therapeutic or diagnostic procedures applied in the course of caring for an illness. This research may not involve any significant risks beyond those presented by medically indicated interventions. Research designed to evaluate new drugs or procedures, however, might present more than minimal risk and sometimes can cause serious or disabling injuries. These types of studies may lead to participant physical risk and thus would be reviewed in the IRB review and via the informed consent. Some of the adverse effects that result from medical procedures or drugs may be permanent, but most are transient. Procedures commonly used in medical research usually result in no more than minor discomfort (for example, temporary dizziness, the pain associated with venipuncture).

Research: Risk of Psychological Harm

Participation in research may result in undesired changes in thought processes and emotion (for example, episodes of depression, confusion, or other cognitive effects resulting from the drugs used; feelings of stress, guilt, and loss of self-esteem). These changes may be transitory, recurrent, or permanent. Most psychological risks are minimal or transitory, but IRBs should be aware that some research has the potential for causing serious psychological harm and should be part of informed consent. Stress and feelings of guilt or embarrassment may occur simply from thinking or talking about one's own behavior or attitudes on sensitive topics such as drug use, sexual preferences, selfishness, and violence. These feelings may be aroused when the subject is interviewed or filling out a questionnaire. Stress may also be induced when researchers manipulate the subjects' environment—such as if emergencies or fake assaults are staged to observe how passersby respond, lighting is changed or noise is used, and so on. More frequently, however, IRBs assess the possibility of psychological harm when reviewing behavioral research that involves an element of deception, particularly if the deception includes false feedback to the research participants or subjects about their own performance.

Invasion of privacy is a risk of a somewhat different character. In the research context, it usually involves either covert observation or participant observation of behavior that the participants or subjects consider private. The IRB must decide the following about the study: (1) Is the invasion of privacy acceptable in light of the participants' reasonable expectations of privacy in the situation under study? (2) Is the research question of sufficient importance to justify the intrusion? The IRB should also consider whether the research design could be modified so that the study can be conducted without invading privacy.

Breach of confidentiality is sometimes confused with invasion of privacy, but it is a different problem. **Invasion of privacy** concerns access to a person's body or behavior without consent; **breach of confidentiality** concerns safeguarding information that has been given voluntarily by one person to another. Some research requires the use of a subject's hospital, school, or employment records. Access to such records for legitimate research purposes is generally acceptable, as long as the researcher protects the confidentiality of that information and the subject is informed of this access. The IRB must be aware, however, that a breach of confidentiality may result in psychological harm to individuals (in the form of embarrassment, guilt, stress, and so forth) or in social harm.

Research: Risk of Social and Economic Harm

Some invasions of privacy and breaches of confidentiality may result in embarrassment within one's business or social group, loss of employment, or criminal prosecution—all representing risk of social and/or economic harm. Areas of particular sensitivity are information regarding alcohol or drug abuse, mental illness, illegal activities, and sexual behavior and identity. Some social and behavioral research may yield information about individuals that could label or stigmatize the participants (for example, as actual or potential delinquents or a person with schizophrenia). Confidentiality safeguards must be effective in these instances. The fact that a person has participated in HIV-related drug trials or has been hospitalized for treatment of mental illness could adversely affect the person's present or future employment, political campaigns, and standing in the community. A researcher's plans to contact these individuals for follow-up studies should be reviewed with care. Participation in research may result in additional actual costs to individuals. Any anticipated costs to research participants should be described to prospective participants during the consent process.

Nurses should be concerned about these issues for two reasons. First, nurses conduct research, and they must follow the same rules as anyone else who uses human participants or even animals used in a study. Secondly, nurses may assist in getting informed consent, data collection, and other aspects of a research study. Nurses also work in areas where clinical research is ongoing. In these situations, the nurse must continue to act as the patient advocate; ensure that the patient's rights are upheld; and should be aware of the study, which should provide as much information as is possible to help the nurse understand the patient's care experience—both aspects related to care and to the research study.

Some student projects are also reviewed to see whether an IRB review is needed for the project. Faculty are responsible for guiding students to determine if the school's (college, university) IRB Committee should make the decision about the need to complete the IRB written requirements or if a clinical site is used for the project must the healthcare organization's IRB be involved.

Knowledge and application of the ethical principles related to research need to be part of practice whenever nurses are directly or indirectly involved in research. **Exhibit 6-4** identifies key points of the Code of Federal Regulations related to research that might affect nurses and nursing care.

Organizational Ethics

In the late 1990s and early 2000s, there were serious breaches of **organizational ethics**. A major stimulus to address this problem occurred in 1994, when it was recognized that the federal government lost 10% of its total healthcare expenditures to fraud, equivalent to $100 billion (U.S. House of Representatives, 1994). Because of increasing corporate healthcare fraud and abuse of patients, the CMS, through legislation, now requires that any healthcare organization that is reimbursed through

---

Exhibit 6-4 Code of Federal Regulations

- Risks to subjects [participants] are minimized.
- The risks to subjects are reasonable in relation to anticipated benefits.
- The selection of subjects is equitable.
- Informed consent must be sought from potential subjects or their legal guardians.

- Informed consent must be properly documented.
- When appropriate, research plans monitor data collection to ensure subject safety.
- When appropriate, privacy of subjects and confidentiality of data are maintained.
- Safeguards must be in place when subjects are vulnerable to coercion.

Reproduced from Schmidt, N., & Brown, J. (2015). *Evidence-based practice for nurses: Appraisal and applications of research*. Burlington, MA: Jones & Bartlett Learning.

for Medicare and/or Medicaid services meet certain compliance conditions to better ensure the organization maintains appropriate organizational ethics. Because it is rare that a hospital does not receive this type of reimbursement to cover care provided to Medicare or Medicaid enrollees, this mandate applies to the majority of hospitals. Organizations must identify a compliance officer, who audits and monitors actions taken to detect, correct, and prevent fraud. Staff must know how to report concerns related to ethical behavior and potential fraud, and they must be provided with education about these critical issues. Reporting methods should ensure privacy for staff, and they should not be penalized for reporting. The federal government established these requirements because it does not want patients abused. In addition, the government is concerned about the major loss of funds that has occurred because of fraud, such as paying for care that was not given, paying more than the typical rate, paying for patients who did not receive care, and so forth.

Whistleblowing can be part of fraud and abuse situations. This action occurs when a person who works for an organization that is committing fraud and abuse reports these activities to legal authorities, sharing extensive information that would be difficult for the authorities to obtain on their own. The False Claims Act, a very old law, protects whistleblowers. This law was passed during the Civil War and amended in 1982 to further shield whistleblowers. Whistleblowers are protected from being sued and from being fired or otherwise penalized by their employer for reporting the organization or staff within the organization. If the federal government pursues the case and recovers funds, the whistleblower is given a portion of the funds. Anyone can be a whistleblower, but the person must have information that could not be obtained otherwise or information that was not public knowledge (such as that reported in a newspaper). This type of legal action is complicated and very difficult to resolve.

One example of whistleblowing occurred in an academic health center in 2016 involving an RN as the whistleblower (Beckers Hospital Review, 2016). The hospital was not following standard procedure to ensure that steps were taken to sterilize equipment used for bronchoscopy and may have led to infections in 100 patients. This also had an impact on monitoring of quality improvement. The nurse tried to get hospital staff to address the problem but was unsuccessful. The nurse then went to an attorney, and the result was a whistleblower civil suit. This case contains many ethical and legal aspects such as a coverup, lack of response to staff feedback about quality care, lack of concern about quality care, and subsequent legal ramifications. It also demonstrates that nurses do take steps to ensure quality and advocate for patients—ethical and legal issues are interconnected in this example.

Stop and Consider #2

Nurses and other healthcare professionals have participated in unethical and illegal practices.

Legal Issues: An Overview

Legal issues are a part of each nurse's practice. Each state board of nursing identifies situations for which licensure could be denied. You can search your state board of nursing's website for this information. Licensure itself is a legal issue that is implemented through the legal system. The nurse practice act in each state is a state law. Legal concerns are also directly related to practice. The following are some examples of nursing-related legal issues:

- When the nurse administers a narcotic medication, specific procedures must be followed to ensure that patients receive medications per healthcare provider orders and that the narcotic drug supply is monitored (counted) to make sure the amounts are correct. If there are errors, it could mean that a criminal act occurred—someone took a narcotic or controlled drug with no right to do so.

- Restraining a patient without a physician's order or not in accordance with the requirements in the order or healthcare organization policy can be considered assault and battery.
- Falsifying medical records can have adverse legal consequences.
- Accessing an electronic medical record for a patient who is not in a specific nurse's care can be questioned.
- Inadequate supervision of patients that leads to serious patient outcomes such as falls with injury or a suicide may have legal consequences.

Critical Terminology

The nurse may encounter the following legal terms as part of his or her practice:

- *Assault:* The threat or use of force on another individual that causes the person to feel reasonable apprehension about imminent harmful or offensive contact. An example is threatening to medicate a patient if the patient does not comply with treatment. This type of threat is not uncommon in behavioral or psychiatric care but should not be made.
- *Battery:* The actual intentional striking of someone, with intent to harm, or in a rude and insolent manner even if the injury is slight. An example of battery is conducting a procedure, such as starting an intravenous line, without asking the patient. If this is an emergency situation and the patient's life is at risk, or if there is risk of serious damage and the patient is not able to provide consent, the event would not be considered battery.
- *Civil law:* This type of statute (law) focuses on private rights.
- *Criminal law:* This type of statute deals with crimes against the public and members of the public, with penalties and all the procedures connected with charging, trying, sentencing, and imprisoning defendants convicted of crimes.

- *Doctrine of res ipsa loquitur:* A doctrine of law in which a person is presumed to be negligent if he, she, or an organization/employer had exclusive control of whatever caused the injury, even though there is no specific evidence of an act of negligence, and without negligence, the accident would not have happened.
- *Emancipation:* A child is a minor, and therefore under the control of his or her parent(s)/guardian(s), until the child attains the age of majority (18 years), at which point he or she is considered to be an adult. In special circumstances, a minor can be freed from control by the minor's parent/guardian and given the rights of an adult before turning 18. In most states, the three circumstances under which a minor becomes emancipated are (1) enlisting in the military (requires parent/guardian consent), (2) marrying (requires parent/guardian consent), and (3) obtaining a court order from a judge (parent/guardian consent not required). A minor can also petition the court for this status if financial independence can be proven and the parents or guardian agree. An emancipated minor is legally able to do everything an adult can do, with the exception of actions that are specifically prohibited if one has not reached the age of 18 (such as buying tobacco). From a healthcare perspective, emancipated minors can sue and be sued in their own name, enter into contracts, and seek or decline medical care.
- *Expert witness:* This is person with specific expertise and knowledge who can provide testimony to prove or disprove the standard of care that is used to support a case. A nurse may serve as an expert witness for nursing care but not for medical care issues. Typically, the nurse is also a specialist in the specific area of care addressed in the legal case. For example, for a case involving the death of a

newborn in a neonatal intensive care unit, the expert witness should be a neonatal nurse.

- *False imprisonment:* Confinement of a person against his or her will is against the law. This can happen in health care—for example, when a patient wants to leave the hospital and is retained (an exception is when a patient is legally committed for medical reasons or held for legal reasons by law enforcement or courts); when a patient is threatened or his or her clothes are taken away to prevent the patient from leaving; or when restraints are used without written consent, appropriate physician order, or a sufficient emergency reason.

- *Good Samaritan laws:* Laws that protect a healthcare professional from being sued when providing emergency care outside a healthcare setting. The provider must provide the care in the same manner that an ordinary, reasonable, and prudent professional would do in similar circumstances, including following practice standards. An example is a nurse stopping on the highway to assist an accident victim and following the expected standard for providing care to a victim with a severe burn to maintain respiratory status under emergency conditions.

- *Respondent superior:* A principal (employer) responsible for the actions of his, her, or its agent (employee) in the course of employment. This doctrine allows someone—for example, a patient—to sue the employee who is accused of making an error that resulted in harm. The patient also may sue the employer, the hospital, because the employer is responsible for supervising the staff member. For example, if a nurse administers the wrong medication, and the patient experiences complications, the nurse may be sued for the action, and the hospital also may be sued for not providing the appropriate education regarding medications and medication administration, for not

ensuring that the nurse received the education, and/or for not providing proper supervision. Typically, in such legal actions, multiple persons and organizations may be sued.

- *Standards of practice:* Minimum guidelines identified by the profession (local, state, national) and healthcare organization policies and procedures. Expert opinion, literature, and research may also be used as standards. Standards are used in legal situations to assess negligence malpractice actions. (See other chapters in this text that include additional information on standards.)

- *Tort:* A civil wrong for which a remedy may be obtained in the form of damages. An example of a tort that is most relevant to nurses and other healthcare providers is negligence, an unintentional tort.

Malpractice: Why Should This Concern You?

Negligence does occur in nursing—for example, medication errors, not adequately providing for patient access to a call light when the patient needs help, a lack of assessment of risk for falls and failure to prevent falls, and failure to implement appropriate interventions when required. Another example of negligence would be failure to communicate information that affects care, which encompasses situations such as not documenting care provided or response to care; not contacting the physician with information that would inform the physician of the need for a change in treatment; and failing to document, such as monitoring data, changes in status, assessment of wound sites or skin status, or malfunctioning intravenous equipment. Negligence may also include inadequate patient teaching, inadequate monitoring and maintenance of medical equipment, lack of identification of an allergy or not following known information about allergies, failure to obtain informed consent, and failure to report another staff member to supervisory staff for negligence or problems with practice. All these examples can lead to malpractice suits.

Malpractice is an act or continuing conduct of a professional that does not meet the standard of professional competence and results in provable damages to the patient. Anyone can sue if an attorney can be found to support the suit; however, winning a lawsuit is not so easy. Often, lawsuits are settled outside of court to reduce costs and prevent negative publicity; in such a case, even if the patient would not have been able to win the lawsuit, the patient may still receive payment of damages.

For a patient or family to be successful with a malpractice lawsuit, all of the following criteria must be met:

1. The nurse (as person being sued) must have a duty to the patient or a patient–nurse professional relationship. The nurse must have provided care to the patient or been involved in the patient's care.

2. The duty must have been breached. This is called negligence, or the failure to exercise the care toward others that a reasonable or prudent person would under similar circumstances. Any of the following could be used as proof: a nurse practice act, professional standards, healthcare organization policies and procedures, expert witnesses (RNs, preferably in same specialty as the nurse sued), accreditation and licensure standards, professional literature, and research.

3. The **breach of duty** must be the proximate (foreseeable) cause or the cause that is legally sufficient to result in liability harm to the patient. There must be evidence that the breach of duty (what the nurse is accused of having done or not done, based on what a reasonable or prudent person would do given the circumstances, such as what other nurses would have done in a similar situation) led directly to the harm that the patient is claiming. There might be other causes of the harm to the patient that have nothing do with the breach of duty.

4. Damages or injury to the patient must have occurred. What were the damages or injury? Are they temporary or permanent? What impact do they have on the patient's life? These questions and many more will be asked about the damages and injury. If the lawsuit is won, this information is also used to assist in determining the amount of damages that will be awarded, although the plaintiff (person suing) will identify an amount when the suit is brought.

These four malpractice elements are illustrated in **Figure 6-2**.

The plaintiff's attorney must prove that each of these elements exists for the judge or the jury to agree to the plaintiff's case, and the plaintiff should be awarded damages. The nurse's attorney will defend the nurse by proving that one or more elements do not exist. If even one element is lacking, malpractice cannot be proved.

Medical malpractice lawsuits have affected healthcare practice and costs. The cases are very expensive to defend, and when the case is won by the plaintiff, awards are often very high. As mentioned earlier, even if the healthcare provider does

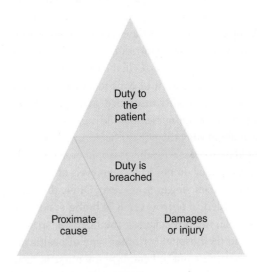

Figure 6-2 Elements of Malpractice

not win the case in a court decision by judge or jury, a settlement may still be made, though typically settlements occur earlier. Collectively, these issues have prompted many healthcare providers to practice "defensive medicine," in which physicians prescribe excessive diagnostic testing and other procedures to protect themselves. This approach increases the costs of care, and if testing or procedures are invasive, it can increase patient risk. Malpractice concerns also increase medical costs because physicians, other healthcare providers, and healthcare organizations must carry malpractice insurance to help cover potential legal costs for malpractice suits; these costs are then passed on to consumers through patient service charges, increasing overall healthcare costs.

Nurses do get sued. A review of closed 516 claims from 2006 to 2010 identified the average total incurred claim was $204,594, with 11 different nursing specialties represented in the cases (Benton, Arm, & Flynn, 2013). The largest number of claims was found in adult medical-surgical care (40.1%), gerontology (18.0%), and obstetrics (10.3%). The cases included 84.5% RNs and 15.5% licensed practical or vocational nurses. The following problems were the focus of these cases: treatment/care (59.6%); medication administration (14.7%); assessment (12.6%); monitoring (6.8%); patient rights, abuse, and professional conduct (5.4%); and scope of practice (1.7%). These examples of categories of lawsuit focus areas provide an overview of the high-risk concerns that require special attention by nurses in their practice.

There are pros and cons to nurses carrying professional liability insurance. Such policies are not expensive for nurses, but the nurse needs to be clear about what the policy offers. A question that could be asked is why nurses would be sued when, typically, they do not have high levels of personal funds. Nurses, however, are sued. Often, the nurse is included in a group that is being sued—for example, the physician(s), the hospital, specific staff in the hospital (or other type of healthcare organization), and others. When a nurse is sued, the nurse should not rely on the nurse's employer's

attorneys to provide a defense; instead, the nurse needs an attorney who represents only the interests of the nurse. Professional liability insurance covers these fees. There are also differences in the types of malpractice insurance that can be obtained. Two of the most common types are (1) claims-made coverage, which covers only those incidents that occur and reported during the policy's effective period, and (2) occurrence coverage, which provides protection for an incident that took place while the policy was in effect even if the claim was not filed until after the policy terminated. When accepting a job, the nurse should explore the pros and cons of carrying personal professional malpractice/liability insurance.

As soon as a nurse learns of a possible lawsuit, the nurse should contact an attorney for advice. If the nurse has liability insurance, the nurse would contact the insurer for legal advice, and the insurer may assign an attorney to the case. In addition, the nurse should recognize that at the conclusion of a lawsuit in which the nurse and the nurse's employer are sued, the employer might then sue the nurse to reclaim damages to cover the nurse's employer's expenses for the lawsuit. Nurses must make informed decisions about whether they would rather have their employer's attorney defend them or seek out the services of an attorney who is covered under their own policy, which is required for some malpractice policies, or a personal attorney. In some instances, if the nurse has a personal attorney or an attorney from the nurse's malpractice policy, the institutional legal team will not assist the nurse.

Nursing students are responsible for their own actions and can be held liable for them. Students are not practicing under the license of their faculty (Guido, 2001). Because of this, students must never accept assignments or do procedures for which they are not prepared. It is also critical that students discuss these situations with faculty or staff if faculty if family are not available rather than acting without guidance.

Stop and Consider #3
Nurses may be sued.

Examples of Issues
with Ethical and Legal Implications

Ethics and legal issues are often interrelated. The following section highlights some of these issues such as privacy, confidentiality, informed consent, rationing care, various patient legal decisions and documents, organ transplants, assisted suicide, and use of social media. All of them relate to nurses and nursing care.

Privacy, Confidentiality, and Informed Consent

Patients have the right to privacy, and this affects multiple situations that might occur during the care process. The obvious is during assessment and examinations. When patients are told about their condition, this should be done in a private area. Rounds are discussed in this text, and privacy is difficult to maintain, particularly when the patient shares a patient room with another patient(s), but we need do what we can to maintain it, such as using curtains to separate the patient area and speaking in lower tones. Privacy is associated with confidentiality and informed consent.

Confidentiality is an issue that is relevant to practice every day; we need to ensure, when possible, that patient information is shared only with those the patient approves or as required for treatment such as the treatment team. The Health Insurance Portability and Accountability Act of 1996 (HIPAA) has had a major impact on information technology and patient information (HHS, 2017). Nurses are required to follow this law to protect patient privacy and confidentiality. Patients are informed about HIPAA when they enter a hospital, visit another type of healthcare facility for care, or receive outpatient care.

Nurses have the responsibility to keep patient information confidential except as required to communicate in the care process and with team members. Patient-centered care also implies that patients have the right to determine who sees their information, and this decision must be honored. It is important to remember that patient information should not be discussed in public areas (for example, elevators, cafeteria, hallways) or any place where the information might be overheard by persons who have no right to hear the information. You will encounter patients and family members who are part of your personal life; however, you must remember that what is known about the patient is private. Nurses who work in the community and make phone calls to and about patients using mobile phones in public places can easily forget that their conversations may be overheard.

It is important to remember that patients drive patient privacy. For example, nurses should not assume that patients want family members to have access to the patient's health information. Instead, patients have to be explicitly asked who can be told about any health information. As a student and as a nurse, you will have access to patient information for only those patients to whom you are directly providing care. You must have a reason related to healthcare provision to access patient information. If you do not adhere to these rules, then you are in violation of HIPAA. Be aware that patients may and do make HIPAA-related complaints to state boards and to educational institutions, in the case of students, about staff or students who do not uphold privacy rules/HIPAA.

Another ethical and legal concern related to confidentiality is consent. Patient care consent occurs when the patient agrees to treatment, and it may be given either orally or in written form. Whenever possible, consent should be informed consent and documented in writing. The patient's physician or other independent healthcare practitioner is required by law to explain or disclose information about the medical problem and treatment or procedure so that the patient can have informed choice. The patient has the right to refuse the treatment. Failure to obtain informed consent puts the practitioner at risk for negligence.

The requirement to obtain informed consent applies to many nurses. An advanced practice registered nurse (APRN), for instance, needs to get informed consent from his or her patients or ensure prior to performing treatments and procedures following required policy. By comparison, the nurse who is not an APRN does not have to get informed consent for every nursing intervention, such as administering a medication. Moreover, this nurse would not be the staff member who obtains patient consent for treatment or procedures. In some cases, the nurse may ask a patient to sign a written consent form, but in doing so, it is assumed that the patient's physician or other healthcare provider has explained the information to the patient. If the patient indicates that this conversation has not occurred, the nurse must talk with the physician or other healthcare provider involved and cannot have the patient sign the form until the patient and the physician have discussed the specific treatment or procedure. If a nurse is required to get informed consent and fails to do so, the nurse is at risk for negligence.

A second type of consent is consent implied by law. This consent is applicable only in emergency situations, when a patient may not be able to give informed consent. If the patient's life is at risk or if major damage or injury to the patient is likely, healthcare providers can provide care. In this case, the assumption is that the patient would most likely give consent if the patient could, based on what a reasonable person would do. Nurses who work in the emergency department encounter this type of consent situation.

Rationing Care: Who Can Access Care when Needed

The United States rations care, albeit not formally. Rationing is the systematic allocation of resources, typically limited resources. In this case, the limited resources are funds to pay for care. Some people receive care, and others do not. Insurers do not cover all care; instead, they determine which care will be provided based on criteria that they identify.

Other forms of healthcare rationing also exist. For example, organ transplantation is a form of rationing—in both the allocation of funds to perform transplants and the allocation of limited organs. Patients are put into a database to receive organ donations, and the order in which patients receive a transplant depends on specified criteria.

Oregon developed a rationing system for Medicaid by identifying the types of treatment that the state would cover, but this approach was not successful. This is an example of a situation in which the ethical principle of justice might be applied because rationing, or allocation of resources, is related to equity. It appears to be more acceptable to say "resource allocation" than "rationing," but in the end, resource allocation and rationing are similar.

Advance Directives, Living Wills, Medical Powers of Attorney, and Do-Not-Resuscitate Orders

Advance directives are now part of the healthcare system. This type of legal document allows a person to describe personal medical care preferences. Often, these documents describe the person's wishes related to end-of-life needs ahead of time, in which case the document is called a **living will**. Patients have the right to develop this plan, and healthcare providers must follow it. Because state requirements vary, it is advised that patients ask physicians if they will uphold the patient's decisions about health care. Any advance directives should be part of the patient's medical record and easily accessible to the healthcare provider. Be aware that end-of-life issues are never simple but should be a critical part of care for these patients.

A **medical power of attorney** document, a type of advance directive, designates an individual who has the right to speak for another person if that person cannot do so in matters related to health care. Another name for this document is durable power of attorney for health care or a healthcare agent or proxy. If a person does not designate a medical power of attorney and the person is married, the spouse can make the decisions if the sick spouse is unable to do so. If there were no spouse, the decision would be made by adult children or parents. People should determine the types of care they prefer and how aggressive that care should be with those who will be their medical powers of attorney. The proxy or agent is not forced to follow the patient's instructions if they are not written in a legal document; if there is no written document, a sick person should trust that the proxy or agent would follow the guide discussed.

Interventions that are typically covered in advance directives include (1) use of life-sustaining equipment, such as a ventilator, respirator, or dialysis; (2) artificial hydration and nutrition (tube feeding); (3) do-not-resuscitate (DNR) or allow-a-natural-death (AND) orders; (4) withholding of food and fluids; (5) palliative care; and (6) organ or tissue donation. The DNR and the AND directives either are forms of advance directives or may be part of an extensive advance directive. Such an order means that there should be no resuscitation if the patient's condition indicates need for resuscitation. A physician may write a DNR/AND order without an advance directive, but the physician must follow hospital policy and procedures regarding this type of decision. It is highly advisable that this situation be discussed with the patient, if the patient is able to comprehend, and with the family. The nurse may be present for this discussion but would not make this type of decision. If there are concerns about how it should be handled, the nurse needs to consult the nursing supervisor/manager. If the organization has an ethics committee, the nurse may consult with the committee, which is typically an interprofessional committee that is prepared to discuss ethical issues

staff and patients encounter and may make recommendations but not final decisions.

Palliative care is now an important healthcare issue, and nurses are involved in this care. Ensuring that patients receive the type of care they want requires nurses to understand the patient's needs and goals and then advocate for them. The decision not to receive "aggressive medical treatment" is not the same as withholding all medical care. A patient may still receive antibiotics, nutrition, pain medication, radiation therapy, and other interventions when the goal of treatment becomes comfort rather than cure. This is called *palliative care*, and its primary focus is helping the patient remain as comfortable as possible. Patients can change their minds and ask to resume more aggressive treatment. If the type of treatment a patient would like to receive changes, however, it is important to be aware that such a decision may raise insurance issues that will need to be explored with the patient's healthcare plan. Any changes in the type of treatment a patient wants to receive should be reflected in the patient's living will (National Cancer Institute, 2000).

Organ Transplantation

As mentioned earlier, organ transplantation is a form of resource allocation. Specific criteria are developed for each type of organ donation, and potential recipients are categorized according to the criteria to determine who might receive a donation and in what order. Organ transplantation registries are a critical component of this process. Nevertheless, it is not always so clear as to who should get a transplant. Many patient factors are considered—such as age, other medical or psychological illnesses, what the person might be able to contribute to society, whether the person is single or married, whether the person has children, comorbidities (other illnesses) such as substance abuse, and ability to comply with follow-up treatment—and some of these factors complicate the decision-making process. Organ transplantation is expensive and may not be covered, or only partially covered, by health insurance. The patient will need lifetime specialized care, which is also costly.

Of course, organ donation must occur first so that organ transplantation is possible. Some people designate their willingness to be organ donors while they are healthy—for example, on their driver's license. However, when the time comes to actually honor this request, family members may be reluctant to consent to it at an emotional time when a loved one has died. Other people may not have identified themselves as organ donors when healthy, but then something happens that makes them eligible to be organ donors, such as an accident. This situation is even more complex, ethically and procedurally. Healthcare providers do ask for organ donations, and hospitals have policies and procedures that describe what needs to be done. It is difficult to approach family members and say that loved ones are no longer able to sustain themselves and then to ask for an organ donation at the same time. With organ donations and transplants, time is a critical element to maintain organ viability, and this complicates the decisions and procedures, occurring when people (patient, donor, family) are stressed and emotional, but also staff are stressed trying to ensure the timelines are met to allow for a healthy transplantation. Nurses do not ask for the donation but may assist the physician in this most difficult discussion with all involved. Later, family members or the patient (if responsive) may want to discuss it further with the nurse.

Assisted Suicide

Assisted suicide is a complex ethical and legal issue, but the nurse's role is very clear: The nurse cannot participate in helping a person end his or her life. In 1997, Oregon passed the first state law pertaining to assisted suicide, the Death with Dignity Act, which allowed terminally ill citizens of Oregon to end their lives through voluntary self-administration

of lethal medications prescribed by a physician for this purpose. The law describes who can be involved and the procedure or steps that must be taken. Two physicians must be involved in the decision. As of 2016, five states (Oregon, California, Vermont, Colorado, and Washington) have legalized physician-assisted suicide by passing legislation, and one state (Montana) has legalized physician-assisted suicide based on a court ruling (ProCon.org, 2016). In other states, this act is considered to be illegal. There has also been an increase in countries that now allow assisted suicides.

The ANA believes that the nurse should not participate in assisted suicide. The organization bases this position on its *Code of Ethics for Nurses with Interpretive Statements* (2015). Nurses, individually and collectively, have an obligation to provide comprehensive and compassionate end-of-life care, which includes the promotion of comfort and the relief of pain, and at times, forgoing life-sustaining treatments (ANA, 2013). In a related topic, the ANA also issued a position statement on the withdrawal of nutrition and hydration (ANA, 2011). This statement indicates that the patient or the patient's surrogate should make this decision, and the nurse should provide expert end-of-life nursing care.

Social Media and Ethical and Legal Issues: A New Concern

Social media or the use of networking web-based instruments or sites such as Facebook, LinkedIn, Instagram, Google+, Flickr, and Twitter has presented nurses with new ethical and legal issues. A critical issue is that social media may lead to problems associated with our professional obligations to protect patient privacy and confidentiality. Nurses should not share information about patients or families, including images. It is not sufficient to limit access using privacy settings. The basic rule is simple: Share no information or image. An example is provided in a recent article on social media and nurses, which offers comments that nurses should be very careful about what they post (Barry, 2017). This can be a slippery slope when we are attached to a patient and then share personal information and thoughts about the patient.

This topic has become very important and organizations such as the NCSBN (2014) have published information on the topic with guidelines for nurses. Many healthcare organizations have also established their own policies on the use of social media that must be followed by students and staff. NCSBN social media guidelines, which support the ANA's principles for using social media, are provided on the organization's website (NCSBN, 2014; Spector, 2012).

The ANA Code of Ethics emphasizes the protection of confidentiality of patient information by nurses. HIPAA also protects patient information, and educational and healthcare institutional policies outline the legal issues related to discussion or sharing of protected information. With expansion in use of online courses, it is important to remember that when patients are discussed in online forums, the same guidelines apply—no specific identifiers should be shared. This should also apply to staff and healthcare organizations—sharing information that can identify a staff person may not be something that staff person would want done—for example, critiquing a staff member or even a healthcare organization.

This chapter presented introductory information about ethical and legal issues in nursing. Nurses must deal with ethical concerns about their patients and encounter numerous issues that could lead to potential legal concerns on a daily basis. A healthcare professional cannot avoid either ethics or legal issues. A nurse cares for patients, families, and communities, and in doing so, must consider how that care affects the feelings and rights of others. From the time a nurse achieves licensure, he or she operates under a legal system through the nurse practice act and other laws and regulations.

Stop and Consider #4

Families of patients do not have the right to be given information about their family member.

CHAPTER HIGHLIGHTS

1. Ethics is concerned with a code of behaviors, whereas bioethics relates to life-and-death decisions.
2. Ethical dilemmas arise when there is conflict among the nurse's, profession's, organization's, and patient's codes for decision making.
3. Principles of ethical behavior fall into four areas: autonomy, beneficence, justice, and veracity.
4. A professional code of ethics guides an entire discipline and is generally set at the national level.
5. State boards of nursing outline the expectations of nurses within their jurisdiction.
6. Reporting unethical, immoral, and unsafe actions is part of a nurse's ethical responsibility to protect the public from harm.
7. Healthcare fraud and abuse involve deliberate deceptive activities to steal funds; both have ethical and legal implications.
8. Research activities require stringent considerations of ethical principles—such as protection of the public from physical, psychological, social, and economic harm—and informed consent for the research protocol offered in language that the research subject understands.

(Continues)

CHAPTER HIGHLIGHTS (CONTINUED)

9. Organizational ethics refers to an institution's ethical expectations of itself as an organization and its employees and the patient's rights.

10. Malpractice and negligence charges can be filed against a nurse. The nurse must understand both of these concepts.

11. Patient privacy and confidentiality are both ethical and legal issues; HIPAA is the federal law that addresses patient protection of privacy and confidentiality.

12. No information or image related to a patient or patient's family should be shared on social media.

ENGAGING IN THE CONTENT

Discussion Questions

1. Describe malpractice and how it applies to nursing care.
2. What is the IRB?
3. Explain the potential harms in research that IRBs are concerned about.
4. How does ethical decision making apply to nursing students?
5. Explain how the profession of nursing incorporates ethics into practice and the profession.

CRITICAL THINKING ACTIVITIES

1. Visit your state board of nursing website and find information about making complaints to the board. Review the information. What is your opinion of this process?
2. Visit https://www.ncsbn.org/3771.htm, the website for the NCSBN, and select one of the topics. Summarize the topic, and discuss why it is relevant to you as a student and would be relevant you as a nurse.
3. Select one of the following topics: confidentiality and informed consent, advance directives, living wills, DNR orders, or organ donation. Explain what it is in language that consumers could understand. What makes the issue you selected an ethical and/or legal issue?
4. NCSBN on Social Media Use: https://www.ncsbn.org/347.htm. View the short video and learn more about guidelines for use of social media by nurses.

ELECTRONIC REFLECTION JOURNAL

Describe an experience you have had in your clinical sessions that was an ethical dilemma for you. Why was it difficult for you? What did you do to cope with it? What will you do if you experience a similar situation in the future?

CASE STUDIES

Case 1

A 5-day-old premature baby was believed to require a blood transfusion because of increasing anemia. The parents were Jehovah's Witnesses and did not wish to have blood or blood products given to the baby. A court order was obtained with the parents' knowledge, and the blood was given. The physician on call the next night did not think he needed to obtain the court's consent for an additional blood transfusion because it had been granted for the earlier transfusion. The blood was ordered, and the nurse was asked to administer the blood. The nurse refused for ethical and legal reasons.

Case Questions

1. What might be the ethical and legal reasons for the nurse to refuse to follow the physician's orders?
2. Which steps should the nurse take?
3. How do you think the nurse should respond to the parents?

Case 2

Following the death of a patient who had received the wrong medication, the patient's family sued the hospital, the physician who ordered the medication, and the nurse who administered the medication. The nurse is very concerned and agrees to legal representation from the hospital attorneys. Weeks go by before she hears from the attorney. The nurse has malpractice insurance, but she is unsure what to do about it. She is frustrated and talks to a friend who is also a nurse. She tells her friend that she feels she should call the patient's family. The following are questions that come up.

Case Questions

1. Is it wise for the nurse to not have her own legal representation? If not, why?
2. What should the nurse do about her malpractice coverage?
3. What does the plaintiff (patient's family) have to prove?
4. Should the nurse call the family? Why or why not?

Working Backward to Develop a Case

Write a brief paragraph that describes a case related to the following questions.

1. I don't understand why we need to discuss this situation as potential fraud.
2. Why would nurses be involved in this issue? We just provide care.
3. Who is the researcher?

REFERENCES

American Nurses Association. (2011). *Position statement: Forgoing nutrition and hydration.* Retrieved from http://www.nursingworld.org/MainMenuCategories/Policy-Advocacy/Positions-and-Resolutions/ANAPositionStatements/Position-Statements-Alphabetically/prtetnutr14451.pdf

American Nurses Association. (2013). *Position statement: Assisted suicide.* Retrieved from http://www.nursingworld.org/euthanasiaanddying

American Nurses Association. (2015). *Code of ethics for nurses with interpretive statements.* Silver Spring, MD: Author.

Bandura, A. (1999). Moral disengagement in the perpetration of inhumanities. *Personality and Social Psychology Review, 3,* 193–209.

Barry, M. (2017, January 11). Social media. Proceed with caution. *The American Nurse.* Retrieved from http://www.theamericannurse.org/2014/01/02/social-media-proceed-with-caution/

Beckers Hospital Review. (2016). *UC health nurse sues health system for covering up scope-related outbreak.* Retrieved from http://www.beckershospitalreview.com/quality/uc-health-nurse-sues-health-system-for-covering-up-scope-related-outbreak.html

Benner, P., Sutphen, M., Leonard, V., & Day, L. (2010). *Educating nurses: A call for radical transformation.* San Francisco, CA: Jossey-Bass.

Benton, J., Arm, D., & Flynn, J. (2013). Identifying and minimizing risk exposures affecting nursing practice to enhance patient safety. *Journal of Nursing Regulation, 3*(4), 5–9.

Burman, M., & Dunphy, L. (2011). Reporting colleague misconduct in advanced practice nursing. *Journal of Nursing Regulation, 1*(4), 26–31.

Fowler, M. (2015). *Guide to the code of ethics for nurses with interpretive statements. Development, interpretation, and application.* (2nd. ed.). Silver Spring, MD: American Nurses Association.

Guido, G. (2001). *Legal and ethical issues in nursing.* Upper Saddle River, NJ: Prentice Hall.

Hyatt, J. (2016). Recognizing moral disengagement and its impact on patient safety. *Journal of Nursing Regulation, 7f*(4), 15–21.

Koloroutis, M., & Thorstenson, T. (1999). An ethics framework for organizational change. *Nursing Administrative Quarterly, 23*(2), 9–18.

National Cancer Institute. (2000). *Fact sheet: Advance directives.* Retrieved from http://www.cancer.gov/search/results

National Commission for the Protection of Human Subjects of Biomedical and Behavioral Research. (1978). *The Belmont report: Ethical principles and guidelines for the protection of human subjects of research.* Washington, DC: Author.

National Council of State Boards of Nursing. (2011). *Filing a complaint.* Retrieved from https://www.ncsbn.org/filing-a-complaint.htm

National Council of State Boards of Nursing. (2014). *Social media guidelines for nurses.* Retrieved from https://www.ncsbn.org/347.htm

Pawderly, H. (2015, December 7). *Biggest healthcare fraud in 2015: Running list.* Retrieved from http://www.healthcarefinancenews.com/slideshow/biggest-healthcare-frauds-2015-running-list

ProCon.org. (2016). *State-by-state guide to physician-assisted suicide.* Retrieved from http://euthanasia.procon.org/view.resource.php?resourceID=000132

Spector, N. (2012). What nurse educators should consider when developing social media policies. *Dean's Notes, 34*(1), 1–2. Retrieved from https://www.ncsbn.org/sep12.pdfc

U.S. Department of Health and Human Services. (1993). *Protecting human research subjects: Institutional Review Board guidebook.* Retrieved from http://www.hhs.gov/ohrp/archive/irb/irb_guidebook.htm

U.S. Department of Health and Human Services. (2014, January 26). *Departments of Justice and Health and Human Services announce record-breaking recoveries resulting from joint efforts to combat health care fraud.* Retrieved from http://www.hhs.gov/news/press/2014pres/02/20140226a.html

U.S. Department of Health and Human Services. (2016). *HEAT task force.* Retrieved from https://www.stopmedicarefraud.gov/aboutfraud/heattaskforce/index.html

U.S. Department of Health and Human Services. (2017). *Health Care Portability and Accountability Act of 1996 (HIPAA).* Health information privacy Pub. L. No. 104-191, 110 Stat. 1998 (1996). Retrieved from https://www.hhs.gov/hipaa/

U.S. Department of Health and Human Services, & National Institutes of Health. (2016, September 21). *Clinical trials registration and results information submission.* Final rule. 42 CFR Part 11, Docket Number NIH-2011-0003, RIN: 0925-AA55. Retrieved from https://s3.amazonaws.com/public-inspection.federalregister.gov/2016-22129.pdf

U.S. Department of Health and Human Services, & Office of the Inspector General. (2011). *Health care fraud and abuse control program report*. Retrieved from http://www.oig.hhs.gov/publications/hcfac.asp

U.S. House of Representatives. (1994, July 19). *Deceit that sickens America: Healthcare fraud and its innocent victims*. Hearings before the Subcommittee on Crime and Criminal Justice of the Committee on the Judiciary House of Representatives, 103rd Congress, second session. Washington, DC: U.S. Government Printing Office.

U.S. Department of Justice. (2016, June 22). *National healthcare fraud takedown results in charges against 301 individuals for approximately $900 million in false billing*. Retrieved from https://www.justice.gov/opa/pr/national-health-care-fraud-takedown-results-charges-against-301-individuals-approximately-900

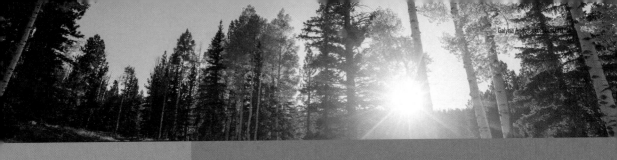

Chapter 7

Health Promotion, Disease Prevention, and Illness: A Community Perspective

CHAPTER OBJECTIVES

At the conclusion of this chapter, the learner will be able to:

- Discuss the *Healthy People 2020* national initiative to improve U.S. health.
- Describe public/community health, expansion of the U.S. healthcare system, and healthcare reform.
- Discuss the continuum of care and continuity of care and its relationship to the individual, family, and community across the life span, as well as health promotion, disease prevention, and healthcare disparities.
- Explain the importance of concepts related to public/community health such as patient-centered care; vulnerable populations; stress, coping, and resilience; aspects of acute illness and population health; chronic illness; the

medical home model; self-management; and health literacy.
- Discuss examples of public/health services: community emergency preparedness, managing population health, migrant and immigrant issues, home health care, school health, rehabilitation, extended care, long-term care, end-of-life and palliative care, case management, occupational health care, complementary and alternative medicine, and genetics.
- Discuss current public/community health problems.
- Critique critical global healthcare concerns and nursing's role in improving global health.

CHAPTER OUTLINE

- Introduction
- A National Initiative to Improve the Nation's Health: *Healthy People 2020*
- Public/Community Healthcare Delivery System
  - Structure and Function of the Public/ Community Healthcare Delivery System
  - Continuum of Care
  - Continuity of Care

- Individual, Family, and Community Health
- Access to Care
- Across the Life Span
- Health Disparities
- Health Promotion and Disease Prevention
  - Health Promotion
  - Disease Prevention

- Important Concepts
  - Patient as Focus of Care and Member of the Healthcare Team
  - Vulnerable Populations
  - Health and Illness
  - Stress, Coping, Adaptation, and Resilience: A Public/Community Perspective
  - Acute Illness
  - Greater Emphasis on Chronic Disease
  - Medical Home Model
  - Self-Management
  - Health Literacy
- Multiple Perspectives of Public/Community Health Services
  - Community Emergency Preparedness
  - Managing Population Health
  - Migrant and Immigrant Issues
  - Home Health Care
  - School Health
  - Rehabilitation
  - Extended Care, Long-Term Care, and Elder Care
  - End-of-Life and Palliative Care
  - Case Management
  - Occupational Health Care
  - Complementary and Alternative Therapies or Integrative Medicine
  - Genetics
    - The Changing Nature of Public/Community Health Problems
  - Violence in Communities
  - Opioid Epidemic
- Global Healthcare Concerns and International Nursing
- Chapter Highlights
- Engaging in the Content
- Discussion Questions
- Critical Thinking Activities
- Electronic Reflection Journal
- Case Studies
- Working Backward to Develop a Case
- References

KEY TERMS

Acute care	Extended care	Primary care provider
Acute illness	Family	Primary prevention
Caregiver	Health	Rehabilitation
Care coordination	Health disparity	Resilience
Case management	Health promotion	Secondary caregiver
Chronic disease	Healthy community	Secondary prevention
Collaboration	Home care	Self-management
Community	Hospice care	Stress
Continuity of care	Illness	Stress management
Continuum of care	Long-term care	Tertiary prevention
Coping	Occupational health care	Vulnerable population
Disease management	Palliative care	
Disease prevention	Population	

Introduction

This chapter provides an introduction to a variety of public/community health issues, such as health promotion and disease prevention, the continuum of care, healthcare disparities, chronic disease, and delivery of care in a variety of settings in the community. Nursing programs provide clinical experiences for students in many of the settings and situations discussed in this chapter, and students also learn about public/community health in more depth in public/community health courses. In this chapter, public/community health is introduced as an important component of healthcare delivery and nursing. Where do patients receive care? Who are the patients? How are health and illness viewed by patients and by nurses, and what impact does this view have on healthcare delivery? Nurses need an understanding of these critical public/community health issues. "Although the United States spends more on health care than any country in the world, its citizens as a whole are the least healthy in the developed world. Nearly 45% of Americans have at least one chronic condition, and chronic conditions are responsible for 70% of the Nation's deaths and 75% of health care spending. Many illnesses associated with chronic conditions are related to unhealthy lifestyle behaviors and can be prevented by increasing access to effective clinical preventive services and promoting community interventions that advance public health. Public health spending has been shown to be particularly effective for lower income, and often higher need, communities, with 21% to 44% greater health and economic effects in low-income communities compared with the average-income community. Increasing public health spending and improving access to preventive care thus holds promise as a cost-efficient way to create healthier communities, reduce the personal and economic burden of chronic illnesses, and improve quality of life while reducing disparities throughout the United States" (U.S. Department of Health and Human Services [HHS], & Agency for Healthcare Research and Quality [AHRQ], 2016). This description indicates that much needs to be done in public/community health and improvement can impact many people.

A National Initiative
to Improve the Nation's Health:
Healthy People 2020

The HHS, its agencies, and other government departments that have responsibilities related to health and healthcare services (federal, state, and local) are charged to develop programs that promote health and prevent disease and illness and provide data to evaluate outcomes. The ultimate measure of success of this health improvement initiative is the health status of the target population. To meet this goal the *Healthy People 2020* (HHS, 2017) is designated as a national prevention initiative that focuses on improving the health of Americans by providing a comprehensive set of disease health promotion and disease prevention goals and objectives with target dates describing a timeline for evaluation of outcomes.

There have been five editions of *Healthy People* (1979, 1990, 2000, 2010, and 2020) (HHS, 2017). Its vision and major goals that should be reached by 2020 include the following:

Vision
A society in which all people live long healthy lives

Mission
Healthy People 2020 strives to:
- Identify nationwide health improvement priorities.
- Increase public awareness and understanding of the determinants of health, disease, and disability and the opportunities for progress.
- Provide measurable objectives and goals that are applicable at the national, state, and local levels.
- Engage multiple sectors to take actions to strengthen policies and improve practices that are driven by the best available evidence and knowledge.
- Identify critical research, evaluation, and data collection needs.

Overarching Goals
- Attain high-quality, longer lives free of preventable disease, disability, injury, and premature death.
- Achieve health equity, eliminate disparities, and improve the health of all groups.
- Create social and physical environments that promote good health for all.
- Promote quality of life, healthy development, and healthy behaviors across all life stages.

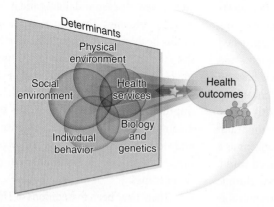

Overarching goals:

- Attain high quality, longer lives free of preventable disease, disability, injury, and premature death.
- Achieve health equity, eliminate disparities, and improve the health of all groups.
- Create social and physical environments that promote good health for all.
- Promote quality of life, healthy development, and healthy behaviors across all life stages.

Figure 7-1 Healthy People 2020

Reproduced from U.S. Department of Health and Human Services. (2017). *Healthy People 2020*. Washington, DC: U.S. Government Printing Office. Retrieved from http://www.healthypeople.gov

Figure 7-1 presents the *Healthy People 2020* model, which emphasizes the critical determinants for a society in which all people live long, healthy lives. These determinants are the physical environment, the social environment, individual behavior, biology and genetics, and health services. All of the determinants affect health outcomes, and the determinants of health interact with one another. The determinants need to be monitored and evaluated to improve the health status of individuals, families, and communities. According to *Healthy People*, health status is determined by measuring birth and death rates, life expectancy, quality of life, morbidity from specific diseases, risk factors, use of ambulatory care and inpatient care, accessibility of health providers and facilities, financing of health care, health insurance coverage, and other factors. Access to health care is critical. This is a complex healthcare issue that affects the health status of individuals and communities. For example, when the causes of death in the United States are examined, there typically is not one single factor or behavior that determines outcomes, but rather multiple factors—such as genetics, lifestyle, gender, and race/ethnic factors; poverty level, education, injury, violence, and other factors in the environment;

and the unavailability or inaccessibility of quality health services.

Healthy People 2020 focuses on topics that are tracked and monitored to assess outcomes. **Exhibit 7-1** describes major topics and identifies their related indicators and objectives, which may change based on monitoring data and outcomes. This plan relates to the annual National Quality and Disparities Report and also to the new National Quality Strategy (NQS). Both of these are discussed in other chapters in this text. The *Healthy People 2020* data indicate that from 2010 to 2014, 14 of the 26 indicators (53.9%) either met their target or have shown improvement (HHS, 2014). Data are typically not up-to-date with the current year as it takes time to collect and analyze the data.

A **community** is defined as "people and the relationships that emerge among them as they develop and use in common some agencies and institutions and share a physical environment" (Williams, 2006, p. 3). The *Healthy People 2020* initiative describes a **healthy community** as one that embraces the belief that health is more than merely an absence of disease; a healthy community includes those elements that enable people to maintain a high quality of life and productivity. A healthy community has

Exhibit 7-1 *Healthy People 2020* Topics and Leading Health Indicators

Topic	Leading Health Indicators
Access to health services	• Persons with medical insurance (percent, <65 years) • Persons with a usual primary care provider (percent)
Clinical preventive services	• Adults receiving colorectal cancer screening on most recent guidelines (age adjusted, percent, 50–75 years) • Adults with hypertension whose blood pressure is under control (age adjusted, percent, 18+ years) • Persons with diagnosed diabetes whose A1c value is >9% (age adjusted, percent, 18+ years) • Children receiving the recommended doses of DTaP, polio, MMR, Hib, hepatitis B, varicella, and PCV vaccines (percent, aged 19–35 months)
Environmental quality	• Air quality index (AQI) exceeding 100 (number of billion person days, weighted by population and AQI value) • Children exposed to secondhand smoke (percent, nonsmokers, 3–11 years)
Injury and violence	• Injury deaths • Homicides
Maternal, infant, and child health	• Infant deaths (per 1,000 live births, <1 year) • Total preterm live births (percent, <37 weeks' gestation)
Mental health	• Suicide (age adjusted, per 100,000 population) • Adolescents with major depressive episodes (percent, 12–17 years)
Nutrition, physical activity, and obesity	• Adults meeting aerobic physical activity and muscle-strengthening federal guidelines (age adjusted, percent, 18+ years) • Obesity among adults (age adjusted, percent, 20+ years) • Obesity among children and adolescents (age adjusted, percent, 2–19 years) • Mean daily intake of total vegetables (age adjusted, cup equivalents per 1,000 calories, 2+ years)
Oral health	• Persons who visited the dentist in the past year (age adjusted, percent 2+ years)
Reproductive and sexual health	• Sexually experienced females receiving reproductive health services in the past 12 months (percent, 15–44 years) • Knowledge of serostatus among HIV-positive persons (percent, 13+ years)
Social determinants	• Students awarded a high school diploma 4 years after starting 9th grade (percent)
Substance abuse	• Adolescents using alcohol or illicit drugs in past 30 days (percent, 12–17 years) • Adult binge drinking in past 30 days (percent, 18+ years)
Tobacco	• Adult cigarette smoking (age adjusted, percent, 18+ years) • Adolescent cigarette smoking in past 30 days (percent, grades 9–12)

Modified from U.S. Department of Health and Human Services. (2017). *Healthy People 2020*. Leading Health Indicators. Retrieved from https://www.healthypeople.gov/2020/Leading-Health-Indicators

the following characteristics: It is safe; provides both treatment and prevention services to all community members; has the infrastructure (roads, schools, playgrounds, and other services) to meet needs; and is a healthy environment (regarding issues of pollution, for example, air and water). Educational and community-based programs need to focus on preventing disease and injury, promoting and improving health, and enhancing the quality of life. According to *Healthy People 2020*, to provide broad access, programs and their services should be located in schools, workplaces, healthcare facilities, and community sites. These programs might offer services for prevention, monitoring, treatment, and rehabilitation focused on the following:

- Chronic diseases
- Injury and violence
- Mental illness
- Oral health
- Tobacco use
- Substance abuse
- Nutrition, physical activity, and obesity

One method that a community might use to develop a healthy community is called "MAP-IT," which is an approach recommended by *Healthy People* to work with community members to plan what needs to be done to improve the community's health. The MAP-IT steps are (HHS, 2010):

- **M**obilize individuals and organizations that care about the health of the community into a coalition.
- **A**ssess the areas of greatest need in the community, as well as the resources and other strengths that planners can tap into to address those areas.
- **P**lan the approach. Community leaders/members start with a vision of where they want to be as a community; they then add strategies and action steps to help them achieve that vision.
- **I**mplement a plan using concrete action steps that can be monitored and will make a difference.
- **T**rack progress over time.

The *Healthy People 2020* initiative not only provides a 10-year plan to improve health care in the United States, but also monitors and reports on progress periodically to determine if the goals and objectives are being met. Data on current outcomes can be found on the *Healthy People* website. When the 10-year time period is completed, all leading indicators are evaluated, and the analysis of the outcome data is then used to develop the goals, objectives, and leading indicators for the next 10 years version 2013 is in preparation.

Stop and Consider #1

Healthy People 2020 is a national initiative that has implications for nursing care.

Public/Community
Healthcare Delivery System

The public/community healthcare delivery system is complex and varied. We have a national system and also state and local systems. This section examines the system and its differences from the acute care system and how they relate to provide an overall health system for members of the community.

Structure and Function of the Public/Community Healthcare Delivery System

Public/community health plays a critical role in improving and maintaining the health of individuals, families, and communities. Public health focuses on issues related to the public health workforce, financing and economics, structure and performance, and information and technology. It is a complicated endeavor, requiring multiple services to meet needs of populations and communities (Robert Wood Johnson Foundation [RWJF], 2012). There is a great need to address multiple complex health problems in communities, such as violence, including domestic, child, and elder abuse; substance abuse and alcohol dependency; tobacco use; injuries; automobile accidents; environmental factors such as air and water quality; food safety and consequent health issues; chronic illnesses; and communicable diseases. Public health has recently become more important with the increasing concern about disaster emergency management, terrorism, and now the growing opioid epidemic. Communities need to develop effective plans to provide healthcare services in major crisis situations. All these concerns require more than just care for individuals who are experiencing these problems; we need to look at populations and communities. Public health incorporates three functions:

- *Assessment:* Assess and diagnose the status of the community's health and identify the needs for services using epidemiology, surveillance, research, and evaluation.
- *Policy development:* Some problems require changes in laws, programs for prevention and treatment, and reimbursement for these services. There is a great need for strategic plans and interventions, and appropriate evaluation of outcomes needs to be developed through the government and its agencies at all levels (local, state, and federal).
- *Assurance:* Ensure universal access to care when it is needed and to health promotion and prevention of disease and illness through community-wide health services.

The public/community healthcare delivery system is complex and can be viewed from the perspectives of the federal, state, and local levels. The HHS, the Centers for Disease Control and Prevention (CDC), Food and Drug Administration (FDA), and the Public Health Service (PHS) have major responsibilities in ensuring the health of the nation. States and local areas vary as to how their public/community healthcare delivery systems are organized and the types of services they provide; however, services typically include immunizations,

environmental health issues (water, air, sanitation), transportation safety, food safety, maintenance of licensure for healthcare providers (such as physicians, nurses, hospitals, long-term care facilities, and others), clinic systems, disaster emergency planning, school health through public schools, and much more. Each state has a public health department or division, and typically counties and other local entities also have their own public/community health services. It is important that all three levels of government public health services collaborate and communicate to ensure effective services; however, this is not always the case. Although the Affordable Care Act of 2010 (ACA) focuses primarily on healthcare reimbursement, which has a direct impact on public/community health, it does have some provisions that relate to public/community health, such as health screening options in insurance plans. Changes in this law may have an effect on these provisions.

Nurses are very active in all types of public/community services, serving in administrative and planning roles at the federal, state, and local levels; assessing service needs; providing services in clinics and other state and local healthcare facilities; providing immunizations; working toward tuberculosis control and control of other communicable diseases, particularly during times of epidemics or unexpected communicable diseases (most recently, for example, the Ebola virus and Zika virus outbreaks; providing human immunodeficiency virus (HIV)/acquired immunodeficiency syndrome (AIDS) care and prevention; developing and implementing health promotion and disease prevention; providing home care and hospice care; working as school nurses and occupational health nurses; conducting research in areas of public/community health; and participating in epidemiology activities). The role of the public health nurse has evolved and includes greater focus on population-based health promotion and prevention (Kulbok, Thatcher, Park, & Meszaros, 2012). This role requires much more collaboration with a variety of organizations, healthcare professionals, and others in the community—community participation is critical to effective public/community health and nursing within the community. Nurses who work in this area need to be able to collect and analyze data, develop plans and interventions, use a variety of interventions such as typical nursing interventions (for example, health assessment, immunizations) and use different interventions (for example, implementing health education focused on population groups, involvement in planning a health fair, working with the city council to develop plans for disasters and other situations, school nursing, work in clinics or even establish nurse managed clinics collaborate with acute care, and so on) (Pilon et al., 2015). Cultural competence is even more important in public/community heath nursing than in acute care. Nurses need greater program planning skills, which requires coordination, communication, and collaboration. When students take public/community health courses, they learn more about this critical area of health care and the roles of nurses and other members of the public/community health team.

Continuum of Care

The **continuum of care** is an important concept in nursing and health care. In 2004, The Joint Commission (then called the Joint Commission on Accreditation of Healthcare Organizations) defined the continuum of care as "matching an individual's ongoing needs with the appropriate level and type of medical, psychological, health, or social care or service within an organization or across multiple organizations" (p. 317). The goal of the continuum of care is to decrease fragmented care and costs. The continuum includes health promotion, disease and illness prevention, ambulatory care, acute care, tertiary care, home health care, long-term care, and hospice and palliative care. The continuum is a view of health care that describes a range of services in a variety of settings so that a patient might receive care at different stages of health and illness.

Some hospitals are evolving into community health networks (Seegert, 2016). This is happening as hospitals are trying to determine how best to deal with a changing payment system, increasing costs, and the need to optimize patient outcomes and improve population health. Collaborating with others in the community—some who provide care and others who provide support services, funding, government structure and functions—may make the difference in meeting goals. Working in isolation from others will not meet the goals. These hospitals are using nurses to help with making greater connection with the community. "Rethinking health care requires a shift in the mindsets and skill sets of all who care for patients. It's less about episodes of care and more about an entire continuum of services" (Seegert, 2016, p. 19). Critical aspects of the continuum include the need for coordination, collaboration, and effective healthcare teams. These topics are discussed in other chapters of this text.

Continuity of Care

"**Continuity of care** is the degree to which a series of discrete events is experienced as coherent and connected and consistent with the patient's medical needs and personal context" (Haggerty, Reid, Freeman, Starfield, Adair, & McKendry, 2003, p. 1219). This definition was developed after a multidisciplinary review of continuity of care literature to determine how different healthcare professionals viewed the concept. It was noted that continuity of care is different from other views of care because it focuses on care over time and on individual patients to ensure connection of treatment to needs as they change. Three types of continuity are important, and they arise at different times, dependent on the care setting.

- *Informational continuity:* Information is very important in health care, across the continuum of care and to continuity of care. This type of continuity focuses on information that is needed to link care from one provider and setting to another—for example, medical information, the patient's preferences, values, and context. As noted in this text, healthcare information technology has become more and more important and now offers greater and faster accessibility to information. In addition, the Internet offers the same to the consumer.

- *Management continuity:* When patients have complex and chronic problems, management of multiple providers ensures that all providers are aware of what each is doing and all are working toward the same outcomes. This requires sharing information and plans and demonstrating flexibility to ensure quality care. A common problem that occurs in these situations is that one provider does not know the medications another provider has prescribed. Often, a home health nurse discovers a lack of coordination when the nurse reviews all the medications (medication reconciliation) a patient is taking that may have been prescribed by different physicians or other providers. Serious medication errors can result from this problem. As more care is provided in the community, there will be increased risk associated with managing clinical problems unless there is improved structure and communication within the community.

- *Relational continuity:* This type of continuity concerns the need for patients to develop relationships with providers, particularly in the community. The **primary care provider** often serves as the entry point into the healthcare system, and if used by the patient, should coordinate the patient's overall care and make referrals to specialists when necessary. Relational continuity emphasizes the need for providers to be familiar with the patient and the patient's history so that when the patient becomes ill, there is someone who has a relationship with the patient and can easily access past medical information.

Nurses are very involved in continuity of care when they transfer and coordinate care over time and focus on consistency of care. Typically, this is done through discharge planning. Nurses who work in the community need to recognize the importance of continuity of care and integrate this into planning for individuals, families, and populations within the community. They need to recognize that care is a continuum and acute care is part of the continuum.

Individual, Family, and Community Health

The usual assumption is to consider the patient as an individual, and most patients are individuals. There are, however, other views of the patient. The family, the community, and specific populations, such as patients with specific chronic diseases, may also be viewed as patients. In public/community health, there is greater emphasis on the health of families, populations, and communities.

A **family** is defined as "two or more individuals who depend on one another for emotional, physical, and/or financial support. Members of a family are self-defined" (Kaakinen, Hanson, & Birenbaum, 2006, p. 322). Functional families are considered healthy families in which there is a state of bio/psycho/socio/cultural/spiritual well-being. A healthy family provides autonomy and is responsive to individual members within the family. In contrast, dysfunctional families have poor communication and relationships with one another and do not provide support to family members.

Nurses work with families in many ways along the continuum of care. The family itself may be the patient, or the nurse may be involved with a family because of one family member's illness. For example, a home health nurse caring for a patient who has uncontrolled diabetes, who is recovering from surgery, and who lives with her daughter and family must be aware of family dynamics, needs, caregiver strain, and other health issues that can impact the identified patient's care and outcomes such as dietary changes.

Family members may also be caregivers. A **caregiver** is someone who provides care to another person. He or she is a nonprofessional healthcare provider. Because many insurance plans provide limited or no coverage for home care, families often need to serve as caregivers for short-term or long-term needs of family members. This is not easy to do when family members work and have other obligations. Serving as a caregiver for a family member on a long-term basis can lead to caregiver psychological, physical, social, and financial problems. The majority of caregivers are women; men are more likely to be cared for by their wives than the reverse because men have a shorter life expectancy (Schumacher, Beck, & Marren, 2006). Caregiver strain is something that the nurse needs to assess periodically to ensure that the caregiver(s), and therefore the family, receive the support needed. Primary caregivers provide the majority of daily aspects of care, and **secondary caregivers** help with intermittent activities (shopping, transportation, home repairs, getting bills paid, emergency support, and so on). Both types of caregiving can put a strain on the caregiver, but primary caregivers are at greater risk. There has been more focus on helping caregivers with information and support. In 2017, Marrelli, a home care nurse expert, developed an Internet-based resource for caregivers. Access to this in depth guide for caregivers will be offered by healthcare providers and insurers to patients and enrollees. This demonstrates the roles that nurses may assume in creating new tools for patients and then collaborating with technology experts to develop the tools (Marrelli, 2017).

Nurses offer many services in communities, and they may focus on an entire community or a specific population that lives in the community. A **population** is "a collection of people who share one or more personal or environmental characteristics" (Williams, 2006, p. 4). Examples of populations within a community include children, the elderly, those with a chronic disease such as diabetes or respiratory disease, and the homeless. A nurse might work in school health, assess needs of the elderly in the home, develop programs to screen for diabetes in people in the community who might be at risk, manage a clinic for the homeless, or develop and implement a community disaster emergency preparedness plan. There are many other ways that a nurse might assist different populations within a community.

Access to Care

Access to care is, of course, the first step in receiving care, and it is not a simple process for many people; for some, there are major barriers. Access to care is a critical public/community health issue at federal, state, and local levels. Many people think of access as solely the ability to physically get to a destination, but access to care actually involves many factors:

- Ability to pay for care, either by insurance or personally
- Transportation to get to care
- Hours of operation at the clinical site
- Waiting time to get an appointment
- Long waits at the time of appointment to see a physician or other healthcare provider
- Ability to get an appointment
- Availability of type of healthcare provider needed
- Ability of the patient and provider to communicate and make use of accommodations for language, hearing, and sight
- Timeliness of laboratory tests
- Handicap provisions at the healthcare site
- Childcare provisions so that family members can go to appointments
- Cultural barriers
- Inadequate information or lack of information
- Lack of provider time (rushed)
- Insurer not covering specific treatment or medications
- Provider not accepting patient's insurance coverage
- Inadequate transportation choices, schedules, and cost

As this list suggests, access is a complex issue, particularly for vulnerable populations.

Access to care has a major impact on the continuum of care. Can the patient get the care that is needed when it is needed? Where is the best location for care? When patients experience barriers to access, they may neglect routine care and put off getting care when it is needed. These patients may then need more complex care and use the safety net, which are services that cover patients who cannot pay for care or who have other access barrier problems. Examples of safety net sites include free clinics, academic health centers, and emergency rooms. This type of care may (or may not) meet the patient's immediate need, and it does not typically support an effective continuum of care and continuity of care. Patients who fall into the safety net often get lost in the system, and their outcomes may not be positive. A *Healthy People 2020* goal focuses on this concern (HHS, 2017). The goal is to achieve health equity, eliminate disparities, and improve the health of all groups.

One approach to improving access to healthcare services is to offer comprehensive and wraparound services. Comprehensive services are best described as "one-stop shopping," in which the patient can go to one place and receive multiple services. These services are typically offered in convenient locations such as neighborhoods, schools, or work sites. Health promotion and illness prevention can also be built into these services. Recognizing that social and economic problems have a major impact on a person's health and access to needed services, wraparound services can be combined with comprehensive health services when the healthcare sites also offer social and economic services (for example, access to a social worker to assist patients with getting food and housing, job issues, and assistance with healthcare reimbursement problems).

Another critical factor that has a major impact on access to care is the ability to pay for care, typically with some type of insurance. The ACA primarily addresses this issue, although its implementation does not mean all citizens will have insurance. The overall goal for the ACA was to reduce the number of people without health insurance in the United States. Using data from the Current Population Survey (CPS), 9.1% of the U.S. population, or 29 million people, were uninsured in 2015, down from 13.3% in 2013 (Kaiser Family Foundation [KFF], 2016). Enrollment is increasing, reducing the number of the uninsured. It is important that the people who enroll in the ACA insurance options represent balanced needs, ideally with a lot of young, healthy people to offset the costs attributable to older, sicker enrollees who require more care. Insurers that are burdened with sicker enrollees without healthier enrollees will have financial problems. This law does not establish a universal healthcare system. If people do not obtain insurance—which is now easier to get, especially given that the law provides some financial support to help some people cover the costs—this law requires persons without health insurance to pay penalties. This carrot-and-stick strategy represents a complex approach to the problem, and this approach may be changed due to the Trump administration's efforts to repeal and replace the ACA. The results of these potential changes will be better known later in the administration. Due to the potential for major changes in the ACA, it is important for nurses to keep up-to-date on changes and consider the impact the changes might have on nurses, nursing care, and health care in general.

Accountable care organizations (ACOs) are recommended in ACA provisions. These organizations attempt to contain healthcare costs by fostering care coordination across disciplines and providing for integrated care delivery. An example of one such ACO is Kaiser Permanente, in which the insurer, physician groups, and healthcare institutions work together to provide integrated services from acute care to community-based care (Accountable Care Facts, 2014). It is important to note that Kaiser Permanente is not a new organization; it existed before the passage of the ACA and it is unclear what affect changes in the ACA might have on such provisions as the one that establishes ACOs.

Across the Life Span

Patients may enter the healthcare system for a variety of needs and services, and they may enter at any point in the life span from:

- Conception
- Birth
- Infancy
- Childhood
- Adolescence
- Young adulthood
- Middle adulthood
- Older adulthood
- End of life

Each of these life-span periods includes specific health concerns and needs, as well as potential disease and illness risks. In addition, social and psychological experiences affect health and wellness. These experiences include situations such as the death of a loved one, change in or loss of a job, beginning school, moving, marriage, birth of a child, divorce, the need to care for a family member who is ill, retirement, and other stressful situations. The federal government collects data about health and illness across the life span. **Exhibit 7-2** provides a list of the leading causes of death that impact public/community health status. The data are updated periodically by the CDC on its website.

Health Disparities

Health disparities have become even more important in the last 10 years. The Institute of Medicine, now known as the National Academy of Medicine (NAM), issued reports in its *Quality Chasm* series of reports with supporting data demonstrating that the U.S. healthcare system has severe problems with health/healthcare disparities (Institute of Medicine [IOM], 2002). A **health disparity** is an inequality or gap that exists between two or more groups. Health disparities are believed to be the result of the complex interaction of personal, economic, societal, and environmental factors. *Healthy People 2020* considers measures of race/ethnicity, gender, physical and mental ability, and geography to be among these factors (HHS, 2017). The national healthcare disparities report is now combined with the quality report and called the National Healthcare Quality and Disparities Report (QDR). Healthcare quality is affected by race, ethnicity, socioeconomic status, age, sex, disability status, sexual orientation, gender identity, and residential location (HHS, & AHRQ, 2015). The 2015 report provides data about disparities related to race and socioeconomic status, for example (HHS, & AHRQ, 2015):

- People in poor households received worse care than people in high-income households for about 60% of quality measures.

Exhibit 7-2 Leading Causes of Death in the United States, 2014 Data *(most frequent to least frequent)*

- Heart diseases
- Cancer
- Chronic lower respiratory diseases
- Accidents (unintentional injuries)
- Stroke (cerebrovascular diseases)

- Alzheimer's disease
- Diabetes
- Influenza and pneumonia
- Nephritis, nephrotic syndrome, and nephrosis
- Intentional self-harm (suicide)

Reproduced from National Center for Health Statistics. (2016). *Health United States, 2015: With special features on racial and ethnic health disparities.* Retrieved from https://www.cdc.gov/nchs/data/hus/hus15.pdf

- Blacks, Hispanics, and American Indians and Alaska Natives received worse care than Whites for about 40% of quality measures.
- Asians received worse care than Whites for about 20% of quality measures.
- For each group, disparities in quality of care are similar to disparities in access to care, although disparities in access tend to be more common than disparities in quality.
- Disparities also varied across NQS priorities:
  - Disparities were more common among measures of person-centered care and care coordination, involving about 60% of comparisons (data not shown).
  - Disparities were less common among measures of patient safety, effective treatment, and healthy living, involving about 30% of comparisons (data not shown).
- Through 2013, about 40% of disparities at baseline for Blacks, Hispanics, and people in poor households were getting smaller. Nearly one-third of disparities for Asians were getting smaller.
- About 20% of disparities at baseline for American Indians and Alaska Natives were getting smaller.
- Disparities that were getting smaller included 24 measures in which a disparity at baseline was eliminated (9% of disparities at baseline), primarily affecting Blacks and Hispanics.
- There were also 16 measures in which a disparity was not present at baseline but developed over time (4% of contrasts in which there was not a disparity at baseline), primarily affecting Asians (data not shown).
- Change in disparities over time also varied across NQS priorities.
  - About 45% of disparities related to care coordination and effective treatment were getting smaller (data not shown).
  - Only about 30% of disparities related to patient safety, person-centered care, and healthy living were getting smaller (data not shown).

Health Promotion and Disease Prevention

The United States spends more on health care; however, its citizens as a whole are least healthy compared to other developed countries (HHS, AHRQ, 2016). Chronic illness is a major factor that affects this outcome; chronic illness also often leads to unhealthier lifestyle behaviors. The American Hospital Association (AHA) developed an initiative that describes a road map for improving America's healthcare system. It focuses on wellness rather than acute care. The goals of this initiative (Health for Life: Better Health. Better Healthcare) are as follows (AHA, 2011):

- Focus on wellness
- Most efficient, affordable care
- The highest quality care
- Best information
- Health coverage for all; paid by all

In addition, the National Quality Strategy promotes health and well-being of communities by promoting healthy living and well-being through (1) community interventions that result in improvement of social, economic, and environmental factors; (2) interventions that result in adoption of the most important healthy lifestyle behaviors across the life span; and (3) receipt of effective clinical preventive services across the life span in clinical and community settings (HHS, AHRQ, 2016).

Health Promotion

Health promotion focuses on changing lifestyle to maximize health and is an important part of primary prevention. This is very difficult for most people to accomplish. An example of efforts to better understand and address health promotion was the 2006 National Prevention Summit, which focused on disease prevention, health preparedness, and health promotion and featured innovative programs that are making a difference in communities across the country to build a healthier country (HHS, &

Office of Disease Prevention and Health Promotion [ODPHP], 2006). These programs examined healthy lifestyle choices—eating a nutritious diet, being physically active, making healthy choices, and getting preventive screenings—to help prevent major health threats and burdens such as diabetes, asthma, cancer, heart disease, and stroke. A special emphasis was the prevention of overweight children and obesity, which have become major problems since 2006 and can lead to long-term chronic diseases such as diabetes (HHS, & CDC, 2011). Another emphasis was on preparing for public health emergencies, such as influenza, biochemical hazards, and natural disasters. The need for this preparation continues in all communities and is discussed later in this chapter.

Many models describe how health promotion might be effective. Pender's health promotion model is a nursing model that has been used in many studies about health promotion (Pender, Murdaugh, & Parsons, 2006). This model does not include fear or threat as a motivator to make people change their behaviors, and it can be used across the life span. Pender's health promotion model includes individual characteristics and experiences; that is, it emphasizes that each person is unique. The following aspects of health promotion have an impact on health and should be considered:

- *Prior related behavior:* The frequency of the same or similar behavior in the past is the best predictor of behavior.
- *Personal factors:* Biological (age, weight, pubertal status, and strength), psychological (self-esteem, coping style, and self-motivation), and sociocultural (race, ethnicity, education, and socioeconomic status) factors may influence the cognitions, affects, and health behavior that are the focus.
- *Behavior-specific cognitions and affects:* These cognitions and affects are very important because nursing interventions can change them, which can in turn move a person toward health-promoting behaviors.

- *Perceived benefits of action:* Whether a person will be active in participating in changing behavior is highly dependent on whether the person sees any benefit in doing so—that is, whether there are perceived benefits. It is important to determine whether perceived barriers are real. If perceived barriers to success are felt by a person, it is much more difficult for that person to change a behavior to a health-promoting behavior.
- *Perceived self-efficacy:* Self-efficacy relates to whether a person feels that it is possible to do what is needed. It does not mean that the person has the competency to do this, but rather centers on whether the person feels that he or she could actually do what needs to be done.
- *Activity-related affect:* Emotions tied to actions are important to recognize, because they can determine whether a person repeats a behavior. Did the person feel good about what he or she did? Did it make the person anxious?
- *Interpersonal influences:* A person is influenced by others, family, friends, co-workers, peers, healthcare providers, and so on. This influence—what it might be and how it might be felt—may or may not be reality based, but it still can influence a person's behavior and the person's ability to change to health-promoting behavior.
- *Situational influences:* A situation or context can influence a person's behavior. If a person smokes and is told that all smoking must take place outside the building in a designated area regardless of the weather, this situation or context may influence a change in behavior.
- *Commitment to a plan of action:* Is a person committed to a specific plan to change to health-promoting behavior? Commitment is not enough; strategies must be laid out that will enable the person to reach the desired outcomes.

- *Immediate competing demands and preferences:* What might interfere with a person changing to health-promoting behavior? Will the family be supportive? Are there other actions that must take precedence (for example, work over exercise)? Each person has alternative behaviors that compete with what the person needs to do to change to a healthier lifestyle.
- *Health-promoting behavior:* This is the outcome, and from this, a person reaches positive health outcomes.

In any context, the social determinants, or the conditions in the environments in which people live, affect an individual's health status. The World Health Organization (WHO, 2011) describes the social determinants of health as geographic region and condition of birth and life, work environment, age, and the health care that is available and accessible. Health is always influenced by access to care—a factor that may be related to an understanding of healthy habits or how to use available health resources, socioeconomic status, and resources that are allocated by governments for the populace (WHO, 2011). When we consider these determinants, we are looking at social policies, cultural and social norms, political issues and systems, diversity, and disparities. We need to use partnerships to address the social determinants—they cross many areas and concerns of society—and we also need to be more prepared—offering more on the determinants in academic health professional programs and to healthcare staff as part of lifelong learning (NAM, 2016).

Disease Prevention

Disease prevention is concerned with interventions to stop the development of disease, but it also includes treatment to prevent disease from progressing further and leading to complications. The major levels of prevention are primary, secondary, and tertiary (Leavell & Clark, 1965).

- **Primary prevention** includes interventions that are used to maintain health before illness

occurs. Health promotion is a critical component of primary prevention. Examples are teaching people (children and adults) about healthy diets before they become obese and encouraging adequate exercise (education about health and healthy lifestyles is an important intervention at this level).
- **Secondary prevention** occurs when a person is asymptomatic after disease has begun. The focus here is on preventing further complications. Examples are breast cancer screening using mammography and blood pressure screening to diagnose hypertension.
- **Tertiary prevention** occurs when there is disability and the need to maintain or, if possible, improve functioning. Examples would be teaching a person with diabetes how to administer insulin and manage the disease or referring a stroke patient for rehabilitation or providing long-term home care.

The ACA mostly focuses on reimbursement for health care, but the law also includes some provisions related to the need for greater services to promote health and prevent disease (though this is not the strength of the legislation). An example is the requirement that insurers pay for certain healthcare screening as part of their covered services; some of these screening services must not be charged to the patient. However, this provision is easy to misunderstand. If the screening is for diagnosis purposes, then it is not free. For example, if a woman notices she has a lump in her breast and has a mammogram to determine if there is a problem, this test would not be covered; in contrast, if she were having a routine annual mammogram (with no notice of a potential problem), then the screening would be free. Over the long term, this change in health plan services will increase the quality of life for many and reduce healthcare costs, but how much improvement and what will improve remain to be determined. In addition, any changes in the law, repeal or replacement, may have an impact on these provisions focused on prevention.

In 2011, the Office of the Surgeon General initiated the National Prevention Strategy, which aims to guide the United States in improving the health and well being of its population. The strategy prioritizes prevention by integrating recommendations and actions across multiple settings to improve health and save lives (HHS, Office of the Surgeon General, 2013). The initiative includes actions that public and private partners can take to help Americans stay healthy and fit and improve the nation's prosperity. It outlines four strategic directions that, collectively, are fundamental to improving the nation's health:

1. *Building healthy and safe community environments*: Prevention of disease starts in communities and at home, not just in the physician's office.
2. *Expanding quality preventive services in both clinical and community settings*: When people receive preventive care, such as immunizations and cancer screenings, they have better health and lower healthcare costs.
3. *Empowering people to make healthy choices*: When people have access to actionable and easy-to-understand information and resources, they are empowered to make healthier choices.
4. *Eliminating health disparities*: By eliminating disparities in achieving and maintaining health, the goal is to improve quality of life for all Americans.

Several initiatives related to health promotion and disease prevention are identified in this chapter, and they are all connected. For example, *Healthy People*, the ACA, and the National Prevention Strategy all focus on both individuals and their communities. Another theme that runs through these initiatives is the need to decrease health disparities—an issue noted in the Surgeon General's strategy, the *Quality Chasm* series of reports on health care, the ACA, *Healthy People 2020*, and the need to provide patient-centered care.

Stop and Consider #2

Nurses can make a positive impact on public/community health.

Important Concepts

Public/community health care includes a number of concepts that may not be found in acute health care or may be viewed differently. For example, the healthcare team may include different members from acute care such as government officials and agencies. The patient may be viewed as more than an individual or family. The following sections discuss some of these concepts.

Patient as Focus of Care and Member of the Healthcare Team

The patient is always the focus of care, even when the larger community is considered. Patients should be viewed as members of the healthcare team and should be involved in decision making about their own care. Patient-centered care means that the patient is the center of that care—receiving the care—and must be involved in care decisions. This point does not just apply to individual patients. In public or community health, the patient may be an individual, family, population, or the community and involve government officials and agencies as well as multiple different types of healthcare delivery services, including the private healthcare sector. All should be part of assessment, planning, and decision making. If this does not happen, the public/community health efforts are at risk for failure. Public/community health initiatives are most successful when community members participate in planning and evaluation of programs and their services. This is demonstrated regularly, for example, in local communities—in their health departments, city and county government meetings that might be discussing pollution, health needs, cost of school nurses, and so on. Community members as elected officials and as taxpayers and voters speak out about issues that relate to health and services in their communities. Patient-centered care is discussed in other chapters in this text.

Vulnerable Populations

A **vulnerable population** is a group of persons who are at risk for developing health problems. These populations often have problems accessing care when they need it, for example, vulnerable populations are children, the elderly, people with chronic disease, immigrants, illegal aliens, migrant workers, people who live in rural areas, homeless people, the serious mentally ill, victims of abuse and violence, pregnant adolescents, and people who are HIV positive. They need careful assessment and monitoring to identify problems early so that complications can be prevented. Typically, complex factors increase risk, such as physiological, psychological, economic, ethnic, religious, social, cultural, and communication factors. There may also be problems related to diet, housing, safety, education, and transportation.

Poverty is an important concern, which has a significant impact on individual and public/community health, as described by the following data (U.S. Census Bureau, 2016a):

- The official poverty rate in 2015 was 13.5%, down 1.2 percentage points from 14.8% in 2014.
- In 2015, there were 43.1 million people in poverty, 3.5 million less than in 2014.
- The 2015 poverty rate was 1.0 percentage point higher than in 2007, the year before the most recent recession.
- For most demographic groups, 2015 poverty rates and estimates of the number of people in poverty decreased from 2014.
- Between 2014 and 2015, poverty rates decreased for all three major age groups. The poverty rate for children under age 18 dropped 1.4 percentage points, from 21.1% to 19.7%. Rates for people aged 18 to 64 dropped 1.1 percentage points, from 13.5% to 12.4%. Poverty rates for people aged 65 and older decreased 1.1 percentage points, from 10.0% to 8.8%.

The poverty rate has been rising since 2000, but dropped by about 2 million people from 2012 to 2015 (U.S. Census Bureau, 2016a). The data are updated annually, though the published poverty rate is typically a few years behind the date reported.

Poverty guidelines are important because financial eligibility for certain federal programs is based on poverty levels; to receive specific services, a person must not have an income higher than the poverty level. An example of current poverty guidelines is found in **Table 7-1**.

Health and Illness

Health and wellness are terms that tend to be used interchangeably. But what does health mean? There is no simple response to this question. A simple definition of **health**, albeit one that is not complete, is to be structurally and functionally whole. Absence of this state is **illness**. Disease and illness are terms that are often used interchangeably. Disease is an indication of a physiological dysfunction or pathological reaction.

The WHO defines health as "a state of complete well-being, physical, social, and mental, and not merely the absence of disease or infirmity" (WHO, 2006). This is a common definition and one that is often quoted. The WHO addresses health and illness from a global perspective and identifies the following principles to guide its work:

- Health is not merely the absence of disease or infirmity.
- The enjoyment of the highest attainable standard of health is one of the fundamental rights of every human being without distinction of race, religion, political belief, or economic or social condition.
- The health of all peoples is fundamental to the attainment of peace and security and is dependent upon the fullest cooperation of individuals and states.
- The achievement of any state in the promotion and protection of health is of value to all.
- Unequal development in different countries in the promotion of health and control of disease, especially communicable disease, is a common danger.

Table 7-1　2017 Department of Health and Human Services Poverty Guidelines

Persons in Family	48 Contiguous States and Washington, DC	Alaska	Hawaii
2	$16,240	$20,290	$18,670
3	$20,420	$25,520	$23,480
4	$24,600	$30,750	$28,290
5	$28,780	$35,980	$33,100
6	$32,960	$41,210	$37,910
7	$37,140	$46,440	$42,720
8	$41,320	$51,670	$47,530
For families/households with more than 8 persons, add this amount per person	Add $4,180 for each additional person.	Add $5,230 for each additional person	Add $4,810 for each additional person.

Reproduced from U.S. Department of Health and Human Services. (2016, January 25). Annual update of the HHS poverty guidelines. *Federal Register, 81*(15), 4036–4037. Retrieved from https://www.federalregister.gov/documents/2016/01/25/2016-01450/annual-update-of-the-hhs-poverty-guidelines. The poverty guidelines are updated periodically in the Federal Register by the U.S. Department of Health and Human Services under the authority of 42 U.S.C. 9902(2).

- Healthy development of the child is of basic importance; the ability to live harmoniously in a changing total environment is essential to such development.
- The extension to all peoples of the benefits of medical, psychological, and related knowledge is essential to the fullest attainment of health.
- Informed opinion and active cooperation on the part of the public are of the utmost importance in the improvement of the health of the people.
- Governments have a responsibility for the health of their peoples that can be fulfilled only by the provision of adequate health and social measures.

Definitions of health should be applicable to all—to those who are well; to those with illness or disease that can be treated; and to those with acquired or genetic impairments that result in a chronic disease or disability. The definition has to be applied to individuals, families, communities, and nations (RWJF, 2000). The determinants of health or factors that have an impact on health are physical, mental, social, and spiritual. Stress and socioeconomic factors are also very important.

According to the Organization for Economic Cooperation and Development (OECD), life expectancy for Americans compared to 33 other countries mostly falls in the lower third performance category with some instances in middle third such as death from cardiovascular disease (OECD, 2015). The United States has long ranked lower in health and healthcare issues when compared by OECD with other countries. Access to care is defined, as availability of healthcare coverage, is also a problem for the United States when OECD compares the United States with other countries. Of the 34 countries, only five countries do not have coverage at the 95% to 100% level, and the United States is one of the five countries. The ACA or possible changes in the law may or may not improve this ranking. However, many other countries have universal health coverage, but this is not the case for the United States, so improvement will be limited.

The U.S. Census Bureau publishes data about health statistics specific for the United States. Life expectancy for the total population is 78.8 years: 76.4 years for men and 81.2 years for women (CDC used 2014 data). Differences in mortality between the Black and White populations persist in the United States, though the gap in life expectancy was reduced to a 3.4-year gap, and the Hispanic population life expectancy increased by 0.2 to a total of 82.8 years. White women have the highest life expectancy. Between 2004 and 2014, the infant mortality rate decreased by 14%, from 6.79 to 5.82 deaths per 1,000 live births. The neonatal mortality rate (among infants under age 28 days) decreased by 13%, from 4.52 to 3.94 per 1,000 live births. Between 2004 and 2014, the post-neonatal mortality rate (among infants aged 28 days through 11 months) decreased 17%, from 2.27 to 1.88 (HHS, & CDC, 2015; U.S. Census Bureau, 2016b). This type of data is used in public/community health to assess status of health in communities and to determine need for health promotion, disease prevention, and treatment services. It also affects other types of services such as projecting housing, education, and employment needs (for example, a community of older persons would require different community services versus a community composed of young families).

Stress, Coping, Adaptation, and Resilience: A Public/ Community Perspective

Stress is a complex experience, which is felt internally. It makes a person feel a loss or threat of a loss. Stress is present in all parts of life. Stress has an effect on current health status and can lead to

health problems—for example, a patient with a cardiac problem can experience more symptoms when experiencing high levels of stress; patients who have socioeconomic problems may not have an adequate diet because of lack of money, or they may experience sleep problems because they work two jobs—all factors that increase stress. Not all persons who experience stress experience negative outcomes. Communities may also experience stress—for example, stress caused by economic problems such as lack of employment and high poverty level, lack of critical healthcare services, increase in violence, or inadequate education for children. Weather can even increase stress in communities; for example, in summer when temperatures may be very high, some urban communities experience more violence among adolescents and young adults and people who may be outside more due to heat experience more risk for violence.

The most effective intervention for stress is **stress management**. Eliminating stress completely is not possible, but helping individuals, families, vulnerable populations, and communities better cope with stress is an important goal in improving health and developing health-promoting behaviors. Effective **coping** can reduce the negative impact of stress and, in many cases, prevent a person, family, or community from experiencing stress. This might be done through identifying stressors or stimuli that cause a person (family, community) to experience stress. Stressors can be biological, sociological, psychological, spiritual, or environmental. Self-assessment to identify stressors is critical to improve coping. Stress management interventions might include education to better understand stress and application of interventions, relaxation techniques, better sleep, healthy diet, exercise, music, and use of assertiveness—community education programs can offer residents information about these methods to reduce stress. Community-oriented interventions might include reducing violence by providing places for teen after-school activities, increasing access to community clinics, increasing jobs, improving transportation to areas where healthcare services are available, providing parenting classes, or increasing exercise classes and social activities in community centers. **Resilience**, or the ability to cope with stress, is an important factor. Communities can develop resilience—sometimes you hear on the news someone interviewed after a disaster such as a tornado and they talk about how the community is coming together, helping one another and they will survive. This is resilience. Adaptation to situations is also important to stress prevention and management. The same principles of stress apply to everyone, including patients—individuals, families, and communities.

Acute Illness

Acute illness is typically self-limiting and occurs over a short period of time—cure is the focus of acute care, though some acute illnesses may not be cured and then result in a chronic illness or death. Some of the care for acute illness takes place in the hospital, commonly referred to as the **acute care** setting, but today, more care is taking place in the patient's home in the community through primary care and ambulatory services or other community services and facilities that are not acute care. Examples of acute illnesses are an infectious disease such as the flu or pneumonia, a broken leg, appendicitis, and a urinary tract infection.

The curative model has long been viewed as the best approach to health; however, this model has come under criticism (RWJF, 2000). Yes, cure is a good goal, but is this the only view that can be applied to the complex area of health? There are other important other goals, as noted by the RWJF:

- Restoring functional capacity
- Relieving suffering
- Preventing illness, injury, and untimely death
- Promoting health
- Caring for those who cannot be cured

These additional goals expand what can be done to help those who need it because cure is not always possible. Moreover, with the increase in the number of people with chronic diseases and the growing elderly population, cure is becoming less important from the patient's daily perspective. There is more focus on functioning at the best possible level. The curative model focuses more on the biological approach, which relies on a hierarchical system of decision making in which physicians make diagnoses and order treatment. Nursing is more involved in other functions, although the nurse certainly participates in providing nursing care that is directed at cure, such as assisting in surgery to repair a fractured hip. The hip can be repaired, but the patient typically has other needs after this surgery that are tied to the other functions. The patient will need help gaining functional capacity, and he or she may never regain full capacity. The patient may require help with health promotion if the cause of the fracture was osteoporosis (for example, lifestyle changes related to diet, vitamins, and exercise). These factors need to be taken into account in follow-up care in the community.

Greater Emphasis on Chronic Disease

Another factor supporting implications for patient-centered care in public/community health is the growing number of patients with chronic diseases who need patient-centered care. In the United States, the total number of persons with chronic diseases has increased, as has the number of people with more than one chronic disease. Many of these diseases are preventable. The following data related to this problem support the need for more focus on chronic disease, which increase healthcare costs and impact quality of life (HHS, & CDC, 2016a).

- As of 2012, about half of all adults—117 million people—had one or more chronic health conditions. One of four adults had two or more chronic health conditions.

- Seven of the top 10 causes of death in 2010 were chronic diseases. Two of these chronic diseases—heart disease and cancer—together accounted for nearly 48% of all deaths.
- Obesity is a serious health concern. During 2009–2010, more than one-third of adults, or about 78 million people, were obese (defined as body mass index [BMI] $\geq$ 30 kg/m^2). Nearly one of five youths aged 2–19 years was obese (BMI $\geq$ 95th percentile).
- Arthritis is the most common cause of disability. Of the 53 million adults with a medical diagnosis of arthritis, more than 22 million say they have trouble with their usual activities because of arthritis.
- Diabetes is the leading cause of kidney failure, lower-limb amputations other than those caused by injury, and new cases of blindness among adults.

Data reported in 2013 indicated that approximately 133 million Americans (45% of the total population) have chronic illnesses. By 2020, this number is projected to increase to 157 million, with 81 million having multiple conditions (National Health Council, 2013).

One reason that the United States has problems with increasing chronic disease is that there is better treatment today, so people with chronic diseases live longer; consequently, there are more people with chronic disease. A second reason is that the United States still needs to improve care provided for chronic disease, particularly for patients with multiple chronic illnesses. Chronic disease is a serious problem not only in the United States, but also worldwide. "We have much to learn about how to structure and furnish health care services for individuals with multiple chronic conditions. And, we need to recognize that countries that perform better in coordinating care invest a higher proportion of their resources than we do in primary care. However, clinical guidelines focused on treating the whole patient, combined with improving the capacity of our primary care providers to better coordinate care, might help us to improve our performance. More importantly, it might result in better outcomes for a vulnerable group of patients" (Bindman, 2016).

Healthcare providers need to understand that care for patients with chronic diseases is different from acute care. In order to ensure that these complex care needs are met, integration of new knowledge and treatment may be required. If a nurse typically cares for patients with sudden-onset illnesses or with injuries for which the cure model is the focus, it may be difficult for the nurse to appreciate the differences in care for chronic diseases and needs of these patients. **Chronic diseases** are diseases for which there is no effective cure; in turn, their treatment focuses on control of symptoms, support, psychosocial issues, and if possible, prevention of deterioration and improved quality of life. Examples of chronic diseases include heart disease, diabetes, stroke, hypertension, rheumatoid arthritis, obesity, and even cancer (cancer survivors live with the long-term effects of the cancer and/or the treatment). Chronic diseases are the leading cause of death worldwide, namely, cardiovascular disease and chronic respiratory disease.

As with adults, chronic illness and disease prevention in children are major health considerations. According to the CDC (CDC used 2015 data), more than 6 million children (under age of 18) had asthma, and it was more common in children in poor families; 8% of all U.S. children aged 3–17 had a learning disability, which affected more boys and children in poor families, and 13% of children had taken a prescription for at least three months. Childhood obesity is also on the rise, increasing the incidence of diabetes, hypertension, and other related complications. Obesity rates have doubled in children and quadrupled in adolescents in the past 30 years (HHS, & CDC, 2011). Obesity has long-term effects on the health and well-being of children, affecting them throughout their lives. These effects include cardiovascular disease, diabetes, and bone and joint problems in addition to self-esteem issues that may lead to social and psychological problems.

Because of the increased recognition of chronic disease, innovations in interventions and services for patients with chronic diseases have increased. Examples from the government payment perspective are important to consider, such as the Centers for Medicare and Medicaid Services (CMS) innovative trial models of care to promote **care coordination**— for example, medical homes. Under this model, patients receive transitional care, care coordination, and comprehensive care management services. Self-management and health literacy are also important to consider when planning services for patients with chronic illness to ensure a comprehensive public/community health program. Methods for delivering care for chronic disease have improved, though much more needs to be done (for example, greater use of disease management, which is another systematic approach to managing a chronic disease). Typically, interventions used in disease management have been tested with large groups; thus they may be more effective than interventions tested in studies with a narrower scope. **Disease management** emphasizes use of interprofessional teams with expertise in the specific disease, use of evidence-based clinical guidelines, clear descriptions of interventions and procedures and application of recommended timelines, patient support and education, and measurement of outcomes. Nurses assume important roles in disease management; specifically, they may be on the team or lead the team. Insurers, hospitals, and other healthcare providers develop and sponsor disease management programs. The major goals are to assist patients in maintaining the best quality of life possible and preventing complications that might lead to deterioration and increased costs of care.

Disease management programs also emphasize prevention, although it is important to emphasize prevention throughout the healthcare system and particularly in community care—not just in special focused programs. Examples of prevention services include tobacco cessation counseling, screening

(breast cancer, colorectal cancer, prostate cancer, diabetes, hypertension, hearing, vision, cholesterol, and so on), and immunizations. Prevention is not always successful. Some of the barriers to its success are related to availability and use of previous services (Peters & Elster, 2002):

- Lack of reimbursement for these services
- Lack of time for services
- Lack of access for populations who need these services
- Inadequate consumer education to support need
- Uncertainty as to effectiveness (from both consumer and provider perspectives)
- Failure to assure empowerment of patients, which leads to effective self-management

Patients with chronic illness need support, as well as information, to become effective managers of their own health. To meet these needs, it is essential for them to have the following resources:

- Basic information about their disease and an understanding of self-management skills
- Ongoing support from members of the practice team, family, friends, and community as part of the self-management process
- Providers who are sensitive to the roles that families, caregivers, and communities assume in different cultures

In general, better patient outcomes are achieved through use of evidence-based techniques that emphasize patient activation or empowerment, collaborative goal setting, and problem-solving skills. The provider team may use standardized assessments of patient self-management needs and activities to enhance their ability to support patients. Such assessments include questions about self-management knowledge, skills, confidence, supports, and barriers (Institute for Healthcare Improvement [IHI], 2011).

A major report titled *Living Well with Chronic Illness: A Call for Public Action* indicates that there is greater interest in chronic illness and meeting the needs of people with these illnesses (IOM, 2012). The report describes this issue as a major public health problem: "Chronic disease is a public health as well as a clinical problem. Therefore, a population health perspective for developing strategies, interventions, and policies to combat it is critical. A population perspective considers how individuals' genes, biology, and behaviors interact with the social, cultural, and physical environment around them to influence health outcomes for the entire population" (IOM, 2012, p. 3). Community-based interventions are an important part of care for chronic illness, with prevention being the first intervention. Communities have many options they use for prevention such as health fairs, immunizations in locations that are easy to access, walking groups in malls, enforcing smoking bans, offering educational opportunities about health, smoking cessation groups, and exercise, as well as screening for diseases, substance abuse, stress, and so on. Establishing places for exercise in parks, walking paths, bike lanes, ensuring healthy diets in school lunches, and so on, help to increase exercise. A new intervention used in some locations is requiring restaurants to post calories for menu items. Community health departments might offer disease management programs and self-help options to benefit citizens. Working closely with an acute care system is critical for all of these efforts.

Medical Home Model

The medical home model, a model supported by the ACA, is a multidimensional solution for planned, clinically integrated care to meet the complex care needs of people with chronic disease; its elements include organizing care around patients, working in teams, and coordinating and tracking care over time (National Committee for Quality Assurance [NCQA], 2017). The focus is on interprofessional primary care teams. A common chronic care model, which is applied in many healthcare organizations, describes two major delivery focus areas: (1) The community needs to have resources and health policies that support care for chronic diseases, and (2) the health system

needs to have healthcare organizations that support self-management and recognize that the patient is the source of control; support a delivery system design that identifies clear roles for staff in relation to chronic disease care; supply decision support, integration of evidence-based guidelines into daily practice; and use of clinical information systems to ensure effective exchange of information and reminder and feedback systems (Wagner, 1998). If all of these elements are in place and effective, the results should be productive interactions with an informed, active patient and a prepared, proactive care team. The ultimate result should then be improved outcomes. The Joint Commission includes use of advanced practice registered nurses (APRN) in its standards for ambulatory care/medical homes. This is a significant change, although there is still disagreement among healthcare professionals over the role of the advanced practice nurse in medical homes (ANA, 2011). Other nurses also have roles in medical homes that should not be ignored.

Self-Management

Self-management is a concept of care that focuses on the patient and the patient's role in managing his or her care with resources provided as needed. It requires that the patient have access to health information (IOM, 2003). Electronic personal health records are useful in facilitating self-management (Mitchell & Begoray, 2010). For example, this record can be used to help patients manage their health through individualized care plans, graphing and recording of symptoms, passive biofeedback, individualized instructive or motivational feedback, aids to assist in decision making about health care, and reminders. Security, privacy, and confidentiality are all critical factors in the use of electronic personal health records. It is important that when these systems are used, the system is able to adjust or meet the health literacy needs of the patient. Public/community health can utilize self-management to support members of the community more support, particularly patients with chronic diseases.

Health Literacy

Health literacy is a factor that has implications in all healthcare settings and for all patients (IOM, 2004). As mentioned elsewhere in this text, diversity is a key element of patient-centered care, but it is important to explicitly recognize it in terms of its relevance to public/community health as well. Patient education—whether from the perspective of individual patients, families, populations, or communities—is influenced by the relevant patient's health literacy. One definition of *health literacy* is "the extent to which an individual is able to access and accurately interpret and evaluate health information," which correlates with the earlier definition in a critical report on health literacy (Mitchell & Begoray, 2010). Effective health literacy improves self-management and engages the patient (individuals, families, populations, communities) in the process. Three key supporting interventions to better ensure health literacy are as follows (Sand-Jecklin, Murray, Summers, & Watson, 2010):

- Identify patients at risk for lack of understanding and not acting on health information.
- Communicate health information and instructions in a way that promotes patient understanding.
- Check for patient understanding.

Stop and Consider #3

Nurses who practice in public/community health need to view the patient as an individual who is part of a family, population, or the community.

Multiple Perspectives
of Public/Community Health Services

The following sections discuss examples of public/community health services that need to be considered and provided to ensure the health of communities and their populations. Many of these services are interrelated and are also needed for effective collaboration and coordination in acute care services.

Community Emergency Preparedness

Communities may be confronted with numerous challenges—natural disasters (for example, fires, floods, severe winter weather, hurricanes, and tornados), infectious diseases, excessive violence, and potential attacks such as bioterrorism or other types of terrorism—that could lead to major community health needs and safety concerns. The AHRQ has developed resources for public health emergency preparedness; more on this topic can be found at the agency's website. Community planning for such events is critical to better ensure the health and safety of the community.

In the last few years, there have been major weather-related disasters in the United States, such as in New Orleans, Oklahoma, and the East Coast, as well as tragic violence and terrorism that have harmed a large number of children and adults. Communities are now more alert to the need to plan for these situations. Nurses are involved both in this planning and in working during the crisis period to help others, either in their regular positions or on specific disaster teams that respond to the immediate and long-term disaster needs. For example, school nurses should participate in planning as part of emergency preparation. **Exhibit 7-3** identifies some critical links that provide more information on this important topic.

There are also community situations that can lead to disasters requiring extensive healthcare services as well as prevention of these problems. A problem that occurred recently is lead in the water system in Flint, Michigan. This is a complex problem that will affect the community, particularly its children, for a lifetime. It requires multiple responses, including provision of immediate water needs, short- and long-term assessment of potential victims, improvement

> **Exhibit 7-3** Sources for Information about Emergency Preparedness
>
> - http://www.ready.gov/
> - http://www.fema.gov/
> - http://emergency.cdc.gov/preparedness/
> - http://www.nursingworld.org/MainMenuCategories/ANAMarketplace/ANAPeriodicals/OJIN
>   /TableofContents/Volume112006/No3Sept06/Overview.htmlhttp://nursingworld.org/MainMenu
>   Categories/HealthcareandPolicyIssues/DPR.aspx

of the water system, health education, short- and long-term treatment, collaboration with education experts to help children who might have disabilities, family support and guidance, mental health services for those suffering from the stress of the experience, and much more. All of this is costly and requires expert healthcare services and guidance. Nurses should be involved at all levels—assessment, prevention, treatment, and follow-up—in multiple settings such as public/community health services, clinics, schools, and other services.

Managing Population Health

There is greater emphasis today on learning how to effectively manage population health to reduce costs and improve outcomes. The first step is to identify the target population (Larkin, 2010). The second step is to assess the health status and needs of the population and then apply prevention and interventions to improve the population's health. This approach can have an impact on overall health care.

What might represent a population? With the increase in number of persons with chronic diseases, focusing on a population with a specific chronic disease, such as arthritis or diabetes, can be useful. Coordinating services across a continuum of care and tracking data about outcomes are important aspects of managing population health within a community. The ACA includes many provisions that emphasize community and population health. For example, the law calls for increased funding for community health centers, development of medical homes and community-based transition grant programs, incentives to reduce readmission rates, outcome measures for chronic diseases and wellness and prevention programs, development of employer wellness programs, and requiring nonprofit hospitals to conduct comprehensive needs assessments every three years and report to the Internal Revenue Service the activities they pursue to address the identified needs. These provisions have been enacted, though if there are changes in ACA funding, some of these provisions may be at risk. To support communities in improving population health, the National Quality Forum (NQF) published a guide, which emphasizes 10 elements (NQF, 2016):

- Collaborative self-assessment
- Leadership across the region and within organizations
- Audience-specific strategic communication
- A community health needs assessment and asset mapping process
- An organizational planning and priority-setting process
- An agreed-upon, prioritized set of health improvement activities
- Selection and use of measures and performance targets
- Joint reporting on progress toward achieving intended results
- Indications of scalability
- A plan for sustainability

The guide is supportive of the NQS, which is discussed in other chapters. The NQS is focused on action to foster healthier people and communities, better health care, and more affordable care. Communities need to use this as a guide for their planning and initiatives to improve overall health.

Migrant and Immigrant Issues

In 2011, the American Nurses Association (ANA) published a policy brief on immigrant health care, *Nursing Beyond Borders: Access to Health Care for Documented and Undocumented Immigrants Living in the United States* (Trossman, 2011). Access to healthcare services for these two populations is weak. Even though this is a complex political issue, it is still important for nurses to understand the needs of these two populations and provide care to them. In health care, they represent a diverse population—representing multiple cultures and languages. This population does not typically increase healthcare expenditures. In fact, its expenditures are lower than care for most adult citizens, and they visit the emergency department less often than U.S. citizens. Based on 2010 data, low-income immigrant children, even those insured, are less likely to see a doctor than children born in United States (Ku & Jewers, 2013). Many of them are employed, but they may not have health insurance coverage. However, they often work in hazardous jobs, such as agriculture and construction, increasing their risk for injuries and illness. There have been increased efforts on the federal level to pass new immigration legislation and need for health insurance coverage, and these issues may become more important and complex with the Trump administration.

Home Health Care

The amount of care provided in the home has increased in the United States. As part of efforts to control costs, patients are discharged earlier and earlier from the hospital. At this point, many patients are not fully recovered or ready to care for themselves. **Home care** provides healthcare services in the home. These services vary as to the type of services, the amount of time that the care provider is in the home, the number of visits per week, and the length of services (for example, provided for a week, three months, and so on). In addition, there is variation in the type of healthcare provider needed: a home health aide who provides assistance with activities of daily living services (bathing, ambulation, simple care, light housekeeping, food preparation); a registered nurse who assesses the patient, develops the care plan, monitors progress, assesses the home environment for safety, and provides more complex care; a physical therapist who helps the patient with exercises to gain strength; or a social worker who assists with obtaining other services that the patient may need, such as Meals on Wheels, payment for healthcare services, and so on. Telehealth is used in some home care situations, using technology to communicate with the patient, assess status, and so on. With this service, health information is sent from one site to another by electronic communication. Given the growing number of persons with chronic disease and the aging population, it is expected that home health care will continue to grow as a community health service.

School Health

School health has changed and expanded in many communities over the years. A critical concern is that it is not uncommon for school health services to be limited due to budget cuts for schools and public/community health services. Typically, decreasing the number of registered nurses in the schools or having school nurses cover several schools are methods used to reduce costs for school health. In some communities, school health services have expanded to full clinics, often covered by pediatric APRNs. This can be particularly important in urban communities that may have limited access to services for children with limited or no health insurance and limited family financial resources or in rural areas that may have limited pediatric services. School nurses can make a major difference in the heath of children and, consequently, their long-term health as adolescents and adults through active use of prevention and appropriate, timely treatment when needed.

Rehabilitation

Rehabilitation is part of tertiary prevention. The goal of rehabilitation interventions is to attain and retain the best possible level of functioning for a person who has an illness or disability that is permanent and irreversible. Rehabilitation can take place in the hospital, in an extended care or long-term care facility, in an ambulatory care facility, or in the home. Rehabilitation therapists assist the patient. The nurse may be the healthcare provider who identifies the need for rehabilitation, or the nurse may be involved by following the rehabilitation plan. A patient may require a specialized therapist, such as a physical therapist, an occupational therapist, a speech-language pathologist, or a vocational therapist. Patients may need to learn how to complete activities of daily living, such as taking care of personal hygiene and dressing; ambulating safely with or without assistive devices such as a walker, cane, or wheelchair; learning basic life skills, such as cooking or driving with a disability; and learning new job skills. Some patients recover more fully than others. Examples of patients who may require rehabilitation are those who have suffered a stroke, severe burns, or major injuries from an automobile accident or a work-related accident, such as a serious fall or being cut, impaled, or crushed by equipment.

Extended Care, Long-Term Care, and Elder Care

The U.S. population is aging, and the need for services to meet this population's needs is growing. Gerontological nursing is an important specialty that focuses on care of the elder population in all settings; however, the most important **extended care** settings involve care in the home. Other services are offered in skilled nursing or intermediate-care and **long-term care**, in which patients receive a range of services from housing, meals, and activities to routine personal care, rehabilitation, and specialized treatment. There is great need within the community for more eldercare services, such as adult day care (a facility where elders may go during the day for socializing and activities), home health care, senior centers, and retirement and assisted-living facilities (these can vary from single rooms to independent living situations with support services as needed).

Older adults can experience health problems in all body systems and psychologically. They may also experience social problems, such as loss of spouse and friends and lessened ability to be mobile, and they may become isolated. Financial problems are not uncommon, and these problems affect food, housing, social activities, transportation, and access to medical care. Community health services for this population must consider multiple factors that impact quality of life.

End-of-Life Care and Palliative Care

Hospice care is a philosophy of care for the terminally ill that involves supporting the quality of one's life as long as possible (end-of-life care). It is not required to be a place, though it can be—for example, a freestanding building in which hospice service is provided. Hospice care can also be provided in the patient's home or in a special unit in an acute care hospital. This philosophy of care includes active participation of the patient and family in all care decisions. Specially trained staff—including physicians, nurses, social workers, and often spiritual professionals, as well as other healthcare providers as needed—support the patient and family during the critical last stages of life. **Palliative care** focuses on alleviating symptoms and meeting the special needs of the terminally ill patient and the family. There is strong support for more nursing leadership and provision of palliative care by nurses. The *Future of Nursing* report (IOM, 2010) identifies nurses as the ideal providers of palliative care. The National Institute of Nursing Research (NINR) provides several resources about palliative care (NINR, 2016). The director of NINR, Dr. Grady, notes "offering interventions and translating our science related to hospice and palliative care can enhance the quality of life for those most in need of symptom management and emotional support" (NINR, 2016). The National Institutes of Health (NIH) collaborates with NINR to expand resources for these critical needs, supporting a partnership among the various institutes and other federal government agencies (NINR, 2017).

Recognizing the growing need to ensure that nurses are prepared to care for patients with palliative care and end-of-life needs, the American Association of Colleges of Nursing (AACN) developed Palliative CARES: Competencies and Recommendations for Educating Undergraduate Nursing Students to support nursing education to ensure this care includes assessment, management of complicated illnesses, monitoring, and providing culturally sensitive care with an interprofessional team approach (AACN, 2016a, 2016b). The competencies include the following (AACN, 2016c):

1. Promote the need for palliative care for seriously ill patients and their families, from the time of diagnosis, as essential to quality care and an integral component of nursing care.
2. Identify the dynamic changes in population demographics, healthcare economics, service delivery, caregiving demands, and financial impact of serious illness on the patient and family that necessitates improved profession preparation for palliative care.
3. Recognize one's own ethical, cultural, and spiritual values and beliefs about serious illness and death.
4. Demonstrate respect for cultural, spiritual, and others forms of diversity for patients and their families in the provision of palliative care services.
5. Educate and communicate effectively and compassionately with the patient, family, healthcare team members, and the public about palliative care issues.
6. Collaborate with members of the interprofessional team to improve palliative care for patients and their families and to ensure coordinated and efficient palliative care for the benefit of communities.
7. Elicit and demonstrate respect for the patient and family values, preferences, goals of care, and shared decision making during serious illness and at end of life.
8. Apply ethical principles in the care of patients with serious illness and their families.
9. Know, apply, and effectively communicate current state and federal legal guidelines relevant to the care of patients with serious illness and their families.
10. Perform a comprehensive assessment of pain and symptoms common in serious illness, using valid, standardized assessment tools and strong interviewing and clinical examination skills.
11. Analyze and communicate with the interprofessional team in planning and intervening in pain and symptom management, using evidence-based pharmacologic and non-pharmacologic approaches.
12. Assess, plan, and treat patients' physical, psychological, social, and spiritual needs to improve quality of life for patients with serious illness and their families.
13. Evaluate patient and family outcomes from palliative care within the context of patient goals of care, national quality standards, and value.
14. Provide competent, compassionate and culturally sensitive care for patients and their families at the time of diagnosis of a serious illness through the end of life.
15. Implement self-care strategies to support coping with suffering, loss, moral distress, and compassion fatigue.

16. Assist the patient, family, informal caregivers, and professional colleagues to cope with and build resilience for dealing with suffering, grief, loss, and bereavement associated with serious illness.

17. Recognize the need to seek consultation (that is, from advanced practice nursing specialists, specialty palliative care teams, ethics consultants, and so on) for complex patient and family needs.*

Case Management

Case management is a system that aims to get the right services to the patient at the right time and avoid fragmented and unnecessary care that can be costly (Finkelman, 2011). It facilitates effective care delivery and outcomes for patients. Case management requires **collaboration** or cooperative effort among healthcare providers and other sources of resources that the patient may require. Coordination is required to organize care so that it is available when needed. Communication is also critical because the case manager must work with many people to ensure the patient gets required care. Case managers frequently do all their work on the telephone and never actually see the patient or family. They are typically employees of an insurance company, a government agency, or a healthcare organization (particularly acute care settings [hospitals]), but they may also work for agencies within the public/community health system. Because one of the employer concerns is cost-effective care delivery, case managers need to have extensive knowledge about reimbursement and understand how to manage the care services in a manner that controls costs. Case managers—who may be nurses, social workers, and other staff who work directly with patients (clients) and their families to assess needs—direct the patient to care when needed and monitor progress.

Typically, care protocols or pathways guide the case manager in making decisions about best care for specific health needs, which are adapted to meet individual patient needs. Hospitals may also use case managers to assist with complex patient needs and plan best care post hospitalization. Case management is a growing area of care delivery that has proved effective in helping patients to get the care they need in an often complex and confusing healthcare system.

Occupational Health Care

Occupational health care may seem a strange topic, but nurses are very active in this setting, providing health promotion; disease and illness prevention; and treatment services, including assessment of risks of illness and injury associated with the work environment. This healthcare service is considered part of public/community health. Providing these services at the work site makes it easier for employees to obtain services with less concern about getting to appointments during work hours. Many employers have found it to be beneficial to provide these services on site for employees, often reducing their potential health risks and providing prompt treatment. All of this can reduce employer health insurance costs and increase work productivity; however, employee privacy continues to be an issue.

Employers may provide a variety of health promotion and prevention services, such as exercise classes or even gym access, stress management resources and classes, diet and weight-loss classes, smoking cessation programs, immunizations, weight management services, and other types of opportunities for employees to maintain a healthy lifestyle. Employers may also consider factors such as the food, and related nutritional factors, served in the cafeteria; environmental health issues; walking areas for employees during breaks; equipment to prevent back injuries while moving patients; air quality at work; noise levels; staff use of ergonomic chairs and desks and other equipment and protective devices

*Reproduced with permission from American Association of Colleges of Nursing (AACN). (2016c). CARES: Competencies and recommendations for educating undergraduate nursing students. Retrieved from http://www.aacn.nche.edu/elnec/New-Palliative-Care-Competencies.pdf

related to lifting; exercise and yoga options on site or external to the work site; and so on.

Complementary and Alternative Therapies or Integrative Medicine

The National Center for Complementary and Alternative Medicine (NCCAM, 2016), which is part of the National Institutes of Health, describes complementary and alternative medicine (CAM) as a group of diverse medical and healthcare systems, practices, and products that are not presently considered part of conventional medicine. Conventional medicine is medicine typically practiced by holders of medical doctor or doctor of osteopathy degrees and by other health professionals, such as registered nurses, physical therapists, and psychologists. Some healthcare providers practice both CAM and conventional medicine. Although there is some scientific evidence supporting use of CAM therapies, for most, there are still key questions that have yet to be answered through well-designed scientific studies—questions such as whether these therapies are safe and whether they work for the diseases or medical conditions for which they are used. The list of what is considered CAM changes continually as therapies that are proved to be safe and effective are adopted by conventional health care and new approaches to health care emerge. Countries in Europe and Asia and in the Middle East, such as Israel, actively use CAM, and these interventions are covered by their universal healthcare plans. Patients typically seek out these interventions in their communities. For example, in San Francisco, California, groups of senior citizens participate in tai chi in the parks.

Many of these interventions are not new, but their use in modern healthcare delivery has increased in recent years. However, many of the CAM interventions still have a long way to go before they become part of conventional medicine. Examples of these interventions are acupuncture, acupressure, massage, light energy, botanical treatment, Reiki, tai chi, and use of a variety of herbs and other supplements, such as garlic, shark cartilage, and ginseng. With the creation of NCCAM, there is now an organized system for clinical trials to gather data about the use of CAM and related outcomes. Nurses may provide some CAM interventions in their practice, and some insurers cover these services, but this is not typical in the United States. As more data are obtained to support their efficacy, there will probably be more inclusion of these interventions in care, and they will gain greater reimbursement coverage.

Genetics

Genetics has become more of a focus in health care, and it will have a long-term effect on public/community services. The U.S. Department of Energy and the National Institutes of Health have funded and led the Human Genome Project, which began in 1990 and was completed in 2003. This project focused on mapping all the loci of the 20,000 to 25,000 genes that make up the human body. The implications of this project are many. We have learned that the interaction of the genetic makeup of an individual and the environment (genomics) often determines whether the person will be healthy or ill for the majority of his or her life. The benefits of this research include the following (U.S. Department of Energy, 2015):

- Improved diagnosis of disease
- Earlier detection of genetic predispositions to disease
- Rational drug design
- Gene therapy and control systems for drugs
- Pharmacogenomics/custom drugs

When this information is used in combination with a family history tool to gather information about diseases in the family, a very thorough risk assessment can be completed (HHS, 2007). If this risk assessment is used in health promotion, the health professional can explain to patients and families not only their risk of a disease because of their genetic profile, but also the interactions between the environment and the person's genomic risk. With the knowledge of how a person's genes interact with drugs, better pain medications may be designed to address individuals. We now have the ability in some cases to fix a bad gene because we know its location. The technology to diagnose diseases and conditions even prenatally is becoming available, giving us the tools to allow a fetus to continue to grow normally instead of having major anomalies at birth. The possibilities are endless for disease prevention and management. We are just at the beginning of a new frontier of health care and related nursing care. The essentials for genetics competencies have already been written for nursing curricula (ANA Consensus Panel, 2008). These are just as critical as the other competencies regarding nursing processes that lead to better patient outcomes and safe care.

Stop and Consider #4

Public/community health services are expanding, and this affects the roles of nurses.

The Changing Nature
of Public/Community Health Problems

Public/community health changes more than acute care, even with all the advancements in medical treatment. It is affected by many factors that are broader—socioeconomic, culture, travel, weather, communicable diseases, community safety, law enforcement and other similar services, education, religion, and much more. The following sections provide a few examples of problems that are primarily focused on the community and for which much of the response must come from the community. This does not mean that acute care is not relevant for many of the problems communities confront. The ideal is to have a system of care that incorporates both acute care and public/community care supporting effective coordination, communication, and collaboration.

Violence in Communities

An example of the changing nature of public/community health is increasing violence in some communities, such as Chicago. This type of violence is not new, but we have times of greater and lesser violence and some communities experience major crises with violence. The National Academy of Medicine published a report on a roundtable it held that examined violence (NAM, 2017). Violence is a social determinant of health and important to consider in public/community health systems and is viewed as a chronic, recurrent disease. Some refer to violence as a contagious disease. This report describes serious problems that result from community violence, even using the descriptor of a "war zone."

We know that violence affects acute care, particularly emergency services, but it also affects other services, police, ambulance, and even (in some cases) the fire department. However, it also affects many other community organizations and groups—schools, transportation, businesses, housing, and community centers and other gathering places such as playgrounds. It even affects home care—for example, how safe nurses feel going into a neighborhood or a home. We cannot deny that ethnic issues—culture, language, and so on are factors that influence what is happening and how we respond.

Violence is an action but also a reaction to situations in which people, often the young people, feel they are trapped, and so they respond with violence and risky behaviors such as using drugs. Domestic violence may also be influenced by the same factors and living environment. The NAM, 2017 report provides a comprehensive analysis of community violence as a population health concern—background, causes, and community interventions. This is a topic that nurses need to understand not only in communities with high levels of violence, but also in any community. Interventions that might be considered are focused on safety first and then prevention. Because violence is such a highly complex issue, it requires understanding multiple variables and the use of interventions covering a broad perspective—safety in housing areas, eliminating empty houses and buildings where gangs can hang out, health services and law enforcement collaborating in planning and implementing interventions, better gun control enforcement, dealing with substance abuse (drugs and alcohol), working in schools to help students—support, safety education, and so on; monitoring areas where children might be at risk such as playgrounds; ensuring the elderly can get needs met when they may be fearful about going out; lighting in public places; and so on. Community members may experience high levels of stress, anxiety, depression, and anger. All of this affects short- and long-term mental health—services are needed for these problems, prevention, and treatment.

Opioid Epidemic

The opioid epidemic is not a common story in our news. Stories such as this one: A city experiences two calls for assistance per hour for overdose patients for 32 hours. The number of overdose calls in 2015 was 4,642; in 2016, it was 6,879 (Hauser, 2017). Data identify five states with the highest rates of death associated to drug overdose—the range is from 28.2 per 100,000 to 41.5 per 100,000—with the CDC reporting 91 deaths due to opioid overdose every day. Many communities across the United States are dealing with this epidemic that is hitting all sectors of society. Narcan is recommended for response to an overdose and can save lives. Emergency services now carry this drug, but getting enough is a problem, as is cost.

In the last few years as concern grew about opioid abuse, several major reports have addressed pain management and also opioid abuse. *Relieving Pain in America* noted that an estimated 100,000 people experienced chronic pain and, as a result, cost $630 billion each year (IOM, 2011). Since this report was published in 2011, the data have changed with opioid use increasing, but the report served as an alert to a growing problem and provided evidence that the United States needed to respond quickly. The message is not that we should not provide treatment for pain, but rather we need to do this carefully, with

an understanding of benefits and consequences and to use methods with the least risk of harm.

This epidemic has led to multiple approaches directed at prevention, treatment, and rehabilitation. Prevention focuses on communication with members of the community about the dangers of abuse and options for getting help. Opioid abuse not only affects the addict, but also families and close associates, employers who must deal with employees who cannot be productive, and criminal activity in a community, and there is a heavy burden on the healthcare delivery system. Education also must be provided to children and adults about the dangers of using this drug. Healthcare providers must also be educated about the risk of prescribing this type of medication. The CDC and the Office of the Surgeon General have developed information and materials to assist in communicating this message and provide approaches to avoid abuse—this initiative is called "Turn the Tide" (HHS, & CDC, 2016b). This information is directed at prescribers; however, all nurses should review this material. The key message is: Do not prescribe opioids as first-line treatment for chronic pain—excluding active cancer, palliative, or end-of-life care. On August 24, 2016, the Surgeon General's information about "Turn the Tide" was sent in a letter and a pocket card for easy use to 2.3 million doctors, nurses, dentists, and other clinicians, asking for their help (Murthy, 2016). This is an example of a broad education effort. In addition, editorials and articles were published in the fall of 2016 in multiple medical journals, supporting the need for greater attention to this problem.

Communities with this problem are working on providing more treatment and rehabilitation options. What is complex about this problem is once someone is addicted, the person has a chronic health problem that can also lead to other health problems. This treatment is costly, and if a person does not have insurance, the situation is even more complex. This may also lead to many other problems such as employment, difficulty with school, problems during pregnancies and for newborns, mental health issues, loss of one's home due to insufficient income, domestic and child abuse, divorce, crime, and much more. These are all major concerns for a community, particularly if they involve many members of the community.

Nurses need to be involved in the plan and responses to the problem along with an interprofessional team that also includes other community leaders such as government officials, law enforcement, religious leaders, education leaders, business owners, and so on. It will take a multipronged approach to improve the health of the community and its residents.

Stop and Consider #5
The problems of violence and opioid use affect all nurses in their practice.

Global Healthcare
Concerns and International Nursing

WHO is the major international health organization that focuses on "building a better, healthier future for people all over the world", and its priorities include (2016, pp. 2–3):

- Advancing universal health coverage: enabling countries to sustain or expand access to all needed health services and financial protection, and promoting universal health coverage.
- Achieving health-related development goals: addressing unfinished and future challenges relating to maternal and child health; combating HIV, malaria, and TB; and completing the eradication of polio and a number of neglected tropical diseases.
- Addressing the challenge of noncommunicable diseases and mental health, violence, and injuries and disabilities.
- Ensuring that all countries can detect and respond to acute pubic health threats under the International Health Regulations.

- Increasing access to quality, safe, efficacious, and affordable medical products (medicines, vaccines, diagnostics, and other health technologies).
- Addressing the social, economic, and environmental determinants of health as means to promote health outcomes and reduce health inequalities within and between countries.

Global healthcare concerns change, and some have become significant both in their impact and their costs. Emerging infections represent a major global health concern, with particular concern about bacteria that are antibiotic-resistant (Cleeson, 2016). Other recent examples of infectious diseases are the Ebola virus and concern about it spreading globally; the Zika virus and concern about long-term impact on infants born when mothers are infected; and war and refugees who need medical care and support services such as housing, food, and so on. All of these situations become complex political situations and problems related to coordination and speed in meeting the needs. The refugee situation is much more complex and will last a long time—affecting multiple countries and a large number of people of all ages.

The International Council of Nurses (ICN) is also involved in global health by providing a voice for nursing throughout the world. Its stated mission is "to represent nursing worldwide, advancing the profession and influencing health policy. The ICN's Strategic Intent is to enhance the health of individuals, populations, and societies by: championing the contribution and image of nurses worldwide; advocating for nurses at all levels; advancing the nursing profession; and influencing health, social, economic and education policy" (ICN, 2014). The ICN and WHO focus on the health of individuals, families, and communities.

Stop and Consider #6
Health and healthcare are global concerns.

CHAPTER HIGHLIGHTS

1. *Healthy People 2020,* coupled with other major reports on the quality of health care, require health professionals to understand the concepts of quality of care, health outcomes, and health indices, as well as to address health disparities in everyday care in the community.

2. The focus of health care is changing to patient-centered care, with the patient in the key decision-making position. This also applies to all types of healthcare settings in the community, across the life span and the continuum of care, to meet healthcare needs within the community and ensure continuity of care.

3. Stress, coping, and resilience have an impact on health promotion, disease prevention, and illness within communities.

4. Continuum of care means that nursing care must be provided in acute care settings, the home, and the community.

5. Vulnerable populations are groups of people who are at risk for developing health problems. Examples include children, the elderly, people with chronic diseases, the homeless, and others.

6. Important concepts to consider in public/community health care are disease prevention, health promotion, life span, vulnerable populations, health and illness, acute illness, chronic disease, self-management, health literacy, continuity of care, and continuum of care.

7. Critical public/community services include community emergency preparedness, managing population health, migrant and immigrant care, home care occupational health care, hospice and palliative care, rehabilitation, extended care, long-term care, elder care, case management, occupational health care, complementary and alternative care, and genetics.

8. Public/community health problems change, probably more than acute care. Two current problems are community violence and the opioid epidemic.

9. The World Health Organization focuses its attention on global health issues, health issues that may have a major impact on multiple countries and a large number of people. The International Council of Nurses is an example of an organization that represents the nursing profession's global interests.

ENGAGING IN THE CONTENT

Discussion Questions

1. What are proposed changes for *Healthy People 2030*? (See https://www.healthy people.gov/2020/About-Healthy-People /Development-Healthy-People-2030)

2. Why is *Healthy People 2020* an important national health initiative?

3. Why is public/community health a critical concern today?

4. Discuss the various views of health and illness presented in this chapter.

5. How does the life span impact the continuum of care in the community?

6. Compare and contrast acute illness and chronic disease related to public/community care.

7. Why are global health issues important considerations for healthcare providers in the United States?

CRITICAL THINKING ACTIVITIES

1. Go to the Take the First Step to Prevention page at the Centers for Disease Control and Prevention's website (http://wonder.cdc.gov /data2010/HU.htm). Search for your state, and review the most current data. Select a specific health indicator, and look at the national data and then data from your own state. How do they compare? Search for data focused on a specific population.

2. Visit the National Center for Health Statistics' website (http://www.cdc.gov/nchs/). Search for current data related to births/natality, infant health, child health, adolescent health, men's health, women's health, and older people's health.

3. Visit http://www.ahrq.gov/clinic/pocketgd .htm to review the current version of the *U.S. Guide to Clinical Preventive Services*. How might you use this information if you were planning services for a community health center?

4. Visit this WHO site: Global Health Estimates http://www.who.int/healthinfo/global_burden _disease/en/index.html What can you learn about global life expectancy, mortality, and the burden of disease? How does the United States compare with other countries?

5. Select one of the vulnerable populations, and discuss issues that would have an impact on the health and illness for that population. Consider issues such as health promotion, disease prevention, and access to care.

6. Analyze the chronic disease model and its relevance to nursing in the community. Institute of Medicine Report: *Living Well with Chronic Illness*: A Call for Action. https://www .nationalacademies.org/hmd/~/media/Files /Report%20Files/2012/Living-Well-with-Chronic -Illness/livingwell_chronicillness_reportbrief.pdf What are the critical elements in coping with chronic illness?

ELECTRONIC REFLECTION JOURNAL

Use your journal to describe your own perspective on health and illness, and explain how this has influenced you as a nursing student compared to your views before becoming a nursing student.

CASE STUDIES

Case 1

Imagine that you are a member of an interprofessional team in a rural county in your state. The team is looking into improving the health status of the community. The community has a high rate of cancer (particularly breast and lung); accidents (farm related); alcohol

CASE STUDIES (CONTINUED)

abuse, particularly among teens; and obesity (adults, but with increasing weight gain in children). The interprofessional team is composed of two registered nurses (one who works in the local hospital, and you, the only school nurse in the area), one physician in private practice, the local hospital administrator, the mayor of the largest town in the area, a psychologist in practice, and a clergyman.

Case Questions

1. Identify the problems that need to be considered by the community.
2. Describe how you think the team should approach these problems based on what you have learned in this chapter.
3. How might you apply information about *Healthy People 2020* in this case?

Case 2

Health literacy has been a long-time problem in health care. Data from a recent community survey completed for your moderate-size city indicate that health literacy problems are increasing and that minority populations have increased in the last five years. Chronic illnesses in these populations have also increased, such as diabetes and hypertension. Clinics and home health agencies have reported an increase in medication errors for patients who are taking medications at home. Many of these errors appear to be due to poor understanding of medication directions and ability to read these directions either in written patient directions or reading medication containers.

Case Questions

1. Consider the following links to get additional information:
   Community Guide: http://www.thecommunityguide.org
   If you were on a task force to improve your community's health, how might you use this website?
2. Given the data provided, identify the key problems and related settings.
3. Research additional information on health literacy and its impact on quality of care.
4. Describe three interventions to address the issues in this community.

Working Backward to Develop a Case

Write a brief paragraph that describes a case related to the following questions.

1. What is the rate of obesity in our community?
2. Why should the school nurses in the county be at our meetings?
3. Do these children receive any health education in school, and if so, what is included in the content?

REFERENCES

Accountable Care Facts. (2014). *Top 10 questions on ACOs and health care delivery reform.* Retrieved from http://www.accountablecarefacts.org/

American Association of Colleges of Nursing. (2016a). *AACN endorses palliative care competencies and recommendations for undergraduate nursing education.* Retrieved from http://www.aacn.nche.edu/news/articles/2016/elnec

American Association of Colleges of Nursing. (2016b). CARES: Competencies and recommendations for educating undergraduate nursing students. *Journal of Professional Nursing, 32*(2), 78–84.

American Association of Colleges of Nursing. (2016c). *CARES: Competencies and recommendations for educating undergraduate nursing students.* Retrieved from http://www.aacn.nche.edu/elnec/New-Palliative-Care-Competencies.pdf

American Hospital Association. (2011). *Health for life: Better health. Better healthcare.* Retrieved from. http://www.aha.org/content/11/11spr-healthforlifeflyer.pdf

American Nurses Association. (2011, May 25). *ANA applauds Joint Commission standards for "medical homes": Patients gain with decision to include nurse-led clinics.* Retrieved from http://nursingworld.org/Especially?For?You/AdvancedPracticeNurses/APRN-News/Joint-Commission-Standards-for-Medical-Homes.aspx

American Nurses Association. Consensus Panel. (2008). *Essential nursing competencies curricula guidelines for genetics and genomics,* 2nd ed. Retrieved from http://www.aacn.nche.edu/education-resources/Genetics__Genomics_Nursing_Competencies_09-22-06.pdf

Bindman, A. (2016). AHRQ Views. *AHRQ's role in improving care for patients with multiple chronic conditions.* Retrieved from http://www.ahrq.gov/news/blog/ahrqviews/ahrqs-role-in-improving-care.html

Cleeson, J. (2016). *Emerging infections: A national patient safety challenge.* Retrieved from https://www.ahrq.gov/news/blog/ahrqviews/emerging-infections.html?utm_source=AHRQ&utm_medium=EN-14&utm_term=&utm_content=14&utm_campaign=AHRQ_EN8_2_2016

Finkelman, A. (2011). *Case management for nurses.* Upper Saddle River, NJ: Pearson Education.

Haggerty, J., Reid, R., Freeman, G., Starfield, B., Adair, C., & McKendry, R. (2003). Continuity of care: A multidisciplinary review. *British Medical Journal, 327,* 1219–1221.

Hauser, C. (2017, February 14). Sudden rise in overdoses for one city in a nationwide epidemic of opioid abuse. *New York Times,* p. A11.

Institute for Healthcare Improvement. (2011). *Self-management support of patients with chronic conditions.* Retrieved from http://www.ihi.org/knowledge/Pages/Changes/SelfManagement.aspx

Institute of Medicine. (2002). *Unequal treatment: Confronting racial and ethnic disparities in health.* Washington, DC: The National Academies Press.

Institute of Medicine. (2003). *Priority areas for national action: Transforming healthcare quality.* Washington, DC: The National Academies Press.

Institute of Medicine. (2004). *Health literacy: A prescription to end confusion.* Washington, DC: The National Academies Press.

Institute of Medicine. (2010). *The future of nursing: Leading change advancing health.* Washington, DC: The National Academies Press.

Institute of Medicine. (2011). *Pain management and prescription opioid-related harms: Exploring the state of the evidence.* Washington, DC: The National Academies Press.

Institute of Medicine. (2012). *Report brief: Living well with chronic illness: A call for public action.* Washington, DC: The National Academies Press.

International Council of Nurses. (2014). *Our mission, strategic intent, core values and priorities.* Retrieved from http://www.icn.ch/about-icn/icns-mission/

Joint Commission. (2004). *Hospital accreditation standards.* Oakbrook Terrace, IL: Author.

Kaakinen, J., Hanson, M., & Birenbaum, L. (2006). Family development and family nursing assessment. In M. Stanhope & J. Lancaster (Eds.), *Foundations of nursing in the community* (pp. 321–340). St. Louis, MO: Mosby.

Kaiser Family Foundation. (2016, September). *Key facts about the uninsured population.* Retrieved from http://kff.org/uninsured/fact-sheet/key-facts-about-the-uninsured-population/

Ku, L., & Jewers, M. (2013, June). *Health care for immigrant families: Current policies and issues.* Migration Policy Institute. Retrieved from http://www.migrationpolicy.org/research/health-care-immigrant-families-current-policies-and-issues

Kulbok, P., Thatcher, E., Park, E., & Meszaros, P. (2012). Evolving public health nursing roles: Focus on community participatory health promotion and prevention. *Online Journal of Issues in Nursing, 17,* 12. Retrieved from http://nursingworld.org/MainMenuCategories/ANAMarketplace/ANAPeriodicals/OJIN/TableofContents/Vol-17-2012/No2-May-2012/Evolving-Public-Health-Nursing-Roles.html

Larkin, H. (2010, October). Managing population health. *H&HN,* 28–32.

Leavell, H., & Clark, A. (1965). *Preventive medicine for doctors in the community*. New York, NY: McGraw-Hill.

Marrelli, T. (2017). *e-Caregiving*. Retrieved from http://e-caregiving.com/

Mitchell, B., & Begoray, D. (2010). Electronic personal health records that promote self-management in chronic illness. *Online Journal of Issues in Nursing, 15*(3). Retrieved from http://www.nursingworld.org/MainMenuCategories/ANAMarketplace/ANAPeriodicals/OJIN/TableofContents/Vol152010/No3-Sept-2010/Articles-Previously-Topic/Electronic-Personal-Health-Records-and-Chronic-Illness.html

Murthy, V. (2016). Ending the opioid epidemic—A call to action. *New England Journal of Medicine, 375,* 2413–2415. Retrieved from http://www.nejm.org/doi/full/10.1056/NEJMp1612578

National Academy of Medicine (2016). *A framework for educating health professionals to address the social determinants of health*. Washington, DC: The National Academies Press.

National Academy of Medicine (2017). *Community violence as a population health issue*. Washington, DC: The National Academies Press.

National Center for Complementary and Alternative Medicine. (2016). *What is complementary and alternative medicine?* Retrieved from https://nccih.nih.gov/health/integrative-health

National Committee for Quality Assurance. (2017). *Patient-centered medical home*. Retrieved from http://www.ncqa.org/programs/recognition/practices/patient-centered-medical-home-pcmh

National Health Council. (2013). *About chronic diseases*. Retrieved from http://www.nationalhealthcouncil.org/NHC_Files/Pdf_Files/AboutChronicDisease.pdf

National Institute of Nursing Research. (2016). *Palliative care*. Retrieved from https://www.ninr.nih.gov/newsandinformation/newsandnotes/category/Palliative%20Care

National Institute of Nursing Research. (2017). *NIH and federal resources in end-of-life and palliative care*. Retrieved from https://www.ninr.nih.gov/researchandfunding/spotlight-on-end-of-life-research/eolpc-externalresources

National Quality Forum. (2016). *Improving population health by working with communities. Action guide 3.0*. Retrieved from http://www.qualityforum.org/Improving_Population_Health.aspx

Organization for Economic Cooperation and Development. (2015). *Health at a glance 2015: OECD indicators*. Retrieved from http://www.oecd-ilibrary.org/social-issues-migration-health/health-at-a-glance-2015_health_glance-2015-en

Pender, N., Murdaugh, C., & Parsons, M. (2006). *Health promotion in nursing practice*. Upper Saddle River, NJ: Pearson Education.

Peters, K., & Elster, A. (2002). *Roadmaps for clinical practice. A primer on population-based medicine*. Chicago, IL: American Medical Association.

Pilon, B., Ketel, C., Davidson, H., Gentry, C., Crutcher, T., Scott, A., Moore, M., & Rosenbloom, S. (2015). Evidence-guided integration of interprofessional collaborative practice into nurse managed health centers. *Journal of Professional Nursing, 31*(4), 340–350.

Robert Wood Johnson Foundation. (2000). *Definition of healthcare*. Retrieved from http://www.rwjf.org/reports/grr/036111.htm

Robert Wood Johnson Foundation. (2012). *A national research agenda for public health services and systems*. Retrieved from http://www.rwjf.org/en/research-publications/find-rwjf-research/2012/05/a-national-research-agenda-for-public-health-services-and-system.html

Sand-Jecklin, K., Murray, B., Summers, B., & Watson, J. (2010). Educating nursing students about health literacy: From the classroom to the bedside. *Online Journal of Issues in Nursing, 15*(13). Retrieved from http://www.nursingworld.org/MainMenuCategories/ANAMarketplace/ANAPeriodicals/ OJIN/TableofContents/Vol152010/No3-Sept-2010/Articles-Previously-Topic/Educating-Nursing-Students-about-Health-Literacy.aspx

Schumacher, K., Beck, C., & Marren, J. (2006). Family caregivers: Caring for older adults, working with their families. *American Journal of Nursing, 106*(8), 40–48.

Seegert, L. (2016). Hospitals evolve into community health networks. *American Journal of Nursing, 116*(2), 18–19.

Trossman, S. (2011). New ANA policy brief: Aiming to help nurses better understand ramifications of immigrants' lack of access to healthcare services. *American Nurse Today, 6*(3), 34–36.

U.S. Census Bureau. (2016a, September). *Poverty*. Retrieved from http://www.census.gov/library/publications/2016/demo/p60-256.html

U.S. Census Bureau. (2016b). *Current population survey, 1960 to 2016 annual social and economic supplements*. Retrieved from www2.census.gov/programs-surveys/cps/techdocs/cpsmar16.pdf

U.S. Department of Energy. (2015). Human Genome Project. *Potential benefits of Human Genome Project Research*. Retrieved from http://www.ornl.gov/sci/techresources/Human_Genome/project/benefits.shtml

U.S. Department of Health and Human Services. (2007). *U.S. Surgeon General's family initiative*. Retrieved from http://www.hhs.gov/familyhistory/

U.S. Department of Health and Human Services. (2010). *Healthy People 2020: MAP-IT*. Retrieved from http://healthypeople.gov/2020/implement/MapIt.aspx

U.S. Department of Health and Human Services. (2014). *Healthy People 2020*. Retrieved from https://www.healthypeople.gov/2020/leading-health-indicators/Healthy-People-2020-Leading-Health-Indicators%3A-Progress-Update

U.S. Department of Health and Human Services. (2017). *Healthy People 2020*. Retrieved from https://www.healthypeople.gov/

U.S. Department of Health and Human Services, & Agency for Healthcare Research and Quality. (2015). *2015 National healthcare quality and disparities report*. Retrieved from https://www.ahrq.gov/research/findings/nhqrdr/nhqdr15/index.html

U.S. Department of Health and Human Services, & Agency for Research and Quality. (2016, March). Priorities in focus. The Issue: Health and well-being of communities. Retrieved from https://www.ahrq.gov/workingforquality/reports/priorities-in-focus-healthy-living.html?utm_source=AHRQ&utm_medium=EN-10&utm_term=&utm_content=10&utm_campaign=AHRQ_EN6_7_2016

U.S. Department of Health and Human Services, & Centers for Disease Control and Prevention. (2016a). *Chronic disease overview*. Retrieved from https://www.cdc.gov/chronicdisease/overview/

U.S. Department of Health and Human Services, & Centers for Disease Control and Prevention. (2016b). *CDC guideline for prescribing opioids for chronic pain*. Retrieved from https://www.cdc.gov/drugoverdose/prescribing/guideline.html

U.S. Department of Health and Human Services, & Centers for Disease Control and Prevention. (2011).

Healthy youth! Health topic: Childhood obesity. Retrieved from http://www.cdc.gov/healthyyouth/obesity

U.S. Department of Health and Human Services, & Centers for Disease Control and Prevention. (2015). *Health United States 2015*. Retrieved from https://www.cdc.gov/nchs/data/hus/hus15.pdf

U.S. Department of Health and Human Services, & Office of Disease Prevention and Health Promotion. (2006). *National Prevention Summit: Prevention, preparedness, and promotion*. Retrieved from odphp.osophs.dhhs.gov/pubs/prevrpt/Volume21/Iss2-3Vol21.pdf

U.S. Department of Health and Human Services, & Office of the Surgeon General. (2013). *National prevention strategy*. Retrieved from http://www.surgeongeneral.gov/initiatives/prevention/strategy/

Wagner, E. (1998). Chronic disease management: What will it take to improve care for chronic illness? *Effective Clinical Practice, 1,* 2–4.

Williams, C. (2006). Community-oriented nursing and community-based nursing. In M. Stanhope & J. Lancaster (Eds.), *Foundations of nursing in the community* (pp. 3–16). St. Louis, MO: Mosby.

World Health Organization. (2006). *WHO Constitution*. Retrieved from http://www.who.int/governance/eb/constitution/en/index.html

World Health Organization. (2011). *Social determinants of health*. Retrieved from http://www.who.int/social_determinants/en/

World Health Organization. (2016). *The global guardian of public health*. Retrieved from http://www.who.int/about/what-we-do/global-guardian-of-public-health.pdf?ua=1

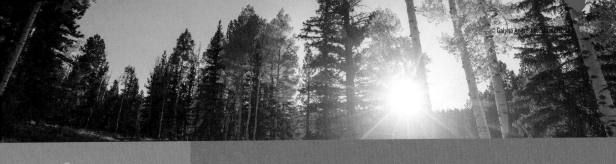

Chapter 8

The Healthcare Delivery System: Focus on Acute Care

CHAPTER OBJECTIVES

At the conclusion of this chapter, the learner will be able to:

- Discuss the corporatization of healthcare delivery by comparing and contrasting for-profit and not-for-profit systems.
- Compare and contrast healthcare organization structure and processes.
- Describe the healthcare provider team and its relationship to nursing.
- Discuss critical elements related to healthcare financial issues and reimbursement.
- Examine how nursing fits into the overall hospital organization.
- Explain the importance of organizational culture.
- Discuss examples of changes in the healthcare delivery system.

CHAPTER OUTLINE

KEY TERMS

Annual limit

Copayment

Corporatization

Deductible

Direct care provider

For-profit

Indirect care provider

Medicaid

Medicare

Not-for-profit

Organizational culture

Process

Reimbursement

Structure

Introduction

Healthcare delivery is a complex process and system. The system includes many types of healthcare provider organizations, such as acute care organizations (hospitals), ambulatory care centers (clinics), private provider offices, public/community health facilities, home care agencies, hospice agencies, extended care facilities, and so on. This chapter focuses on the largest type of healthcare organization (HCO): the acute care hospital. This does not mean that other types of HCOs are not important; however, nursing students typically spend more of their clinical time in hospitals. Many of the organizational elements of a hospital are similar to those of other HCOs but may vary depending on the organization and purpose. The content in this chapter explores current issues related to hospitals, hospital organization and function, and the hospital provider team, and provides an introduction to healthcare financial issues and nursing organization and functions within the hospital.

Many factors affect hospitals, leading them to change their services, collaborate with others in their communities, realign their organization with other organizations, close because of financial issues, meet quality improvement requirements, and so forth. Examples of factors that influence hospitals today:

- Increase in healthcare costs
- Shortage of healthcare providers (may be geographic or HCO specific)

- Uninsured and underinsured patients who are unable to pay for their care
- Compromised access to care for some individuals, leading to healthcare disparities
- Advances in medical technology that can improve care but may be costly and require special staff training and may not be accessible to those who cannot pay for them
- Impact of quality improvement data and requirements that may lead to changes
- Greater use of informatics in documentation and for other healthcare informational purposes
- Growing diversity in patients and the healthcare workforce—for example, increasing need for interpreter services and greater representation of ethnic groups in the healthcare workforce
- Increasing consumerism—more knowledgeable patients who demand more information and participation
- Hospital mergers and closings, altering access to services
- Changing number of available beds; changing specialty services (for example, increasing the number of intensive care beds, eliminating obstetric services, offering home health services)
- Changes in patient demographics that require reassessment of which services to offer and how those services are provided (for example, increasing services for the elderly, immigrants, and single parents; expanding clinic hours to facilitate access; and so on)
- Legislation such as the Affordable Care Act of 2010 and possible changes to this law

Examples of key influences on health care are highlighted in **Figure 8-1**. **Exhibit 8-1** identifies examples of organizations that influence healthcare delivery.

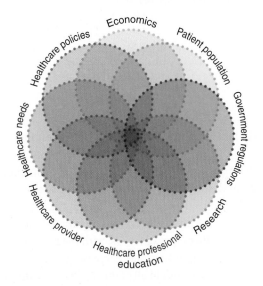

Figure 8-1 Influences on Healthcare Delivery

Corporatization of Health

Care: How Did We Get Here?

Using the term **corporatization** or *business* when referring to a hospital may seem strange; however, health care is a business—a very large business. It provides services to most of the population at some time during a person's life, from birth to death. Hospitals have a very large employee pool, with nurses representing the largest percentage. Hospitals provide jobs for many people—both professionals and nonprofessionals; thus, they represent one of the largest employment sectors. Within a community, HCOs also usually own or lease a large amount of property, purchase a great number of supplies and equipment, and pay taxes—all activities that bring income into a community. Typically, healthcare leaders hold significant positions in the business sector and the community. Health care consumes the largest amount of federal and state dollars through healthcare reimbursement programs such

---

Exhibit 8-1 Examples of Organizations Important to the Healthcare Delivery System

- National Association of Children's Hospitals and Related Institutions: http://www.childrenshospitals.org
- American Academy of Hospice and Palliative Medicine: http://www.aahpm.org
- American Association of Homes and Services for the Aging: http://www.leadingage.org
- American Association of Retired Persons: http://www.aarp.org
- American Health Care Association: http://www.ahcancal.org/Pages/Default.aspx
- American Hospital Association: http://www.aha.org/aha/about
- American Nurses Association: http://www.nursingworld.org
- Nursing Specialty Organizations: http://www.nursingcenter.com/library/JournalArticle.asp?Article_ID=623779
- American Public Health Association: http://www.apha.org
- Arthritis Foundation: http://www.arthritis.org
- American Diabetes Association: http://www.diabetes.org/?loc=404page
- The Joint Commission: http://www.jointcommission.org
- National Association of Public Hospitals: https://essentialshospitals.org
- National Committee on Quality Assurance: http://www.ncqa.org
- National Health Council: http://nationalhealthcouncil.org

as Medicare and Medicaid, as discussed in other chapters.

It is not uncommon to refer to hospitals as for-profit or not-for-profit. The terms **for-profit** and **not-for-profit** can be confusing. The first critical point is that every hospital needs to make a profit, which means the HCO needs to have money left over after expenses are paid. The distinguishing characteristic between for-profit and not-for-profit organizations is what the organization does with its profit. The assumption by most is that all hospitals are not-for-profit organizations, but this is not correct. Many large HCOs are for-profit corporations. Some of their profit must go to their stockholders/shareholders or to their owners. However, even for-profit organizations must cover their operation costs and reinvest money in the hospital for maintenance, expand space and renovate, develop new services, purchase equipment and supplies, and so on. Not-for-profit organizations do not have stockholders/shareholders, but these hospitals still need to make a profit for the same reasons that for-profit organizations need a profit.

Knowing whether the hospital you work for is a for-profit or not-for-profit organization can help you understand why and how decisions are made. For example, if a hospital is burdened with a high number of nonpaying patients, the hospital may eventually spend more than it is making and thus be "in the red" when its debt increases. When this happens, the hospital may cut staff, limit new equipment purchases, control use of supplies, fail to maintain equipment effectively, neglect facility maintenance needs and renovation, attempt to reconfigure services to attract paying patients, decrease staff education, and make other changes to improve the hospital's financial condition. All HCOs have to be concerned with cost containment, but when the financial situation is weak, the organization will need to use cost containment more. A for-profit HCO must always have funds to pay stockholders or owners, and this consideration can have an impact on the availability of money for other purposes that affect nurses and nursing.

Stop and Consider #1

Healthcare delivery is a business.

The Healthcare
Organization

Hospitals are one type of HCO, and the largest. Other types of HCOs are identified in **Exhibit 8-2**. Descriptions of HCO should include information about the organization's structure, processes, staff, and organizational culture. Although the majority of registered nurses (RNs) work in hospitals, many work in other types of HCOs, with the percentage RNs working in hospitals decreasing over recent years. Nurses work in all of the healthcare settings identified in Exhibit 8-2. Data from 2015, and still most current data available at the end of 2016, indicated that 61% of RNs worked in state, local, and private hospitals; 7% in nursing and residential care facilities; 7% in physician offices; 6% in home healthcare services; and 6% in government healthcare services (U.S. Department of Labor, 2015).

The organization of hospitals varies, but there are some standard types of organization. In the past, it was more common for hospitals to operate as single organizations. Now, more hospitals have formed complex organizations consisting of multiple hospitals. In some cases, these systems also include other healthcare entities such as home care agencies, rehabilitation centers, long-term care facilities, and freestanding ambulatory care centers. Most of the reasons for this change in organization structure are related to financial issues and the survival of the organization—to keep patients in the system, increase services, and expand the continuum of care. Some communities have seen multiple changes in their local hospitals, with hospitals merging with

Exhibit 8-2 Types of Healthcare Organizations

- Substance abuse treatment/rehabilitation centers (inpatient and outpatient)
- School health clinics
- Diagnostic centers
- Ambulatory care surgical centers
- Dental offices and clinics
- Long-term care facilities
- Skilled nursing facilities
- Occupational health clinics
- Rehabilitation centers
- Acute care hospitals
- Physician offices
- Medical homes
- Advanced practice registered nurses practice sites, such as nurse-managed clinics
- Specialty hospitals (for example, pediatric, psychiatry-mental health)
- Long-term care hospitals (for example, psychiatric)
- Urgent care centers
- Home health agencies
- Hospice care
- Ambulatory care/clinics
- Clinical practices, such as family practice, specialty (for example, orthopedics, dermatology)
- Retail clinics

other hospitals or others trying to go it alone. The critical message is hospitals are changing their overall organization, and it is not clear what the future holds.

Small hospitals with 100 or fewer beds and hospitals in rural areas are particularly vulnerable. They often have difficulty getting enough admissions, and therefore, they often lose money. In addition, they must keep costly equipment current by purchasing new equipment and maintaining their equipment and physical facilities. Hospitals have to maintain a certain level of staff: This is not a business that can easily flex staffing numbers and use a lot of temporary staff, and it takes time to orient new staff. These vulnerable hospitals may also have problems recruiting RNs for their workforces because many RNs prefer to work in urban centers and in large, up-to-date hospitals. Schools of nursing in states with large rural areas are increasingly partnering with rural hospitals to improve student enrollment from these areas and, they hope, increase the RN pool in the workforce for these geographic regions. Such partnerships provide courses and clinical experiences in rural healthcare settings and may use distance education to facilitate the nursing programs, making it easier for students and reducing student travel time to campus.

The U.S. healthcare delivery system has an estimated $750 billion in wasted resources in the system. This money is lost, so it cannot be spent on improving healthcare outcomes. A recent report on healthcare in the United States indicates that there is need to focus on the best care at a lower cost, not a higher cost (Institute of Medicine [IOM], 2013). The report *Best Care at Lower Cost: The Path to Continuously Learning Health Care in America* describes the system in this way: "Health care in America presents a fundamental paradox. The past 50 years have seen an explosion in biomedical knowledge, dramatic innovation in therapies and surgical procedures, and management of conditions that previously were fatal, with ever more exciting clinical capabilities on the horizon. Yet, American health care is falling short on basic dimensions of quality, outcomes, costs, and equity" (IOM, 2013, p. 1).

Compared to other countries, the United States is paying more for less, resulting in poorer healthcare outcomes than are found in other industrialized nations. The complex U.S. healthcare delivery system must manage costs while simultaneously ensuring quality, evidence-based care. Trying to achieve this balance will lead to more changes in the healthcare delivery system and impact nursing.

Structure and Process

One way to describe a hospital is to consider its structure and process. A hospital's **structure** is based on how the organization is configured, and the best source for a view of a hospital's structure is its organizational chart. **Figure 8-2** is an example of a hospital organizational chart, which displays the components of the hospital in a vertical structure. The chart identifies to whom staff report, or rather, who is a staff member's manager or supervisor. Organizations that focus more on this type of structure tend to be more bureaucratic and highly centralized with key persons in the organization making decisions. Bureaucratic organizations typically have the following characteristics:

- *Division of labor:* descriptions of jobs that include clearly defined tasks
- *Defined hierarchy:* clear description of the reporting relationships

- *Detailed rules and regulations:* greater emphasis on policies and procedures; expectation that these will be followed and guide decision making
- *Impersonal relationships:* expectation that staff will do their jobs and supervisors will ensure that jobs are done as expected

Hospitals typically have hierarchical management levels. The top level consists of the board of trustees or board of directors. This board typically includes members of the community and community leaders who are not directly involved in health care. The board is responsible for developing the overall direction of the hospital and ensuring that the goals of the organization are met. The board hires the hospital's chief executive officer (CEO—also sometimes called the organization's president), and this person reports to the board. The CEO then hires the other major leaders for the hospital, such as the chief financial officer (CFO) and the nursing leader. The nursing leader may be called the chief nursing executive (CNE), the chief nursing officer (CNO), or in some cases, the vice president for nursing or patient services. This last title may also reflect the person's oversight of nursing and other disciplines or ancillary services,

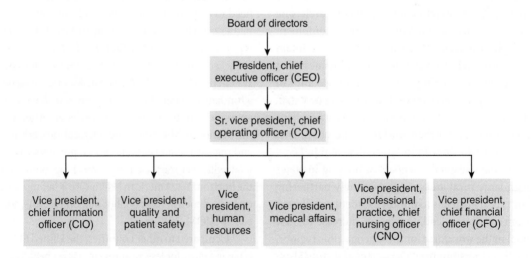

Figure 8-2 Example of a Hospital Organizational Chart

such as occupational therapy, physical therapy, or nutrition. Often, the board approves these hires. Because the board has ultimate responsibility for the budget, it has significant influence over matters that impact nurses, such as staffing and other resources important to nursing.

Although bureaucratic organizations are less common today, many hospitals still use this approach, emphasizing a vertical structure that includes these elements but is less rigid than the structure of past formal bureaucratic organizations. Line authority, or chain of command, is very important, in that each staff member knows to whom to report, and it is expected that this order will be followed. A true bureaucratic organization does not expect or want much staff input regarding decisions, but this does not apply in most organizations today, with administration encouraging more staff commitment and thus engagement in the organization. Another element of organizational structure is span of control, or the number of staff managed by each supervisor or manager. The more staff a manager supervises the more complex that supervision becomes.

A horizontal structure is decentralized, with emphasis placed on departments or divisions; decisions are made closer to where work is done. Departments or divisions focus on special functions such as those related to nursing, laboratory, pharmacy, and dietary/patient food services. This is referred to as departmentalization. Later in this chapter, examples of common hospital departments or services are discussed.

The matrix organization structure is newer and less clear than the traditional bureaucratic organization that is centered on departments. In a matrix organization, staff might be part of a functional department, such as nursing services, but if the nurse works in surgery, the nurse may also be considered a staff member in the surgical services/department. This type of organization is considered flatter because decisions do not flow clearly from the top down.

Process, the other dimension of organizations, focuses on how the organization functions. How would a staff member gain an understanding of a hospital's process? The hospital's vision, mission statement, and goals are a good place to begin to find out what is important to the organization and how the hospital describes itself and its functions. Other sources of information relevant to process include policies and procedures, communication systems and expectations, decision-making processes, delegation process, implementation of coordination (teams), informatics, and evaluation methods (quality improvement [QI]). The key question is *how does the work get done?*

Classification of Hospitals

Hospitals can be classified using a variety of descriptors. The following are some of these descriptors:

- *Ownership:* Is the hospital for-profit (investor owned), not-for-profit, part of a corporate system, faith based, or governmental (state, federal)? Government hospitals include Veterans Administration (VA) hospitals, military hospitals, state mental health hospitals, the National Institutes of Health Clinical Center, and Indian Health Service hospitals.
- *Number of beds:* Bed size or the number of beds can vary widely from hospital to hospital.
- *Licensure:* State health departments are responsible for hospital licensure, which ensures hospitals in the state meet state standards. Licensure and accreditation are not the same, though they both are concerned with quality. Licensure comes from a government agency. Accreditation is a process to determine whether a hospital meets certain minimal standards; this process is voluntary and provided by a nongovernmental organization. For hospitals to receive Medicare and Medicaid reimbursement—and this is an important source of income for hospitals—they must be certified or given authority by the Centers for Medicare and Medicaid Services (CMS) to provide services to Medicare and Medicaid

recipients. Meeting all these requirements and participating in the surveys take staff time, which is costly, but it is very important for the overall financial status of an institution. In addition, hospitals that do not meet these requirements cannot be used as sites for healthcare professional students' clinical practice experiences (nursing, medicine, and others). Professional licensure and related regulation are discussed in other chapters.

- *Teaching:* A hospital is classified as a teaching hospital if it offers residency programs for physicians. The expansion of nurse residency programs may also become a method for classifying hospitals in the future, although this is not certain at this time and few hospitals have such programs. Some hospitals are referred to as academic health centers (AHCs). These hospitals are associated with academic institutions that offer healthcare profession education, primarily medicine, but typically if the university has a nursing program or other programs such as pharmacy, they will also be associated with the AHC. In these hospitals there may be cross-administration—for example, the Dean of Medicine and Dean of Nursing might have positions in the hospital as well as some of the faculty. This is a more formal arrangement than referring to a hospital as a teaching hospital where students come for clinical experience.

- *Length of stay:* Length of stay refers to how long patients typically stay in a hospital, a measure given as a range or average length of stay. Fewer than 30 days is referred to as short stay, and more than 30 days is long term. Length of stay has been decreasing in the last 15 years because of decreasing reimbursement for hospital care and a greater push to provide more healthcare services outside the hospital.

- *Multihospital system:* Since 1991, there has been growth in large hospital systems that include multiple hospitals. These systems often provide more than just acute care services; for example, they may offer ambulatory care (clinics, surgery), hospice care, home care, long-term care, and other services. This partnering provides the hospitals with a continuum of services, from acute care to long-term care, to meet the needs of their patients. In a sense, the system does not lose the patient; the patient just goes on to a different part of the system for additional care needs and may return to the system for other services if needs change. For example, suppose a patient has been in a hospital intensive care unit for complications related to chronic obstructive pulmonary disorder. The patient returns home after discharge and receives home care from the hospital's home care agency. One week after discharge, the home care nurse assesses the patient and decides that the patient needs to be rehospitalized because of pneumonia. The patient is then admitted to the same hospital.

Typical Departments in a Hospital

As was discussed in relation to the structure of organizations, hospitals are made up of departments, divisions, and/or services. This structure has existed for a long time. Students need to be familiar with these departments because nurses interact with all of them at some point in their practice, and they need to know how to coordinate care by using services from a variety of departments and collaborate with interprofessional staff. What are some of the departments found in an acute care hospital? Titles may vary from hospital to hospital, but the functions described here are typical and part of daily hospital operations:

- *Administration:* This is the leadership for the hospital, the central decision-making source—for example, the CEO or administrator; assistant administrators; financial services and budget staff; the CNO, CNE, or vice president for nursing or patient services; department heads; and others.

- *Nursing:* This is the largest department in terms of employee numbers. Often it is called patient services, which is a title used by many hospitals since the early 1990s. This does not mean that patients receive only nursing care; many other departments are directly involved in patient care, such as laboratory, dietetic services, respiratory services, pharmacy, and others. However, nursing service is the 24/7 coordinator of patient care and provides the largest percentage of direct care to patients.

- *Medical staff:* Physicians who practice in a hospital, if not part of a training program such as a residency or fellowship, must be members of the medical staff. Their credentials are reviewed, and they are given admitting privileges. This is done to ensure that standards are met. A director or chief of medical staff leads the medical staff. Medical staff may or may not be employees of the hospital. If a college of medicine is partnered with the hospital, the organization may be more complex, as noted earlier with AHCs.

- *Admission and discharge:* This department manages all aspects of admission and discharge for patients, including paperwork, reimbursement, patient room assignments, and in some cases, assignment of physicians. Case management may be part of this department or part of patient services.

- *Medical records:* Documentation is a critical part of all aspects of care. The medical records department provides oversight of documentation, whether paper documentation or information in a computerized system. This complex function requires nursing input to ensure that nursing documentation is recognized and nursing care information is included.

- *Information management:* This department ensures that required information is collected, analyzed, monitored, and summarized—typically administrative and clinical data. Its function is directly related to medical records and documentation. Another area in which information management is important today is for QI efforts. Staff need ongoing training to ensure effective use of digital information systems (electronic medical/health records). Health information technology (HIT) is a rapidly expanding area in healthcare organizations.

- *Quality improvement:* This department is charged with ensuring that the hospital has a QI program, implements active QI efforts, evaluates its outcomes, and makes changes to improve care. Nurses often are part of the staff in this department because they have much to offer with their experience and knowledge in providing and assessing quality care. Nurses should be actively involved in these activities throughout the hospital and in their daily practice. Additional discussion on QI is found in other chapters.

- *Infection control:* This function has become increasingly important, influenced by a greater need to provide services that decrease infection risk for patients and staff. Nurses are typically active staff members in this department; they develop and implement policies and procedures, monitor infection rates, and train staff.

- *Research and evidence-based practice (EBP):* Many hospitals, particularly AHCs, have research departments. The department's purpose is to conduct research studies and review and approve studies prior to their implementation through the institutional review board (IRB). Typically, professionals in medicine lead this department, although nurses often participate in research studies and may lead their own nursing studies. The nursing department may have its own designated nurse researchers. In some healthcare organizations, research and EBP are combined, or there may be a separate EBP service or department. The EBP department is one of the newest in hospitals, and not all hospitals have this department. Some hospitals are incorporating the management of EBP—both medicine and nursing—into other departments. The EBP functions may be part of nursing or patient services, QI, or evidence-based medicine related to medical staff organization. Additional information on research and EBP is found in other chapters.

- *In-service or staff development:* This is the department that implements orientation and ongoing education for staff.
- *Environmental services (housekeeping):* Staff from this department interacts with nurses in the patient care areas to ensure that areas are clean for patients.
- *Dietary:* This department is responsible for ensuring patients' nutritional needs are met through meals that conform to individual patient dietary requirements and offer other dietary interventions.

Other departments focus on specific health needs, such as pharmacy, respiratory therapy, clinical laboratory, infusion therapy, occupational therapy, radiology, physical therapy, and social services. Nurses get involved in all these services. Hospitals are typically organized around clinical areas (units, services, and in some cases, departments) such as medicine, surgery, intensive care (medical intensive care unit [MICU], surgical intensive care unit [SICU], cardiac care unit [CCU], and neonatal intensive care unit [NICU]), post-anesthesia unit (PACU), labor and delivery (L&D), postpartum, nursery, gynecology, pediatrics, emergency department (ED), urgent care, psychiatric or behavioral/mental health, ambulatory care, ambulatory care

surgery, and dialysis. Clinical areas may also be specific to a specialty, such as medical units for the post-cardiac care unit may be referred to as step-down units, oncology units, or other internal medicine subspecialties; surgical units might focus on orthopedics, urology, and so on.

Stop and Consider #2
Organization structure and process affect healthcare organizations.

Healthcare Providers:
Who Is on the Team?

The hospital healthcare team providing care is composed of a variety of healthcare providers, both professional and nonprofessional. All are important in the care process. In addition, many other staff are critical to the overall operation of a hospital, such as office support staff, dietary staff, housekeeping staff, facilities management and maintenance staff, patient transportation staff, medical records staff, communications (HIT) staff, equipment maintenance and repair staff, and many others. For our purposes, the focus is on staff that provides care, either direct or indirect patient care. A staff member who provides **direct care**, such as a nurse, comes in contact with the patient. An **indirect care provider** might be someone who works in the lab to complete a lab test, but this provider may never actually see the patient. However, the work done in the lab is very important to the patient's care.

The group of staff who provide care to a patient is referred to as a team. They have a common purpose: providing patient care. Interprofessional teamwork is one of the five recommended core competencies for all healthcare professionals and is discussed in other chapters. Nurses work together with other nursing staff (licensed vocational nurses [LVNs]/licensed practical nurses [LPNs] and nursing/patient care assistants on teams) to provide care; however, today there is also greater emphasis on the need for interprofessional teams in which nurses collaborate and coordinate with members of multiple disciplines, such as physicians, pharmacists, social workers, and many other members.

The following are some of the major team members and their functions. Not all patients require services from all these healthcare professionals; instead, services are based on individual patient needs.

- *Registered nurse (RN):* Nurses are the backbone of any acute care hospital. They work in a variety of positions and departments, not just the nursing department; for example, they work in medical records, QI, infusion therapy, case management, staff development, radiology, ambulatory care, and other departments. Some nurses are in management positions and do not provide direct care.
- *Licensed practical/vocational nurse (LPN/LVN):* An LPN/LVN is a member of the nursing staff who has completed a 1-year nursing program, successfully passed the LPN/LVN licensing exam, and licensed by state in which they practice. They are supervised by RNs and are important team members. The state board of nursing determines what care they may provide, although not all states use the LPN/LVN designations. It is important for RNs to know what LPNs/LVNs are allowed to do including familiarity with their position descriptions and provide supervision for this care. RNs can delegate to LPNs/LVNs, but the reverse is not true.
- *Patient care assistant or nursing assistant:* Patient care assistants or certified nursing assistants may have a variety of titles. They are nonprofessional nursing staff who have a short training period (typically a few months) that prepares them to provide direct care, such as assisting with activities of daily living (bathing, taking vital signs, and so on). They are supervised by RNs or, in some cases, by

LPNs/LVNs and are important members of the team.

- *Advanced practice registered nurse (APRN):* A nurse practitioner is an RN with a master's degree in a specialty. In some states, APRNs may provide some services independent of physician orders, such as prescribing certain medications and treatment procedures. APRNs may work in clinics and typically do not work in acute care units, although this situation is changing. In some states, APRNs may have admitting privileges along with their prescriptive authority (that is, the right to prescribe medication). As discussed in content on nursing education, the future plan is APRNs will get a doctor of nursing practice (DNP) degree instead of a master's degree.
- *Clinical nurse specialist (CNS):* A CNS is an RN with a master's degree. This nurse is prepared to provide care in acute care settings and guides the care provided by other RNs. Examples of CNS specialties are cardiac care and behavioral health (psychiatry), where they would work with staff to improve care and assist in educating staff and focusing more on EBP.
- *Clinical nurse leader (CNL):* This nurse has a master's degree and is a provider and a manager of care at the point of care to individuals and cohorts (groups of patients) but is not in an administrative or manager position. The CNL may be involved in team leadership by improving information management; determining patient risk; collecting outcomes data for QI; providing clinical leadership; applying EBP; advocating for patients, the community, and the care team; and providing other related activities (American Association of Colleges of Nursing [AACN], 2013). The CNL is involved in care planning and coordination and working with the nursing team and interprofessional teams to better ensure quality care and outcomes.

- *Certified nurse–midwife (CNM):* A nurse–midwife has a master's degree and is prepared to provide women's health services and services to obstetric patients (L&D, postpartum, and obstetric clinics). In some states, CNMs have admitting privileges. Their scope of practice may be regulated under either the medical or nursing practice act, depending on the state.

- *Certified registered nurse anesthetist (CRNA):* This nurse anesthetist has a master's degree and is prepared to provide services to patients requiring anesthesia, which is done in many hospitals today for inpatient and ambulatory care surgery or for procedures that require anesthesia. As discussed in other chapters, the CRNA is transitioning to a DNP degree rather than a master's degree.

- *Doctor of nursing practice (DNP):* An RN with a DNP has a terminal doctoral practice degree. This nurse is prepared to carry out roles similar to the traditional APRN and CNS, in addition to focusing at the systems level on EBP, QI, leadership, and financing expertise. These nurses may hold a variety of positions in a hospital.

- *Physician:* A physician has a medical degree and typically has a specialty such as surgery, medicine, pediatrics, or obstetrics and gynecology; some physicians may even have a subspecialty. For example, a physician with a specialty in internal medicine may subspecialize in rheumatology, dermatology, oncology, or neurology. A surgeon may subspecialize in orthopedics, oncology (and even more specifically in breast surgery), and so on. In a teaching hospital, which has medical students and residents, and in AHCs, the typical team includes faculty/attending physician, the chief resident, residents, interns, and medical students. They are responsible for the medical aspects of patient care and have oversight of overall care requirements.

- *Physician's assistant (PA):* A PA is prepared to practice some aspects of medicine under the supervision of a physician. The PA conducts physical examinations, performs diagnostic workups, makes diagnoses, prevents and treats diseases, assists with procedures, and may have some prescribing privileges.

- *Pharmacist:* The pharmacist has completed professional education and ensures that pharmaceutical care is appropriate for patient needs. Given the growing concern about medication errors, pharmacists are important members of the team, and nurses should work closely with them. Some hospitals have a centralized pharmacy department with all pharmaceutical services coming from a central unit. Others have moved to include pharmacists as direct team members on units, providing an invaluable service and staff education about pharmaceutical agents at the point of care.

- *Occupational therapist (OT):* OTs are not present in every hospital, but they provide important services for patients with rehabilitation needs because of impaired functioning, such as patients who have had a stroke or patients who have experienced a serious automobile accident. Another type of a therapist, who might be used especially for patients who have had a stroke, is a speech-language pathologist. These types of therapists are commonly found in rehabilitation services, but these services can also be provided in all types of settings, such as in hospitals, long-term care facilities, and home care.

- *Physical therapist (PT):* PTs provide musculoskeletal care to patients, such as assisting with teaching patients how to walk (for example, stroke patients or post-hip replacement), use crutches, or use of other assistive devices. They also help design exercises to ensure or increase patient mobility and may train nurses to assist in providing physical therapy for patients as they provide daily patient care.

- *Registered dietitian:* Dietitians work with patients to help resolve dietary and nutritional needs. Nurses work with dietitians as patient dietary needs are identified and implemented.

- *Respiratory therapist:* Respiratory therapists provide care to patients who have a variety of respiratory problems. They are trained to provide specific types of treatments, such as oxygen therapy, inhalation therapy, intermittent positive-pressure ventilators, and artificial mechanical ventilators. Respiratory therapists go to the patient's bedside for these treatments, and some respiratory therapists may be assigned to work solely in intensive care units, where there is great need for these treatments. Respiratory therapists are also part of the team that responds to codes when patients experience cardiac or respiratory arrests.

- *Social worker:* Social workers have professional degrees and assist patients and their families with such issues as reimbursement, discharge concerns, housing, transportation, discharge plans, and other social services. Nurses work with social workers to identify patient issues that need to be resolved in order to decrease stress on patients and families. Social workers (and nurses) may serve as case managers, and they may be important resources in providing effective discharge plans.

Medical care in acute care has been examined over the last few years with several problem areas noted that have led to changes in some hospitals. Two of the newest members of the healthcare team are the hospitalist and the intensivist. The hospitalist position usually is a doctor of medicine (MD), although APRNs and CNSs may hold this position

in some hospitals. The hospitalist is a generalist who coordinates the patient's care, serving as the primary provider while the patient is in the hospital. In this case, the patient's primary provider outside the hospital is not involved in the inpatient care, and the patient returns to that provider in the community after discharge. This reduces the time that the primary care provider (internist, family practitioner, pediatrician) needs to devote to inpatient care. Thus, the primary care provider (PCP) has more time to focus on patient outpatient needs. In addition, the hospitalist is more current with acute care and the treatment required. The intensivist is similar to the hospitalist, but because this MD focuses on care of patients in intensive care, he or she is providing more specialized patient care, care that requires physicians who are up-to-date on critical information and intensive care procedures. The hospitalist and intensivist positions were developed to increase coordination and continuity of care in the hospital. Both of these providers are paid by the hospital as hospital employees. A major disadvantage of this model of medical care is that the patient has no relationship with the hospitalist or the intensivist prior to hospitalization and will not have any contact after hospitalization. Some patients may not be satisfied with a nurse in this role. Patient choice is always an important factor to consider as this has a direct impact on patient satisfaction.

Stop and Consider #3

Nurses need to understand the roles of the multiple healthcare providers.

Healthcare Financial
Issues

Healthcare financial issues can be viewed from three perspectives. The first perspective is the macro view, or the status of healthcare finances viewed from a national or a state perspective. The second is the micro view, which focuses on a specific HCO and its budget. A third perspective is reimbursement for healthcare services.

The Nation's Health Care: Financial Status (Macro View)

The macro view is important because it encompasses the major financial support for the U.S. healthcare system. The United States spends a lot of money on health care, yet not everyone has been covered by healthcare insurance. In 2016, national spending for health care averaged more than $10,000 per person. By 2025, health care spending is expected to be 20% of the total economy; in 2015, it was 17.8%. Medicare enrollment is also increasing, and by 2025, one of every five Americans will be enrolled in Medicare, spending an average of nearly $18,000 a year per Medicare enrollee; in 2015, this amount was $15,000 (Pear, 2016). Looking into the future, further national healthcare spending is expected to increase from 2016 through 2025 by 5.6% per year, with a projection of $5.5 trillion in 2025 (Ellison, 2017). This is a projected vision of the future of healthcare financial status, and changes in healthcare delivery and reimbursement that might be made by the Trump administration will have an impact on these projections. As discussed in other content on QI, it is noted that efforts to improve care may reduce costs; for example, national efforts to reduce hospital-acquired conditions resulted in 125,000 fewer deaths and saved more than $28 billion from 2010 to 2015 (U.S. Department of Health and Human Services [HHS], Agency for Healthcare Research and Quality [AHRQ], 2016a). This is a good example of the critical importance of QI for better patient outcomes and reducing costs.

Reimbursement issues impact the status of health care and coverage of these expenses. **Figure 8-3** describes the nation's healthcare dollar—how much Medicare and Medicaid spent on different categories of services. **Figure 8-4** provides information on Medicare benefit payments by type of service for 2012. These expenditures are changing, and they are increasing.

The National Quality Strategy (NQS), discussed in more detail in other chapters, includes long-term goals related to affordability of healthcare, recognizing that cost is associated with quality care (HHS, AHRQ, 2016b):

1. Ensure affordable and accessible high-quality health care for people, families, employers, and governments.
2. Support and enable communalities to ensure accessible, high-quality care while reducing waste and fraud.

The goals apply to health care across the continuum of care from acute care to public/community health and services. The NQS now tracks outcomes related to these goals by using data from the National Quality and Disparities Report (QDR) and other sources. It is clear that costs are rising. The QDR report describes the status of affordability. These reports usually represent data that are at least 1 year behind the current year.

The Individual Healthcare Organization and Its Financial Needs (Micro View)

The hospital budget is used by hospitals to manage their financial issues—to plan, monitor expenses and revenue, and then make adjustments to ensure financial stability. The budget is prepared for a specific time period, usually a year. In addition, a longer-term plan covering several years is prepared, although this plan must be adjusted over time because of changes in the organization's financial status and other factors that affect the organization and its services. The budget describes expected expenses, such as staff salaries and benefits, equipment, supplies, utilities, pharmaceutical needs, facility maintenance, dietary needs, administrative services, clinical care, HIT, QI, staff education, legal fees, insurance coverage,

THE NATION'S HEALTH DOLLAR ($3.2 TRILLION), CALENDAR YEAR 2015: WHERE IT CAME FROM

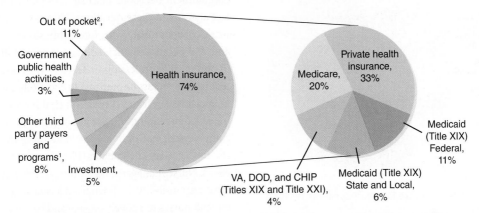

Out of pocket[2], 11%

Government public health activities, 3%

Health insurance, 74%

Other third party payers and programs[1], 8%

Investment, 5%

Medicare, 20%

Private health insurance, 33%

Medicaid (Title XIX) Federal, 11%

VA, DOD, and CHIP (Titles XIX and Title XXI), 4%

Medicaid (Title XIX) State and Local, 6%

[1] Includes worksite health care, other private revenues, Indian Health Service, workers' compensation, general assistance, maternal and child health, vocational rehabilitation, Substance Abuse and Mental Health Services Administration, school health, and other federal and state local programs.
[2] Includes co-payments, deductibles, and any amounts not covered by health insurance.
Note: Sum of pieces may not equal 100% due to rounding.

THE NATION'S HEALTH DOLLAR ($3.2 TRILLION), CALENDAR YEAR 2015, WHERE IT WENT

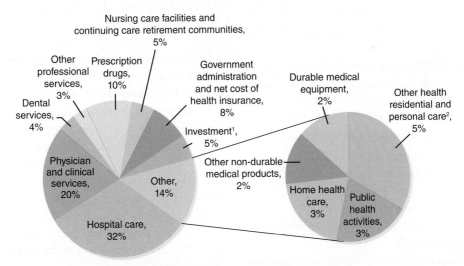

Nursing care facilities and continuing care retirement communities, 5%

Other professional services, 3%

Prescription drugs, 10%

Dental services, 4%

Government administration and net cost of health insurance, 8%

Durable medical equipment, 2%

Other health residential and personal care[2], 5%

Physician and clinical services, 20%

Investment[1], 5%

Other non-durable medical products, 2%

Other, 14%

Home health care, 3%

Public health activities, 3%

Hospital care, 32%

[1] Includes Noncommercial Research (2%) and Structures and Equipment (3%).
[2] Includes expenditures for residential care facilities, ambulance providers, medical care delivered in non-traditional settings (such as community centers, senior citizens centers, schools, and military field stations), and expenditures for Home and Community Waiver programs under Medicaid.
Note: Sum of pieces may not equal 100% due to rounding.

Figure 8-3 The Nation's Health Dollar, Calendar Year 2015, Where It Went

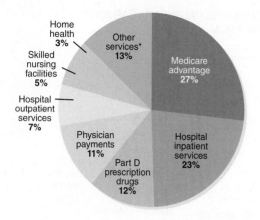

Figure 8-4 Medicare Benefit Payments by Type of Service

Reproduced from Kaiser Family Foundation. (2016). An overview of Medicare. Retrieved from http://kff.org /medicare/issue-brief/an-overview-of-medicare/. Reprinted with permission. Data from Congressional Budget Office, 2016 Medicare Baseline (March 2016).

parking and security, and so on, and also includes any major expenses outside of operating expenses such as expansion or renovation. The budget also includes projected revenue or money coming into the organization.

It is very important that nursing management participate in the budget process because the budget has a major impact on nurses and nursing care. Reimbursement and other aspects of healthcare finance affect nursing care and responses to questions such as these:

1. Are there enough nursing staff?
2. Are there sufficient and effective support services for nurses so that they are free to provide care and not do nonpatient duties?
3. Are the most up-to-date supplies and equipment available?
4. Is there an efficient computerized documentation system?
5. Is orientation sufficient for new staff?
6. Do nursing staff receive the training they need?
7. Are nurse managers provided with effective training and education?

All of these are critical questions, and more, are of interest to nursing staff. Nursing leaders in an

organization should be actively involved in cost containment decisions because these decisions affect answers to these questions. Nurses should also work collaboratively with interprofessional leaders and staff because financial decisions are not limited to one specific profession or service. This, however, requires that nurses be prepared to effectively consider financial issues. More content on health economics is needed in nursing education programs to develop competencies not only for graduate programs, but also for baccalaureate students (Platt, Kwasky, & Spetz, 2015). Nurse managers and administrators have the most responsibility for financial decisions; however, for staff nurses to actively engage and be effective in the organization, they too need to have some understanding of this area and provide input when needed.

Nurses are not usually directly involved in the development of budgets unless they are in a management position; however, it is important for nurses to understand what a budget is and why it is important. Nurse managers need to ask their nursing staff for input when unit budgets are developed and need to share budget outcomes with staff. The nurse leader of the nursing department should consult with department nurse managers as budgets are developed and monitored.

The hospital board of directors approves the final budget. After a budget is approved and implemented, it is important that budgetary data are monitored on a regular basis, and this information should be shared with the healthcare organization's managers throughout the year. This monitoring is done to better ensure that the budget goals are met and facilitate early recognition of budget issues that may require adjustment in the budget and in the workplace.

Reimbursement: Who Pays for Health Care?

Reimbursement is a critical, complex topic in health care. It represents the third perspective on healthcare financial issues. Nursing students may wonder why this topic is relevant to them or even to nurses in general. Basically, reimbursement pays the patient's bill for services provided, and this payment in turn covers costs of care, such as staff salaries and benefits, drugs, medical supplies, physician fees, facility maintenance and upgrades, equipment, general supplies, and much more. These monies then provide healthcare providers with funds to pay their bills and cover their services. So, for example, reimbursement dollars eventually become the dollars that pay staff salaries in hospitals, clinics, physician practices, homecare agencies, and so on.

Hospitals that do not bring in enough money to pay their bills are said to be operating "in the red," and this is not a good position for a hospital. It means the hospital cannot pay all its bills. Most hospitals are operating in the red, but how far in the red can make the difference between modernizing or filling staff positions or not doing so—and whether the hospital stays open for business. Some hospitals in this country have closed. Particularly hard hit have been hospitals in rural areas and small hospitals that are not able to compete for patients. Their closing may have a major impact on access to care. Some patients may not have access to a local hospital for needed services, or even for emergency services, or people may have to travel long distances for obstetric care or specialized care for children (pediatrics, neonatal care for newborns), mental health services, oncology (diagnosis and treatment), complex surgical procedures, and many other services.

The United States is experiencing a serious crisis in its safety net hospitals, which are hospitals that serve populations with limited or no resources to pay for service. The government defines safety net hospitals as hospitals with the highest number of inpatient stays that are paid by Medicaid or for which there is no insurance coverage (HHS, AHRQ, 2016b). Healthcare Cost and Utilization Project (HCUP) data for 2014 indicate that one quarter of these hospitals accounted for 33% of all inpatient stays, 50% of stays covered by Medicaid,

45% of uninsured stays, and 43% of all mental health-related stays (HHS, AHRQ, HCUP, 2016). Often, these hospitals are teaching hospitals and AHCs. This does not mean these hospitals do not or could not serve patients with excellent reimbursement; however, it is typically the case that the majority of their patients cannot provide sufficient reimbursement and in some cases potential patients with insurance do not want to go to these hospitals. Patients with limited or no reimbursement also tend to be more complex in terms of their care: low income, medically vulnerable, with complex social needs, and have had limited preventive care. Some have chronic medical conditions that have not been treated. Other complications include socioeconomic problems, language issues, and immigrant status, all of which contribute to the need for complex healthcare treatment. The safety net hospital system struggles to operate effectively to meet the complex medical and social services for vulnerable populations, but they need sufficient reimbursement for services to cover their operating costs (Dewan & Sack, 2008). "As providers of last resort, safety net systems offer services that are expected by their communities and required by state and local governments, regardless of whether adequate revenue streams exits to support these services" (VanDeusen et al., 2015, p.1). These systems require changes to meet the needs of patients, provide quality care, and also to remain financially stable.

It is important for nurses to understand basic information about reimbursement. Patients today frequently worry about payment for care. Questions that arise are: Do patients have insurance coverage? How much of their care will be covered by insurance? Will they get the treatment they need from the providers they prefer? Experiencing an illness is difficult for any patient and the patient's family, and to add worry about payment for services adds to this stress and can have an impact on a patient's health as well as the patient's response to the health problem. This stress can affect whether patients can follow treatment recommendations. Can the patient afford needed medications, or would the costs compromise the patient's ability to buy food or pay rent? Can the patient afford to take a bus or taxicab to a doctor's appointment? Can the patient afford to take off work for an appointment? None of this is simple.

The Third-Party Payer System

The U.S. healthcare delivery system is funded primarily through a third-party payer system (insurance) that is primarily employer based, with healthcare services paid by someone other (insurer) than the patient and services provided mostly in private sector healthcare organizations, but also in some public or government healthcare organizations. This means if your employer does not offer an insurance benefit, you must purchase your own insurance, apply for Medicaid if you are eligible, apply for Medicare if you are eligible, or go without insurance. Under the Affordable Care Act, going without insurance means you have to pay a penalty; however, this penalty may change with Trump administration initiatives. Examples of third-party payers include Blue Cross and Humana. Medicare and Medicaid, though government programs and not employer based, are also third-party payers. The patient pays for part of the care, but the payment for most patients goes through another party, the insurer (the third-party payer). Typically, the patient or enrollee in the insurance policy is covered as part of a group, most likely through the enrollee's employer healthcare policies as an employee benefit. Some employers allow employees to choose from certain policy plans of varying cost and covered services.

The Patient Protection and Affordable Care Act (ACA) established insurance exchanges (at the federal level and in some states as well). An individual can buy personal health insurance through these exchanges when he or she does not have access to employer healthcare insurance (for example, someone who is self-employed or whose employer does not provide insurance). The new legislation also provides some financial support and reduced costs for people who have to buy insurance through the exchanges, but they must meet certain criteria to obtain this support. The launch of this system was accompanied by numerous problems—particularly technological problems, but also issues related to the insurance plans and some people having to change coverage, which in some cases was more costly or required a change in providers. It is unclear what the long-term results of these changes will be because the Trump administration plans on making changes; details are not yet known.

Fee-for-service is the most common reimbursement model in the United States. In this model, physicians or other providers, such as hospitals, bill separately for each patient encounter or service that they provide, rather than receiving a salary or a set payment per patient enrolled. The third-party payer actually pays the bills, but the enrollee usually has some payment responsibilities that vary from one policy to another. This is a complex area, so nurses, as consumers of health care and as healthcare providers, need to understand the basics. Enrollees (patients) may pay any or all of the following:

- *Deductible:* The **deductible** is the part of the bill that the patient must pay before the insurer will pay the bill for the services. If the patient reaches the total amount allowed per year, the patient pays no additional deductible for that year.
- *Copayment and coinsurance:* The **copayment** is the fixed amount that a patient may be required to pay per service (physician visit, lab test, prescription, and so on), and this amount can vary among insurance policies. For example, for a physician visit, the patient may pay a small amount at the time of the visit or be billed by the physician. The insurer pays the rest of the bill. Health plans vary as to the amount of this copay per service.

Both the deductible and the copayment represent the patient's annual out-of-pocket expenses, in addition to the annual fee or premium, that the employee pays for the coverage. These expenses have been steadily increasing for consumers, some years more than others: "In 2016, the average annual workplace family health premiums rose a modest 3% to $18,142; more workers enrolled in high-deductible plans with savings options over the past 2 years; average deductible rose 12% to $1,478 annually" (Kaiser Family Foundation [KFF], 2016a). These costs are expected to increase. Employers also pay a portion of the annual insurance fee. Fees vary from policy to policy and from one employer to another. There has long been no requirement in the United States that every employer provide healthcare insurance coverage, although this changed with the ACA in that there are other insurance options. The ACA also increases the number of employers who offer insurance to employees by basing requirement to offer insurance on how many employees the employer has, but if the law is repealed and new legislation passed, this may or may not be the case in the future.

Annual limits are also important as they define the maximum amount that enrollees have to pay; after that level is reached, they no longer have to contribute to the payment. For example, suppose the employee or enrollee has bills exceeding $5,000, and the annual limit is $5,000. This enrollee or patient would not have to pay any more for care that year after paying $5,000; the patient is 100% covered for care for the remainder of that year.

Employees may include their families on their employer insurance coverage. The ACA now makes it a requirement that insurers allow families to include uninsured adult children up to age 26 on their insurance, even if the adult child is no longer dependent on the parents. This has been very popular and may or may not continue with changes the Trump administration may make. Typically, employees have to pay more per year for family insurance, and there may be different requirements for the family (for example, a higher annual out-of-pocket limit) than for an individual employee.

Another critical element of reimbursement is preexisting conditions. A preexisting condition is a medical condition that a person developed before the person applies for a particular health insurance policy; this condition could affect the person's (enrollee or employee) ability to get coverage or how much the enrollee has to pay for it. What is considered a preexisting condition? Differences in how policies answer this question have long been a problem; however, the ACA has had an impact on the preexisting condition requirement in that insurers are no longer able to use a preexisting condition as a reason to deny insurance coverage. This is an important part of ACA that most Americans like, and it may or may not be maintained at current level due to potential changes in healthcare reimbursement legislation.

Government Reimbursement of Healthcare Services

State and federal governments cover a large portion of the healthcare costs in the United States, but there is no universal coverage, meaning that not all citizens have healthcare coverage. The United States is one of the few industrialized countries that do not have universal coverage. The ACA does not support full universal healthcare coverage, although more people are now able to get coverage and all are required to have coverage or pay a penalty, but the government does not cover insurance for everyone. The Trump administration does not plan on implementing universal healthcare coverage.

There are several types of government-sponsored reimbursement. The largest programs are Medicare and Medicaid, which are managed by the CMS as part of HHS. In 1965, Title XVIII, an amendment to the Social Security Act, established **Medicare**. Medicare is the federal health insurance program for people aged 65 and older, persons with disabilities, and people with end-stage renal disease. Medicare had 55,504,005 beneficiaries in 2015, and this number increases each year (KFF, 2016b). The need for Medicare coverage is growing because of the increase in the population older than age 65. There are several parts to Medicare: Part A covers hospital services; Part B covers physician and outpatient care; Part C, referred to as Medicare Advantage, offers Medicare approved private insurance plans that cover Part A and B services, but Medicare enrollees may choose one of these plan—the plans may charge different fees; and Part D provides coverage for prescriptions. Enrollees have to pay a portion of costs for Part B and prescriptions (Part D). Medicare does not pay for long-term care but does cover some skilled nursing and home health care for specific conditions.

The CMS sets standards and monitors Medicare services and payment. Medicare covers many patients in acute care today. It is a very important part of the U.S. healthcare delivery system that supports older citizens and other populations; however, there is concern about financing this program in the future because of the increase in the number of citizens who will be 65 and older, and this will increase costs. The CMS is also concerned about quality care, as discussed in other chapters in this text.

Medicaid, established in 1965 by Title XIX of the Social Security Act, is the federal/state program for certain categories of low-income people. Medicaid covers health and long-term care services for more than 51 million Americans, including children, the aged, the blind, disabled persons, and people who are eligible to receive federally assisted income maintenance payments. The number of people enrolled in Medicaid is increasing, and this has been influenced by the ACA, as more people are now eligible for Medicaid due to changes in the program made by the ACA to increase insurance coverage for many. Pre-ACA average monthly enrollment was 56,392,477, and in 2016, total monthly Medicaid/CHIP enrollment was 74,369,888 (KFF, 2016b). Government data are typically 1–2 years behind the current year. This program may also experience major changes in the Trump administration healthcare initiatives.

The Medicaid program is funded by both federal funds and state funds, but at this time, each state sets its own guidelines and administers the state's Medicaid program. The federal poverty guidelines (described in the *Health Promotion, Disease Prevention, and*

Illness chapter), which establish the annual income level for poverty defined by the federal government, are important in identifying people who meet coverage criteria for Medicaid reimbursement.

Covered Medicaid services include inpatient care (excluding psychiatric or behavioral health); outpatient care with certain stipulations; laboratory and radiology services; care provided by certified pediatric and family nurse practitioners when licensed to practice under state law; nursing facility services (long-term care) for beneficiaries aged 21 and older; early and periodic screening, diagnosis, and treatment for children younger than age 21; family planning services and supplies; physician services; medical and surgical care; dental services; home health care for beneficiaries who are entitled to nursing facility services under the state's Medicaid plan; certified nurse–midwifery services; pregnancy-related services and services for other conditions that might complicate pregnancy; and 60 days' postpartum pregnancy-related services.

A second group of persons is also eligible for Medicaid: the medically needy. These are persons who have too much money (which may be in savings) to be eligible categorically for Medicaid but who require extensive care that would consume all their resources. Each state must include the following populations in this group: pregnant women through a 60-day postpartum period; children younger than the age of 18; certain newborns for 1 year; and certain protected blind persons. States may add others to this list. The federal government requires that each state cover, at a minimum, persons who qualify for Aid to Families with Dependent Children, all needy children younger than age 21, those who qualify for old-age assistance, those who qualify for Aid to the Blind, persons who are permanently or totally disabled, and those older than 65 who are on welfare.

The government also reimburses care through the following organizations and methods:

- *Military health care:* In this system, the government not only pays for the care for all in military service, but also is the care provider through military hospitals and other healthcare services. The military also covers care of dependents whose care may or may not be provided at a military facility.

- *U.S. Department of Veterans Affairs:* The VA provides services to veterans at VA facilities and covers the cost of these services. VA hospitals are found across the country and provide acute care; ambulatory care; and pharmaceutical, rehabilitation, and specialty services. In some cases, the VA provides care at long-term care facilities. The VA does not cover healthcare services for families of veterans.
- *Federal Employees Health Benefit Program:* Federal law mandates federal employee health insurance. More than 21,995,000 federal employees, retirees, and their dependents are covered (Jeffrey, 2015). Enrollees choose from a variety of healthcare insurance plans as part of the Federal Employees Health Benefit Program. This is just a reimbursement or insurance program; it does not provide healthcare services.
- *State insurance programs:* States offer health insurance to their state employees. Typically, the state government is the largest employer in a state, and therefore, the state's largest insurer. State employees choose from a variety of plans and contribute to the coverage in the same way that non–state employees pay into their employer health programs.

The Uninsured and the Underinsured

The United States has a large population of people who are not insured or who are underinsured (that is, they do not have enough insurance coverage to pay for their needs). As more Americans register for insurance as required by the ACA, the number of uninsured decreases, but the problem of uninsured will not be eliminated. The ACA has had an impact

and continues to do so. "The current enrollment numbers (as of February 2016) are roughly: 12.7 million in the marketplace, and very roughly 20 million total between the ACA between the Marketplace, Medicaid expansion, young adults staying on their parents plan, and other coverage provisions. The 2016 uninsured rate remains at an all time low with the uninsured rate at 11.9% for Americans 18–64 and 8.6% for all Americans. 8.6% is down from 9.1% as of 4th quarter 2015, and 15.7% before the Affordable Care Act was signed into law" (Obamacare Facts, 2016). The uninsured rate is dropping and now is under 10%. Data such as the number of uninsured are always a few years behind the current year with current data found at the U.S. Census Bureau website. Data change as more Americans move in and out of the health insurance pool, and changes in ACA will affect the number of uninsured.

The uninsured and underinsured are in great need of healthcare services—preventive, ongoing, acute, and chronic care. They also have complex needs related to employment, housing, finances, food, transportation, and education. Discharge planning to meet these needs should include a thorough assessment of the patient's needs at home and a plan to ensure that patients receive the care they need post-hospitalization. Complex and vulnerable populations need care and are at serious risk for not being able to access the care and other services they need.

Stop and Consider #4
The United States does not have a universal healthcare reimbursement system.

The Nursing Organization
Within the Hospital

RNs are members of the nation's largest healthcare profession, and they practice wherever people need nursing care. There has been a serious shortage of all types of nurses in the United States in recent years. Although this trend slowed down somewhat, it is expected to increase again as more nurses retire and the population ages requiring more care. The shortage of nursing faculty continues to be a major, long-term problem, as discussed in content on nursing education in this text, and this affects the number of students nursing programs may admit.

Nurses assume critical roles in a variety of healthcare settings—a topic explored throughout this text. The focus in this chapter is on hospitals as one example of a HCO. Nursing services may be organized differently in hospitals. The traditional nursing organization—which is still the most common type—is a nursing department. In this model, nursing staff (RNs, LPNs/LVNs, patient care/nursing assistants) are part of the nursing department, which includes unit support staff or a unit clerk (secretary and other titles) and other support administrative staff as well. The title for the unit clerk position varies, but this is the person or persons who help with clinical unit administrative issues such as records, supplies, reception at the central desk area, and so on.

The second and newer organization model is a patient services department. In this case, the department focuses on the function of multiple patient services, not just nursing. Other patient care services might include medical records, respiratory therapy, infusion therapy, infection control, and so on. The configuration varies widely from one hospital to another. **Figures 8-5** and **8-6** provide examples of this type of organization. **Figure 8-7** describes a hospital unit structure.

An RN is the designated leader as noted in Figures 8-5 through 8-7, which illustrate department models. An RN must be the overall leader of nursing services to meet The Joint Commission accreditation standards. The nurse leader title has changed over time. Director of nursing (DON) was the title most commonly used in the past, and some hospitals still use this title today. The traditional DON

just focused on nursing, and the DON had little, if any, input into the functioning of the hospital as a whole and no input into the budget. Today, even if the nurse leader is called a DON, the DON has much more input into all aspects of the hospital administration and the budget. This is an important change. Given that nurses account for the largest percentage of hospital staff and provide most of the direct care, it is critical that a nurse leader represents the nurses in the organization. This nurse leader needs to be recognized in the organization as an important HCO leader and participate in major HCO decision making.

In the 1970s and 1980s, directors of nursing began to gain more power, and their titles changed to vice president for nursing or patient services in recognition of their organization leadership role—but the focus was still on nursing. During this time, increasing numbers of nursing leaders began to complete graduate degrees. It was recognized that they were running large, complex departments that represented a significant portion of the overall hospital budget. Gradually, the vice president of nursing (VPN) was included in the hospital's budget process as an equal partner. The next change was the evolution of the vice president of patient services position, in which the nurse leader is responsible for more than just nursing services. This was a major shift, but the idea that a nurse could manage other healthcare disciplines changed very slowly. As is true for all such information about hospitals, there is great variation from one hospital to another. The size of the hospital has an impact on how the nursing services are organized.

More nurses today are also taking positions in hospital administration that are not related to just nursing; for example, a nurse could be the chief operating officer or CEO. This is a major shift, but there are not many nurses in these positions. Nurses are also serving on boards of directors for a variety of healthcare organizations in acute care and in community organizations. Today, any nurse who serves

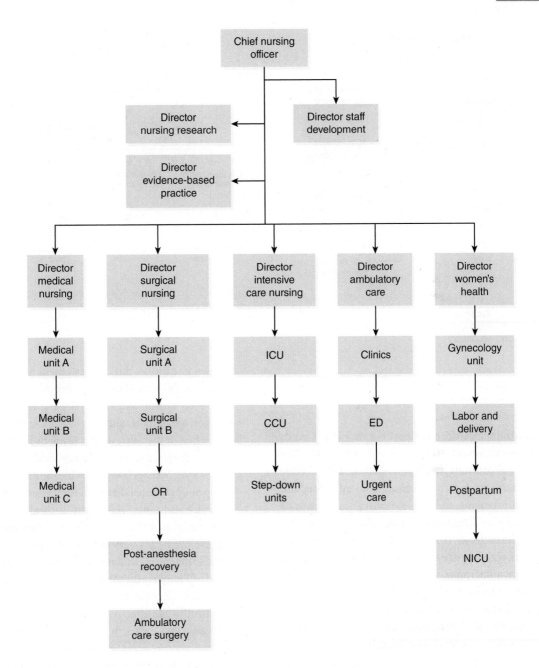

Figure 8-5 An Example: Nursing Department Organizational Chart

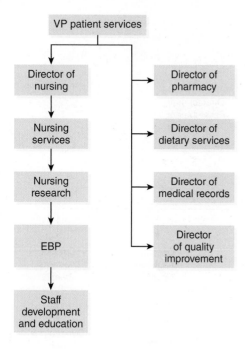

Figure 8-6 An Example: Patient Services Organizational Chart

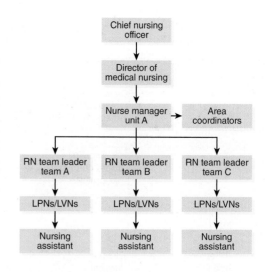

Figure 8-7 An Example: Medical Nursing Unit Organizational Chart

in a nursing leadership position in a HCO needs to be competent in administrative responsibilities such as planning, budgeting, staffing, QI, effective decision making, communicating, coordinating, and public speaking, and he or she must also demonstrate leadership. The nurse administrator must involve others in decision making, support teamwork, and work with other healthcare professionals to support effective interprofessional teamwork to ensure quality care and a healthy work environment.

The nursing organization or department includes a variety of nursing management staff. Typically, there are three levels of management:

- *Upper level:* Responsible for establishing goals, objectives, and strategic plans for the organization. The highest-level nurse leader (DON, VPN, vice president of patient services positions) is in upper-level management.
- *Middle level:* Supervise first-level managers. For example, there may be directors of specific

types of services—director of women's health, director of surgical services, director of behavioral health, and so on. These directors supervise multiple units that have a common function or specialty, such as women's health (for example, gynecology, obstetrics).

- *First level:* Managers who provide the day-to-day or operational direction for the nursing service and units. This group is composed of supervisors and managers. Titles for these managers vary. Some examples are nurse manager, head nurse (not used much today), nursing unit manager, and nursing or nurse coordinator. These managers are critical to the effectiveness of any hospital because they deal with the daily functioning of patient care areas, quality care and safety for patients and staff, budget implementation and use of resources, staffing, staff issues and morale, teamwork, coordination, and communication. They work with multiple disciplines to ensure that patients get the care they need. Nurse managers do not typically provide direct care.

Participation in nursing committees and inter-professional committees provides opportunities for nurses to be directly involved in decision making and have an impact on care delivery. Some of the committees typically found in hospitals focus on policies and procedures, QI, staffing, staff development/education, medical records and documentation, pharmacy, EBP, and research. Some committees are special task forces that address specific issues—for example, preparing for change to a new computerized documentation system.

Stop and Consider #5

The organization of nursing services has an impact on its staff.

Organizational Culture

Typically, culture refers to an individual person's culture, the culture of a group in a country, or a country's culture, but there is also **organizational culture**. Curtin described organizational culture in this way: "There is in each institution an implicit, invisible, intrinsic, informal, and yet instantly recognizable weltanschauung that is best described as 'corporate culture.' Like most important things, it is difficult to define or even describe. It is not 'corporate climate,' 'organizational climate,' or 'corporate identity.' The corporate culture embodies the organizational values that implicitly and explicitly specify norms, shape attitudes, and guide the behaviors of the members of the organization" (2001, p. 219).

Organizational culture has an impact on nursing staff and their practice. The overall HCO has a culture. Nursing within an organization also has a culture; the nursing department and even separate divisions or units may have different cultures. New staff members need to get to know the culture of the organizations that they are considering for employment. Students may be able to identify organizational cultural issues in the units where they have clinical experiences.

Two terms are often used to describe organizational culture: dissonant and consonant. Hospital leaders need to be aware of which label applies to their organization's culture. A dissonant culture means that the organization is not functioning effectively. Such organizations have the following characteristics (Jones & Redman, 2000, p. 605):

- Unclear individual staff and department expectations. (Staff do not know what they should be doing and how they should be working.)
- Lack of consistent measurement of quality of service. (Data from monitoring quality may lead to improvement, but a dysfunctional organization is not as interested in improvement or may not have effective processes to monitor quality.)
- Organized to serve the staff (providers of care) instead of serving the consumers (patients). (Consumers are less important, and thus services will not focus on consumer needs.)
- Limited concern for employee welfare. (Employees are viewed only as workers and not as part of the team and not valued.)
- Limited education and training of staff. (Educated staff members lead to better care and improvement, but the dysfunctional organization is not interested in improvement and better patient outcomes or has difficulty providing education that is of benefit to the staff.)
- Frequent disagreements among staff that relate to control (turf battles). (This situation indicates a high stress level among staff and thus affects effective staff functioning and can impact quality of care—for example, increase in errors.)
- Lack of patient involvement in decision making. (Lack of interest in consumers affects the care provided, patient satisfaction, and quality; this in turn may have financial

implications if patients do not want to receive care in the HCO.)

- Limited recognition of staff accomplishment. (The organization does not value staff.)

Today, there is growing concern about staff incivility and bullying with one another—nurse to nurse and nurse to other healthcare staff. This is a symptom of a dissonant culture. Additional information on incivility is discussed in other chapters in this text. Healthcare organizations are taking strong stands against this type of behavior.

The goal is to develop and maintain a consonant culture, or a functional and effective organization—one that would have the opposite of each of the characteristics of a dissonant organization. People do not like to go to work in stressful environments and want to work in organizations that are effective, creative, and productive. How does an organization attain these characteristics? The hospital's formal framework lays the groundwork for an effective, healthy workplace. This includes the hospital's structure and functions, chain of command, rules and regulations, and policies and procedures. The hospital's vision and mission statements are important. The vision statement describes the hospital's values and its view of the future and provides direction for the organization. The mission statement describes the hospital's purpose. The mission describes the current state of the organization, and the vision is what the organization aspires to be. Hospitals also identify goals and objectives that flow from the vision and mission statements. These statements are part of the organization's process and are very important to the organization's culture. The vision, mission, goals, and objectives should not be documents that are filed away, but rather their messages should be implemented in the hospital's processes and in its structure.

It is not always easy to describe an organization's culture. The first response to an organization's culture takes the form of a gut feeling that a patient has when the patient enters the hospital and observes its physical appearance, how staff respond, the ease of finding one's way around, services set up for the consumer, and so on. The following are other considerations that staff should recognize as important to the organization culture:

- The organization's structure and process
- Communication (types, effectiveness, who is included in communication, level of secrecy, information overload, timeliness of communication, and so on)
- Acceptance of new staff (who become members of the organization)
- Willingness of staff to listen to new ideas
- Inclusion of staff in decision making
- Morale
- Vacancies and turnover
- Acceptance of students (all types of healthcare professions)
- Positive feelings by patients about their care experiences
- Welcome feeling by visitors

Nurses usually know which hospitals are functional (consonant) organizations in the communities in which they live and practice. They share this information with colleagues, and this can have an impact on recruitment of new staff.

Workforce diversity and patient diversity both influence the hospital's culture. All the people who work in the organization and all the people who interact with the organization, such as the patients and their families, public/community healthcare organizations, and community members and representatives, affect organization culture. Workforce diversity has become a critical issue in health care—specifically, there is need for greater diversity in all of the healthcare professions. Labor laws affect this diversity. Title VII of the Civil Rights Act of 1964 and Executive Order 11246 prohibit employer discrimination on the basis of race, color, religion, sex, or national origin. The Americans with Disabilities Act of 1990 prohibits discrimination as a result of disability, including mental illness, if the person can complete the job requirements. These federal laws apply to any hospital (or any type of HCO) that receives any federal funds such as Medicare or Medicaid reimbursement. On a practical level, this means nearly all hospitals are subject to these requirements because few do not provide services to patients covered by these two payment systems or receive other types of federal funding/payment. Language is another issue that is related to diversity. Hospitals need to have access to interpreters to communicate with patients if staff cannot do so.

Another critical aspect of the hospital's culture is its effectiveness. Since 2001, there has been more interest in whether or not the environment is a healing environment. This is just as difficult to define or describe as organizational culture. Some of the factors considered when assessing the environment are (1) privacy, (2) air quality, (3) noise levels, (4) views from windows, and (5) visual characteristics. The needs of patients can vary and, in turn, affect the type of healing environment needed. The elderly may require more safety measures to prevent falls, but if restraining patients is used to accomplish this, the person's (patient, family) may then have a negative view of the environment and healthcare delivery. Restraining a patient may prevent injury, but the patient may also feel imprisoned and punished or abused. Its use should be based on assessment and identification of the best intervention—but at no time should restraining be a long-term intervention without routine assessment as to the patient's status and continuing need. Older adults may have problems hearing and can tolerate more noise. Others may not be able to tolerate a lot of noise and may complain that they cannot sleep in the hospital. From a historical perspective, Florence Nightingale's view of care was associated with healing and the patient's need for fresh air, cleanliness, quiet, diet, and light. Other aspects of a healing environment include physical environment—use of color, sameness or variety, sense of warmth in furnishings, type of artwork on the walls, and so on. Some colors are more peaceful than others. Put simply, is the architecture and furnishings patient-centered and safe? More attention needs to be paid to the physical environment and consideration of changes that improve the environment—leading to a healing environment.

Planetree is a nonprofit organization concerned with the environmental impact of the delivery system on health care. It is one example of a model of healing in healthcare environments. The focus in this model is on body, mind, and spirit, with active patient and family involvement. Hospitals that meet specific criteria can be designated as Planetree hospitals. This patient-centered healing environment model emphasizes the need to consider the healthcare organization's cultural transformation, patient activation, leadership development, and performance improvement with a focus on "patient-centered care is the right thing to do" (Planetree, 2014). Many hospitals are now designated as Planetree hospitals when they meet criteria that emphasize a healing environment as proposed by Planetree.

Stop and Consider #6

An organization's culture has an impact on every nurse on the staff, and nurses have an impact on the organization's culture.

Changes in Healthcare
Delivery

Historically, hospitals have experienced many changes. In the past, hospitals had a significant role in nursing education, but their most important role—then and now—is the provision of healthcare services in their communities. What has been the history of hospitals? The reengineering of health care—that is, the redesigning of how care is provided and how the organization functions—has led to major changes in healthcare organizations. Many healthcare organizations have undergone some level of reengineering in the last decade. This might include restructuring, developing new services, improving processes and systems, or perhaps decreasing services. A common response to periods of healthcare worker shortages has been to redesign how work is done and by whom. If there are not enough providers, the organization needs to consider how staff and management are working and how work processes and resources can be improved to be more effective. As hospitals change, many factors influence the need for change and how it occurs. Some of these factors were highlighted earlier in Figure 8-1.

Change is inevitable in any type of organization today, but particularly in health care. Science and knowledge have driven some of this change, such as development of technology that has affected diagnosis and treatment options and increased digital options, but there are other factors to consider. Change is a process that is driven by forces that motivate a person or an organization to consider what needs altering. The key is to be clear about this need and understand the *why* before taking the next steps. It is also important to consider whether staff are ready for the change. Staff can act as either barriers to or facilitators of change. Staff members are typically tired of changes and feel that there are too many. They often also feel left out of the decision process that leads to changes. In such a case, they may become critical of the change or feel no commitment to the success of change. This attitude, in turn, becomes a major barrier to successful change; for example, if staff do not understand the need behind a decision to

change a form in the medical record, it will be more difficult to train them in the use of the form, and it may be difficult to get them to even use the form or to use it correctly. The complexity of the change and how frequently changes are made can lead to overload for staff. The goal is to have staff behind the change and committed to it; they will then be facilitators of change. Understanding resistance to change can help in preparing for the change and in developing any training that might be required. When changes are planned within a hospital, planners need to consider the impact that the changes may have on policies and procedures; accreditation and regulation requirements; financial issues; the structure of the organization; the ways in which staff do their work; patients, visitors, and students (for example, nursing, medical, other); and much more. Other chapters in this text discuss change and its implications, such as QI, which often identifies change needs.

This chapter focused on healthcare organizations, with acute care hospitals as the major example of a HCO. Understanding how hospitals are structured and their processes (functions) helps the nurse practice in this setting. The departments and team members assume important roles in how the organization functions. The U.S. healthcare system has been undergoing many changes. This will continue due to important legislation such as the ACA and any subsequent legislation that may be initiated. Nurses are very much involved in these changes and should participate in the change process.

Stop and Consider #7

Healthcare delivery is not static; there are frequent factors that change and then impact health care.

CHAPTER HIGHLIGHTS

1. Healthcare delivery is a complex process and system that includes multiple delivery sites: acute care organizations (hospitals), ambulatory care clinics, private provider offices, community health facilities, home care agencies, hospice agencies, extended care facilities, and so on.

2. Many factors affect hospitals and cause changes in their services and how they collaborate with others, realign their organization with the external environment, or even close because of financial issues.

3. Health care is a business; it provides services to a population.

4. Healthcare entities may be for-profit or not-for-profit organizations, depending on what they do with their revenues.

5. Healthcare organizations may differ depending on their structure and process. For example, a bureaucratic structure receives little input from staff as part of its decision-making processes.

6. Horizontal structure is decentralized, with an emphasis on departments or divisions; decisions are made closer to where staff members do the work.

7. The matrix organization structure is newer and less clear than the traditional bureaucratic organization centered on departments. A matrix organization is flatter (that is, decisions do not flow from the top down).

8. The process of an organization focuses on how it functions.

9. Classification of hospitals varies greatly and may reflect the hospital's mission focused on teaching or research, length of stay, ownership, and so on.

10. The hospital healthcare team is composed of a variety of healthcare providers, both professional and nonprofessional.

11. Hospitalists and intensivists are generally physicians who specialize in acute in-hospital care, although some hospitals use APRNs and CNSs in these roles.

12. Healthcare finances can be viewed from a macro, micro, or reimbursement perspective.

13. The 1965 Title XVIII established Medicare, which is an amendment to the Social Security Act. It is the federal health insurance program for people aged 65 and older, persons with disabilities, and people with end-stage renal disease.

14. The 1965 Title XIX of the Social Security Act established Medicaid, which is the federal–state program for certain categories of low-income people, children, the disabled, blind persons, and so forth.

15. The number of uninsured and underinsured individuals has been growing in the United States, but implementation of the Affordable Care Act of 2010 (ACA) should reduce this number—although changes in this law may have a negative impact on this outcome. (*This may change based on possible future changes in the legislation or new legislation.*)

16. Nursing within an organization is a critical component of healthcare delivery.

17. Organizational culture reflects the mission, core values, and vision of the entity—the goal is consonant cultures.

18. Healthcare delivery systems may be viewed as a healing environment.

19. Changes in healthcare delivery have an impact on hospitals, and staff members need to understand and participate in the change process.

ENGAGING IN THE CONTENT

Discussion Questions

1. What is the difference between organizational structure and process? Identify examples for each.
2. If you were not a nursing student, what other healthcare team member would you want to be and why? Does this healthcare team member have something in common with nursing?
3. Compare and contrast the three financial perspectives—macro, micro, and reimbursement.
4. Describe ways to organize nursing services in a hospital, key roles of nursing services, and nursing services' relationship to other departments.
5. What does organizational culture mean, and why is it important?
6. What is your opinion of the healing environment model? How do you think the designation of a Planetree hospital might affect nursing care?

CRITICAL THINKING ACTIVITIES

1. What is your reaction to the corporatization of health care? Discuss with a student team.
2. Search the Internet for a hospital website. See if you can find information on that hospital's vision, mission, goals, and objectives. Many hospital websites include this information. After you find an example, review the information. How does this information apply to nursing? Discussion team members could select different HCO websites, and then compare and contrast the information they gather.
3. Visit the website for the American Hospital Association (http://www.aha.org). What is the American Hospital Association? Click on "Advocacy Issues" and select one of the key initiatives to explore. What have you learned about the issue? Student teams should select different issues to review and then share what they learned. Consider the implications for nursing.
4. Search the Internet for information about one type of healthcare team member to learn more about the profession.
5. Visit the consumer site for Medicare (http://medicare.gov). If you were a Medicare beneficiary, how helpful would this site be? What information can you find? Click on Compare Hospitals in Your Area (www.hospitalcompare.hhs.gov/) and review hospitals in your area from the perspective of a consumer who is 70 years old and needs to have a hip replacement.

ELECTRONIC REFLECTION JOURNAL

Write a description of a healthcare organization where you have had a clinical experience. Consider the information in this chapter as you describe the organization. Reflect on its culture and how you felt while being in the organization. How do you think staff, patients, and families might feel? What could be improved in the organization based your experience? When you first entered the hospital and one of its units, what did you feel like? Consider all your senses in your response.

CASE STUDIES

Case 1

It is time to interview for you first hospital job. You are not sure what you should do in the interview and what questions you should ask. You are having lunch with fellow students, and all of you are focused on this issue.

Case Questions

1. How should we prepare for our interviews?
2. Tell me what questions you think are critical to ask?
3. Why is it important to talk to several nurses who work in the hospital?

Case 2

You are a staff nurse on a surgical unit. The nurse manager has formed a task force to provide input on the budget for the unit. She asks you to serve on the task force. You tell her you do not feel competent because you have been a nurse for only 1 year, but she says she wants fresh input. Now, you find yourself at the first meeting. The chair opens the meeting with some questions. How would you respond to them?

Case Questions

1. What type of budget do we have for our unit?
2. What types of expenses do we have? If we find that some of these expenses have been increasing, what interventions and/or changes might we suggest to lower the expenses (cost containment)? Why should staff get involved in unit budget planning?

Working Backward to Develop a Case

Write a brief paragraph that describes a case related to the following questions and comments.

1. What is the status of our unit and organization culture?
2. What needs to be improved? What is effective?
3. How does the culture impact nurses and nursing in the organization?

REFERENCES

American Association of Colleges of Nursing. (2013). Competencies and curricular expectations for clinical nurse leader education and practice. Retrieved from http://www.aacn.nche.edu/publications/white-papers/cnl

Curtin, L. (2001). Healing healthcare's organizational culture. *Seminars for Nurse Managers, 9,* 218–227.

Dewan, S., & Sack, K. (2008, January 8). A safety-net hospital falls into financial crisis. *The New York Times,* pp. A1, A18–A19.

Ellison, A. (2017, February 15). CMS projects next decade of health expenditures: 5 takeaways. Retrieved from http://www.beckershospitalreview.com/finance/cms-projects-next-decade-of-health-expenditures-5-takeaways.html

Institute of Medicine. (2013). *Best care at lower cost: The path to continuously learning health care in America.* Washington, DC: The National Academies Press.

Jeffrey, T. (2015, September 8). Government workers now outnumber manufacturing workers by 9,932,000. Retrieved from http://www.cnsnews.com/news/article/terence-p-jeffrey/government-workers-now-outnumber-manufacturing-workers-9932000

Jones, K., & Redman, R. (2000). Organizational culture and work redesign: Experiences in three organizations. *Journal of Nursing Administration, 30*(12), 604–610.

Kaiser Family Foundation. (2016a). Average annual workplace family health premiums. Retrieved from http://kff.org/health-costs/press-release/average-annual-workplace-family-health-premiums-rise-modest-3-to-18142-in-2016-more-workers-enroll-in-high-deductible-plans-with-savings-option-over-past-two-years/?utm_campaign=KFF-2016-September-EHBS&utm_content=39585919&utm_medium=social&utm_source=twitter

Kaiser Family Foundation. (2016b). Total number of Medicare beneficiaries. Retrieved from http://kff.org/medicare/state-indicator/total-medicare-beneficiaries/?current Timeframe = 0

Obamacare Facts. (2016). American healthcare coverage continues to rise. Retrieved from http://obamacarefacts.com/sign-ups/obamacare-enrollment-numbers

Pear, R. (2016, July 14). National health spending to surpass $10,000 a person in 2016. *The New York Times.*

Retrieved from https://www.nytimes.com/2016/07/14/us/national-health-spending-to-surpass-10000-per-person-in-2016.html?_r=0

Planetree. (2014). The formula. Retrieved from http://planetree.org/

Platt, M., Kwasky, A., & Spetz, J. (2015). Filling the gap: Developing health economics competencies for baccalaureate nursing programs. *Nursing Outlook, 64*(1), 49–60.

U.S. Department of Health and Human Services. Agency for Healthcare Research and Quality. (2016a). National patient safety efforts save 125,000 lives and nearly $28 billion in costs. Retrieved from http://www.ahrq.gov/professionals/quality-patient-safety/pfp/2015-interim.html?utm_source=AHRQ&utm_medium=PSLS&utm_term=&utm_content=14&utm_campaign=AHRQ_NSOHAC_2016

U.S. Department of Health and Human Services. Agency for Healthcare Research and Quality. (2016b). Chartbook on care affordability. National healthcare quality and disparities report (2015). Retrieved from https://www.ahrq.gov/sites/default/files/wysiwyg/research/findings/nhqrdr/chartbooks/careaffordability/qdr2015-chartbook-careaffordability.pdf

U.S. Department of Health and Human Services. Agency for Healthcare Research and Quality. Healthcare Cost and Utilization Project. (2016, October). Characteristics of safety net hospitals. Statistical Brief #213. Retrieved from https://www.hcup-us.ahrq.gov/reports/statbriefs/sb213-Safety-Net-Hospitals-2014.pdf

U.S. Department of Labor. (2015, December 17). Bureau of Labor Statistics, *Occupational outlook handbook, registered nurses.* Retrieved from https://www.bls.gov/ooh/healthcare/registered-nurses.htm#tab-3

Lukas, C. V., Holmes, S. K., Koppelman, E., Charn, M. P., Frigand, C., Gupte, G., & Neal, N. (2015, June) *System redesign responses to challenges in safety-net system: Summary of field study research.* Rockville, MD: Agency for Healthcare Research and Quality. Retrieved from http://www.ahrq.gov/professionals/systems/system/systemredesign safetynet/index.html

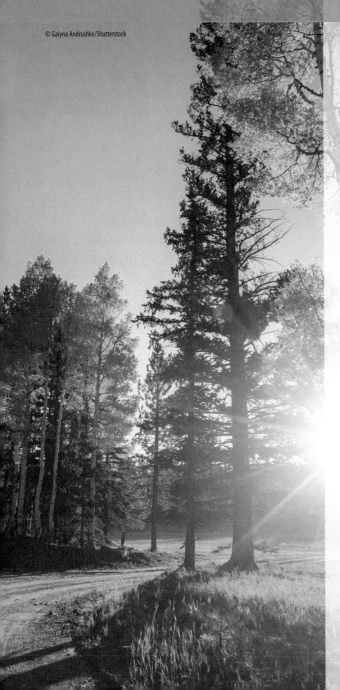
© Galyna Andrushko/Shutterstock

Section 3

Core Healthcare Professional Competencies

In its 2003 report, Health Professions Education, *the Institute of Medicine (IOM) identified core competencies for all healthcare professionals. These are not the only competencies, but rather they form the core competencies that should be addressed in all healthcare professionals' education: nurses, physicians, pharmacists, allied health professionals, and healthcare administrators. These competencies are based on the need to improve the quality of health care and the recognition that healthcare professional education was not effectively including these five critical competencies. The five core competencies are summarized here:*

- *Provide patient-centered care: Identify, respect, and care about patients' differences, values, preferences, and expressed needs; relieve pain and suffering; coordinate continuous care; listen to, clearly inform, communicate* with, and educate patients; share decision making and management; and continuously advocate disease prevention, wellness, and promotion of healthy lifestyles, including a focus on population health.

- Work in interprofessional teams: *Cooperate, collaborate, communicate, and integrate care in teams to ensure that care is continuous and reliable.*

- Employ evidence-based practice: *Integrate best research with clinical expertise and patient values for optimal care and participate in learning and research activities to the extent feasible.*

- Apply quality improvement: *Identify errors and hazards in care; understand and implement basic safety design principles, such as standardization and simplification; continually understand and measure quality of care in terms* of structure, process, and outcomes in relation to patient and community needs; and design and test interventions to change processes and systems of care, with the objective of improving quality.

- Utilize informatics: *Communicate, manage knowledge, mitigate error, and support decision making using information technology.*

These competencies are interrelated, and all should be applied in most clinical interactions. This competency-based approach to healthcare education should lead to improved quality because educators should be able to gather data about learning outcomes that could then be associated with better patient care, the desired goal.

Source: Institute of Medicine. (2003). *Health professions education* (p. 4). Washington, DC: The National Academies Press.

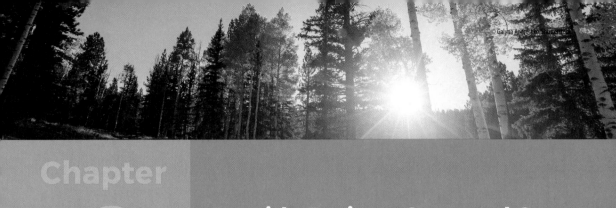

© Galyna Andrushko/Shutterstock

Chapter 9

Provide Patient-Centered Care

CHAPTER OBJECTIVES

At the conclusion of this chapter, the learner will be able to:

- Describe the competency: Provide patient-centered care and its relationship to nursing.
- Discuss the importance of consumerism in health care.
- Explain the relationship of culture, diversity, and disparities to health and healthcare delivery.
- Support the need for patient advocacy.
- Summarize processes that nurses use to ensure better care coordination.
- Apply critical thinking/clinical reasoning and judgment to patient-centered care.
- Explain the need for self-management of care.
- Discuss the impact of the therapeutic use of self on the nurse–patient relationship.

CHAPTER OUTLINE

KEY TERMS

Bias	Diversity	Patient advocacy
Care coordination	Ethnicity	Patient-centered care
Concept/care map	Ethnocentrism	Prejudice
Consumer/customer	Health literacy	Race
Culture	Macro consumer	Stereotyping
Discrimination	Micro consumer	Therapeutic use of self
Disparities	Nursing process	

Introduction

This chapter begins the discussion of the five healthcare profession core competencies for all healthcare professionals. The first core competency focuses on **patient-centered care**. The U.S. healthcare system is patient centered, but it is not at the level it should be. This content describes patient-centered care, relevant nursing theories, consumerism in health care, diversity and disparities, patient advocacy, care coordination to meet patient-centered care needs, self-management of care, and therapeutic use of self in the nurse–patient relationship. As you enter your nursing education program, it is assumed that you are in a nursing program because of your concern about patients; however, providing patient-centered care does not come naturally. It requires knowledge and caring, time, critical thinking, and clinical reasoning and judgment to ensure that care is coordinated and the implementation process focuses on patient-centered care. This all must be done during a time of many changes in health care. As a reminder, some of the changes related to patient-centered care are as follows:

- The U.S. population is becoming older and more diverse.
- Preventive care and chronic care are increasingly joining curative and acute primary care as the focus of health care.
- Chronic disease management is more prominent in many medical practices.
- More patients want active involvement in their health care.
- The financial mechanisms that support health care are changing.
- There is greater concern about the interrelationship of access, cost, quality, and outcomes.

The Competency: Provide
Patient-Centered Care

In 2003, five key core competencies were identified for all healthcare professionals. This chapter focuses on the first core competency: *provide patient-centered care*: "Identify, respect, and care about patients' differences, values, preferences, and expressed needs; relieve pain and suffering; coordinate continuous care; listen to, clearly inform, communicate with, and educate patients; share decision making and management; and continuously advocate disease prevention, wellness, and promotion of healthy lifestyles, including a focus on population health" (Institute of Medicine [IOM], 2003a, p. 4). On the surface, this definition may seem simple, but it is not; patient-centered care includes multiple factors and activities—all aimed at making the patient the

center of care and an active decision maker, if the patient chooses to be active. The content in this chapter focuses on the key elements of the core competency as illustrated in **Figure 9-1**.

Support of Patient-Centered Care

Why is patient-centered care included in the core competencies? What is the basis for emphasizing patient-centered care? All of the core competencies are interrelated, as seen in **Figure 9-2**. The central focus in this figure is on *providing patient-centered care*. Evidence-based practice, quality improvement, and use of informatics all affect patient-centered care, and interprofessional teams encircle all and bring care to the patient.

Crossing the quality chasm: A new health system for the 21st century (IOM, 2001) describes

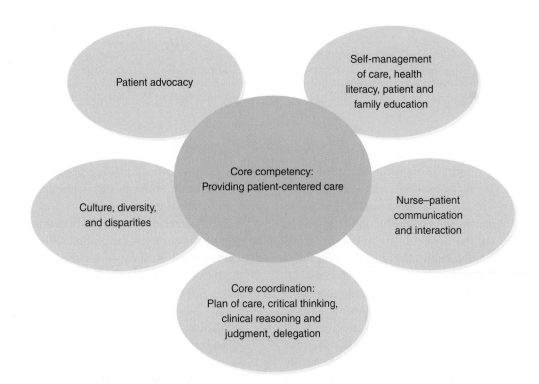

Figure 9-1 Providing Patient-Centered Care: Key Elements

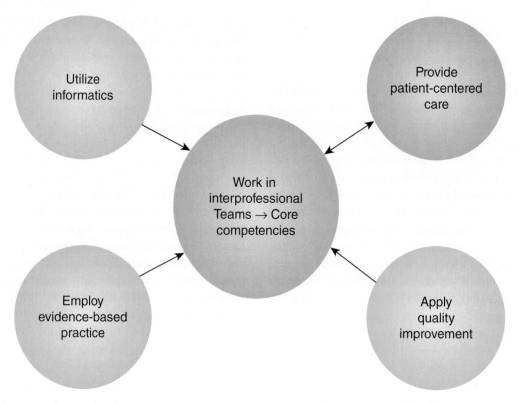

Figure 9-2 IOM Relationship Core Competencies

Reproduced from Interprofessional Education Collaborative Expert Panel. (2011). *Core competencies for interprofessional collaborative practice: Report of an expert panel.* Washington, D.C.: Interprofessional Education Collaborative.

10 rules for redesigning patient care and presents a vision for the U.S. healthcare delivery system. The first four rules specifically apply to patient-centered care, supporting the need to include patient-centered care in the core competencies and focus on the need for continuous health relationships, individualized care, patient engagement in decision making, and sharing of information. The other six rules are not directly related to patient-centered care. They are, however, a major part of the framework to improve the quality of care and are discussed in the quality improvement content in this text. Improving

health care requires improved competencies in all healthcare professionals, beginning with providing patient-centered care.

Patient-centered care is a critical part of the six domains of quality. A description of the skills required to provide patient-centered care expand on the meaning of patient-centered care (IOM, 2003a, pp. 52–53):

- Share power and responsibility with patients and caregivers (family, significant others) (for example, involve the patient in care, make the patient the center of care and decision making; work to increase patient understanding, acceptance, and cooperation; help caregivers as they provide care to a family member [education for patient and family]; support self-management; provide comfort and emotional support; manage pain and suffering; relieve anxiety; provide expert care to manage symptoms).

- Communicate with patients in a shared and fully open manner (for example, patients have access to information, communication with healthcare providers [including nurses], and use of technology to communicate).
- Take into account patients' individuality, emotional needs, values, and life issues (for example, culture, religion, family, language, profession).
- Implement strategies to reach those who do not present for care on their own, including care strategies that support the broader community (for example, underserved members of the community, vulnerable populations).
- Enhance prevention and health promotion (for example, population focus, risk factors, health promotion, and prevention strategies).

As hospitals focus more on patient-centered care, the inevitable question is, how do we accomplish effective patient- and family-centered care? Three key elements in a hospital organization make a major difference in reaching this goal (Balik, Conway, Zipperer, & Watson, 2011):

- Emphasis on an integrated system
- Effective leadership at the executive, middle, and front-line levels
- Effective, engaged teams

Patient-centered or person-centered care is the key focus for all nurses and the care they provide. Hagenow comments, "This care alleviates vulnerability in all of its forms. That care should and must then be delivered at the right time, at the right level, in the right place, and so on. If care were on a compass, it would be true north and all other functions would

stand in line to provide added value and service to that fact" (2003, p. 204). However, it is important to recognize that patients should not be passive in the care process but rather need to be active, engaged, and empowered to speak out and participate in decision making. Nursing has long supported this view of patients (Pelletier & Stichler, 2013).

Levels of Patient-Centered Care

There are three levels of concern when discussing patient-centered care. The first relates directly to the identification of patient-centered care as the core healthcare professional competency, focusing on the care provided by an individual healthcare professional. The necessary knowledge base for each healthcare professional, such as a nurse, in order to provide patient-centered care is discussed in this chapter. The second level focuses on the organizational level and the ways in which healthcare organizations situate themselves to be patient-centered organizations. The third level is the macro focus—how the healthcare system, as viewed from the local, state, and national perspectives, ensures that it is patient centered. Strategies to ensure the third level are primarily healthcare policy concerns.

There is consensus about the key attributes describing patient-centered care at the healthcare system level. In an analysis of nine models and frameworks used to define patient-centered care, the following six core elements were identified most frequently (Shaller, 2007):

- Education; shared knowledge
- Family and friends involvement
- Collaboration and team management
- Sensitivity to nonmedical, spiritual dimensions of care
- Respect for patient needs and preferences
- Accessibility of information

Shallar also identifies the following factors as contributing to the six core elements, which has an impact on patient-centered care at the organizational level (2007):

- Leadership, chief executive officer and board of directors, committed, engaged in a common mission
- A strategic vision communicated to all staff members
- Involvement of patients and families at multiple levels throughout the organization
- A supportive work environment for caregivers
- Systematic, continuous measurement and feedback
- A supportive, nurturing physical space and design for patients, families, and employees
- Supportive technology engaging patients and families directly in the care process; facilitating information access and communication with their caregivers

The Agency for Healthcare Research and Quality (AHRQ) now offers resources for healthcare organizations and providers on using patient- and family-centered innovations to improve care (U.S. Department of Health and Human Services [HHS] & Agency for Health Research and Quality [AHRQ], 2016a). This website provides multiple examples of innovations such as redesigning bedside change-of-shift reporting, using a patient and family advisor rounding program, and improving outpatient rehabilitation with better patient education and resources, for example AHRQ toolkits (for example, a patient-centered improvement guide, recommendations for including patients and families on committees and task forces, engaging patients and families in quality improvement, and so on). There is a clear message that healthcare organizations and providers can makes changes to improve patient-centered care. An example of a more commonly used method by healthcare organizations is to include families in rounds, if the patient agrees. Some hospitals have also expanded visiting hours and even moved to 24/7 family presence in patient rooms. A recent study indicates that increased opportunity for family presence improves patient satisfaction,

though 70% of hospitals continue to have restrictive visiting policies (Gasparini, Champagne, Stephany, Hudson, & Fuchs, 2015). Some hospitals are now allowing families to be present during resuscitation. Nurses have mixed reactions to this change. Typical concerns from healthcare providers are: (1) The family will see and hear things that may be disturbing to them; (2) there is concern the team will not function well, and the family will see this; and (3) the family may become disruptive and interfere with treatment (Twibell et al., 2008). Despite these concerns, there has been movement toward changes to allow more family presence—all require careful thought and planning with nursing input and preparation of staff.

An example of an approach to improve patient-centered care within healthcare organizations is the Planetree model, discussed in other chapters in this text (Planetree, 2014). The Planetree Institute is a nonprofit membership organization that partners with hospitals and health centers to develop and implement patient-centered care in healing environments. These healthcare organizations meet certain criteria to be designated as a Planetree institution, demonstrating effective healing environments.

Does a Patient-Centered Healthcare System Exist in the United States?

Throughout the *Quality Chasm* reports, patient-centered care is emphasized by the IOM, now known the National Academy of Medicine. "Research shows that orienting health care around the preferences and needs of patients has the potential to improve patients' satisfaction with care as well as their clinical outcomes. Yet, one of five American adults reports that they have trouble communicating with their doctors and one of 10 says that they were treated with disrespect during a healthcare visit. Patients often report that test results or medical records were not available at the time of a scheduled appointment or that they received conflicting information from their providers" (Commonwealth Fund, 2008).

Patients want to be partners in their care, but why? This approach offers benefits in the following areas:

- Provider–patient communication
- Patient educational materials about health concerns
- Self-management tools to help patients manage their illness or condition and health and make informed decisions
- Access to care (timely appointments, off-hours services, and so on) and use of information technology (for example, automated patient reminders and patient access to electronic medical records)
- Continuity of care
- Post-hospital follow-up and support
- Management of drug regimens and chronic conditions
- Access to reliable information about the quality of physicians and healthcare organizations, with the opportunity to give feedback

"Ensuring that all patients have a medical home would be an important first step toward creating a patient-centered care system" (Commonwealth Fund, 2008). People need a regular place to receive care and the opportunity to develop a relationship with healthcare providers. The benefits noted above have a greater chance of occurring when a patient has a regular source of care.

Throughout this text quality improvement is discussed, and we need to consider it with patient-centered care. It is, however, not easy to measure. The National Database of Nursing Quality Indicators (NDNQI), the only monitor of nursing-sensitive indicators, which is discussed in other chapters, needs more inclusion of a performance measure on patient and family engagement (Pelletier & Stichler, 2013). Having data about outcomes on this measure would be very helpful in improving care. The National Healthcare Quality and Disparities Report (QDR) does include person- and family-centered care measures (HHS & AHRQ, 2015a). Data for 2014 indicate person-centered care is improving. Current report data can be obtained at the AHRQ website.

A serious difficulty in developing and maintaining a patient-centered healthcare system is insufficient insurance reimbursement for patient-centered care. For example, insurers do not cover care coordination; it is just considered a natural part of care delivery. However, this really does not account for the time that staff must spend on coordinating care, communicating with team members, and so on. In addition, alternative communication methods are not typically covered, such as communication with patients over the Internet or telephone. To really change the system, this critical issue of reimbursement must be addressed. Insurers, however, are telling providers they need to be more productive and yet they have less time to spend with patients; less time to be patient-centered. Meeting the latter demand requires more—not less—time with patients. When there is a nursing shortage (which has fluctuated over the last few years and may occur in certain geographic regions or individual healthcare organizations), this affects providing patient-centered care. Nurses may feel overburdened with work if staffing is not at the level it should be, and this may then have an impact on nurses' ability to provide this care—less time, more stress, more acutely ill patients requiring more time, increase in risk of errors, and so on. This may also lead to staff conflict and frustration and a poor working environment.

How can this goal of patient-centered care be reached at the same time that insurance coverage, access to care, and quality of care need to be improved in the United States? To better ensure patience-centered care, all healthcare professionals need to be competent and also understand how to support patient-centered care. The following attributes of patient-centered care indicate what needs to be done to reach this goal (Davis, Schoenbaur, & Audet, 2005, p. 954), with examples as to how they might be described:

- *Improved access to care* (for example, patients can easily make appointments; wait times for appointments are reasonable; off-hours service is available or patients know whom to contact)

- *Greater patient engagement in care* (for example, patients have the option of being informed and engaged partners in their care; patients participate in treatment planning and are updated; self-care and counseling assistance are provided)
- *Clinical information systems that support high-quality care, practice-based learning, and quality improvement* (for example, healthcare organizations maintain patient databases and monitor adherence to treatment; patients receive decision support and information on recommended treatments)
- *Care coordination* (for example, coordinated care across the continuum and settings; monitor and prevent errors that occur when multiple healthcare providers are involved; provide post-hospital follow-up and support)
- *Integrated and comprehensive team care* (for example, free flow of communication among physicians, nurses, and other health professionals)
- *Routine patient feedback to physician/healthcare providers* (for example, Internet-based patient surveys used to obtain patient feedback and ensure patient input into treatment plans; there is follow-up if patients provide negative feedback)
- *Publicly available information* (for example, patients have access to accurate, standardized information about healthcare providers [physicians, hospitals] to help them choose where they will get their care)

The following is a summary of strategies from experts and researchers that emphasizes the key points in improving and maintaining patient-centered care: (1) share power and responsibility with patients and caregivers and (2) engage in an ongoing discussion with patients to increase understanding, acceptance, cooperation, and identification of common goals and related care plans (Gerteis, Edgman-Levitan, Daley, & Delbanco, 1993; Halpern, Lee, Boulter, & Phillips, 2001; IOM, 2001, 2003a; Lewin, Skea,

Entwistle, Zwarenstein, & Dick, 2001; Pew Health Professions Commission, 1995; Stewart, 2001).

To reach, the goal of significantly improved patient-centered care within a healthcare organization requires redesigning care processes to improve care delivery. It necessitates partnerships among practitioners, patients, and patients' families as appropriate. We also need stronger partnerships between schools of nursing and clinical organizations to enable students to gain more experience and better understanding of the complexity of patient-centered care and the impact of care processes (Finkelman & Kenner, 2012). The *Quality Chasm* reports indicate that it is more common for the patient to have to adapt to the healthcare delivery system than the system adapting to the patient's needs and preferences. This approach needs to change. Patients who are involved in their own care tend to have better outcomes. Important methods that should be used to change the system to a more patient-centered approach are greater use of rounds, care at the bedside, services in one location at a clinic rather than asking the patient to go to other locations for tests, and so on.

There is greater and greater access to information among healthcare providers, which in turn means patients also have more potential access to information. Information provides more power and control—not just for healthcare providers, but for patients as well. It is, however, important to recognize that just providing information is not enough for effective shared decision making with patients (Hargraves, LeBlanc, Shah, & Montori, 2016). We need to talk with patients, not just give information—that is, have a conversation. For example, if patient rounds are conducted with conversation "over the patient" rather than with the patient, then this cannot be called patient-centered care. We also need to include expected outcomes in treatment planning that the patient identifies (Lavalleel et al., 2016). These methods lead to a greater patient empowerment, a topic discussed further in this chapter in the sections on consumerism and self-management.

There is a great need to develop patient-centered models that focus on particular populations, such as persons with chronic illness, rural and urban populations, minority groups, women, children, the elderly, persons with special needs, and patients at the end of life. Focusing on certain populations better ensures that unique patient-centered needs will be met. Nurses assume major roles in these new models and will continue to be active as additional models are developed for hospitals and in public/community health settings. Despite barriers mentioned in this chapter and in healthcare literature, Davis, Schoenbaum, and Audet comment, "The concept of patient-centered health care is beginning to take hold. Increasingly, patients expect physicians to be responsive to their needs and preferences, to provide them with access to their medical information, and to treat them as partners in care decisions. But despite being named one of the key components of quality health care by the IOM, 'patient-centeredness' has yet to become the norm in primary care" (2005, pp. 953–954).

Related Nursing Theories

Nursing theories are discussed in other content in this text, but in this chapter, we examine theories that are particularly relevant to patient-centered care. Examples include Watson's theory on caring, Orem's self-care theory, Leininger's cultural theory, Peplau's interpersonal theory, and some theories related to learning.

- *Watson's theory on caring:* This theory focuses on caring. Patient-centered care includes an emphasis on caring—how the patient receives care, how the patient perceives care, and how nurses and other healthcare providers perceive their roles and implement care.
- *Orem's self-care theory:* This theory focuses on providing support and guidance to patients so that they can be actively involved in their own care, or self-management of care.

- *Leininger's cultural diversity theory:* This theory focuses on cultural issues and their importance in health and healthcare delivery. The definition of patient-centered care includes cultural aspects of care, and as discussed in early *Quality Chasm* reports, disparities in health care are a critical concern now monitored by the annual National Healthcare Quality and Disparities Report.
- *Peplau's interpersonal relations theory:* This theory emphasizes the importance of the nurse–patient relationship and communication. It is difficult to discuss or provide patient-centered care without considering the patient–provider relationship and communication.
- *Learning theories: Knowles's adult learning and the health belief model:* These two theories particularly relate to a patient-centered approach and patient education. Patient and family education about health and illness is a critical part of patient-centered care. This education emphasizes the active role of the patient in the care delivery process and the patient as a decision maker, with greater emphasis on self-management. If a patient does not have adequate information and/or necessary skill to care for self, this diminishes patient-centered care. Adult learning theory emphasizes adult learners are different from younger learners—a factor that must be considered in any educational endeavor with adults (Knowles, 1972). Patient education certainly includes children; however, there are more adult patients who have complex needs. Often, adult education is approached in a paternalistic manner in which patients are not treated as adult learners, and this is ineffective patient education.

Another view to consider with patient-centered care is the health belief model, which is also referred to as the theory of reasoned action and focuses on health promotion (Hochbaum, 1958). This model was developed to predict if a person would follow medical recommendations and to gain a better understanding of patient motivation. According to this model, Masters comments that a person's response to a health threat is based on the following factors (2009, p. 173):

- The person's perception of the severity of the illness
- The person's perception of susceptibility to illness and its consequences
- The value of the treatment benefits (for example, do the cost and side effect of treatment outweigh the consequences of the disease?)
- Barriers to treatment (for example, expense, complexity of treatment, access to care)
- Costs of treatment in physical and emotional terms
- Cues that stimulate taking action toward treatment of illness (for example, mass-media campaigns, pamphlets, advice from family or friends, and postcard reminders from healthcare providers)

By assessing these factors, nurses can develop more effective patient education plans that are patient-centered.

Stop and Consider #1

Patient-centered care is the central concern today in healthcare delivery.

Consumerism: How Does
*It Affect Health Care
and Nursing?*

Consumerism might seem a strange term to use in a nursing text. It is commonly encountered in business, particularly in advertising. However, consumerism in health care has become a very important concept, and it relates directly to patient-centered care. As far as nursing is concerned, nursing has long viewed the patient as an integral part of the nursing process. What does this really mean, and has nursing grasped the concept of consumerism so that it is not only spoken about but also incorporated as a critical part of the implementation of nursing care? With the growing number of advanced practice registered nurses, many may be in their own practices or hold roles where consumerism is even more relevant to them.

Patients expect more and more to be active in their own care at all levels. They do not like it when they are ignored and left out of decision making. Families are also becoming much more assertive. Both patients and families are more concerned about quality and costs. A *Quality Chasm* report on safety led to greater recognition of the major safety problem in health care in the United States (IOM, 1999). When this report was published, the media widely shared the report's information via newspapers, radio, television, and the Internet. The statistics in the report about the high level of errors were frightening to consumers and, consequently, alerted the public (consumers) to the need to be more vigilant.

The U.S. Department of Health and Human Services (HHS) also now provides more resources to engage consumers. One example is the AHRQ initiative to develop and test a healthcare safety hotline (HHS & AHRQ, 2016b). There has been extensive work done to get data from healthcare providers about adverse events, errors, and unsafe conditions in healthcare settings, and now there is more effort being made to include patient data—from patients. This would be done on a secure website or toll-free phone number. This AHRQ report discusses how this could be done. There are other national opportunities for patients to provide input on specific healthcare issues. Patients can report healthcare providers (individuals and organizations), insurers, or any other related healthcare entity for failure to meet HIPAA requirements, which are violations of the law (HHS, 2017). This can be done online or in writing via the HHS website. Both of these approaches empower patients beyond filling out a patient satisfaction survey; however, it is important that consumers know they can make these reports and how to report concerns.

Who Are the Consumers or Customers?

There are two major types of **consumers/customers** in health care. **Macro consumers** are the major purchasers of care: the government and insurers. They pay for care, and therefore, are consumers in that they have expectations of the product (the care delivered) and can influence that care. The **micro consumer** is the patient. Patient families and significant others, when the patient agrees that the family may have a role in the patient's care and/or decision-making process, are also micro consumers. Patients are turning more to nurses and asking questions about their health care and the healthcare delivery process. In the past, nurses knew little about reimbursement and the delivery process, but today's nurses need to be prepared to answer patient questions or to direct patients to resources for answers.

Customer-centered health care means that the nurse must be more aware of customer/consumer/patient needs, but this is not a simple process. Typically in retail and business, one thinks of the statement, "The customer is always right"; however, in health care, this may not always be the case. The patient may not have all the information necessary to make an informed decision and may require the expertise of healthcare professionals to meet his or her needs. Nurses need to find a balance—meeting patient needs, including the patient, respecting the patient's opinion, and applying their professional nursing expertise. Leebov identifies customer service goals that are important in the healthcare system and related to nursing (2008, pp. 21–23):

- *Caring with compassion:* This is not an unusual concept for nurses; it is part of the traditional view of nursing.

- *Making sure caring comes across:* It is easy to wonder why caring should even be discussed in relation to nursing because caring is so much a part of nursing and its image. Key questions, however, we need to ask: Does the patient perceive the caring? Do nurses say and do things that do not support caring?
- *Paying quality attention:* Focusing on quantity improvement requires engagement of staff who understand how to participate in quality improvement, but we are not yet clear on how we measure staff attention and impact it might have on the patient. The skill of presence or mindfulness involves controlling attention. This allows the persons (patient, family, others) who are on the receiving end of the care to feel like the center at that moment. The nurse is not distracted, and the patient connects; the result should be better quality care that is focused on the patient.
- *Reducing patient anxiety:* This is a major part of daily nursing practice in any setting. One can view this goal differently from what might occur with typical customers. For example, retail store sales staff want to make customers happy, but nurses and other healthcare staff want to reduce patient anxiety and support them. Making patients feel happy is not a bad result, but it may not actually reduce anxiety or provide support; may not be the critical outcome, but it is important.
- *Your personal calling:* Are you committed to improvement and caring, and how do you demonstrate this in your practice?

It is important to understand what patients want and what they think their care outcomes should be. In the face of increasing out-of-pocket patient expenses, patients are compelled to know more about their needs and care and want to influence care decisions. If one compares this to shopping for a product such as an automobile, the buyer (customer) typically wants the best quality for the best price. Consumers are expressing concerns about the limits in their healthcare choices (for example, employers offering fewer choices of health plans, offering plans with restricted or limited services, or placing restrictions on provider use). Although healthcare consumers may have changed over the years, quality of care and access to services remain important consumer issues. When managed care was the major approach used in healthcare reimbursement, it actually became a stimulus for increasing consumer engagement with the healthcare system. Consumers became more active in their complaints about the changes made by managed care healthcare reimbursement. Over time, this had an impact on the system, adjusting use of managed care strategies—for example, consumers insisting on more patient choice in healthcare providers. Today we see increased consumer activism as changes are considered in the Affordable Care Act (ACA).

Patient Rights

Healthcare providers and many consumers commonly understand patient rights, but we do not have a clear statement of patient rights that is applied in all situations (American Organization of Nurse Executives & National Alliance for Quality Care, 2012). The American Hospital Association (2017) first published a Patient Bill of Rights in the 1970s; it was updated in its "Patient Care Partnership" brochure. The U.S. Congress has considered multiple versions of national patient rights legislation, with none approved. The U.S. Advisory Commission on Consumer Protection and Quality published a version in 1998, which is often referenced. The ACA provides a new version in is provisions, which focuses on rights to treatment and reimbursement (FamiliesUSA, 2011). The rights noted are ensuring coverage for people with preexisting conditions, ensuring the right to choose a doctor, ensuring the right to fair treatment of emergency care, making sure insurance policies cannot be canceled unfairly, ending annual and lifetime limits, enhancing access to preventive services, ensuring the right to appeal

health plan decisions, ensuring health coverage for young adults, and protections under "grandfathered plans." If the Trump administration makes changes in reimbursement and healthcare delivery, these rights may also change. The Centers for Medicare and Medicaid Services support these rights for its beneficiaries (U.S. Department of Health and Human Services & Centers for Medicare and Medicaid Services, 2017). Many national organizations (such as the American Cancer Society, National Institutes of Health clinical trials) provide their own bill of rights.

The Patient Self-Determination Act of 1990 is a law that significantly affects patient information and process and relates to patient rights. It applies to all healthcare organizations that receive Medicare or Medicaid reimbursement; thus, because few healthcare organizations do not receive this form of reimbursement, this law applies to most healthcare organizations. It requires that all these organizations or providers give their patients certain information that relates to confidentiality; consent; the right to make medical decisions, be informed about diagnosis and treatment, and refuse treatment; and supports use of advance directives. As yet, no federal legislation has been passed that specifically addresses a general statement of patients' rights, although several attempts have been made. Individual healthcare organizations publish a list of patient rights that are shared with their patients and that staff are expected to follow. However, patient-centered care can best be actualized with the patient–healthcare provider (nurse) relationship, and patient rights must be part of this relationship.

Information Resources and Consumers

Today, technology provides easy access to information not only for healthcare providers, but also for consumers. The chapter on informatics discusses this trend in more detail, but it is mentioned in this chapter because healthcare informatics and technology also relate to patient-centered care. Through the use of new technologies, providers have multiple ways to communicate with current customers/consumers/patients, such as email, Internet, and cell phones, and extensive methods to collect, manage, and use healthcare information. Patients use such information to self-manage their health and care, expanding their knowledge of self-care and wellness. They seek medical advice, learn about their treatment options, and obtain information about reimbursement. Patients also increasingly obtain information to help them evaluate providers (physicians, hospitals, and so on), such as "report cards" about healthcare organizations and outcomes, which are now more widely available to the public.

Patient Satisfaction

Kennedy comments, "When the subject of patient satisfaction surveys is raised among RNs working in hospitals, most will argue that the findings are either inapplicable or skewed. They'll say that patients' expectations of care are unrealistic and not achievable. They'll say that such surveys, especially follow-up surveys, don't accurately reflect the quality of care because they don't ask the right questions and don't take into account myriad of other issues that might have affected patients' experiences" (2015, p. 7). Nurses think that patients are often more concerned with issues that do not really affect quality. Hospitals are focusing more on patient ratings—but not necessarily in a positive way—mostly to make their overall ratings higher rather than care better. When hospitals receive low patient satisfaction scores, the response is often to look for easy fixes and not really address problems. Patient satisfaction is heavily associated with nurses and nursing care. What is patient satisfaction, and how do we measure it effectively? Or can we measure it, and how does it relate to patient-centered care?

Patient satisfaction is a critical topic in most healthcare organizations. Hospitals expend a great deal of energy and monies to assess how patients feel about their services. Companies external to

healthcare organizations, such as Press Ganey, may assist in data collection and analysis. Patient satisfaction data can be helpful, but this information must be viewed carefully and should be used as one source of data to assist in assessment of quality care. Zimmerman identifies the following as examples of myths related to satisfaction data that are important to consider, with additional comments provided as to the validity of the myth (2001, pp. 255–256):

- *Patient satisfaction is objective and straight-forward.* This is not true. Patient surveys are difficult to develop, and they are often poorly designed.
- *Patient satisfaction is easily measured.* Satisfaction is complex and not easily measured. Patient expectations influence the process, and many factors can affect patient responses that are not always easy to identify.
- *Patient satisfaction is accurately and precisely measured.* This is not possible at this time; attitudes are difficult to measure.
- *It is obvious who is the customer.* A healthcare organization actually has many different types of customers—more than just patients. For example, families, physicians, insurers, and internal staff are also customers (staff within the organization become customers to other staff; for example, the laboratory provides services to the units and thus nursing staff on the units are also the laboratory's customers).

A complete customer satisfaction analysis should include multiple types of customers in the healthcare organization. **Exhibit 9-1** identifies examples of key consumer or patient tips to better ensure safe health care and outcomes and influence patient satisfaction.

Healthcare organizations are making more efforts to engage patients in their care and in quality improvement to implement strategies to improve the patient's healthcare experience. One method that healthcare organizations are using more to improve patient satisfaction is structured hourly rounds. Nursing staff routinely go to patients every hour to

> ## Exhibit 9-1 Consumer Tips for Safe Health Care
>
> - Ask questions if you have doubts or concerns.
> - Keep and bring a list of all medications you take.
> - Get the results of any test or procedure.
>
> - Talk to your doctor about which hospital is best for your health needs.
> - Make sure you understand what will happen if you need surgery.

Data from U.S. Department of Health and Human Services. Agency for Health Resources and Quality. (2014). Five Steps for Safer Care. Patient Fact Sheet. Retrieved from https://archive.ahrq.gov/patients-consumers/care-planning/errors/5steps/index.html

check on a variety of factors—for example, "pain level, need for toileting or elimination, assessment of the environment including temperature, proximity of personal items, safety hazards, and positioning of the patient or need to change the patient's position" (Brosey & March, 2015, p. 153). Hospitals that use this type of rounds find that patient satisfaction is higher—patients do not have to ask for help as much when staff assess routinely. This increases patient trust in staff to be there when the patient needs help. Another benefit of this rounding is to prevent errors and improve patient outcomes—for example, identify a safety hazard in the room before a patient falls; assist the patient to the bathroom so that the patient does not get frustrated calling for help and gets out of bed without assistance; ensure pain medication is given in the most effective time period to reduce patient pain level.

When it comes to quality of care, there is no clear universal definition of quality of care. Patient-centered care implies that not only is the patient the focus of care, but also is the focus of evaluation of that care. Patient-centered care implies a contract and partnership between the patient and all healthcare providers (individuals and organizations). This means we are required to include the patient in the assessment of the care process and outcomes. A patient often sees quality of care and services differently than a nurse or physician might view care quality. The insurer also has a different view—mostly from a cost perspective. This makes it difficult to analyze satisfaction data objectively—you get a snapshot of

one view. It is important to not assume that when a healthcare provider has a positive view of care quality and patient satisfaction the patient will agree. For example, patients receiving ambulatory care usually express different views of quality than do hospitalized patients. In examining the issues in this example, ambulatory care patients may be concerned with access to care, accessible and safe parking, wait time for appointments, amount of time the provider spends with the patient, interaction with the provider, response from office or clinic staff, follow-up, access to information, or patient outcomes while the healthcare provider in the clinic may focus only on patient outcomes. Assumptions should also not be made about what patients want or who they want to know about their health care. A hospitalized patient may have different views of quality, such as how many times the doctor visits them, noise level, food quality, staff routinely use hand washing, getting pain medication when need, call light answered in a timely manner, sharing of information, staff attitudes, whether they feel better or worse, and much more, and again hospital healthcare providers may focus on patient outcomes.

Over time, a variety of data collection methods will undoubtedly emerge, but right now there are only a few reliable sources of data, such as Hospital Consumer Assessment of Healthcare Providers and Systems (HCAHPS): "survey is the first national, standardized, publicly reported survey of patients' perspectives of hospital care. HCAHPS (pronounced 'H-caps'), also known as the CAHPS Hospital

Survey, is a survey instrument and data collection methodology for measuring patients' perceptions of their hospital experience. While many hospitals have collected information on patient satisfaction for their own internal use, until HCAHPS there was no national standard for collecting and publicly reporting information about patient experience of care that allowed valid comparisons to be made across hospitals locally, regionally and nationally" (U.S. Department of Health and Human Services [HHS], Centers for Medicare and Medicaid Services [CMS], & Hospital Consumer Assessment of Healthcare Providers and Systems [HCAHPS], 2013). This survey is an important resource for data about hospitals and patients and includes 21 patient perspectives on care and patient rating items—for example, communication with doctors, communication with nurses, responsiveness of hospital staff, pain management, communication about medications, discharge information, cleanliness of the hospital environment, noise level in the hospital environment, and transition of care (HHS, CMS, & HCAHPS, 2017). Current information about the survey is found on the HCAHPS website.

Stop and Consider #2
A patient is a consumer.

Culture, Diversity,
and Disparities in Health Care

The growing **diversity** of patients also demands more patient-centered care. Diversity is a key driver of change in healthcare delivery today. Along with the changes in diversity is the grave concern about disparities in health care, with some populations receiving different care than others; as noted by the *Quality Chasm* reports on diversity, treatment is all too often unequal (IOM, 2003a). *Healthy People 2020* identifies four major goals for the health of U.S. citizens, one of which emphasizes cultural diversity: "Achieve health equity, eliminate disparities, and improve the health of all groups" (HHS, 2010). This

goal also indicates that providers throughout the healthcare system, including nurses, need to know more about culture and its impact on healthcare needs and delivery of care. The definition of patient-centered care includes culture as one of its elements.

Culture

Culture is "the accumulated store of shared values, ideas (attitudes, beliefs, values, and norms), understandings, symbols, material products, and practices of a group of people" (IOM, 2003b, p. 522). Nurses view patients through their personal experiences with culture and their personal histories. This may lead to problems, such as misinterpretation of communication and behavior that result in limitations in planning and implementing patient-centered care that meets the patient's needs. Culture and language may influence the following aspects of care (U.S. Department of Health and Human Services [HHS] & The Office of Minority Health [OMH], 2008):

- Health, healing, and wellness belief systems
- Patient/consumer perception of causes of illness and disease
- Patients/consumer behaviors and their attitudes toward healthcare providers
- Provider perceptions and values

In the United States, the diversity of racial and ethnic communities and linguistic groups is growing. Each of these subpopulations, with its own cultural traits and health profiles, presents a challenge to the healthcare delivery system and providers. The provider and the patient bring their individual learned patterns of language and culture to the healthcare experience, which in turn affects the care process and may further increase healthcare disparities. Demographic data indicate that more nurses are caring for patients from different cultural, racial, and ethnic backgrounds. In some areas, there are clusters of specific cultural populations, such as Blacks, Hispanics/Latinos, Native Americans, and Asians. In 2015, data indicate the following about the total U.S population: White 61%, Hispanic/Latino Americans 18%, Blacks 12%, Asian American 6%, and American Indian/Alaska Native 1% (Kaiser Family Foundation, 2015, according to March 2016 U.S. Census Bureau). Areas of the United States that typically have the highest diversity (in order of size) are the South, the West, the Northeast, and the Midwest. The presence of such diversity requires greater emphasis on providing care that is respectful of, and responsive to, the health beliefs, practices, and cultural and linguistic needs of the various patient populations.

Cultural Competence

Schools of nursing and healthcare organizations are working to improve students, faculty, and staff cultural competence. This trend has been driven by the *Quality Chasm* reports, which discuss the presence of significant healthcare disparities in the healthcare delivery system. Competence "implies having the capacity to function effectively as an individual and as an organization within the context of the cultural beliefs, behaviors, and needs presented by consumers and their communities" (Anderson, Scrimshaw, Fullilove, Fielding, & Normand, 2003, pp. 68–69). There are three conceptual approaches to cross-cultural education: (1) focus on attitudes (cultural sensitivity/awareness approach), (2) knowledge (multicultural/categorical approach), and (3) skills (cross-cultural approach) (IOM, 2003b, p. 19). Implementation of all three approaches is necessary for improvement. As discussed in other chapters of this text, schools of nursing include content on culture, diversity, and disparities to ensure that pre-licensure and graduate students meet cultural competencies (National League for Nursing, 2016; American Association of Colleges of Nursing [AACN], 2006, 2008, 2011).

Disparities in Health Care

Disparities in health care are defined as "racial or ethnic differences in the quality of healthcare that are not due to access-related factors or clinical needs, preferences, and appropriateness of intervention"

(IOM, 2003b, pp. 3–4). The IOM examined two issues when determining the existence of disparities in health care. The first is how the U.S. healthcare system functions and which legal and regulatory issues may make it difficult for patients to get equal care. The second issue relates to discrimination at the patient–provider level. **Discrimination** is defined as "differences in care that result from bias, prejudices, stereotyping and uncertainty in clinical communication and decision-making" (IOM, 2002, p. 4). What are some of the key terms related to diversity?

- **Bias**: Predisposed to a point of view
- **Ethnicity**: Shared feeling of belonging to a group—peoplehood
- **Ethnocentrism**: Belief that one's group or culture is superior to others
- **Prejudice**: Making assumptions or judgments about the beliefs, behaviors, needs, and expectations of patients or other healthcare staff of a different cultural background than one's own because of emotional beliefs about the population; involves negative attitudes toward the different group
- **Race**: A biological designation of a group; belonging to the group based on biological factor(s)
- **Stereotyping**: A "process by which people use social groups (such as sex and race) to gather, process, and recall information about other people . . . these are labels" (IOM, 2002, p. 475) (It is natural for people to organize information, and organizing information about people is part of this. This process, however, can be negative if it involves unfairly classifying people or using incorrect information about an individual who may or may not meet the characteristics.)

After the *Quality Chasm* report on healthcare disparities indicated there were problems in the United States, it was recognized that it is necessary to have more effective monitoring of diversity and disparities in health care. In 2001, the National

Healthcare Disparities Report was created. This annual report, which was later combined with the National Quality Report, focused on five critical areas of measurement (IOM, 2002, p. 2):

- Socioeconomic status in disparities research
- Disparities in healthcare services and quality
- Disparities in healthcare access
- Geographic units in disparities research
- Subnational data sets

Critical issues of socioeconomic status, service and quality, and access, as well as geographic issues, are covered in this annual report. Healthcare disparities occur consistently across a variety of illnesses and delivery services and are associated not with specific types of illnesses but with a broad spectrum of characteristics.

In 2010, the AHRQ, which serves as the administrator for the national annual the healthcare quality and disparities report, asked the IOM to review past national quality and disparity reports and provide a vision to improve the annual reports. A committee was formed, the Committee on Future Directions for the National Healthcare Quality and Disparities Reports, to address this task. Through research and deliberations, the committee concluded that while the disparity reports alone will not improve the quality of health care, the report results assist in better understanding of issues to close the gap between current performance levels and recommended standards of care. The committee recommended that the AHRQ take the following steps (HHS & AHRQ, 2010):

- Align the content of the reports with nationally recognized priority areas for quality improvement to help drive national action.
- Select measures that reflect healthcare attributes or processes that are deemed to have the greatest impact on population health.
- Affirm through the contents of the reports that achieving equity is an essential part of quality improvement.

- Increase the reach and usefulness of the AHRQ's family of report-related products.
- Revamp the presentation of the reports to tell a more complete quality improvement story.
- Analyze and present data in ways that inform policy and promote best-in-class achievement for all actors.
- Identify measure and data needs to set a research and data collection agenda.

This is a good example of how an initiative such as the original recommendation for national monitoring of healthcare quality and disparities can be expanded and must be reviewed periodically to see if the process needs to be improved. The first annual disparities report was completed in 2003, but now due to this review, subsequent annual reports are combined with the annual quality report (National Healthcare Quality and Disparities Report [QDR])—recognizing that healthcare disparities have a major impact on quality care. The 2015 report's content related to patient-centered care comments on the following (HHS & AHRQ, 2015b, p. 1).

- Access to care has improved dramatically.
- Quality of care continues to improve, but wide variation exists across the National Quality Strategy (NQS) priorities:
  - Effective treatment measures indicate improvements in overall performance and reductions in disparities.
  - Care coordination measures have lagged behind other priorities in overall performance.
  - Patient safety, person-centered care, and healthy living measures have improved overall, but many disparities remain.
- Despite progress in some areas, disparities related to race and socioeconomic status persist among measures of access and all NQS priorities.
- Improvements in access were led by sustained reductions in the number of Americans without health insurance and increases in

the number of Americans with a usual source of medical care.

- Care affordability measures are limited for summarizing performance and disparities.
- Disparities in access tend to be more common than disparities in quality.

The QDR is always a few years behind the current year because it takes time to collect and analyze the data.

The HHS publishes information on its website about culture and health care. It describes health disparities as the persistent gaps between the health status of minorities and non-minorities in the United States (HHS, 2008). Health services involve "providing care that does not vary in quality because of personal characteristics such as gender, ethnicity, geographic location and socioeconomic status" (IOM, 2001, p. 6). Despite ongoing advances in health care and technology, racial and ethnic minorities continue to experience more disease, disability, and premature death than non-minorities. African Americans, Hispanics/Latinos, American Indians and Alaska Natives, Asian Americans, Native Hawaiians, and Pacific Islanders have higher rates of infant mortality, cardiovascular disease, diabetes, human immunodeficiency virus infection/acquired immunodeficiency syndrome, and cancer, as well as lower rates of immunizations and cancer screening. Two major factors influence these results:

- *Inadequate access to care:* Barriers to care can result from economic, geographic, linguistic, cultural, and healthcare financing issues.
- *Substandard quality of care:* Even when minorities have similar levels of access to care, health insurance, and education, the quality and intensity of health care they receive are often poor. Lower-quality care has many causes, including patient–provider miscommunication, provider discrimination, stereotyping, and prejudice. Quality of care is now usually rated using the IOM-recommended measures: safe, timely, effective, equitable, efficient, and patient-centered (STEEEP).

The HHS developed a disparities action plan that focuses on reducing racial and ethnic health disparities: "With the HHS Disparities Action Plan, the Department commits to continuously assessing the impact of all policies and programs on racial and ethnic health disparities. It will promote integrated approaches, evidence-based programs and best practices to reduce these disparities. The HHS Action Plan builds on the strong foundation of the Affordable Care Act and is aligned with programs and initiatives such as Healthy People 2020, the First Lady's Let's Move initiative, and the President's National HIV/AIDS Strategy" (HHS & OMH, 2016). The goals of the plan are to (1) transform health care; (2) strengthen the nation's health and human services infrastructure and workforce; and (3) advance the health, safety, and well-being of the American people, advance scientific knowledge and innovation, and increase the efficiency, transparency, and accountability of HHS programs. This is an example of the connection between legislation (for example, ACA) and changes (the HHS Disparities Action Plan), but it may also be something that would change if there were changes in or repeal of legislation.

Disparities: Examples and Importance

The QDR identifies some of the current major quality and disparities issues. Data provided in the 2015 report indicate that overall quality and access are improving, but disparities related to race and socioeconomic status continue to be a problem (HHS & AHRQ, 2015b). This report was completed prior to implementation of the first major changes dictated by the ACA, which were initiated in late 2013 and early 2014. These changes—particularly the expansion of insurance coverage among the U.S. population—made some difference in reducing disparities. The QDR correlates with *Healthy People 2020*, the National Partnership for Action, and the NQS to end health disparities.

It is not possible to totally eliminate disparities in health care; however, much can be done to improve care for all persons and better ensure equity in health care. Ensuring access is critical. Can patients get the care they need from experts in a timely manner? Access involves multiple factors, such as appointments, transportation to appointments, availability of qualified staff, wait times, service hours, and so on. Disparity issues require that all healthcare professionals actively consider patient values and preferences (a critical component of patient-centered care). These values and preferences can vary between groups and within groups. It is easy to stereotype and assume that everyone in a specific ethnic group is the same, but this is not the case. Monitoring data on disparities is important to assist in identifying current status and to develop and improve effective interventions to reach desired outcomes.

Diversity in the Healthcare Workforce

The Sullivan Commission report, which is discussed in other chapters, examined disparities in health care from a different perspective (Sullivan, 2004). This commission concluded that a key contributor to the growing healthcare disparity problem is disparities in the U.S. health professional workforce. This is one factor that limits minorities' access to health care and to healthcare providers who understand their needs. The commission suggested that there should be an increase in the number of minority health professionals. This recommendation came at a time when there was a shortage of nurses and other healthcare providers.

There is a continuing need to increase minority admissions to nursing programs and retain minority students. The federal government provides grants to encourage schools of nursing to increase minority enrollment, develop student support services, and also increase minority enrollment in graduate school to increase the number of minority nursing faculty. It will take time to improve the level of minority participation in nursing. The U.S. Census Bureau

in 2012 reported that ethnic and racial minorities accounted for approximately 37% of the U.S. population. In 2013, the National Council of State Boards of Nursing (NCSBN) and the Forum of State Nursing Workforce Centers reported that only 19% of all U.S. registered nurses (RNs) were members of an ethnic or racial minority (2013 data) (AACN, 2015). Data from AACN also indicate that 48.4% of White RNs complete nursing degrees beyond the associate degree level, but the number is significantly higher or equivalent for minority nurses: African American (52.5%), Hispanic (51.5%), and Asian (75.6%) nurses. RNs from minority backgrounds recognize the importance of higher levels of nursing education beyond the entry level.

The AACN and the Robert Wood Johnson Foundation (RWJF) partnered together to launch an initiative entitled Doctoral Advancement in Nursing. The project aims to attract more minority students to PhD and DNP programs. These organizations also support another joint initiative, the RWJF New Careers in Nursing Scholarship Program, which focuses on providing monies for minority students in accelerated programs. The Campaign for the Minority Nurse Faculty Scholars Program, co-sponsored by the AACN and Johnson & Johnson, focuses on preparing minority nurses for faculty roles (AACN, 2017). These are just a few of the initiatives that are directed at the ongoing shortage of minority nurses and nursing faculty.

The American Organization of Nurse Executives is an important organization for nurses in leadership and management positions. This organization's principles include diversity: "the success of nursing leadership is dependent on reflecting the diversity of the communities nurses serve . . . diversity is one of the essential building blocks of a healthful practice/work environment," and a belief that healthcare organizations should apply these principles (American Organization of Nurse Executives, 2011, pp. 1–2):

1. Strive to develop internal and external resources that support patient-centered care and meet

the needs of the diverse patient and workforce populations served.

2. Establish a healthful practice/work environment that is reflective of diversity through a commitment to inclusivity, tolerance, and governance structures.

3. Partner with universities, schools of nursing, and other organizations that educate healthcare workers to support development and implementation of policies, procedures, programs, and learning environments that foster recruitment and retention of a student population that reflects the diversity of the United States.

4. Collect and disseminate diversity-related resources and information.

Stop and Consider #3
We do not provide equal care in the United States.

Patient Advocacy

Patient advocacy has always been a major aspect of the nursing role, and effective advocacy requires leadership skills. Nursing standards developed by the American Nurses Association, nursing specialty organizations, and healthcare organizations, as well as those developed by accrediting organizations and other healthcare professional organizations, support advocacy and consumerism. Throughout the care delivery process, nurses participate in and support actions that emphasize patient advocacy. The standards support patient and family education, patient satisfaction, the complaint process, efforts to improve care, and increasing patient participation in healthcare decision making.

As each nurse provides care, he or she has numerous opportunities to serve as the patient's advocate. The nurse coordinates care and, in doing so, represents the patient, but the nurse needs to recognize the patient's values and preferences in this process, thereby supporting patient-centered care. This

means that the nurse must know about the patient's values and preferences—for example, cultural issues and how they might affect the patient. This should lead to an improved collaborative relationship with the patient. Collaboration is working with others to arrive at the best outcome. When the nurse acts as the patient advocate, the nurse remembers that the patient must be involved. Advocacy does not mean that the nurse makes the patient dependent on the nurse. The nurse must also be persuasive with other healthcare team members to ensure better care for the patient that meets the patient's needs to reach the desired outcomes. Advocacy means that the nurse respects the patient and the patient's rights and ensures the patient has the necessary information to understand treatment and care needs and is informed about patient rights. Support is also given to the patient and family. When the patient makes a treatment decision, the nurse does not judge the patient's decision, even though the nurse may disagree with that decision.

Stop and Consider #4
As a nurse, you are a patient advocate.

Care Coordination:
A Plan of Care

Care coordination is recognized as an important part of the care process. The purpose of care coordination is "to establish and support a continuous healing relationship, enabled by an integrated clinical environment and characterized by a proactive delivery of evidence-based care and follow-up" (IOM, 2003a, p. 49). To accomplish this, healthcare providers, including nurses, need to provide patient-centered care. The goal is care coordinated across people, functions, activities, and sites (including the community and home) so that the patient receives effective care. A critical issue today is the need to improve interprofessional teamwork in the care planning process for patients, and care coordination is a part of effective teamwork and quality care. This particular content is discussed in other chapters.

The NQS includes care coordination in its priorities: Promote communication and coordination of care. As a result of this inclusion in NQS, care coordination is now monitored in the QDR, focused on three long-term goals (HHS & AHRQ, 2016c, p. 2):

1. Improve the quality of care transitions and communications across care settings.
2. Improve the quality of life for patients with chronic illness and disability by following a current care plan that anticipates and addresses pain and symptom management, psychosocial needs, and functional status.
3. Establish shared accountability and integration of communities and healthcare systems to improve quality of care and reduce health disparities.

These goals are also important for healthcare organizations and nurses who want to improve care coordination for all patients. The measures that are used to determine care coordination typically focus on transitions of care, preventable emergency department visits, potentially avoidable hospitalizations, integration of medication information, and use of electronic medical records (HHS & AHRQ, 2016c, p. 3).

Stop and Consider #5
Patient-centered care requires care coordination.

Application of Critical

Thinking and Clinical Reasoning and Judgment

For a long time, nurse educators have included critical thinking in curricula; however, the content itself and the means by which it is taught need to be revised to include clinical reasoning and judgment, as discussed in other chapters in this text. It is

important to recognize in this chapter that the processes of critical thinking and clinical reasoning and judgment relate to planning, implementing, and evaluating patient-centered care. Critical thinking and clinical reasoning and judgment should be used throughout the nursing process. These competencies are important to effective nursing practice, but it takes time and experience to develop them and to use them effectively.

Nursing Process

The **nursing process** is a systematic method for thinking about and communicating how nurses provide patient care. It is a step-by-step tool that guides nurses as they plan and provide care in a variety of clinical settings. Students are asked to use this process often by developing extensive care plans for patients and applying critical thinking and clinical reasoning and judgment. As students become RNs and move into practice, this process is adapted for daily use with multiple patients. The nursing process is similar to the problem-solving process in that there is a concern that requires more information to determine the best approach to solve it. In the nursing process, there are five steps, as described in **Figure 9-3**.

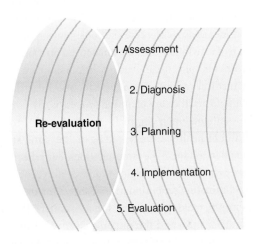

Figure 9-3 Nursing Care Process

Assessment

Information or data about the patient is required to describe the patient's health status and needs. This information is collected during assessment by multiple methods, such as a description of the patient's health history, interviews, observation, physical examination, and review of medical records.

The nursing process is not linear; it is ongoing, and one step leads to the next step and then the process begins again. Assessment is the initial step in the process; however, assessment is also ongoing because a patient's health status and needs change, which may require a change in diagnosis, in plan, and in how a plan is implemented. This also affects outcomes and evaluation. During assessment, the nurse must evaluate the quality of the information to determine if additional information is needed and the best method to obtain the information. It is during this step that the nurse begins to establish the nurse–patient relationship.

Patient-centered care means that the patient's values, preferences, needs, culture, and history are important factors to consider in the care plan. The nurse needs to document the assessment in a manner that is clear and informs other staff. In today's healthcare settings, interprofessional teams typically deliver more effective care. This means that the nursing plan of care should not be separate from other aspects of the patient's care needs. The team needs to consider all aspects of care and collaborate. A patient plan of care rather than a plan focused on a specific profession's plan of care, such as the nursing care plan or medical care plan, is more effective. Regardless of the focus, the care planning process is the same.

Patients often complain that many staff from different healthcare disciplines or the same staff members ask them the same questions. Some healthcare organizations are trying to address this problem by eliminating repetition in assessment forms—for example, making sure that the assessment forms physicians use and the nursing assessment forms are not repetitive unless a sufficient rationale exists for the repetition. Some healthcare organizations

have been more successful than others in controlling unnecessary repetition.

It is important during assessment to communicate to patients that they are the center of concern. Achieving this goal requires attention on the part of the nurse. Patient rights—for example, maintaining privacy during the assessment, ensuring confidentiality of information obtained, and explaining to the patient the process and the patient's rights—are also important.

Diagnosis

Diagnosis occurs as the nurse analyzes and interprets the information/data to determine the patient's nursing problems and needs—actual and potential. Nursing diagnoses have been identified and categorized through a system referred to as the North American Nursing Diagnosis Association (2017). Patient problems and needs change throughout the care process and thus lead to changes in the plan.

Planning

The care plan directs the care that will be given, promotes communication and sharing of information, and provides a record of the plan. The plan identifies the interventions or actions that the nurse may take to manage or resolve problems, monitor the patient, decrease risks of injury or illness, promote health or prevent injury or illness, support patient self-management, and provide patient-centered care. Interventions may be direct or indirect care. Examples of direct care are administering medication, helping the patient get out of bed, changing a dressing, teaching the patient, and assessing or monitoring patient status—all interventions or actions that include the patient and the nurse. Examples of indirect care are documenting in the medical record; preparing medications; giving a report to other staff on a patient's status; talking to the physician about the patient; reviewing medical orders; and delegating care to unlicensed assistive personnel, such as explaining what needs to be done for the patient during daily care—all interventions or actions in which the patient is not directly involved in the process. Classification of nursing care and interventions includes the following categories: (1) dependent care—most nurses cannot legally prescribe medications or act without a physician order (after the physician orders the medical intervention, the nurse follows the orders unless the nurse assesses the situation and determines the physician needs to be consulted before implementing the orders); (2) independent care—the nurse may make decisions about use of nursing interventions to prevent, reduce, or alleviate a problem; and (3) interdependent care—includes care in which both the nurse and the physician collaborate. State nurse practice acts identify the types of care that are independent, dependent, and interdependent within each state. There is now greater interest in using interprofessional care plans; in such cases, nursing plans would be part of the treatment team's plan.

Planning takes time and must be connected to assessment data and diagnoses/problems identified for the patient. The patient needs to be part of the planning and the identification of care needs, which should include an explanation of the care plan. This approach supports patient-centered care. The final decision about treatment is really up to the patient, unless the patient is not physically able to make decisions.

The plan identifies interventions, responsibility for implementing interventions, a timeline, and expected outcomes, and the plan should be based on best evidence. Outcomes are particularly important in evaluation. Some schools of nursing and some hospitals may use standardized nursing interventions and outcomes. The common source for this is the Nursing Intervention Classification (University of Iowa, College of Nursing, Center for Nursing Classification and Clinical Effectiveness, 2017).

Implementation

The plan is developed so that the patient can receive the care required, which is achieved through implementation of the plan. Change may be required at any time during this process, and the patient should be included in decision making. It is possible that as the plan is implemented, the patient's status might change, or perhaps an intervention might not be effective. Many factors affect implementation, such as the nurse's competency, the strategy used for delegation, staffing levels, acuity levels of all the patients whom the nurse is caring for at the time, availability of supplies and resources, the number of interruptions, the needs of the patient's family, patient cooperation and acceptance of the plan, time management and priorities, and much more. Throughout the implementation step, it is critical that the nurse coordinates, collaborates, and communicates with the interprofessional team and other nursing staff. Delegation is part of implementation, which is discussed in content about teams.

Evaluation

Evaluation focuses on each of the nursing care process steps. The following questions are asked (the applicable nursing process step or steps follow each question in parentheses):

- Was the assessment adequate? (assessment)
- Are there changes in the patient's status that require attention? (assessment)
- Are there new diagnoses/problems? Incorrect identification of problem(s)? (diagnosis)
- What are the outcomes for the identified nursing diagnoses/problems? (diagnosis, evaluation)
- Were the interventions completed, and what were the outcomes? (planning, implementation, evaluation)
- Are new interventions required? (planning, implementation, evaluation)

Reevaluation takes place throughout the process as the patient's health status changes. This may require that the nurse return to a previous step in the nursing process.

Getting patients involved in their own care can be challenging. Most patients want to be involved, and nurses must use strategies to support patient-centered care. It is important to be aware of

---

Exhibit 9-2 Strategies to Help Healthcare Providers Encourage Patient Participation in the Critical Thinking/Clinical Reasoning and Judgment Process

- Stay in the room. Don't talk to patients from the doorway.
- Pay attention to your body language and to the patient's body language.
- Sit down so that you are at eye level with the patient.
- Use open questions and comments such as "Tell me about . . ." instead of closed questions that imply you expect a short answer.
- Touch patients, but be respectful of their space and cultural norms.
- Use collaborative thinking language, such as "We should think this through," "Let's look at some possible conclusions," and "Can we analyze this together?"

- Use phrases that let the patient know that the patient's situation is not so unusual that the patient cannot discuss it. For example, "Some people feel anxious when . . ."
- Address patients respectfully. Find out if they prefer Mr. or Mrs., Doctor, Professor, Reverend, and so on. Do not use affectionate terms to address the patient, such as "sweetheart," "dear," and so on.
- Do not look at your watch, no matter how busy you are.
- Be direct and honest. For example, tell patients when the schedule is backed up and why.
- If you feel like avoiding a patient, reflect on why you feel that way.

Reproduced from Rubenfeld, M., & Scheffer, B. (2015). *Critical thinking tactics for nurses.* Burlington, MA: Jones & Bartlett Learning.

---

your attitude and tone of voice when you speak with adult patients. Some nurses approach all patients as if they were children, which is not helpful in engaging adult patients in their care. For example, when patients are recovering from anesthesia, the nurse speaks to the patient in "baby tones"; this is not appropriate.

Exhibit 9-2 provides some examples of strategies to help encourage patient participation in the critical thinking/clinical reasoning and judgment process. A new concern today is use of electronic devices with patients—the staff member may be documenting in the computer and not paying attention to the patient, missing important observations and acting as a barrier to patient-centered care.

Care/Concept Mapping

The traditional format for the nursing care plan, which focuses on the five steps just outlined, has

been used for a long time; however, it has been the subject of some criticism. Its length is an issue, particularly with students. This approach may also limit student critical thinking and clinical reasoning, and judgment because of its rigid format. Another approach to care planning is the **concept/care map**, defined by Schuster as follows: "The concept map care plan is an innovative approach to planning and organizing nursing care. In essence, a concept map care plan is a diagram of patient problems and interventions. Your ideas (concepts) about patient problems and treatments are the 'concept' that will be diagrammed" (2007, p. 2). Using concept mapping for care plans develops your critical thinking and clinical reasoning. Follow these steps to develop a concept map plan:

- *Develop the basic skeleton diagram.* Begin with the patient's reason for care (often the medical diagnosis), putting it in the center of the page or diagram. Around this central point, identify general problems (nursing problems). This represents the first concept map.

- *Analyze and categorize data.* In this step, the focus is on the information (assessment data) that is known; categorization provides evidence for the medical and nursing diagnoses. The information is obtained from history, assessment, medical records, and interviews with the patient. This information is added to the care map—problems/diagnoses with related data.
- *Analyze nursing diagnoses relationships.* Using the data map with the problems and related data assists in making connections by analyzing relationships among the diagnoses, drawing lines to identify the relationships, and numbering each problem/diagnosis. The goal is to achieve a holistic view of the patient.
- *Identify goals, outcomes, and interventions.* On a separate page, identify the patient's goals and outcomes. Next, identify interventions to meet these goals and outcomes for each of the problems/diagnoses numbered on the care map. This step is similar to the planning process in the nursing care process.
- *Evaluate the patient's responses.* On the page with the goals, outcomes, and interventions for each of the problems, add the patient's outcomes to each intervention after it has been implemented and evaluated. This information is then used in documentation.

When using a concept map, you create a diagram describing the care and can add to it as needed. This document is similar to the traditional nursing care plan format in that all the components of care are included. The concept map, however, allows for more creative thinking as you create a visual depiction of the patient's status, care needs, and the plan for care. It also may serve as student study tool.

Stop and Consider #6
The nursing process guides nursing practice.

Self-Management of Care

Regardless of whether healthcare providers accept it, patients are very active in managing their own care, as discussed in public/community health content. Even if they choose not to receive health care, they have made a decision about their health and what they want to do about it. In some cases, the patient is pushed into greater personal responsibility for care; for example, the patient may have inadequate reimbursement or no reimbursement at all or may not have support from family and others. It is recognized that critical strategies in preventing health problems and reducing healthcare costs are self-management, health promotion, and disease and illness prevention. When patients use self-management effectively and are supported by healthcare providers to use it, the outcomes are (1) greater collaboration with healthcare providers, (2) better understanding of treatment choices and patient and healthcare provider responsibilities, and (3) improved follow-up to treatment. Patients who are involved in their healthcare decisions are more satisfied with their health care and health status. Self-management of care is "the systematic provision of education and supportive interventions to increase patients' skills and confidence in managing their health problems, including regular assessment of progress and problems, goal setting, and problem-solving approach" (IOM, 2003b, p. 52). The Institute for Health Improvement website provides many self-management resources for healthcare providers and organizations to assist patients who might use self-management.

Health Literacy: A Barrier

Health literacy is important to effective self-management and for healthcare in general as noted in other chapters, as well as to reducing healthcare disparities (IOM, 2004). Nearly 90 million Americans (almost half of all adults) have difficulty understanding and using health information. This serious problem has increased the rate of hospitalizations and the use of emergency services, and it increases healthcare costs. If a patient cannot understand directions or does not follow recommended directions, the patient may need more intensive care, including hospitalization. A patient who does not understand the diabetic diet or know how to use insulin correctly will have more health problems; that person may then seek out help in the emergency room and consequently need to be hospitalized.

Healthcare literacy includes reading, writing, and arithmetic skills; listening and speaking abilities; and conceptual knowledge—how patients get information, analyze it, and then understand it so they can use it. Even educated people can find themselves with a health literacy problem and not understand medical information. The Joint Commission (2008) notes that communication problems are the most common root cause of healthcare errors. Safety and errors are discussed in more detail in other content in this text, but it is important in this discussion to recognize the connection between patient-centered care and healthcare literacy, self-management, and errors.

With the increase in the number of patients from diverse backgrounds, healthcare organizations are seeking more language interpreters, particularly those who speak Spanish, but also other languages. Families are not the best interpreters because they are not trained in medical terminology and they may influence the communication and decision-making processes due to their personal connection to the patient. An interpreter interprets only the language or words and is not involved in how the patient should respond. Some healthcare organizations have bilingual staff that can be a useful source of interpreting services if they are easily accessible and still able to complete their usual work.

The HHS Office of Minority Health offers a guide to help healthcare organizations implement effective language access services and improve care for patients with limited English skills. This report, *A patient-centered guide to implementing language access services in healthcare organizations*, offers a practical and basic step-by-step approach to implementing language services (HHS & OMH, 2005).

In 2011, the AHRQ announced that low health literacy in older Americans is linked to poorer health status and a higher risk of death, more emergency room visits, and more hospitalizations. The agency noted that more than 75 million English-speaking adults in the United States have limited health literacy. In 2016, the AHRQ published the second edition of its *Health literacy universal precautions toolkit*; its goals are (HHS & AHRQ, 2016):

- Simplify communication with and confirming comprehension for all patients so that the risk of miscommunication is minimized.
- Make the office environment and healthcare system easier to navigate.
- Support patients' efforts to improve their health.

The toolkit offers a variety of resources that can be used by healthcare providers and organizations. To improve health literacy jargon needs to be reduced and information needs to be provided in easy-to-understand written information, clear forms, and straightforward information on websites. Verbal communication with all patients also needs to improve.

Nurses are in direct contact with patients daily and encounter many patients who are experiencing health literacy problems. This has an impact on how effective nurses can be in providing care; assisting patients with self-management of their care; and teaching patients what they need to understand about their health, illness, and care needs. Nurses should be involved in healthcare organization efforts to address health literacy throughout the organization.

Patient/Family Education: Inclusion in the Plan of Care

Patient and family education has long been a part of nursing, but it is not easy to provide such education effectively. If we expect patients to be engaged in their care, then they need to be prepared to do this. One can look at patient education from two perspectives: (1) helping the patient understand the illness experience and how to cope with it effectively and (2) providing information and direction for self-management of care.

One of the major nursing interventions is patient education. It is not an intervention that the nurse can delegate unless the learning need is best addressed by another healthcare professional—RNs cannot delegate patient education to non-RN nursing staff such as a licensed practical nurse or a nursing assistant. It is not easy to provide effective patient education. The barriers to meeting patient education needs may include the following:

- Inadequate assessment of the patient's education needs
- Inadequate patient education plan
- Impact of patient factors such as medical status, cognitive status, and language
- Lack of time to provide the education required
- Interruptions that limit concentration
- Medical status of the patient (inability of the patient to adequately participate)
- Unclear assessment of the role of the family/significant others (whether the patient wants the family to participate in the education as this is the patient's decision)
- Patient education in settings such as ambulatory care typically not reimbursed; less emphasis placed on education as a result (not reimbursed in acute care either but there is more emphasis placed on it, mostly to get the patient ready for discharge)
- Confusion regarding who is responsible for patient education
- Lack of effective learning strategies and tools to meet individual patient education needs
- Lack of nursing staff (nurses view other aspects of their job nursing as more important)
- Lack of follow-up and evaluation of patient outcomes related to the education provided

Given the realities of the healthcare workplace today, it is difficult to plan and implement education for patients and their families. This can be very frustrating for both the nurse and the patient. Patients are discharged earlier today, but they are often still sick. While in the hospital, they may not be able to concentrate on what they need to learn, and then they are sent home and feel at a loss. Home care is one solution, but most home care is not provided around the clock, and patients still need to know about their illness or injury and treatment. Home health nurses provide patient education, but patient education needs to be provided in the hospital as well—and not all patients receive homecare services. Caregivers need a lot of information and support, but also we need more guidance for nurses who work in home care, an expanding area of practice (Marrelli, 2016).

When nurses are rushed, the typical scenario is to hand the patient and/or family written information. The nurse may ask if there are questions. This is not effective patient education. Effective education includes the patient in the entire process, a process that includes the following:

- The nurse assesses the patient's education status and needs. What does the patient need to know? How much does the patient know?
- The nurse identifies (diagnosis) learning needs. For example, the patient may need to know how to administer insulin and how to plan a diet.
- The nurse develops a patient education plan with specific interventions. These interventions are based on expected outcomes. The nurse identifies who is responsible for providing the learning intervention and creates the timeline. Here, the nurse must consider the patient's values and preferences, age, family support, religion, cultural background and issues, and health literacy. For example, the nurse teaches the diabetic patient about equipment and where to get it; how to draw

up insulin, including checking dosage and so on; how to prepare the skin; and how to administer the medication. The nurse talks with the patient about complications and aftercare needs and how to track insulin administered and store insulin. The nurse plans several sessions with the patient and uses a variety of teaching–learning strategies, such as discussion, visual aids, equipment, demonstration, and return demonstration; today, more technology is used so that patients can easily access information. The family is included as appropriate and with permission of the patient. The patient needs time to ask questions and express concerns. Rushing patient education is the greatest barrier to its success.

- The nurse implements the plan. Typically, this responsibility is not delegated unless assigned to another RN. Many of the barriers mentioned earlier come into play when implementing the plan. It takes planned effort to make sure the patient gets the education that is needed at the proper time.

- The nurse evaluates the plan/interventions and documents. Were the expected outcomes met? This should not be done in a threatening way, as if it was a test. Evaluation is commonly a weak link in the process, often because the patient goes on to another healthcare setting or home. It is important, whenever possible, to assess outcomes, such as through questions, return demonstrations, teach-back (the nurse asks the patient to repeat information included in the patient education experience), and so on, and also to ask the patient how he or she feels about the process and outcomes. Often, however, the patient is discharged, preventing complete evaluation of patient education. In some situations, the patient may be called after discharge, but this should be done only with the patient's permission.

For nursing care to be patient centered, with each patient developing effective self-management for their health and care needs, the patient needs information and skills to meet his or her individual needs.

Stop and Consider #7
Effective self-management requires health literacy.

Therapeutic Use
of Self in the Nurse–Patient Relationship

When you are a nurse and begin to care for patients, eventually you realize that the relationship is different from other relationships that you have experienced. It is not a parent–child relationship, a teacher–student relationship, or a personal or friend relationship. As you progress in the nursing program and then become an RN, this difference becomes even more evident. In the beginning, students often try to make the nurse–patient relationship into something it is not (for example, in many cases, the student tries to be friends with the patient). The key difference between the nurse–patient relationship and a friendship is that in a friendship, there is an expectation, on both sides, that friends will help each other, listen to each other, and be there for each other. This is not the case in a nurse–patient relationship. There should not be any expectation that the patient will listen to the nurse's concerns, feelings, or problems, nor is the patient there to support the nurse. The nurse is expected to listen to the patient, work with the patient (even if the nurse does not really like the patient), and meet the patient's care needs. This is difficult to learn, but it does come with experience.

The nurse–patient relationship has been described as therapeutic. *Therapeutic* means treatment. Using this term to describe this special relationship emphasizes that this relationship is part of the care process. **Therapeutic use of self**, a concept that was developed in the past to describe the nurse–patient relationship, "requires the nurse to use his/her personality consciously and in full awareness in an attempt to establish relatedness and to structure nursing intervention. . . . This requires self-insight, self-understanding, an understanding of the dynamics of human behavior, ability to interpret one's own behavior, as well as the behavior of others, and the ability to intervene effectively in nursing situations" (Travelbee, 1971, p. 19). The importance of this relationship should not be minimized. Parker notes that "Professional successes, especially at the bedside, are most often measured objectively through such sources as patient outcome data, length of stay, response to treatment, patient satisfaction, and the like. But other measurements, which are often therapeutic but less tangible, cannot be discounted as measures of success. These patient outcomes may take the form of relief in a troubled countenance, tears of joy, or a peaceful, pain-free sleep" (2006, p. 28).

In this relationship, the patient expects the nurse to be competent and have expertise in nursing care. There is no such expectation of the patient. The nurse plans and initiates care for the patient with the patient. The center of the nurse–patient relationship is the patient. Even when a patient asks about the nurse's personal reactions, the patient is still more focused on self. Through the nurse–patient relationship, the patient is given support and guidance in coping with the illness experience and/or health wellness process. Patients with acute illness recover, but they still need help with coping during their illness, and they may need time to reflect on their illness after recovery. As has been discussed, more and more people have chronic illnesses that are not resolved. These patients need to receive support and learn coping skills that can help them during the ups and downs of their illness process, and the therapeutic relationships supports this process.

The National Council of State Boards of Nursing (NCSBN, 2014) identifies key information about boundaries in the nurse–patient relationship. A professional boundary is an invisible line that provides limits to a nurse's behavior and focuses professional nurse–patient behavior so that the patient is the center. The patient expects that the nurse will act for the patient and respect his or her values and preferences. There should be no personal gain for the nurse. The NCSBN identifies the guiding principles with additional comments added (2014, p. 6):

- The nurse's responsibility is to delineate and maintain boundaries. *(It is not the patient's responsibility to know the boundaries or enforce them.)*
- The nurse should work within the zone of helpfulness. *(The zone of helpfulness falls between under involvement or over involvement with the patient. The most common boundary issue involves over involvement.)*
- The nurse should examine any boundary crossing, be aware of its potential implications, and avoid repeated crossings. *(For example, if a patient offers the nurse a gift, the nurse should not accept the gift. The nurse should analyze the situation and may consider discussing this situation with a supervisor, mentor, or colleague to get feedback and assistance in best response.)*
- Variables such as the care setting, community influences, patient needs, and nature of therapy affect the delineation of boundaries. *(For example, patients in mental health settings are particularly vulnerable to boundary issues, and nurses have to be clear about the boundaries.)*
- Actions that overstep established boundaries to meet the needs of the nurse are boundary violations. *(For example, the nurse does not describe his or her personal problems to patients, does not accept money or individual gifts from patients, and does not give money or gifts to patients.)*

The nurse should avoid situations where the nurse has a personal or business relationship, as well as a professional one. *(For example, the nurse should not date a patient, develop a friendship outside the nurse–patient relationship, or have a business transaction with a patient.)*

- Post-termination relationships are complex because the patient may need additional services and it may be difficult to determine when the nurse–patient relationship is truly terminated. *(Post-care personal relationships with patients are not recommended.)*

Figure 9-4 illustrates a continuum of professional behavior described in the NCSBN guide (2014).

How does a nurse know that there may be a boundary violation with a patient (NCSBN, 2014, p. 9)?

- Discussing intimate or personal issues with a patient

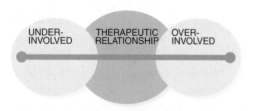

Figure 9-4 Continuum of Professional Behavior

- Engaging in behaviors that could reasonably be interpreted as flirting
- Believing you are the only one who truly understands or can help the patient
- Spending more time than is necessary with a particular patient
- Speaking poorly about colleagues or your employer with the patient and/or family
- Meeting a patient in settings besides those used to provide direct patient care or when you are not at work

All nurses need to watch for these situations of potential boundary violations and respond to them by altering communication and behavior.

Communication is a critical component of the nurse–patient relationship. The nurse needs to be clear and consistent with the patient and provide explanations about the care. Both verbal and non-verbal communication are integrated throughout the communication process. Nurses need to be aware of their own communication patterns and nonverbal messages, as well as those of the patient and people around the patient (family, friends, and other members of the healthcare team). **Exhibit 9-3** identifies some examples of therapeutic communication responses.

Exhibit 9-4 identifies examples of validation remarks that promote patient participation in

Exhibit 9-3 Therapeutic Communication Responses

- Using silence
- Accepting others for who they are
- Giving recognition
- Offering self
- Using broad openings
- Offering general leads
- Placing an event in time or sequence
- Making observations
- Encouraging description or perceptions
- Encouraging comparison
- Restating

- Reflecting
- Focusing
- Exploring more fully
- Seeking clarification
- Presenting reality
- Voicing doubt
- Verbalizing the implied, then asking for validation
- Attempting to translate words into feelings
- Formulating a verbal contract
- Assessing, evaluating with the patient

Exhibit 9-4 Validation Remarks to Promote Patient Participation in Decisions

- Here's what I think; do you agree?
- What would you say is going on here?
- How is all of this affecting you?
- Does it seem that way to you? It does to me.
- Let's think about this together for a minute.
- Only you know your daily living situation, so how do you think it might affect the care plan after you are discharged?
- Can we find a way through this together?

- Let me explain my thinking to you.
- What do you think?
- Does this feel okay?
- Do you agree with this?
- This is what I'm thinking; what do you think?
- I'm interested in your take on all of this.
- If you could change this, what would be different?
- If you had a magic wand, what would you have it do?

Reproduced from Rubenfeld, M., & Scheffer, B. (2015). *Critical thinking tactics for nurses.* Burlington, MA: Jones & Bartlett Learning.

decisions. These communication examples illustrate how communication, the nurse–patient relationship, and patient-centered care are interrelated.

The AHRQ data on person- and family-centered care include communication with providers. In the 2017 review of the QDR data, the AHRQ reported that poor communication between adult patients and healthcare providers decreased significantly for all ethnic groups from 2002–2013 (HHS & AHRQ, 2017). The measures used to collect the data are:

- Poor communication with adult and child healthcare providers in offices/clinics
- Poor communication with doctors and nurses in hospitals
- Provider–patient communication among adults receiving home health care, by language and by race/ethnicity
- Providers asking patients to assist in making treatment decisions, by insurance, education, number of chronic conditions, and ethnicity

Stop and Consider #8
A nurse is not a patient's friend.

CHAPTER HIGHLIGHTS

1. The competency—provide patient-centered care—refers to considering the patient's needs, cultural values, preferences, and unique situation instead of centering on the provider's prospective.

2. Four rules underpin patient-centered care: (1) care is based on continuous health relationships, (2) care customization is based on patient needs and preferences, (3) patients are the source of control, and

(Continues)

CHAPTER HIGHLIGHTS (CONTINUED)

(4) there is shared knowledge and free flow of information.

3. Patients who are involved in their care have better outcomes.

4. Examples of four nursing theories related to patient-centered care are Watson's theory on caring, Orem's self-care theory, Leininger's cultural diversity theory, and Peplau's interpersonal relations theory.

5. Macro consumers of health care are government and insurers.

6. Micro consumers of health care are the patient and family.

7. Patient satisfaction is a key factor that many healthcare institutions measure as a part of their delivery of care, although it is difficult to effectively quantify satisfaction.

8. The health disparities problem includes issues related to access to care, level of care, and equality of care across races and ethnic groups.

9. Strategies to overcome disparities include addressing access-to-care issues—such as wait times, appointment availability, and hours of service—to better meet the needs of the population served. Another strategy is to include patient values and preferences in the delivery of care.

10. Patient advocacy means the nurse is active in respecting patient rights and ensuring that the patient has the knowledge necessary to understand his or her treatment and care needs.

11. Care coordination is an important part of high-quality, patient-centered care, but it is an aspect of care that is not generally reimbursable. Effective interprofessional teamwork includes coordination.

12. Clinical reasoning and judgment is different from critical thinking. It focuses on putting the care needs within the context that the patient presents—environment, values, and preferences—as gathered in the assessment.

13. The nursing process is a systematic method for thinking about and communicating how nurses provide patient care.

14. A concept map care plan is a diagram of patient problems and interventions that offers a more interactive plan than the traditional care plan.

15. Healthcare literacy includes reading, writing, and arithmetic skills; listening and speaking ability; and conceptual knowledge. Lack of healthcare literacy can present a barrier to care because patients may not understand aspects of their care.

16. Nurses provide patient and family education to allow patients to more actively participate in their care and care decisions and to encourage effective self-management of health and illness.

17. A professional boundary is an invisible line that places limits on a nurse's behavior.

18. Effective communication is an important component of patient-centered care.

ENGAGING IN THE CONTENT

Discussion Questions

1. What does *patient-centered care* mean, and why is it relevant to nursing?
2. Describe a nursing theory that relates to patient-centered care.
3. How is diversity related to patient-centered care?
4. Explain consumerism in health care and its relevance to nursing.
5. Describe healthcare disparity and its importance.
6. What is health literacy?
7. Why is patient advocacy important?
8. What is self-management of care?
9. Discuss the importance of patient education.

CRITICAL THINKING ACTIVITIES

1. The National Healthcare Quality and Disparities Report monitors our health care (https://www.ahrq.gov/research/findings/nhqrdr/index.html). Go to the site. What can you learn about current disparities in health care? What measurements are used?

2. Watch an episode of a favorite TV show, including the commercials. This program does not have to be a health-related TV show. As you watch the show, keep notes describing ethnic, racial, and culture issues that arise. Who is playing which types of the roles? Also note the communication, clothing, attitudes, values, and any other factors related to diversity. Do the same for the commercials. Share your findings in an online course discussion forum, and relate your findings to the content in this chapter about diversity and disparities.

3. Review the material on health literacy found at the following site: http://nnlm.gov/outreach/consumer/hlthlit.html. In a team discussion, consider the identified vulnerable populations and their relevance to health literacy.

4. Visit The Joint Commission website to review the report on diversity in hospitals (http://www.jointcommission.org/assets/1/6/ARoadmapforHospitalsfinalversion727.pdf). Visit http://www.crculturevision.com/commissionupdate.aspxlearn. What does this organization emphasize about diversity in health care and its cultural competency standards? What can you learn that might help you be more culturally competent? How might this type of information improve health care?

ELECTRONIC REFLECTION JOURNAL

Consider the following in your journal by clearly and briefly responding to the following questions:

- How would you describe yourself ethnically/racially/culturally? Has your view of ethnicity/race/culture changed over time? If so, how?
- Do you think people are treated differently because of race or ethnicity? If so, describe an example.
- Have you been treated differently because of your own ethnicity or race? If so, how?
- When did you first become aware that people were different ethnically or racially?
- If you were or are a member of a minority group, would you want to have a healthcare professional who is a member of that minority group care for you? Why?

CASE STUDIES

Case 1

A 45-year-old woman fell during an ice storm. She went to the emergency department because she thought she might have broken one or more ribs. When the X-ray results came back, the physician told the patient and her husband that they showed a carcinoid tumor in one lung. The patient had never smoked and was healthy. There was no history of lung cancer in her family. The couple left devastated, with a list of specialists for follow-up. They spent 3 weeks in testing. Both the patient and her husband assumed from the term *carcinoid* that she had malignant lung cancer. The patient and her husband had college degrees and held management positions. The physician in the emergency department did not discuss what "carcinoid" meant. The couple's anxiety rose with each passing day. At a later appointment, it became evident that the couple was not clear on what "carcinoid" meant and that the couple's interpretation included more life-threatening implications than necessary.

What does *carcinoid* mean? The National Cancer Institute (NCI) in the National Institutes of Health (NIH) defines "carcinoid" as a slow-growing type of tumor usually found in the gastrointestinal system (most often in the appendix) and sometimes in the lungs or other sites. Carcinoid tumors may spread to the liver or other sites in the body, and they may secrete substances such as serotonin or prostaglandins, causing carcinoid syndrome. This patient's tumor was localized, and it was removed.

Case Questions

1. What do you think could have been done differently?
2. What role might a nurse have assumed, and what specifically might the nurse have done?

CASE STUDIES (CONTINUED)

3. Is this an example of health literacy? If so, how is it an example?
4. How might patient-centered care be applied to this case? Be specific.

Case 2

A nurse on a medical unit was caring for an elderly woman. The patient's family visited frequently. The nurse, patient, and family spent a lot of time together, and the nurse was very helpful to the family. The nurse shared with the patient and family that her husband was out of work and her family was experiencing a difficult time. Her husband had applied for a job at many businesses, and in the course of the conversation, the nurse realized that her husband had applied to the patient's son-in-law's business. He had never been called for an interview.

After the patient left the hospital, the family sent flowers to hospital unit for the nurse. The nurse was surprised and happy to receive the flowers, which she took home. A week later, her husband received a call for an interview at the business owned by the patient's son-in-law; he received a job offer one week later. The couple was very happy.

Case Questions

1. How were professional boundaries crossed in this case?
2. Describe how this case relates to nurse–patient (and family) relationships as described in this chapter.
3. What should the nurse have done when she experienced issues related to professional boundaries?

Working Backward to Develop a Case

Write a brief paragraph that describes a case related to the following questions.

1. Why does management expect us as nurses to contribute to plans for the redesign of the lobby of the hospital and the admissions office?
2. I think we should ask our patients about the unit.
3. What should be the main focus of the design of our unit?

REFERENCES

Agency for Healthcare Research and Quality. (2011). *Low health literacy linked to higher risk of death and more emergency room visits and hospitalizations.* Retrieved from http://www.ahrq.gov

American Association of Colleges of Nursing. (2006). *The essentials of doctoral education for advanced nursing practice.* Washington, DC: Author. Retrieved from http://www.aacn.nche.edu/dnp/Essentials.pdf

American Association of Colleges of Nursing. (2008). *The essentials of baccalaureate education for professional nursing practice*. Washington, DC: Author. Retrieved from http://www.aacn.nche.edu/Education/pdf/BaccEssentials98.pdf

American Association of Colleges of Nursing. (2011). *The essentials of masters education for nursing*. Washington, DC: Author. Retrieved from http://www.aacn.nche.edu/education-resources/MasEssentials96.pdf

American Association of Colleges of Nursing. (2015). *Enhancing diversity in the workplace*. Retrieved from http://www.aacn.nche.edu/media-relations/fact-sheets/enhancing-diversity

American Association of Colleges of Nursing. (2017). *Johnson & Johnson campaign for nursing-American Association of Colleges of Nursing minority faculty scholars program 2017–2018 academic year*. Retrieved from http://www.aacn.nche.edu/students/scholarships/2017-J-J-Call-for-Applications.pdf

American Hospital Association. (2017). *The patient care partnership*. Retrieved from http://www.aha.org/advocacy-issues/communicatingpts/pt-care-partnership.shtml

American Organization of Nurse Executives. (2011). *AONE guiding principle for diversity in healthcare organizations*. Retrieved from http://www.aone.org/resources/diversity.pdf

American Organization of Nurse Executives, & National Alliance for Quality Care. (2012). *Guiding principles for patient engagement*. Retrieved from http://www.aone.org/resources/patient-engagement.pdf

Anderson, L., Scrimshaw, S., Fullilove, M., Fielding, J., & Normand, J. (2003). Culturally competent healthcare systems: A systematic review. *American Journal of Preventive Medicine, 24*(3S), 68–79.

Balik, B., Conway, J., Zipperer, J., & Watson, J. (2011). *Achieving an exceptional patient and family experience of inpatient hospital care*. IHI Innovation Series white paper. Cambridge, MA: Institute for Healthcare Improvement. Retrieved from http://www.ihi.org/resources/Pages/IHIWhitePapers/AchievingExceptionalPatientFamilyExperienceInpatientHospitalCareWhitePaper.aspx

Brosey, L., & March, K. (2015). Effectiveness of structure hourly nurse rounding on patient satisfaction and clinical outcomes. *Journal of Nursing Care Quality, 30*(2), 153–159.

Commonwealth Fund. (2008). *Patient-centered care: An overview*. Retrieved from http://www.commonwealthfund.org/Program-Areas/Archived-Programs/Delivery-System-Innovation-and-Improvement/Patient-Centered-Coordinated-Care.aspx

Davis, K., Schoenbaum, S., & Audet, A. (2005). A 2020 vision of patient-centered primary care. *Journal of General Internal Medicine, 15*, 953–957.

FamiliesUSA. (2011). *Affordable Care Act: Patients' bill of rights and other protections*. Retrieved from http://familiesusa.org/sites/default/files/product_documents/Patients-Bill-of-Rights.pdf

Finkelman, A., & Kenner, C. (2012). *Teaching the IOM: Implications of the IOM reports for nursing education* (3rd ed., Volumes I and II). Washington, DC: American Nurses Association.

Gasparini, R., Champagne, M., Stephany, A., Hudson, J., & Fuchs, M. (2015). Increased family presence and the impact on patient- and family-centered care adoption. *Journal of Nursing Administration, 45*(1), 28–34.

Gerteis, M., Edgman-Levitan, S., Daley, J., & Delbanco, T. (Eds.). (1993). *Through the patient's eyes*. San Francisco, CA: Jossey-Bass.

Hagenow, N. (2003). Why not person-centered care? The challenges of implementation. *Nursing Administration Quarterly, 27*, 203–207.

Halpern, R., Lee, M., Boulter, P., & Phillips, R. (2001). A synthesis of nine major reports on physicians competencies for the emerging practice environment. *Academic Medicine, 76*, 606–615.

Hargraves, I., LeBlanc, A. Shah, N., & Montori, V. (2016). Shared decision-making: The need for patient–clinician conversation, not just information. *Health Affairs, 35*(4), 627–629.

Hochbaum, G. (1958). *Public participation in medical screening programs: A sociological study*. Public Health Service Publication No. 572. Washington, DC: U.S. Government Printing Office.

Institute of Medicine. (1999). *To err is human*. Washington, DC: The National Academies Press.

Institute of Medicine. (2001). *Crossing the quality chasm: A new health system for the 21st century*. Washington, DC: The National Academies Press.

Institute of Medicine. (2002). *Guidance for the national healthcare disparities report*. Washington, DC: The National Academies Press.

Institute of Medicine. (2003a). *Health professions education*. Washington, DC: The National Academies Press.

Institute of Medicine. (2003b). *Unequal treatment*. Washington, DC: The National Academies Press.

Institute of Medicine. (2004). *Health literacy: A prescription to end confusion*. Washington, DC: The National Academies Press.

The Joint Commission. (2008). *Facts and figures*. Retrieved from http://www.jointcommission.org/NewsRoom/PressKits/Health_Literacy/facts_figures.htm

Kaiser Family Foundation. (2015). *Population distribution by race/ethnicity*. Retrieved from http://kff.org/other/state-indicator/distribution-by-raceethnicity/?currentTimeframe=0

Kennedy, M. (2015). Revisiting patient satisfaction surveys. Are hospitals using the results properly. *American Journal of Nursing, 115*(8), 1.

Knowles, M. (1972). *The modern practice of adult education.* New York, NY: Associated Press.

Lavalleel, D., Chenok, K., Love, R., Petersen, C., Holve, E., Segal, C., & Franklin, P. (2016). Incorporating patient-reported outcomes into health care to engage patients and enhance care. *Health Affairs, 35*(4), 575–582.

Leebov, W. (2008). Beyond customer service. *American Nurse Today, 3*(1), 21–23.

Lewin, S., Skea, Z., Entwistle, V., Zwarenstein, M., & Dick, J. (2001). Interventions for providers to promote a patient-centered approach to clinical consultations. *Cochrane Database System Review, 4,* CD003267.

Marrelli, T. (2016). *Home care nursing: Surviving in an ever-changing care environment.* Indianapolis, IN: Nursing Knowledge International.

Masters, K. (2009). *Role development in professional nursing practice* (2nd ed.). Burlington, MA: Jones & Bartlett Learning.

National Council of State Boards of Nursing. (2014). *A nurse's guide to professional boundaries.* Retrieved from https://www.ncsbn.org/ProfessionalBoundaries_Complete.pdf

National League for Nursing. (2016, February). *Accreditation standards for nursing education programs.* Commission for Nursing Education Accreditation. Retrieved from http://www.nln.org/docs/default-source/accreditation-services/cnea-standards-final-february-201613f2bf5c78366c709642ff00005f0421.pdf?sfvrsn=4

North American Nursing Diagnosis Association. (2017). *Nursing diagnoses.* Retrieved from http://nanda.org

Parker, D. (2006). Establishing a passion for nursing: The role of the nurse leader. *Nurse Leader, 4*(5), 28–32.

Pelletier, L., & Stickler, J. (2013). Action brief: Patient engagement and activation: A health reform imperative and improvement opportunity for nursing. *Nursing Outlook, 61*(1), 51–54.

Pew Health Professions Commission. (1995). *Critical challenges: Revitalizing the health professions for the twenty-first century.* San Francisco, CA: UCSF Center for the Health Professions.

Planetree. (2014). *The formula.* Retrieved from http://planetree.org/

Schuster, P. (2007). *Concept mapping: A critical thinking approach to care planning.* Philadelphia, PA: Davis.

Shaller, D. (2007). *Patient-centered care: What does it take?* New York, NY: Commonwealth Fund. Retrieved from http://www.commonwealthfund.org/publications/publications_show.htm?doc_id=559715

Stewart, M. (2001). Towards a global definition of patient-centered care. *British Medical Journal, 322*(7284), 444–445.

Sullivan, L. (2004). *Missing persons: Minorities in the health professions: A report of the Sullivan Commission on diversity in the healthcare workforces.* Washington, DC:

Sullivan Commission on Diversity in the Healthcare Workforce. Retrieved from http://www.aacn.nche.edu/media-relations/SullivanReport.pdf

Travelbee, J. (1971). *Interpersonal aspects of nursing.* Philadelphia, PA: Davis.

Twibell, R. et al. (2008). Nurses' perceptions of their self-confidence and the benefits and risks of family presence during resuscitation. *American Journal of Critical Care, 17*(2), 101–111.

University of Iowa, College of Nursing, Center for Nursing Classification and Clinical Effectiveness. (2017). *CNC—Overview: Nursing interventions classification (NIC).* Retrieved from https://nursing.uiowa.edu/cncce/nursing-interventions-classification-overview

U.S. Census Bureau. (2012). *2012 census.* Retrieved from http://www.census.gov/newsroom/releases/archives/population/cb13-112.html

U.S. Department of Health and Human Services. (2008). *National partnership for action to end healthcare disparities.* Retrieved from http://minorityhealth.hhs.gov/npa/

U.S. Department of Health and Human Services. (2010). *Healthy People 2020.* Washington, DC: U.S. Government Printing Office.

U.S. Department of Health and Human Services. (2017). *Filing a complaint.* Retrieved from https://www.hhs.gov/hipaa/filing-a-complaint/

U.S. Department of Health and Human Services, & Agency for Healthcare Research and Quality. (2010). *Future directions for the national healthcare quality and disparities report.* Retrieved from https://www.ahrq.gov/sites/default/files/wysiwyg/research/findings/final-reports/iomqrdrreport/iomqrdrreport.pdf

U.S. Department of Health and Human Services, & Agency for Healthcare Research and Quality. (2015a). *Chartbook on care person- and family-centered care. National healthcare quality and disparities report.* Retrieved from https://www.ahrq.gov/research/findings/nhqrdr/2014chartbooks/personcentered/index.html

U.S. Department of Health and Human Services, & Agency for Healthcare Research and Quality. (2015b). *National healthcare quality and disparities report.* Retrieved from https://www.ahrq.gov/research/findings/nhqrdr/nhqdr15/executive-summary.html

U.S. Department of Health and Human Services, & Agency for Healthcare Research and Quality. (2015c). *Health literacy universal precautions toolkit* (2nd ed.). Retrieved from ttps://www.ahrq.gov/professionals/quality-patient-safety/quality-resources/tools/literacy-toolkit/healthlittoolkit2.html

U.S. Department of Health and Human Services, & Agency for Healthcare Research and Quality. (2016). *AHRQ health literacy universal precautions toolkit.*

Retrieved from https://www.ahrq.gov/professionals /quality-patient-safety/quality-resources/tools/literacy -toolkit/index.html

U.S. Department of Health and Human Services, & Agency for Health Research and Quality. (2016a). *Patient- and family-centered innovations to improve care*. Retrieved from https://innovations.ahrq.gov/node/8383?utm _source=issueanc&utm_medium=email&utm _campaign=20160720

U.S. Department of Health and Human Services, & Agency for Health Research and Quality. (2016b). *Developing and testing the healthcare safety hotline: A prototype consumer reporting system for patient safety events.* Retrieved from https://www.ahrq.gov/professionals /quality-patient-safety/patient-family-engagement /hotline/index.html

U.S. Department of Health and Human Services, & Agency for Health Research and Quality. (2016c). *Chartbook on care coordination. National healthcare quality and disparities report.* Retrieved from https://www.ahrq .gov/sites/default/files/wysiwyg/research/findings /nhqrdr/chartbooks/carecoordination/qdr2015-chart book-carecoordination.pdf

U.S. Department of Health and Human Services, & Agency for Health Research and Quality. (2017). *AHRQ chartbook on person- and family-centered care reports on communication*. Retrieved from https://www .ahrq.gov/research/findings/nhqrdr/chartbooks /personcentered/index.html

U.S. Department of Health and Human Services, Centers for Medicare and Medicaid Services, & Hospital Consumer Assessment of Healthcare Providers and Systems. (2013). *HCAHPS: Patients' perspectives of care survey*. Retrieved from http://www .cms.gov/Medicare /Quality-Initiatives-Patient-Assessment- Instruments /HospitalQualityInits/HospitalHCAHPS.html

U.S. Department of Health and Human Services, & Centers for Medicare and Medicaid Services. (2017). *Patient's bill of rights*. Retrieved from https://www.cms.gov /CCIIO/Programs-and-Initiatives/Health-Insurance -Market-Reforms/Patients-Bill-of-Rights.html

U.S. Department of Health and Human Services, Centers for Medicare and Medicaid Services, & Hospital Consumer Assessment of Healthcare Providers and Systems. (2017). *HCAHPS: Home*. Retrieved from http://www.hcahpsonline.org/home.aspx

U.S. Department of Health and Human Services, & The Office of Minority Health. (2005). *A patient-centered guide to implementing language access services in healthcare organizations*. Retrieved from https://minorityhealth .hhs.gov/omh/content.aspx?ID_4375

U.S. Department of Health and Human Services, & The Office of Minority Health. (2008). Retrieved from http:// minorityhealth.hhs.gov/

U.S. Department of Health and Human Services, & The Office of Minority Health. (2016). *HHS disparities action plan*. Retrieved from https://minorityhealth.hhs.gov /omh/browse.aspx?lvl=2&lvlid=10

Zimmerman, P. (2001). The problems with healthcare customer satisfaction surveys. In J. Dochterman & H. Grace (Eds.), *Current issues in nursing* (6th ed., pp. 255–260). St. Louis, MO: Mosby.

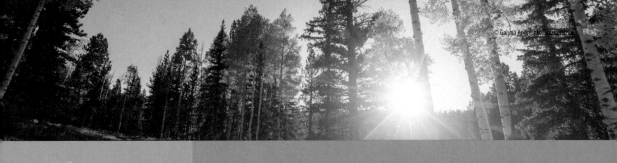
© Galyna Andrushko/Shutterstock

Chapter 10

Work in Interprofessional Teams

CHAPTER OBJECTIVES

At the conclusion of this chapter, the learner will be able to:

- Discuss the core competency: Work in interprofessional teams.
- Examine team leadership, teamwork, types of teams, relationship to effective team functioning, and improving teams by using TeamSTEPPS®.
- Discuss communication and its relationship to patient care and teams.
- Examine the knowledge and competencies needed for effective team functioning.
- Discuss effective team decision making.
- Examine collaboration and its relationship to patient care and teams.
- Explain how coordination relates to patient care and teams.
- Examine the problem of incivility in the healthcare work environment and approaches to resolving the problem.
- Apply the delegation process.
- Analyze the change process and implications for health care and teams.
- Explain conflict and conflict resolution and implications for nursing.
- Discuss power and empowerment in the healthcare delivery system.

KEY TERMS

Assertiveness
Call-out
Check-back
Checklist
Clinical protocol/pathway
Collaboration
Communication
Conflict
Conflict resolution
Coordination
Delegatee

Delegation
Delegator
Empowerment
Followers
Interprofessional team-based care
Interprofessional teamwork
Microsystem
Mindful communication
Plan-do-study-act (PDSA) cycle

Power
Situation-background-assessment-recommendations (SBAR)
Team
Team leader
Teamwork
Types of power
Unlicensed assistive personnel (UAP)

Introduction

This chapter focuses on working in teams—both nursing teams and interprofessional teams. Throughout this content, when the term **team** is used, it applies to both interprofessional teams and nursing staff teams. Nurses are members of interprofessional teams and also members of nursing teams (nursing teams include nursing staff such as registered nurses (RNs), licensed practical/vocational nurses, and unlicensed assistive personnel (UAP).

This is a critical competency for every nurse. The content includes an explanation of the healthcare professions core competency, teams and teamwork, and critical components of effective teams:

communication, collaboration, and coordination. Incivility is a problem that many healthcare organizations and staff are experiencing, and this behavior leads to ineffective teamwork. In addition, delegation is a part of the daily work for every nurse and is part of planning care and **teamwork** or how a team functions. Teams must cope with change and learn to make effective change decisions. Conflict and conflict resolution are issues that all teams face. Power and empowerment are also discussed in this chapter as they relate to staff and teams.

Through its assessment of the U.S. healthcare system, the IOM (2001) described the healthcare system as a system "in need of fundamental change. Many patients, doctors, nurses and healthcare leaders are concerned that the care delivered is not, essentially,

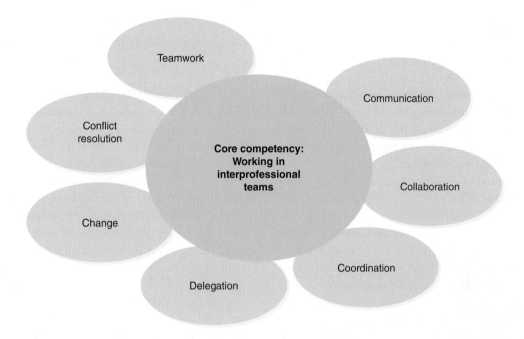

Figure 10-1 Working Interprofessional Teams: Key Elements

the care we should receive. The frustration levels of both patients and clinicians have probably never been higher. Yet the problems remain. Healthcare today harms too frequently and routinely fails to deliver its potential benefits" (p. 1). This description continues to be relevant today. Technology, new drugs, and many other care advances can improve health and health care, but something is wrong with the care delivery models. This set of problems is what drove the need to it identify the five healthcare professions core competencies. This chapter examines the core competency that most directly addresses the need for changes in the care delivery models: Work in interprofessional teams. **Figure 10-1** highlights the key elements for this competency.

The Core Competency:
Work in Interprofessional Teams

The first of the healthcare professions core competencies is "provide patient-centered care." This

chapter covers the second core competency, "work in interprofessional teams." The competency is described as: "cooperate, collaborate, communicate, and integrate care in teams to ensure that care is continuous and reliable" (IOM, 2003, p. 4). As a reminder, these core competencies were developed for all healthcare professions, not just nursing; however, this chapter focuses on nurses who are members of interprofessional teams and also members of nursing teams.

One has to ask why there is such emphasis on this core competency. After all, it makes sense that teams are important—why would anyone question this? The critical issue is whether healthcare professionals are prepared to participate effectively in teams, particularly interprofessional teams, but the conclusion is they are not. Healthcare professional education takes place in isolation; each healthcare profession provides its own education, with limited reference to other healthcare professionals. The result is that nursing, medicine, pharmacy, and allied health students (for example, physical therapists, occupational therapists, and so on) have limited, if any, contact with one another in their educational programs. As a consequence, they have limited knowledge of roles of the other professions and the ways in which they must collaborate and coordinate care to provide patient-centered care. This is a serious problem because when healthcare professionals graduate and meet licensure requirements, they are expected to work together.

In 2009, the Interprofessional Education Collaborative (IPEC) was formed to address the need for competencies that were not profession-specific (IPEC, 2011). The collaborative emphasizes that all healthcare organizations need to develop effective interprofessional teamwork and maintain these efforts. In 2016, IPEC published an update of its work (IPEC, 2016). Since 2009, recognizing the importance of interprofessional teams more education accreditors for different healthcare professions are including the IPEC competencies in their accreditation requirements. The American Association of Colleges of Nursing (AACN) is a founding member of IPEC and supports its approaches in AACN accreditation. Endorsement of IPEC content, standards, model, and so on from many healthcare professional accreditation bodies ensures greater integration in healthcare profession education and inclusion in professional literature, including textbooks and other professional literature to share with students. The 2016 update of the 2011 report on interprofessional competencies also included significant changes in health care, such as greater inclusion of quality improvement and references to changes related to the Affordable Care Act of 2010 (ACA), with greater emphasis on population health at the local, state, national, and global levels. Since 2011, there are more interprofessional education activities—for example, in 2011, 76% of schools of medicine offered these activities, and in 2014, 92% included these learning activities (IPEC, 2016).

IPEC also now offers a website to provide resources for faculty. Changes were made in the description of the core competencies: (1) The interprofessional collaborative domain is a domain in and of itself to assist in integrating population health competencies, and (2) there is emphasis on the Triple Aim (improve patient experience—quality and satisfaction, improve health of populations, and reduce costs). Additional content on the IPEC and its competencies is found in this text's content on nursing education, for example, as described in an earlier figure, **Figure 3-2**. The 2016 IPEC update of the interprofessional collaborative practice core competency domains continue to support the World Health Organization (WHO) perspective on the need for and the impact of interprofessional education leading to effective interprofessional teams.

In addition, nurses need to know how to work on nursing teams whose focus is nursing care. In most cases, this, too, leads to isolation and limited recognition of the need for greater reaching out to other healthcare disciplines. Nurses tend to focus on the nursing care plan to the detriment of the total plan of care for the patient—a nursing care plan, as opposed to a patient-centered care plan. Nursing education reinforces this perspective by emphasizing the nursing care plan. This is not to say that the same scenario does not exist in other healthcare professions because it does. Nursing students need a broader view of health care along with the nursing perspective (Barnsteiner, Disch, Hall, Mayer, & Moore, 2007). Nurses also work together on teams related to service and healthcare delivery in general, such as committees and task forces. These teams require the same competencies as teams focused on patient care.

All healthcare providers should be focused on delivering patient-centered care—care that "alleviates vulnerability in all of its forms. That care should and must be delivered at the right time, at the right level, in the right place, and so on. If care were on a compass it would be true north and all other functions would stand in line to provide added value and service to that focus" (Hagenow, 2003, p. 204). Because one individual healthcare profession cannot do it all alone, interprofessional teams are best suited to achieve this patient-centered care.

Stop and Consider #1

All nurses should be competent in serving on interprofessional teams.

Teamwork

With the increasing complexity of care and concerns about the fragmented healthcare system, interprofessional teams are even more important. In addition, the complex needs of patients with chronic illness, providing critical acute care, geriatric care, and care at the end of life require effective planning to ensure improved outcomes. Patients who require such care have multiple, complex needs. The types and complexity of settings, multiple types of healthcare providers, and need to share information and planning across settings require more teamwork. Use of interprofessional teams tends to result in improved quality care and a decrease in healthcare costs (IOM, 2003a).

Clarification of Terms

The term *interdisciplinary* is used in the core competency (IOM, 2003), although recently the more widely accepted term has been *interprofessional*. In the literature and in practice, nurses encounter other terms that seem similar, such as *multidisciplinary*. Multidisciplinary refers to "a team or collaborative process where members of different disciplines assess or treat patients independently and then share information with each other" (McCallin, 2001, p. 420). The core competency recognizes that "team members integrate their observations, bodies of expertise, and spheres of decision making to coordinate, collaborate, and communicate with one another in order to optimize care for a patient or group of patients" (IOM, 2003, p. 54). This description

is further supported in recent work that examined the need for greater interprofessional education and identified two key definitions (IPEC, 2011, p. 2):

- **Interprofessional teamwork**: The levels of cooperation, coordination, and collaboration characterizing the relationship between professions in delivering patient-centered care.
- **Interprofessional team-based care:** Care delivered by intentionally created, usually relatively small work groups in health care, who are recognized by others as well as by themselves as having a collective identity and shared responsibility for a patient or a group of patients—for example, rapid response team, palliative care team, primary care team, operating room team.

The key difference between these two descriptors for teams is that multidisciplinary focuses on how individual team members do their work and encourages sharing of information with others who are providing care. For example, nurses share information about the nursing care plan with physicians and social workers, and vice versa. This typically is what has been done in health care, but it is not what is recommended in this core competency. The descriptor *interprofessional* is much more involved, emphasizing collective action and in-depth collaboration in planning and implementing care. Less emphasis is placed on what individual team members do, and more emphasis is placed on what individual members can do together to contribute to the joint team plan and initiatives. Use of interprofessional teams improves care delivery, for example, these teams may:

- Decrease fragmentation in a complex care system.
- Provide effective use of multiple types of expertise (for example, medicine, nursing, pharmacy, allied health, social work, and so on).
- Decrease utilization of repetitive or duplicate services.

- Increase creative or innovative solutions to complex problems.
- Increase learning for team members about different roles and responsibilities, communication and coordination, and ways to better plan care.
- Improve motivation and increased self-esteem in team and individual performance.
- Allow for greater sharing of responsibility.
- Empower team members to speak up.

Microsystem

Another way to describe the clinical team is to refer to its role as a **microsystem** (Nelson et al., 2008). A microsystem in a healthcare system has been described as follows: "[A] small group of people who work together on a regular basis to provide care to discrete subpopulations including the patients. It has clinical and business aims, linked processes, [and a] shared information environment and produces performance outcomes. [Microsystems] evolve over time and are (often) embedded in larger organizations. As a type of complex adaptive system, they must: (1) do the work, (2) meet staff needs, and (3) maintain themselves as a clinical unit" (Dartmouth College, 2010). Clinical microsystems serve as direct care or front-line units where there is interaction among patients, families, and care teams. Clinical staff, support staff, processes, technology, communication and information, staff behavior and attitudes, and outcomes are factors that influence microsystems, which should be patient centered. The major focus is to provide care and as care is provided and work is done the team needs to consider the elements of quality, safety, reliability, efficiency and innovation, patient satisfaction, and staff morale.

Team Leadership

Teams typically have designated **team leaders**. For a nursing team, the leader is an RN. Interprofessional teams may have different leaders, and in some cases, the leader may be a nurse. Regardless of who is the leader, all team members are critical to the success of a team. To be effective, a team leader must first recognize that it is the work of the team that is critical. The leader should not focus on personal success as a leader or on the success of any individual team member. Effective team leadership is demonstrated through the effectiveness of the entire team.

Leaders need to know when to guide, when to let the team function, and when to be directive. If the team is on task as planned, direction is not as critical. In contrast, if the team is floundering and not able to get work done, the leader needs to be more active in directing the team, engaging the team to assume more responsibility. Leaders need to encourage and accept members' ideas and actively seek information and ideas from team members. Some of the responsibilities of team leaders are as follows:

- Lead the team—at meetings and in the team's work. Represent the team when the organization requires someone from the team to speak for the team and its activities—for example, with management, committee meetings, and so on.
- Determine or clarify the team's purpose and operating rules or guidelines. Some of this may be predetermined by the organization.
- Select team members. In many cases, someone other than the team leader or the organization's policies determine who will serve on a team; for example, team members may be assigned to a unit or a particular patient.
- Orient team members to the team, including coaching and training new members.
- Determine the plan of action with team members' participation. After the team reviews information, discusses issues, and arrives at team decisions, the team leader ensures that there is an effective plan of action. If it is a clinical team, keep the focus on the patient(s).

- Determine how to make the team more effective given the time constraints.
- Provide resources and information to the team as needed.
- Update the team as necessary.
- Ensure that the team's plan of action is implemented as designed.
- Recognize the team's work as well as the work of individuals.
- Resolve conflict when it occurs.
- Evaluate the team's outcomes; include input from all team members; strive for improvement. This information then feeds into the organization's quality improvement program.
- **Encourage team learning to improve effectiveness.**
- Ensure that required information about team functioning, decisions, and actions implemented is documented.
- Accept feedback from team members and others who may be involved.
- Provide feedback to team members and the team as a whole.
- Ensure that the team effectively uses collaboration, coordination, communication, and delegation.

Development of Effective Teams

The word *team* implies there is a group of people, but how do they develop into a team? To just say, "Today this group of staff is a team," does not mean that the group is actually functioning as a team. It takes time to develop a team. The term *team* does not include the letter *I*, and this is important to note. Teams are about groups of people who work collaboratively, not about individuals. However, it takes effort and time to move a team to a state where it is truly functioning as a team and not as a group of individuals (Weinstock, 2010). The most common scenario is that team members work in "silos" most of the time and then come together periodically to collaborate and communicate. Unfortunately, this pattern leads to problems and errors, which may then affect team functioning. The development of an effective team is critical to the success of new and innovative methods such as briefings before handoffs, checklists, and time-outs before surgery, such as the Situation–background–assessment– recommendations (SBAR; a standardized communication method), TeamSTEPPS®, and others. Organizations that just use these methods without working on developing effective teams to be effective will not be as successful, but using them in combination with teamwork creates a more effective organization and improved care outcomes. These methods are described in this chapter and other chapters.

TeamSTEPPS is an evidence-based teamwork system aimed at optimizing patient outcomes by improving communication and teamwork skills among healthcare professionals. It was developed by the Department of Defense, and now the Agency for Healthcare Research and Quality (AHRQ) assists in making this resource available to healthcare organizations (HHS, AHRQ, 2017). The system and its resources include a comprehensive set of ready-to-use materials and a training curriculum to successfully integrate teamwork principles into any healthcare system (HHS, AHRQ, 2016). **Figure 10-2** describes the TeamSTEPPS model, and **Figure 10-3** provides an overview of the TeamSTEPPS action planning.

Within a team, members have informal and formal roles, and some members may assume multiple roles at different times as team members interact. Heller (1999, p. 42) defines some of these roles:

- *Coordinator:* Pulls together the work of the team
- *Critic:* Keeps an eye on the team's effectiveness
- *Idea person:* Encourages the team to be innovative
- *Implementer:* Ensures that the team's functioning is effective
- *External contact:* Looks after the team's external contacts and relationships
- *Inspector:* Ensures that standards are met
- *Team builder:* Develops the team spirit

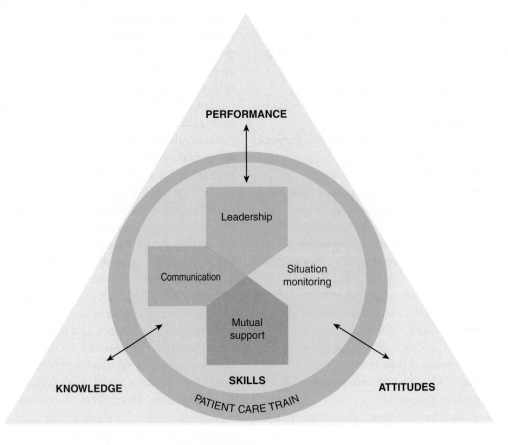

The TeamSTEPPS triangle logo is a visual model that represents some basic but critical concepts related to teamwork training as explained below.

Individuals can learn four primary trainable teamwork skills. These are:

1. Leadership.
2. Communication.
3. Situation monitoring.
4. Mutual support.

If a team has tools and strategies it can leverage to build a fundamental level of competency in each of those skills, research has shown that the team can enhance three types of teamwork outcomes:

1. Performance.
2. Knowledge.
3. Attitudes.

Figure 10-2 TeamSTEPPS®

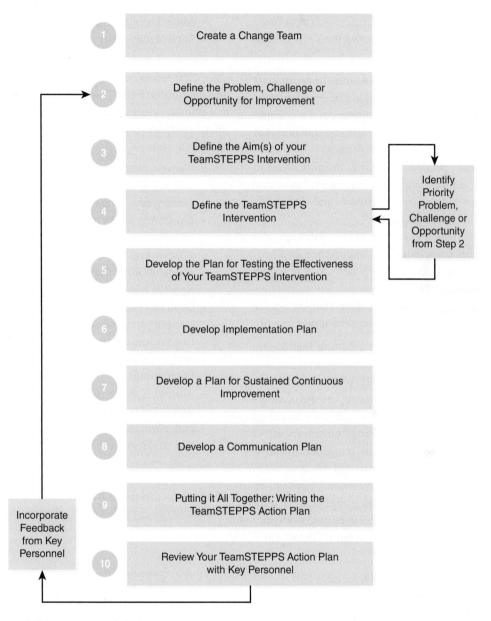

Figure 10-3 TeamSTEPPS®: Action Planning At-a-Glance

Reproduced from Agency for Healthcare Research and Quality (AHRQ). (October 2014). The quick reference guide to TeamSTEPPS® action planning. Retrieved from http://www.ahrq.gov/professionals/education/curriculum-tools/teamstepps/instructor/essentials/implguide3.html

The four areas of particular concern that need to be considered when evaluating team effectiveness are (IOM, 2001, p. 132):

1. Team makeup, such as having the appropriate team size and composition of members and the ability to reduce status differences (for example, between the nurse manager and staff nurses or between nurses and physicians).
2. Team processes, such as communication structure, conflict management, leadership that emphasizes excellence, and clear goals and expectations.
3. Nature of team tasks, such as matching roles with knowledge and experience and promoting cohesiveness when work is highly interdependent.
4. Environment context, such as obtaining needed resources and establishing appropriate rewards.

"Effective teams have a culture that fosters openness, collaboration, teamwork, and learning from mistakes" (IOM, 2001, p. 132). Healthcare delivery tends to overemphasize personal accountability of healthcare professionals such as nurses and physicians, and this may negatively affect teamwork. Teams often resort to uncoordinated or sequential action rather than collaborative work, which is required for effective teams. TeamSTEPPS identifies the following barriers to effective to team performance. These barriers can be used to identify areas to assess and improve team performance (HHS, AHRQ, 2014a):

- Inconsistency in team membership
- Lack of time
- Lack of information sharing
- Hierarchy
- Defensiveness
- Conventional thinking
- Varying communication styles
- Conflict
- Lack of coordination and follow-up
- Fatigue
- Workload

- Misinterpretation of cues
- Lack of role clarity

Because there is more focus on quality improvement (QI) teams need to be concerned with QI, on a continuous basis. TeamSTEPPS recommends that team structure can be used to support patient safety, particularly in the following areas (HHS, AHRQ, 2014a):

- *Communication*: Structured process by which information is clearly and accurately exchanged among team members.
- *Leadership*: Ability to maximize the activities or team members by ensuring that team actions and are understood, changes in information are shared, and team members have the necessary resources.
- *Situation monitoring*: Process of actively scanning and assessing situational elements to gain information or understanding, or to maintain awareness to support team functioning.
- *Mutual support*: Ability to anticipate and support team members' needs through accurate knowledge about their responsibilities and workload.

Stop and Consider #2
Teamwork makes a difference in effective teams.

Improving Team
Communication

Communication is important throughout the healthcare system, but it is critical for teams. They cannot function without communication, and *effective* communication makes a difference in team functioning. An important role for team leaders is to lead the team's activities, and much of this is done through team discussion and also discussion with non–team members. The process of leading discussions can be informal or formal. When the team leader seeks out individual team members to discuss team issues and the team's work, this is informal discussion. In this situation, the leader is seeking an open discussion of issues and sharing of ideas. Such an exchange can help the leader to better understand team members and identify issues that are important to the team's functioning and activities. Informal discussion can also be used for the team members to get to know the leader on a different level. Formal communication typically takes place in meetings and through written communication methods.

Overview of Communication

All nurses communicate—with other nurses, other staff, patients, families, and others who impact patient care. The assumption is that individuals know how to communicate effectively, and this is not always true. Nurses have an ethical mandate to become skilled communicators; doing so is an essential standard of practice (O'Keefe & Saver, 2014; Kuppeschmidt, Kientz, Ward, & Reinholz, 2010). What is important is the effectiveness of this communication. Teams must communicate, too. The effectiveness of team communication may also vary, but it is clear that communication makes a difference in results, decreases errors, and improves the work environment.

Individuals have communication styles, and understanding one's style is important. Some people are more passive; others use more nonverbal communication; others prefer to see important information in writing; and so on. Using professional jargon often creates a barrier, limiting clear communication. This is why using structured communication practices such as SBAR, call-out, and check-back is important in reducing communication barriers. Within these methods, all healthcare providers use the same terminology and process so that they do not have to take time to figure out the process or what someone else means.

Communication is the sharing of a message between one person or group and another. It is important to know if the message was received as sent. Interpretation has a major impact on effective communication, and sometimes interpretation confuses or changes the original message. Nonverbal communication also has an impact on the message sent. If a team member verbally affirms commitment to an action but the team member's facial expression shows a lack of interest (such as no eye contact or a hurried manner), the message of commitment may be viewed as noncommitment. As team members get to know one another, they learn each other's communication styles, including nonverbal methods. This knowledge confers an advantage in that it can improve and speed up communication. Nevertheless, in some cases, team members may jump to conclusions, and communication may not be clear. The same could be applied to student communication in the classroom or in team discussions.

The Joint Commission analyzed data related to healthcare quality from 2004 to 2012 and concluded that communication issues were the major reasons for deaths related to a delay in treatment. Data from 2010 to 2012 indicated that communication was the third highest root cause of sentinel events (The Joint Commission, 2013; O'Keeffe & Saver, 2014). Not communicating is the major issue in communication breakdown. Situations that are most at risk for communication breakdown include those involving broken rules or taking shortcuts (workarounds), mistakes or use of poor clinical judgment, lack of support, incompetence, poor teamwork, disrespect, and micromanagement when someone abuses authority (Maxfield, Grenny, McMillan, Patterson, & Switzler, 2005). Clearly, effective communication is critical for delivery of quality health care and something that must be frequently monitored and improved.

The relationships and communication between nurses and physicians have long been important healthcare issues because they have an impact on the quality of care and work satisfaction. One small study that included 20 medical and surgical residents examined their attitudes toward nurses (Weinberg, Miner, & Rivlin, 2009). In this study, 19 of the 20 residents shared examples of poor communication or problematic relationships with nurses, but the important result was the residents did not feel such issues presented a problem for patient care because the nurse's role was to follow orders and nothing more. The residents did say that when nurses were knowledgeable and collaborative, such qualities had positive effects on the residents and on patient care—which, of course, contradicts their view of the importance of nurses' contribution to health care. Knowledgeable and collaborative nurses were able to anticipate and respond to needs of and then work with residents to identify patient needs and interventions. This working relationship was part of the residents' positive comments; however, this was not the common experience. This type of result indicates that residents view nurses with more education and experience in a more positive light, suggesting there might be a more collaborative relationship formed in this circumstance. Because this study focused on residents, transferring these results to experienced physicians is not possible; they represent a different sample. This study also did not examine nurses' views of the medical residents.

In reality, this is not a one-sided perspective, and blame for poor communication with nurses cannot just be placed on nurses, medical residents, or any other specific type of staff. Nurses have responsibilities in the communication process, and their role in this partnership is complicated, too. There is more of a power struggle today because of the increased number of female physicians, increased number of nurse practitioners, increased nursing autonomy, and decreased perception of physician esteem due to accessibility of information online (Nair, Fitzpatrick, McNulty, Click, & Glembocki, 2012). It is easy to stereotype and to frequently complain about doctors; however, this is not helpful.

Researchers tend to focus on physician–nurse communication, but there is much more to communication in healthcare settings—for example, nurse to nurse, nurse to unlicensed personnel, nurse to other healthcare professionals, and nurse to administrators/managers. All of these communication processes are critical to effective functioning of the healthcare delivery systems, yet problems occur in all of these interaction combinations.

Another recent study that focused on quality care reached an interesting conclusion related to the issue of interprofessional teamwork (Curry et al., 2011). This study examined factors that may be related to better performance in care of patients with an acute myocardial infarction diagnosis, which the study measured by assessing risk-standardized mortality rates. The sample included 11 hospitals and 158 staff members. The high-performing hospitals demonstrated organizational cultures that supported improved care for this patient population. The conclusion was that evidence-based protocols and processes are important but not sufficient to reach high hospital performance. These hospitals had clear organizational values and goals, senior management was involved, communication and coordination were evident in broad staff presence and expertise, and problem solving and learning were important. These are all elements of effective teamwork, which does make a difference in patient outcomes, and depending on the effectiveness of the team, it can be negative or positive.

Formal Meetings

Formal meetings are an important part of teamwork, and the team leader or someone designated by the leader usually leads these meetings. Besides participating in team meetings, team members and leaders may participate in a variety of meetings: staff meetings, committees, task forces, staff education sessions, and so on.

Formal meetings can be held in a variety of settings. The most common site is a conference room in the healthcare setting. The setting should be private and conducive to fostering communication.

Space should be provided for team members to sit and take notes. In clinical settings, telephone access is important, although members should be encouraged to keep interruptions to a minimum—with the increasing use of cell phones this can be a challenge.

Another method for conducting meetings today is virtual conferencing, including conference calls, video conferencing, and Internet conferencing. These methods also require planning and equipment. Members must be informed about access requirements, and technological support may be needed to assist with possible connection problems. The following guide recommends steps for conducting formal team meetings:

- *Planning the meeting*: Planning before the meeting is important. Avoid scheduling meetings just to have a meeting. Time is too limited. Staff will be reluctant to attend and may not be productive in meetings they feel are not worthwhile. Before completing the final agenda, the leader might survey members via email for additional agenda items.
- *Steps before the meeting*: Arrange for meeting space and any technology required. Send out the agenda, any necessary handouts, and minutes from the last meeting. Allow time for this material to be reviewed. Typically, these items are now sent electronically. If there is no designated "minutes taker" or secretary, the leader may ask a member to assume this role.
- *Meeting time:* Meetings should begin and end on time. All members should make an effort to be on time, come prepared, and follow the agenda. The leader should guide the meeting to ensure the agenda is followed. At the beginning of the meeting, minutes should be reviewed and approved—the minutes are the team's documentation. The leader is responsible for making sure all members have the opportunity to participate. If the discussion digresses from the agenda or

becomes volatile, the leader needs to guide the discussion back to the topic and away from personal reactions. Decisions should be clearly identified. The minutes should reflect action items, persons responsible for those items who may or may not be team members, and timelines for completion. Planning and conducting a meeting in an orderly fashion indicates that a team member's time is valued and accountability for actions is an expectation.

- *After the meeting:* Minutes are finalized. The leader and members complete actions that require follow-up or as designated in the team's decision plan timeline. A report of these actions should be addressed at the next meeting or may be sent to members to report progress as needed.
- *Evaluation of meetings:* Consider these questions: (1) Did the meeting have a clearly defined purpose (agenda)? (2) Were there measurable outcomes (do the minutes provide data, and were they met)? (3) What was the attendance level? (4) Did members participate in the meeting(s), or was the leader doing all of the talking? (5) Is it easy to identify actions taken?

Another type of meeting that is common among clinical teams is the patient care planning meeting. Such meetings may take place daily, each shift, or several times a week. The purpose of these meetings is to assess patient care and determine the patient plan of care. This type of meeting is typically less structured than the formal meeting (for example, no structured agenda or minutes). However, the team leader does need to plan the topics for discussion. The team may develop a common order in which patient issues are discussed. Notes should be kept, although they need not be formal minutes. The team may add changes to the patient's plan of care or other standard clinical documents. The responsibilities noted earlier for team leaders remain the same for the clinical planning team as for other types of teams. In this type of meeting staff are typically anxious to get to their work so a focused meeting is critical.

In many hospitals, patient rounds are also used for planning. Staff members as a team go to the patient's bedside to talk with the patient and assess needs. The patient should be an active participant in the rounds, although this is not always the case. Rounds may be interprofessional (the ideal method) or focused on a specific profession (such as nursing rounds or physician rounds). Patient rounds are discussed in this text in quality improvement content.

Debriefing

Effective teams need to incorporate debriefing as one of their routine communication methods. It can improve team and individual provider performance. *Debriefing* is defined as "a dialogue between two or more people; its goals are to discuss the actions and thought processes involved in a particular patient care situation, encourage reflection on those actions and thought processes, and incorporate improvement into future performance. The function of debriefing is to identify aspects of team performance that went well, and those that did not. The discussion then focuses on determining opportunities for improvement at the individual, team, and system level" (HHS, AHRQ, PSNet, 2016). It is important that debriefing is used as a learning tool and not to take punitive steps to identify individuals who may have made an error. There are three common phases to debriefing.

1. *Description or reactions*: The leader asks team members for their perspectives.
2. *Analysis*: The analysis phase prioritizes concerns and rationales discussed. This phase, as is true for all phases, requires an environment in which staff feel comfortable in being direct with one another and respect other perspectives.

3. *Application*: This phase focuses on summarizing the key points learned so that they can be applied as needed.

Effective debriefing demonstrates clear communication, clear and known roles and responsibilities, understanding of the context of the problem or situation, sharing of workload, and continuous monitoring.

Assertiveness

Assertiveness is a communication style that is often confused with aggression and, therefore, may be viewed negatively. Assertiveness, however, is important, though many nurses have to learn how to use it effectively. Using assertiveness, a person stands up for what he or she believes in but does not push or control others. The assertive nurse uses *I* statements when communicating thoughts and feelings and *you* statements when persuading others (Fabre, 2005).

Fabre also recommends that nurses need to approach situations calmly, reducing emotional responses. When problems occur, delaying response usually is not helpful; however, if emotions are high a "cool down" period may be advised. As discussed in other content in the text on communication we need to consider our audience and use terminology that others can understand.

Nurses need to break the code of silence (Fabre, 2005). Nurses are often silent, keeping their opinions to themselves rather than being open with the treatment team and management. This pattern of not communicating most likely reflects low self-esteem of the profession as a whole, which has a very negative impact—namely, loss of valuable nursing input. Speaking up may be risky, but the results can be worthwhile. It may take time for team members to value one another's opinions and expertise. If done in a professional manner with the goal of collaboration and coordination, over time most team members begin to respect and trust one another;

they see value in the team's diversity of multiple healthcare professionals and variety in experience.

Listening

Listening is an important skill to develop. Most people think they listen when they really do not do so effectively. Effective listening is important when delivering care—to the patient and family, in working in teams, and with colleagues. Most people probably would say that they listen, but listening takes practice. There are also a number of barriers to effective listening:

- Anxiety and stress
- Distractions and interruptions
- Too many tasks to do
- Fatigue and hunger
- Lack of self-esteem
- Anger
- Overwork
- Reaction from the past
- Confusing message

In addition, the team member may not think individual team members' opinions are valued, leading the member to tune out or exhibit a lack of concern or respect for the communicator. The opposite can also occur with the team member thinking he or she knows enough and thus does not need to listen.

When you recognize that you are not listening, you should think about what is interfering with your listening. What is the barrier(s) at the moment? Through this self-examination, you can learn more about the listening process and improve your listening skills—and, in turn, your communication skills. Fabre (2005, p. 80) identifies why listening is important beyond generally improving communication; it is critical to effective identification and description of problems:

- Listening exposes feelings—those invaluable, but sometimes inconvenient, traits that make us truly human.

- Listening jump-starts the solution process because answers may pop up during candid conversations.
- Listening relieves stress. Bottling up thoughts and feelings simply depletes our energy.
- Active listening is more than hearing; it requires communicating to the other person that you are listening.
- Just saying "yes" and "no" is not active listening.
- Paraphrasing communicates that you have listened.

Nurse–physician communication has long been an important topic, probably more so in nursing than in medicine. In addition to the studies mentioned earlier, other studies have examined this issue and the impact of collaboration on care (Baggs et al., 1999; Fairchild, Hogan, Smith, Portnow, & Bates, 2002; Higgins, 1999; Thomas, Sexton, & Helmreich, 2003). These studies indicate communication problems can affect collaboration and, consequently, patient outcomes. In one study, two nurses and one physician conducted a study using focus groups of nurses and physicians. They identified methods to improve nurse–physician communication (Burke, Boal, & Mitchell, 2004). The researchers noted that some communication problems require major organizational changes—system changes. Suggested methods that are not as system focused but rather are steps individual nurses could take to improve are:

- Develop a personal connection, which helps to increase colleagueship.
- Use humor.
- Make the assumption that you are on the same team.
- Recognize that team members are equal in their expertise, which can be important to patient care.
- If you speak frequently to a physician over the phone, arrange to meet in person; a face-to-face interaction may improve your communication over the phone.

- Report good news about patients—improvements, not just problems.
- Recognize that conflict will occur, but this does not mean that communication and collaboration cannot be maintained.
- Discuss preferred methods of communication (telephone, email, pager, in person, voice message) and under which circumstances they should be used.
- Ask for parameters regarding when the physician wants to be called.
- Plan ahead for meetings or times of contact so that you are prepared with information and know what you want to communicate. Provide clinically pertinent information.
- Work with the physician to determine the best methods for communicating with the family, and determine who should contact whom and for what purposes.

Mindful Communication

Mindful communication is a process by which actively aware individuals engage in communication that is meaningful, is timely, and responds continually as events unfold (Anthony & Vidal, 2010; O'Keefe & Saver, 2014, p. 9). It is easy to assume that one is communicating and participating in an active way by talking—but more needs to be done about how we communicate, verbally and nonverbally, and why. Then we consider what needs to be communicated and, finally, whether we really did communicate the message we wanted to send. This all requires us to consider the receiver of the message. Many factors affect how our message will be received and even if it will be received as intended. In healthcare settings, these factors are even more complex. Patients are sick, and their communication may not be at the patient's usual level. The same can be said for families and significant others. Many factors in the work setting, such as stress, miscommunication, power, past problems and current ones, supervisory inadequacies, policies and procedures, understaffing, staff not prepared, workload, and so

on, all impact communication—staff to staff, staff to patients and families, and others. Use of mindful, more conscious communication can make a difference in clear communication, sent and received in a timely manner. Consider emails—how often do we quickly write an email without thinking about the content or tone and hit the send button only to realize then or later that we could have done better. This applies to all forms of communication—oral, written, and electronic. Mindfulness is discussed in other chapters in this text.

SBAR

The **situation–background–assessment–recommendations (SBAR)** is a structured communication method that is used to improve team communication (typically, interprofessional, such as physician to nurse, but also other types of teams, such as nursing teams). It focuses on critical information about a patient that requires immediate attention and action. To ensure more effective communication, a consistent process is used that includes the following steps (IHI, 2011a):

- **S**ituation: What is going on with the patient?
- **B**ackground: What is the clinical background or context?
- **A**ssessment: What do I think the problem is?
- **R**ecommendation: What would I do to correct it?

This process includes use of the call-out and the check-back. The **call-out** is used to communicate important or critical information that lets all team members hear the information at the same time and clarifies responsibilities. The **check-back** provides assurance that the team members heard and understood the information from the sender. **Exhibit 10-1** offers an example of SBAR in action.

Checklists

Dr. Atul Gawande (2009) wrote *The Checklist Manifesto* to address safety in the surgical arena. His document mandates that all staff working in

Exhibit 10-1 SBAR Example

This is an example of how SBAR might be used to focus the message in a telephone call between a nurse and a physician. The nurse would not wait for the physician to ask these questions, but rather would routinely provide the information in clear statements as indicated by SBAR.

Situation: What is going on with the patient? A nurse finds a patient on the floor. She calls the doctor: "I am the charge nurse on the night shift on 5 West. I am calling about Mrs. Jones. She was found on the floor and is complaining of pain in her hip."

Background: What is the clinical background or context? "The patient is a 75-year-old woman who was admitted for pneumonia yesterday. She did not complain of hip pain before being found on the floor."

Assessment: What do I think the problem is? "I think the fall may have caused an injury. Her pain is level 7 out of 10. Vital signs are normal."

Recommendation: What would I do to correct it or respond to it? "I think we need to get an X-ray immediately and have her seen by the orthopedic resident."

---

the surgical arena should follow a **checklist**. This checklist itemizes a list of activities that should be examined by the team *before* surgery takes place to ensure clear communication and certainty about actions to be taken. Gawande based his work on the checklist approach used by pilots to ensure safety during takeoff, landing, and during other critical points in a flight. We now see checklists used in different areas of health care to ensure processes are followed and identify potential risks or near misses before they lead to harm and improve care. Checklists are not just associated with improving care—reducing errors, but effective use of checklists is connected to how a team might function. A study examined whether perceptions of teamwork predicted use of checklist (Singer et al., 2016). In this study, the checklist was used in surgery in only 3% of the surgical cases. When it was used, the team leader, the surgeon, had a significant impact on this use—the leader believed in the use of the checklist and provided clinical leadership, clear communication, and effective teamwork.

Stop and Consider #3
Improving your communication is an ongoing process.

Healthcare Team
Members: Which Knowledge and Competencies Do They Need?

Team members may be viewed as **followers**. This is not a negative term. If there were no members or followers, there would be no team. There may be times when a follower, leader of a subgroup, or another member must assume the leadership role, such as in the absence of the team leader; however, in most cases, team members are followers. The follower role should not be a passive one, but rather a very active one. Each member needs to feel a responsibility to participate actively in the work of the team and feel that the members have the right to help the team determine its rules, structure, and activities.

Effective teams need members who engage with one another as the team works. This requires ability to effectively communicate, negotiate, and delegate. Team members need to assess their own dynamics and use time management to get their work done, which requires sharing information in timely manner with staff who need it. Sometimes team members are not in the same site, and in this case, the team needs to determine how they will work together to communicate and coordinate so that outcomes can be met. It is inevitable that teams may experience conflict, either within the team or with persons or teams external to the team. This requires use of conflict resolution, which is discussed later in this chapter. Effective teamwork takes time and effort, but the results can be much better than individual's functioning alone.

Recent work that has sought to clarify ways to ensure interprofessional team education has identified key competencies for all healthcare professions related to teamwork (IPEC, 2011, pp. 19, 21, 23, 25). The following competencies might look like they form a to-do list. In a way they do because these are the expected actions/competencies of the healthcare team:

- Work with individuals of other professions to maintain a climate of mutual respect and shared values.
- Use the knowledge of one's own role and the roles of other professions to appropriately assess and address the healthcare needs of patients and populations served.
- Communicate with patients, families, communities, and other health professionals in a responsive and responsible manner that supports a team approach to the maintenance of health and treatment of disease.
- Apply relationship-building values and the principles of team dynamics to perform effectively in different team roles to plan and deliver patient/population-centered care that is safe, timely, efficient, effective, and equitable.

Accomplishing these competencies requires greater emphasis on interprofessional education for all healthcare profession students.

Stop and Consider #4
Followers are as important to teams as are leaders.

Teams and Decision
Making

Teams make decisions about the work that they need to do and use problem solving as they make decisions. The amount and quality of information that is required and the number of possible solutions for a problem affect decisions. The schedule is very important; for example, is an immediate decision required, or can time be taken to consider options carefully? Many clinical teams must act quickly in response to clinical problems. These teams need to develop quick thinking and analytic skills (depending on the expertise of team members), trust one another, weigh benefits and risks, and move to a decision. At other times, teams may have more time to fully analyze an issue or problem, brainstorm possible solutions, and develop a consensus regarding the best decision—for example, a decision made by a committee. Teams must recognize that there may not be a perfect solution (there rarely is) and that there is risk, but decisions need to be made. Not making a decision is really making a decision—to do nothing is a decision. Several decision-making styles may be used (Milgram, Spector, & Treger, 1999, p. 42):

- *Decisive decision making* depends on minimal data to arrive at a single solution or decision.
- *The integrative style* uses as much data as possible to arrive at several reasonable solutions or decisions.
- *The hierarchic style* uses a large amount of data and organizes the data to arrive at one optimal decision.
- *The flexible style* relies on minimal data but generates several different options or will shift focus as the data are interpreted.

A team leader and the team typically use more than one decision-making style, depending on the issue or problem. It is important to understand styles used by team members and the team leader, who is also a team member.

Key questions that are asked during decision-making are: (1) What is the issue, problem, or task to be done and the desired outcome? (2) What type of data do we need? (3) How complicated and substantial is the issue, problem, or task? (4) How many possible solutions or approaches are there, and what are they? (5) Can the desired outcome(s) be met with acceptable cost–benefit standards? (Note that cost is more than financial; it could refer to the patient's health status if an outcome is not achieved or risk of an error due to a decision-making problem, and so on.) **Figure 10-4** illustrates team thinking. **Exhibit 10-2** provides an example of a team-thinking inventory that teams can use to assess their thinking.

Stop and Consider #5
Team decision making never stops.

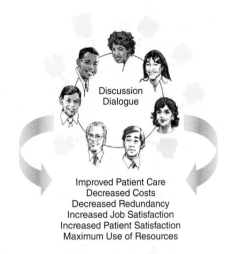

Discussion
Dialogue

Improved Patient Care
Decreased Costs
Decreased Redundancy
Increased Job Satisfaction
Increased Patient Satisfaction
Maximum Use of Resources

Figure 10-4 Interprofessional Team Thinking

Reproduced from Rubenfeld, M. & Scheffer, B. (2015). *Critical thinking tactics for nurses.* Burlington, MA: Jones & Bartlett Learning.

Exhibit 10-2 Team-Thinking Inventory

- Which strategies are used to help team members think about the big picture as well as the parts?
- Which strategies are used to help team members see the situation from different perspectives?
- Which strategies are used to help team members see their biases and assumptions?
- Which strategies help team members think about patterns and interrelationships of issues and parts of problems?
- Which strategies are used to help team members think beyond cause-and-effect consequences?
- Does the thinking that occurs in the team resemble simple sharing of information or discussion/dialogue? Why? How can you move in the direction of discussion/dialogue?
- What is done to encourage team members to share their thinking or feel comfortable enough to talk about it?
- How is conflict managed in the team to promote thinking instead of discouraging it?

- Which other sources of gratification, besides interprofessional teamwork, are available for team members to socialize, obtain recognition, and interact?
- How were the interprofessional team members prepared for their thinking roles?
- How does the team deal with ambiguity? How long can team members tolerate not having a solution?
- How does the team examine its own thinking processes (for example, how it works, not what it is doing), and who is doing it?

From Rubenfeld, M. & Scheffer, B. (2015). *Critical thinking tactics for nurses.* Burlington, MA: Jones & Bartlett Learning. Data adapted from Senge, P. (1998). *The fifth discipline: The art and practice of the learning organization.* New York, NY: Doubleday; Bensimon, E. & Neumann, A. (1993). *Redesigning collegiate leadership: Teams and teamwork in higher education* Baltimore, MD: Johns Hopkins University Press; and Brookfield, S. & Peskill, S. (1999). *Discussion as a way of teaching: Tools and techniques for democratic classrooms.* San Francisco, CA: Jossey-Bass.

Collaboration

Collaboration is an integral part of patient-centered care and safe, quality care. When staff or team members work in a collaborative environment, it is a satisfying work experience with limited conflict. **Collaboration** means that all the people involved are listened to and decisions are developed together. Views are respected; however, at some point, decisions must be made, and not all views or opinions will be part of the final decision. Compromise is part of effective collaboration. The goal is to arrive at the best possible decision. Working with others increases the possibility of having the best decision because there is greater availability of ideas and dialogue about ideas and solutions. Though diversity may cause barriers, it can also improve decision-making by providing different viewpoints to better understand an issue.

The American Nurses Association (ANA) standard on collaboration states, "the registered nurse collaborates with the healthcare consumer and other key stakeholders in the conduct of nursing practice" (2015a, p. 73). The standard supports patient-centered care. It requires nurses to communicate, collaborate with the plan of care, promote conflict management, build consensus, engage in teamwork, cooperate, and partner with others to effect change and produce positive outcomes while adhering to professional standards and codes of conduct. Effective collaboration requires understanding who are the potential stakeholders or partners; their expertise, level of power and influence and common goals.

Another factor that influences collaboration that is not always considered is space and environment (Gum, Prideaux, Sweet, & Greenhill, 2012). What does this mean? In most clinical units, there is a space that is central to coordinating work. In many hospitals, this space is called the nurses' station; however, this title may act as a barrier to improving interprofessional collaboration. The title for the

space should not focus on one profession. This is changing but is still a problem in some healthcare organizations. Teams need space in which they can collaborate, discuss issues and patients, plan, and so on. This then means the space needs to be conducive to privacy and quiet, with limited interruptions. The station as described here does not usually meet these criteria—it is noisy, offers little privacy, and is often crowded and stressful. Nurses and others need to consider the space in which they work and collaborate.

Collaboration requires that open communication take place and team members feel comfortable expressing their opinions even when they disagree. Team members of different healthcare professions must work across professional boundaries to develop a team culture of working together. The goal is not to make an individual's profession look good, but rather to focus on the team as a whole. Even when the team is composed of members from the same healthcare profession, such as a nursing team, the focus is on the team, not individuals. This does not mean that conflicts will not occur, but some can be prevented. When conflict does occur, the team uses effective methods for coping to reach a common goal.

Stop and Consider #6

Healthcare delivery requires more and more collaboration.

Coordination

Nurses coordinate patient care through planning and implementing care, and they have been involved in the development of care **coordination** throughout its evolution (Lamb, 2013). "Care coordination involves deliberately organizing patient care activities and sharing information among all of the participants concerned with a patient's care to achieve safer and more effective care. This means that the patient's needs and preferences are known ahead of time and communicated at the right time to the right people, and that this information is used to provide safe, appropriate, and effective care to the patient" (HHS, AHRQ, 2014b). Effective coordination needs to be interprofessional. Coordination and collaboration should be interconnected. Care is complex, and patients require healthcare providers with different expertise to meet these needs. With this type of situation, the different providers need to collaborate to reach a plan and then implement care in a manner that makes sense—meeting the timeline required, with minimal conflict and confusion.

Although the need for care coordination is clear, there are obstacles within the U.S. healthcare system that must be overcome to provide this type of care. Redesigning a healthcare system in order to better coordinate patients' care is important for the following reasons (HHS, AHRQ, 2014b):

- Current healthcare systems are often disjointed, and processes vary among and between primary care sites and specialty sites.
- Patients are often unclear about why they are being referred from primary care to a specialist, how to make appointments, and what to do after seeing a specialist.
- Specialists do not consistently receive clear reasons for the referral or adequate information on tests that have already been done. Primary care physicians do not often receive information about what happened in a referral visit.
- Referral staff deal with many different processes and lost information, which means that care is less efficient.

Coordination through team effort—working to see that the pieces and activities fit together and flow as they should—can help to meet patient outcomes. "Conscious patient-centered coordination of care not only improves the patient experience, it also leads to better long-term health outcomes, as demonstrated by fewer unnecessary trips to the hospital, fewer repeated tests, fewer conflicting

prescriptions, and clearer advice about the best course of treatment" (HHS, 2013).

Patients often complain about the number of care providers that interact with them. They may not know who is responsible for which aspects of their care, and they receive confusing and often conflicting communication and information. The patient needs to have an anchor—a healthcare provider to whom the patient can turn for support and knowledge of the plan. Basically, patients are saying that they are not the center of care and their care is fragmented. This leads to an increased risk of errors and decreases the quality of care. Care is coordinated through the implementation of the care plan, documentation of care, and teamwork. Healthcare teams that recognize these concerns can help patients more, engaging patients in the care and as a member of the care team. All of this increases opportunities to improve care and reach outcomes.

Barriers and Competencies Related to Coordination

Coordination is not easy to achieve even when team members want to achieve it. Some of the barriers to effective coordination are listed here:

- Failure of team members to understand the roles and responsibilities of other team members, particularly members from different healthcare professions
- Lack of a clear interprofessional plan of care
- Limited leadership
- Overwork and excessive burden of team member responsibilities
- Ineffective communication, both oral and written
- Lack of inclusion of the patient and family/significant others in the care process
- Competition among team members to control decisions

Despite these barriers, coordination can be achieved through use of effective interventions.

First, the team must recognize that coordination is critical and strive to ensure that it is used. The team needs to understand the purpose and goals of coordination and work to achieve them. To do so, the team must evaluate its work and be willing to identify weaknesses and figure out methods to improve coordination. Team members need to communicate openly and in a timely manner. Teams that effectively solve problems together will improve their coordination. Delegation, discussed elsewhere in this chapter, is an important part of coordination. One person cannot do everything (and that one person may not even be the best person for the task or activity). Coordination requires team members who understand the different roles and expertise of the members, determine the best member to deliver care to meet the timeline, and then evaluate the outcomes.

Tools to Improve Coordination

Health care has developed a variety of tools and methods to increase coordination. From a chronic illness perspective, disease management is a process used to improve coordination and collaboration, typically using practice guidelines and clinical protocols or pathways. A **clinical protocol** or **pathway** is a written guide to provide direction for specific clinical problems. The pathway content includes interventions, timeline, and resources needed; identifies expected outcomes; and provides a sequencing of interventions to reach the outcomes. **Figure 10-5** provides examples of information categories that might be found in a clinical pathway.

Pathways are developed in a number of ways. In some situations, healthcare organizations may create them by identifying focus areas based on needs commonly found in their patients—for example, pathways that focus on the care of a diabetic patient who has been hospitalized, a patient who needs a hip replacement and then rehabilitation, or

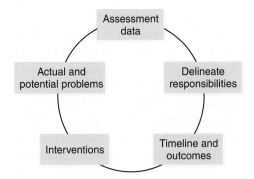

Figure 10-5 Categories of Information Found in Clinical Pathways

a patient who is severely depressed and suicidal. An interprofessional team of experts then develops the pathway describing expected care and outcomes. Current literature and evidence from research should be used when developing pathways, and examples from other hospitals or examples found in professional literature may be used. In other situations, the healthcare organization may decide to use a published clinical pathway rather than develop one for the organization. After the clinical pathway is developed or selected, staff members need training about the pathway and its use. Pathways can be used to evaluate care and outcomes by collecting data about their use and the patients' outcomes. The question to be addressed during evaluation is simple: Does the pathway, or specific interventions within a pathway, make a difference? Are expected outcomes met?

There are a number of advantages to using clinical protocols or pathways. First, this type of tool improves team coordination and increases the likelihood of meeting outcomes. Because clinical protocols or pathways are written and based on evidence, there is a care standard and greater consistency in care provided, which should enhance quality of care and facilitate evidence-based practice. However, whenever a pathway is used, the team must review the standard pathway to ensure that it meets the individual needs of the patient and then adapt it accordingly. Other advantages of using clinical protocols or pathways include more effective use of expertise and resources, better management of healthcare costs, improved collaboration and communication, decreased errors, improved patient satisfaction (because patients feel that their care is organized and they are more informed), improved care documentation (because it follows a consistent plan), improved identification of responsibilities, and a clear statement of interventions.

Stop and Consider #7
Coordination is a major responsibility of teams.

Incivility in Healthcare
Work Environment

Nurses work closely with physicians, and this relationship has a long history of conflict. Often it is stereotyped as "us versus them," which is an unhealthy approach. With the greater emphasis on teamwork, nurses and physicians are slowly being forced into improving their work relationships. This change in attitude really needs to begin at the student level. Organizations need to stand behind efforts to improve team collaboration, coordination, and communication. One area that has received special attention is abuse—usually verbal—from physician to nurse. Unfortunately, this is also a problem from nurse to nurse—incivility or bullying among nurses is now found in healthcare organizations as well as in schools of nursing.

In schools of nursing, incivility is found among students and faculty, in both student–faculty and student–student interactions. Students may also experience bullying with nurses during their clinical experiences or observe it. In 2008, the National Student Nurses Association published an article about incivility in its journal (Luparell, 2008). Involvement in this type of behavior may lead to physical and emotional responses, even causing the victim to feel traumatized, powerless, or stressed; lose sleep; and develop anxiety and depression. People may try to avoid one another for fear of another negative encounter leading to distrust. When students and faculty are in situations where evaluation occurs, distrust on both sides may prevent objective faculty evaluation of students and student evaluation of faculty. This behavior can be disruptive in the classroom and in clinical experiences, interfering with student learning both for the students directly involved and for the students on the sidelines. The community of learning then becomes a place where no one wants to be.

Incivility demonstrates disrespect. When this type of behavior occurs, decreasing the escalation of the behavior is critical. Many times, incivility occurs from misunderstanding, so trying to talk about the issue—in a calm manner—is important. Students may feel that they have no power. If the issue cannot be worked out directly with those involved, all schools should have a process for discussing difficult issues, and these guidelines should be followed.

Before you go to talk to the person (another student or faculty member) about the situation that you found unacceptable, think about what you will say and even practice before the discussion. Doing so will help you cope with your emotions because you do not want to have a repeat of the uncivil behavior. Another method for dealing with verbal abuse is to try to remove the emotion from the situation—step back for a breather and then discuss the issue or problem on a factual basis. This strategy may require a third party to act as a neutral mediator in the discussion. This is not easy to do when parties are emotional and often tired and stressed, but it does make a difference. Such an approach provides time to gain more objective perspective.

When students observe or are involved in uncivil encounters in clinical experiences, this has a negative impact on their professional socialization and learning. Such behaviors are all connected to communication, ability to compromise and listen, and respect and trust, which in turn affect the ability to work collaboratively as a team member. Students begin to learn about healthy interactions with others when they are students, lessons that should then be carried into their practice to reduce incivility in the workplace.

Organizations associated with health care have made statements about the problem of incivility. In 2008, The Joint Commission issued a sentinel alert on incivility for its accredited healthcare organizations. As the problem increased, the Commission now requires that these healthcare organizations have standards in place to address this type of behavior. The American Association of Critical Care Nurses also issued a statement about healthy work environments (American Association of Critical Care Nurses, 2005; Dixon, 2008). The ANA published a position statement on incivility in the workplace. It emphasizes the ANA Code of Ethics as a base for preventing and resolving incivility so that the workplace is one in which healthcare organizations can "create an ethical environment and culture of civility and kindness, treating colleagues, coworkers, employees, students, and others with dignity and respect" (ANA, 2015b, p. 4). The position statement examines incivility, bullying, and violence in the workplace (ANA, 2015c). All of this affects nursing practice. It also has financial ramifications because incivility reduces productivity and may have a negative influence on staff retention as well as recruitment. This all can lead to health problems for nurses and interfere with career development.

Concern has also emerged about the impact of verbal abuse and disruptive behaviors among team members on patient care. Examples of disruptive behaviors include verbal abuse, negative behavior, and physical abuse (for example, profanity, innuendo, demeaning comments); reprimanding or insulting another person in public and inappropriately; threatening; telling racial or ethnic jokes; undermining team cohesion; scapegoating; silence (not speaking to a team member); and assaulting another person, throwing objects, and outbursts

of rage (Lower, 2007). One study sought to explore the impact of work relationships on clinical outcomes (Rosenstein & O'Daniel, 2005). This research was published in a nursing journal, although a physician and a healthcare administrator conducted the study. This was a follow-up to an earlier study that examined the impact of disruptive behavior on job satisfaction and retention (Rosenstein, 2002). In the 2005 study, 1,500 surveys from nurses and physicians were evaluated. Nurses were reported to exhibit disruptive behavior as frequently as physicians. Both groups felt that disruptive behavior (which included verbal abuse) negatively affected relationships and created stress, leading to frustration, lack of concentration, poor communication, and inability to effectively collaborate and provide effective information transfer in the workplace. Given that this chapter discusses the need for greater use of effective interprofessional teams to provide quality, patient-centered care, it is easy to see how these results may be perceived as disturbing. The participants also felt that disruptive behavior was adversely affecting patient safety, patient mortality, the quality of care, and patient satisfaction. These concerns further emphasize the need to improve teamwork and professional relationships. The researchers recommended that organizations should take the following steps to improve workplace relationships beginning with an assessment to determine the extent of the problem and sharing results with staff (Rosenstein & O'Daniel, 2005). The HCO needs to support open, safe communication among all staff members. To ensure this occurs staff require education about the problem of disruptive behavior and how to respect and communicate with one another even during stressful situations. HCOs must ensure that collaboration, communication, teams and teamwork, and conflict management are part of the culture and also included in staff ongoing education. To augment these strategies policies and procedures need to be developed and effectively implemented to guide staff in their actions.

All of these organization strategies should promote better patient care and clinical outcomes.

There are also strategies that individual staff should consider to respond or reduce incivility. Gessler, Rosenstein, and Ferron identify examples of these strategies (2012, p. 11):

- Be assertive and confront the person(s) who is involved in the uncivil behavior.
- Use "I" language when talking to the involved person(s).
- If direct conversation about the situation does not work, then staff should report the occurrence as expected in the organization process. Identify critical information such as date, time, who was involved, and what occurred.

Many organizations now have zero-tolerance policies related to this type of abuse. Some healthcare organizations, as well as schools of nursing, have identified codes of conduct that staff or, in the case of a school of nursing, faculty, students, and staff are expected to follow (Lewis & Malecha, 2011). However, the existence of a written policy does not guarantee on its own that attitudes and behaviors will automatically improve. Staff need to know about the policy content and the consequences of violating the policy, and these consequences must be applied when necessary. Some healthcare organizations are using the term "Code Pink" (Trossman, 2014). Nurses who are experiencing incivility use the code to alert others to these negative experiences and ask for support. It is important for staff to have a structured method to ask for help. Nursing leaders as well as other leaders in the organization need to commit to reducing these problems (Lewis & Malecha, 2011). In addition, as noted earlier, this is not just an issue for the workforce. As noted in this content, students experience incivility, and they also need to know how to cope with it when they enter the workforce. Given these concerns, the ANA has resources for nurses and students on its website (ANA, 2014).

In summary, it is very easy to say that poor attitudes and abusive behaviors are all the physicians'

fault when, in fact, they are not. Many nurses enter the profession with a negative attitude toward physicians and feel that they do not want to be controlled by physicians. The better approach is for new nurses to enter the profession with a positive attitude toward nursing as a profession, be knowledgeable about the nursing role and responsibilities, be competent, and possess a reasonable level of self-esteem. Nurse–nurse incivility is all too prevalent and a serious problem; thus the problem involves more than just nurse–physician incivility. What is needed to prevent incivility is someone who wants to work with others, not against others, and someone who approaches issues and problems with an open mind and who is not tied to an "I know better" mindset. If all healthcare professionals approached practice in this manner, then collaboration, coordination, and communication would improve. There would also be less incidence of verbal abuse, and the work environment would be positive and healthy for all team members.

Stop and Consider #8
Incivility in the healthcare workplace is a major problem.

Delegation

Delegation is part of daily work of nurses. Care is planned and coordinated to meet patient needs, but at some point the registered nurse (RN) may need to delegate work to others. Much of the work is done in a team model, in which it is not cost-effective for all care to be provided by the RN. **Delegation** involves giving another staff member the responsibility and authority to complete a task or activity. Before an RN can delegate, the RN needs to have responsibility and authority, or the power over the activity or task. An RN cannot delegate something that is outside approved nursing practice as determined by the nurse practice act in the state where the nurse practices. An extreme example is that an RN cannot delegate prescriptive authority (prescribing of medications) because an RN typically cannot do this activity. An advanced practice registered nurse may have prescriptive authority because this nurse has met special requirements and the state allows it, but even this nurse cannot delegate prescriptive authority.

When an RN delegates to another staff member, such as **unlicensed assistive personnel (UAP)** or a licensed practical nurse/licensed vocational nurse (LPN/LVN), the RN is not avoiding work and is still held accountable for the outcomes, but the care is provided in a more efficient manner. Accountability is "being responsible and answerable for actions or inactions of self or others in the context of delegation" (ANA, NCSBN, 2006). The UAP is an unlicensed staff member who is trained to function in an assistive role to the licensed nurse in the provision of patient activities as delegated by the nurse. The UAP may have several different titles, such as nursing assistant or nurse's aide. There is no national standard that is accepted and enforced in every state as to employment requirements, training, or position descriptions for the UAP. The RN (the delegator) is still responsible for supervising the work (activity, task) that the other staff member (the delegatee) is to do.

Supervision and *assignment* may be confused with *delegation*; however, they are related to one another. When a nurse is monitoring patient care and work performance, this is supervision. The nurse may be in a formal management position, such as a nurse manager, a team leader, or an RN staff nurse who has delegated work and then ensures that a task is done effectively. Assignment is the process that moves an activity from one person to another, including the responsibility and accountability. For example, the nurse manager might assign an RN to lead a team or to administer medications to the patients. An assignment can be given only to staff that have the required qualifications to complete the task and can assume the responsibility and accountability; however, the accountability is still shared. The person doing the activity has the accountability

for the actual action or activity, whereas the person who made the assignment is responsible for the assignment decision.

Importance of Delegation

Why is delegation important, and why is it part of care coordination and teamwork? One RN or one team member cannot always do everything that is required for a patient. There must be effective use of staff resources—expertise and time. Delegation is a critical part of providing cost-effective, quality care. In some situations, it is more cost-effective if care can safely be provided by a UAP or a licensed practical nurse, whose salary is lower than that of an RN, with the RN providing overall supervision. Quality care requires that patient outcomes be achieved with no harm to the patient. Through delegation, the RN determines the tasks that should be done, by whom, when, and how.

Communication and information are critical elements of delegation. If communication is not effective or there is inadequate information, delegation may then be ineffective. This can in turn lead to problems for the patient and interfere with the team's ability to achieve the desired patient outcomes. It is often difficult to provide clear communication in rushed, stressful healthcare environments, but doing so has never been more important if care is to be improved. Mindfulness—staying alert to key information and evaluating and updating that information as necessary—is an active process that can improve communication during delegation, as discussed earlier. The goal is not to share as much information as possible, but rather to share the critical information—that is, information that has meaning in the situation. Anthony and Vidal (2010) comment, "When mindful communication is integrated as a principle of delegation, it involves more than knowing the facts regarding the care plan. Mindful communication practice is recognizing the significance of the facts and how they pertain to the patient situation. When nurses engage in mindful communication, information processing is redirected, resulting in a unique set of decisions and actions. Historically, RNs have relied on job descriptions and delegated skills lists to guide delegation practices . . . hospitals value standardization as a means to improve safety through consistent practices. Paradoxically, however, overreliance on standards that results in routine interpretations and behaviors may jeopardize patient safety when nurses do not engage in mindful communication about the task at hand."

The National Council of State Boards of Nursing (NCSBN) has identified delegation standards and described the delegation process. The NCSBN defines *delegation* as "transferring to a competent individual authority to perform a selected nursing task in a selected situation. The nurse retains the accountability for the delegation" (ANA, NCSBN, 2006).

This definition really says the following:

- *Transferring* means the RN can do something that will be passed on to someone else to do. The RN has the right to do transfer tasks; however, the RN cannot delegate something that the RN has no right to do as an RN. (For example, suppose a patient needs a bed bath. The RN can do the bed bath, but it is more efficient to have the UAP complete the bed bath while the RN assesses the patient's overall status at the beginning of a shift.)
- The RN transfers this activity to a *competent* person—someone who can complete the task because that person has the skills and experience to do so. (For example, the UAP has been trained to give bed baths and report to the nurse any problems encountered.)
- In the delegation process, the delegator or RN is giving the delegatee the authority or power to do the act or task. (For example, RNs have overall responsibility and authority for all nursing care—from basic care, such as a bed bath, to complex care needs. The RN determines who is the best staff member is to

complete a task. In some cases, the RN may decide that because of the critical status of the patient and the need for intensive interaction and assessment, the RN should complete the bed bath; alternatively, the RN may decide that the UAP is best suited to handling this task.)
- The delegatee must then do something—this action is specific and attached to a specific situation. (For example, the UAP completes the bed bath for a patient, documents the care if required, and informs the RN that there was nothing unusual to report.)

Five Delegation Rights

It is natural to wonder who is responsible for the care in delegation. The **delegatee** is responsible for the care that the delegatee provides or the delegatee performance, and the **delegator** is responsible for the delegation process. This process is not a simple one and requires experience. The RN must consider the five rights of delegation (ANA, NCSBN, 2006).

- *Right task:* The task must be delegatable for a specific patient or situation. If the RN or delegator is not clear about what the task is, the RN will not be able to clearly identify what needs to be done and by whom.
- *Right circumstances:* The appropriate setting, available resources, and other relevant factors need to be considered. Perhaps the RN needs to tell the delegatee where to complete the task and identify which supplies, equipment, and other resources are needed to complete the task effectively.
- *Right person:* The right person delegates the right task to the right person, to be performed by the right person. The RN must consider the best staff member to complete the task (type of staff, experience and skills, availability of time to complete task without negatively impacting other work, and so on).
- *Right direction/communication:* Providing a clear, concise description of the task, including

its objective, limits, and expectations, is part of effective delegation. The delegator must explain to the delegatee what is to be done, how to do it (if that is not already clear), the time frame, outcomes, and so on. The delegatee needs to feel comfortable asking questions for clarification or expressing concern about the delegatee's inability to complete the task. The delegator must be an effective communicator and must be sensitive to concerns and issues to establish a communication environment that allows for open discussion. This is critical to ensure patient-centered care that is focused on quality. If the delegatee is afraid of speaking up and saying, "I do not know how to do something" or "Would you explain more about what you want done?" then this is an ineffective delegation process that may harm the patient. The delegatee may need help in organizing work and setting priorities, or the delegatee may need to be told what to report to the RN and when. The delegator needs to ask directly if there are questions or concerns and be open to the response. All of this is part of providing clear directions and guidance.

- *Right supervision:* Appropriate monitoring, evaluation, intervention (as needed), and feedback are part of delegation. The RN as a delegator does not just delegate a task and then forget about it. Instead, the RN needs to supervise as required. Monitoring methods include observation, verbal feedback, written feedback, and review of records in which the delegatee documents what was done. In some situations, supervision is minimal; in other situations, there may be a greater need for monitoring. Factors such as the expertise of the delegatee, the patient's status, the complexity of the task, and timing may all affect the monitoring process.

Another factor that cannot be ignored during delegation is how comfortable the delegator feels

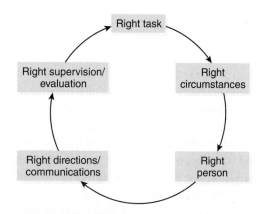

Figure 10-6 Five Rights for Effective Delegation

in delegating and how well the delegator knows the delegatee. New RNs may be very nervous about delegating; trusting another person to complete a task can be risky. Some new RNs may be overly concerned because they feel that they could perform the task better. In both situations, the result could be excessive hovering or overmonitoring; the delegatee may interpret the delegator's behavior or attitude as indicating a lack of confidence in the delegatee. This message can have a negative impact on team relationships. Finding the right balance takes experience. New RNs need time to learn how to delegate effectively and need to seek guidance from their own supervisors or mentors to assess their delegation competencies. **Figure 10-6** highlights the five delegation rights that all who delegate need to apply.

Delegation Principles

The American Nurses Association (ANA) and the NCSBN collaborated to identify the key delegation principles that should be applied by every RN (ANA, NCSBN, 2006, pp. 2–3):

- The RN takes responsibility and accountability for the provision of nursing practice.
- The RN directs care and determines the appropriate utilization of any assistant involved in providing direct patient care.

- The RN may delegate components of care but does not delegate the nursing process itself. Nursing judgment cannot be delegated.
- The decision of whether to delegate or assign is based on the RN's judgment concerning the condition of the patient, the competence of all members of the nursing team, and the degree of supervision that will be required of the RN if a task is delegated.
- The RN delegates only those tasks that the RN believes the other healthcare worker has the knowledge and skill to perform, taking into consideration training, cultural competence, experience, and facility/agency policies and procedures.
- The RN individualizes communication regarding the delegation to the nursing assistive personnel and patient situation, and the communication is clear, concise, correct, and complete. The RN verifies comprehension with the nursing assistive personnel and ensures that the assistant accepts the delegation and the responsibility that accompanies it.
- Communication must be a two-way process. Nursing assistive personnel should have the opportunity to ask questions and clarify expectations.
- The RN uses critical thinking and professional judgment when following the five rights of delegation.
- Chief nursing officers are accountable for establishing systems to assess, monitor, verify, and communicate ongoing competence requirements in areas related to delegation.
- There are both individual accountability and organizational accountability for delegation. Organizational accountability for delegation relates to providing sufficient resources.*

It is important for the RN, as the delegator, to thank the delegatee and recognize the work that the delegatee has done. The RN should provide positive feedback when work is done well and constructive feedback as needed; the RN should not criticize work negatively, but rather discuss the work and outcomes and make recommendations for improvement. It is easy to take things for granted and not recognize the work of team members. It really takes little time to give positive feedback and a "thank you," and this step can go a long way toward building teams and individual staff competence.

Will there be times when the RN as delegator must change a decision about delegation? If so, why would this occur? In the monitoring process, the delegatee may ask for help. The RN needs to listen to this request and intervene. There may be times when the patient's condition changes, and someone else, including the RN, may be better suited to complete the task. The RN may recognize that the delegatee is not as qualified to complete the task as originally thought. The RN must be aware of the need to avoid being negative, hurting the delegatee's self-confidence, or embarrassing the delegatee in front of others. How the RN communicates and intervenes can make the situation a positive learning experience for the delegatee. In addition, the RN must recognize the impact on the patient—how the patient views the change of assignment and if the patient wonders what is going on.

Supervision is a critical part of delegation. The ANA and the NCSBN have similar definitions of supervision. The ANA defines *supervision* as the "active process of directing, guiding, and influencing the outcome of an individual's performance of a task" whereas the NCSBN defines it as "the provision of guidance or direction, oversight, evaluation and follow-up by the licensed nurse for the accomplishment of a delegated nursing task by assistive personnel" (ANA, NCSBN, 2006). It is important to note that supervision does not necessarily mean that the RN is in a management position. RNs who are not in management positions must also supervise when they delegate. **Figure 10-7** describes the decision tree for delegation that should be applied by staff when using delegation.

Step One — Assessment and Planning

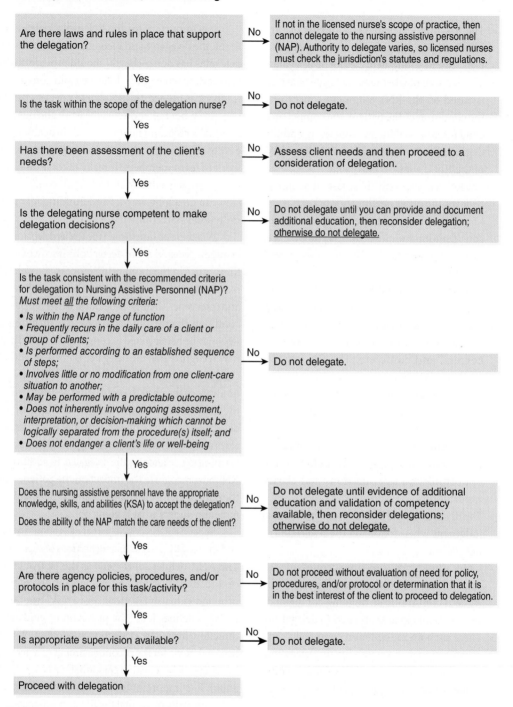

Are there laws and rules in place that support the delegation?	No →	If not in the licensed nurse's scope of practice, then cannot delegate to the nursing assistive personnel (NAP). Authority to delegate varies, so licensed nurses must check the jurisdiction's statutes and regulations.

↓ Yes

Is the task within the scope of the delegation nurse?	No →	Do not delegate.

↓ Yes

Has there been assessment of the client's needs?	No →	Assess client needs and then proceed to a consideration of delegation.

↓ Yes

Is the delegating nurse competent to make delegation decisions?	No →	Do not delegate until you can provide and document additional education, then reconsider delegation; otherwise do not delegate.

↓ Yes

Is the task consistent with the recommended criteria for delegation to Nursing Assistive Personnel (NAP)? *Must meet all the following criteria:*

- *Is within the NAP range of function*
- *Frequently recurs in the daily care of a client or group of clients;*
- *Is performed according to an established sequence of steps;*
- *Involves little or no modification from one client-care situation to another;*
- *May be performed with a predictable outcome;*
- *Does not inherently involve ongoing assessment, interpretation, or decision-making which cannot be logically separated from the procedure(s) itself; and*
- *Does not endanger a client's life or well-being*

No → Do not delegate.

↓ Yes

Does the nursing assistive personnel have the appropriate knowledge, skills, and abilities (KSA) to accept the delegation? Does the ability of the NAP match the care needs of the client?	No →	Do not delegate until evidence of additional education and validation of competency available, then reconsider delegations; otherwise do not delegate.

↓ Yes

Are there agency policies, procedures, and/or protocols in place for this task/activity?	No →	Do not proceed without evaluation of need for policy, procedures, and/or protocol or determination that it is in the best interest of the client to proceed to delegation.

↓ Yes

Is appropriate supervision available?	No →	Do not delegate.

↓ Yes

Proceed with delegation

Figure 10-7 National Council of State Boards of Nursing Decision Tree for Delegation to Nursing Assistive Personnel

Evaluation of Effective Delegation

How does the RN evaluate delegation? The first focus is the role of the delegator. Were the right tasks delegated, and why were they delegated? The second concern is the directions. Were the directions clear? The RN should consider to whom the task was delegated and the delegatee's strengths and limitations. Did the delegatee have the resources to complete the task? Did the delegatee have the time to complete the task? What impact did performing the specific task have on other responsibilities that the delegatee may have had? Did the delegatee have the authority to complete the task? Were the expected outcomes met? Was the delegator available to the delegatee if questions arose or problems occurred? This availability is more than just physical; it concerns not only whether the delegatee is able to reach the delegator, but also whether the delegator is able to listen and hear the delegatee and then respond effectively.

RNs want to be effective delegators, and all new RNs struggle with how to delegate. The following are some characteristics of effective delegation (Milgram, Spector, & Treger, 1999, p. 245):

- Do not give employees just menial tasks; include tasks that offer opportunities for learning and growth.
- Distribute tasks with an understanding of each employee's position description and job status, abilities, and total workload.
- Delegate when there is someone skilled available or when the task can be completed by a subordinate whose time is less expensive.
- Use benchmarks to monitor progress along the way; having only a final deadline can be overwhelming. (This applies to activities or tasks that take a longer time to complete.)
- Do not micromanage subordinates. Experienced employees usually have the skills necessary for managing complex tasks on their own (particularly if the tasks are typically done by them).

- Establish what needs to be done, and then provide support to the employee so that the employee can decide how to effectively accomplish the activity or task.

The focus of this discussion thus far has been on RNs delegating to other nursing staff—staff that are not RNs. It is important to recognize that RNs may assign work or tasks to other RNs. A team may include several RNs, and one may be the team leader. The nurse manager or nurse coordinator of a unit assigns work to RN staff routinely.

Effective delegation takes practice; it does not "just happen." There are barriers to delegation. Staff may be uncomfortable with delegating and with criticism, depending on whether they are the delegator or the delegatee. This can interfere with effective delegation and positive outcomes. RNs typically delegate to UAPs. Consequently, RNs need to know about UAP roles and job responsibilities. UAPs cannot do the following or be delegated these activities: health counseling, teaching, and activities that require independent, specialized nursing knowledge, skills, or judgment. The ANA (1997) identified the UAP direct and indirect patient care activities as follows:

- *Direct patient care activities* assist the patient in meeting basic human needs (settings may be hospitals, home, long-term care, and other). Activities include assisting with feeding, drinking, ambulation, grooming, toileting, dressing, and socializing. Collection, reporting, and documentation of data related to these activities are important. UAPs need to report data to RNs; data then are used to make clinical judgments about patient care.
- *Indirect patient care activities* support the patient and the patient's environment, such as providing a clean, efficient, and safe patient care milieu. Activities might include companion care; simple meal preparation; housekeeping; providing transportation; and clerical, stocking, and maintenance tasks. Many of these activities would take place in the patient's home,

where UAPs may be working one-on-one with patients through a home health agency or some type of community agency.

Generally, tasks that can be delegated are those that have the following characteristics (ANA, NCSBN, 2006):

- Frequently occur
- Are considered technical by nature
- Are considered standard and unchanging
- Have predictable results
- Have minimal potential for risks

Figure 10-8 illustrates the key to delegation and highlights the key aspects of delegation.

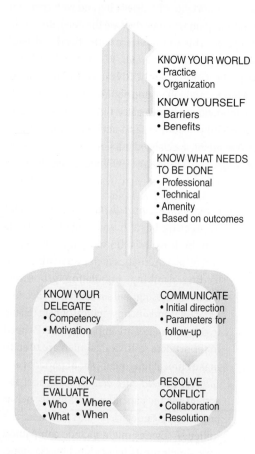

KNOW YOUR WORLD
• Practice
• Organization

KNOW YOURSELF
• Barriers
• Benefits

KNOW WHAT NEEDS TO BE DONE
• Professional
• Technical
• Amenity
• Based on outcomes

KNOW YOUR DELEGATE
• Competency
• Motivation

COMMUNICATE
• Initial direction
• Parameters for follow-up

FEEDBACK/ EVALUATE
• Who   • Where
• What   • When

RESOLVE CONFLICT
• Collaboration
• Resolution

Figure 10-8 The Key to Delegation

Reproduced from Hansten, R., & Jackson, M. (2004). *Clinical delegation skills: A handbook for professional practice.* Burlington, MA: Jones & Bartlett Learning.

Stop and Consider #9
Effective delegation is not easy to learn.

Change

Change can be discussed in relation to changes in the healthcare delivery system, but change is also a part of collaboration and coordination, which are difficult to accomplish without some change; change may be required from an individual team member, the entire team, a unit, or the organization. Patients are asked to change all the time. Why do team members often not like change? They may be fearful of the results, particularly of the unknown; they may fear losing something of value, such as control, job responsibility, and so on; or they may have a belief that change will not make things better. The other view of change is its potential as an opportunity for improvement. Sometimes, however, change does not lead to positive outcomes. This situation has to be dealt with, but not changing means stagnation and lack of improvement. The change process includes the following steps:

- Identify the issue or problem/need for change and factors that influence the need for change.
- Engage staff when possible in the planning process.
- Gather information to better understand the need and possible solutions.
- Identify stakeholders and barriers to and support for the change.
- Describe solutions to solve a problem or to improve one.
- Select the solution to implement.
- Prepare staff for the change (inform them about the change, the reasons for the change, the timeline, planning and implementation, and training staff if needed; engage them in the implementation).
- Implement the change (the solution).
- Evaluate the results (including staff feedback).

- Determine whether any adjustments are needed (ongoing); ideally, include relevant staff early in the process to enhance staff commitment.

The **plan–do–study–act (PDSA) cycle** is used more today by healthcare professionals and teams to assist in decision-making, make changes, and ensure better coordinated care (IHI, 2011b). This cycle is used to test changes. During the first step (*plan*), the team identifies the objective(s) and discusses predictions as to what might happen and why; the team then develops a plan to implement the change. In the next step (*do*), the team institutes the change and collects and analyzes outcome data. In the third step (*study*), there is more in-depth analysis of the outcome data and relationship to the problem. In the last step (*act*), the change may be modified and then fully initiated.

What methods can be used to decrease barriers to change and increase team involvement in change? Explanation and education about the issue or problem and the need for change is the first step. Including team members in the discussion about the need for change and possible solutions allows members to buy into the change process. They will participate more fully and be more invested in the results. Change is stressful; this stress needs to be recognized, and when possible, implement interventions to reduce stress. Experiencing too many changes at one time or too quickly can make effective change difficult. Sometimes there are situations in which change is dictated. When this occurs, team members still need an explanation and should be included in the change process. Asking for feedback and listening are important. Change is risky—and sometimes it will fail. Teams need to learn from their errors and ineffective decisions and then move on. Effective collaborative teams do not place blame on individuals; rather, they look at results in an objective manner and realize that the team works together and sometimes can make mistakes.

Stop and Consider #10
Change can be positive or negative.

Conflict and Conflict
Resolution

Conflict is inevitable; however, what is important is how it is handled. In many cases, conflict can be prevented. It is natural for misunderstandings to occur among people who work together, such as in teams. Often, causes of conflict relate to whether resources are shared equitably, insufficient explanation of expectations, questioning someone's performance, unexplained changes that disturb routines and process and for which team members are not prepared, and stress resulting from changes that team members do not understand and may see as threatening or ineffective. Each of these causes can be prevented from developing into conflict. Engaging in clear, timely communication and including team members in the process can reduce conflict.

There is another cause of conflict that is more difficult to manage: an individual's personal responses and behavior that may increase team conflict. Examples include the team members who do not do expected work, are late to meetings, do not listen to others, complain, are overly critical of others, do not know how to communicate effectively, want to be the star and take all the credit, and so on. **Figure 10-9** describes a conflict flowchart that can be applied to better understand what happens during a conflict.

Conflict resolution requires leadership and participation from team members. When difficult issues or problems arise, it is best to deal with them rather than postpone decisions (which usually means that the problem has time to get worse). Using threats and negativity with little positive feedback can lead to more conflict, so these approaches need to be avoided. Listening can go a long way toward preventing conflict, and if conflict does occur, resolving it. When team members treat one another

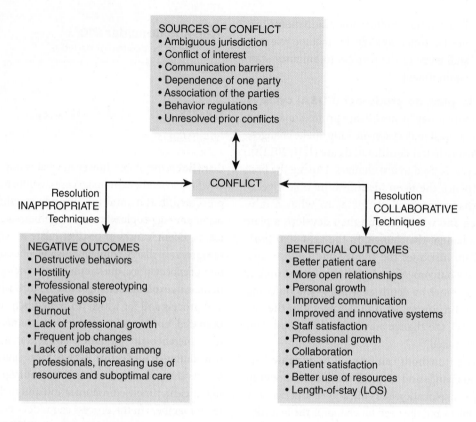

Figure 10-9 Conflict Flowchart

Reproduced from Hansten, R., & Jackson, M. (2004). *Clinical delegation skills: A handbook for professional practice.* Burlington, MA: Jones & Bartlett Learning.

with respect and communicate clearly, conflict can be decreased. Respect means to recognize another's right to have opinions and listen and discuss these opinions. Nonverbal communication can give important clues as to when conflict is increasing. When teams or individual members experience stress, the risk of conflict increases. Open communication is key to resolution of conflict, and it is key to preventing conflict when possible.

When conflict occurs, it is important to provide opportunities to identify the facts, determine the purpose of the actions or activities at the time, and review team member perspectives. When members are emotional, this factor can interfere with effective resolution, so sometimes the best first approach is to step back and allow some time for all parties involved

to temper their emotional reactions. However, the issue needs to be resolved, so this time period needs to be monitored—it should not go on too long. Sometimes one or two members need to be persuaded to reexamine the issue. This effort may or may not be successful. Teams need to understand that individual team members do not always get their viewpoint accepted by all. Compromise is required; however, when this occurs, it must be done in a manner that respects divergent opinions and does not use negativity or reduce self-esteem. All of these facets of conflict resolution require leadership—on the part of the designated team leader and from the members who commit to the team and its effectiveness. **Figure 10-10** describes a collaborative resolution method.

Use of describe–express–suggest–consequences (DESC) is an example of a structured approach to address a conflict (O'Keefe & Saver, 2014, p. 12). The goal is to arrive at consensus and keep the discussion on track. The DESC script includes the following elements:

- **D**escribe the specific conflict situation or behavior using concrete data.
- **E**xpress how the situation made you feel or identify your concerns.
- **S**uggest alternatives and seek agreement.
- **S**tate consequences in terms of effects on team goals; strive for consensus.

Stop and Consider #11
Nurses encounter conflict in the workplace.

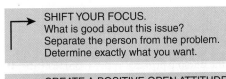

SHIFT YOUR FOCUS.
What is good about this issue?
Separate the person from the problem.
Determine exactly what you want.

CREATE A POSITIVE OPEN ATTITUDE.
Listen and restate what the other party wants.
Be certain he or she feels heard.
Reflect and respect feelings expressed.

STATE YOUR PERCEPTION.
Use assertive language.
Express what it is you want from a factual viewpoint.
Determine what you are willing to do, or give up, to get what you want.

ESTABLISH MUTUAL GOALS.
Determine what the other party is willing to do, or give up, to get what he or she wants.
Propose a solution that reflects your understanding of both parties' needs/desires.
Summarize each party's agreed-on actions.

Figure 10-10 Hansten & Washburn's Collaborative Resolution Method

Reproduced from Hansten, R., & Jackson, M. (2004). *Clinical delegation skills: A handbook for professional practice.* Burlington, MA: Jones & Bartlett Learning.

Power and Empowerment

As people work together, the issue of power arises. Simply put, **power** can be described as when healthcare provider A wants something that healthcare provider B has and may or may not need or want as much; healthcare provider B then has more power in the relationship. Typically, there is not a balance of power in a team, particularly when it is first formed. This is most commonly seen with nurses and physicians; physicians typically have more power because of their profession, experience, and history. This balance, however, can shift and should change as the team develops, with members recognizing one another's value and experience. Nevertheless, an imbalance can be difficult to overcome and makes the work situation stressful.

How a person feels about his or her work and job has an impact on how that person functions on a team. Herzberg's theory, as described in **Figure 10-11**, identifies job maintenance factors

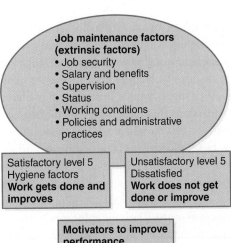

Figure 10-11 Herzberg's Theory on Job Satisfaction

Exhibit 10-3 Types of Power

Type of Power	Description
Legitimate/formal power	Power that originates from serving in a formal position (for example, a team leader, nurse manager, or chief nursing officer).
Referent/informal power	Power that originates from others' recognizing that an individual has leadership qualities and choosing to follow that person.
Informational power	Power that originates from information a person has and others need.
Expert power	Power that originates from a person's expertise, which can be useful to others and enable the person to provide guidance (for example, a nurse clinical specialist).
Reward power	Power that originates from a person's ability to reward others (for example, the ability to grant a salary increase, promotion, or assign an interesting project) if they agree to do something.
Coercive power	Power that originates from a person's ability to punish others (for example, the ability to assign an unpleasant task or project, or deny a promotion) if they do not do what is asked.

or extrinsic factors that influence job satisfaction; however, there is more to job satisfaction than these hygiene factors, as Herzberg calls them. The motivator factors (intrinsic factors) must also be considered. Herzberg suggested that because of these factors, organizations that increase accountability, create teams, remove controls, provide feedback, introduce new tasks, allocate special assignments, and grant additional authority might increase staff motivation (Michalopoulos & Michalopoulos, 2006). Staff may then feel increased personal achievement and more **empowerment**. The same authors noted that the factors to increase staff motivation are part of the need for nurses to "increase responsibility, control over their work, and the opportunity to use their own initiative, all of which are offered in team nursing and the nursing process" (pp. 54–55). **Exhibit 10-3** describes the **types of power**.

Empowering teams means that the leader of the team needs to be less assertive over time and gradually allow the team to lead itself. The team needs to find the best solutions by using the expertise of all the members and then assuming more leadership. This actually strengthens the team leader's leadership—with the result of better team outcomes. Power and empowerment are discussed in other content in this text, particularly in content related to nursing leadership.

Stop and Consider #12
Empowerment allows you to practice fully as a nurse.

CHAPTER HIGHLIGHTS

1. The essential features of the interprofessional team include examination of self as it relates to the team effort, interprofessional communication and conflict resolution, and the impact of the team's efforts on quality, safety, patient-centered care, and overall delivery of care.

2. Healthcare professional education takes place in isolation, with each healthcare profession providing its own education with limited regard to other healthcare professionals. This has limited the development of effective interprofessional teams.

3. A team leader must first recognize that it is the work of the team that is critical and avoid focusing on personal success as a leader.

4. Communication is the sharing of a message between one person or team/group and another. It is important to know if the message was received as sent. Interpretation plays a major role in effective communication, and sometimes interpretation confuses or changes the original message sent. Practices such as SBAR and checklists help to reduce communication problems.

5. Formal meetings are an important part of teamwork.

6. Listening is critical to effective communication.

7. Team members need knowledge and competence that assist them in being effective team members.

8. Teams participate in decision making.

9. Collaboration means that all people involved are listened to and that decisions are developed together—interprofessionally. Effective teams value openness and collaboration.

10. Coordination—working to see that the pieces/activities fit together and flow as they should—can help to meet desired patient outcomes and is part of interprofessional teams.

11. A clinical protocol or pathway is a written guide that provides direction for specific clinical problems; considers the interventions, timeline, and resources needed; and identifies expected outcomes—improving care coordination.

12. Incivility in the healthcare workplace is a growing problem.

13. Delegation refers to the process of transferring responsibility for a task to another person. The person delegating must have the authority to transfer this task; the task must then be handed off to someone whose scope of responsibilities includes this work. There are five rights of delegation: right task, right circumstances, right person, right direction, and right supervision.

14. Change is part of collaboration, coordination, and teamwork, which are difficult to accomplish without some change; change may be required from an individual team member, the entire team, a unit, or the organization. The plan–do–study–act (PDSA) cycle is one method for planning and implementing change that a team might use.

15. Causes of conflicts may relate to inequitable sharing of resources, insufficient explanation of expectations leading to performance being questioned, unexplained changes that disturb routines and process and for which team members are not prepared, and stress resulting from changes that team members do not understand and may see as threatening. Resolving conflict requires leadership and participation from team members.

16. Empowering teams means that the leader of the team must be less assertive over time and allow the team to lead.

ENGAGING IN THE CONTENT

Discussion Questions

1. Explain the healthcare core competency "work in interprofessional teams." Why is this issue important to address in healthcare education? What is its impact on practice?

2. What is a team? How does it function? Would a nursing team and an interprofessional team function differently? If so, how?

3. How does collaboration influence team effectiveness?

4. Why is coordination a key activity of a clinical interprofessional team? Of a nursing team?

5. Explain the communication process.

6. Discuss the five delegation rights. How would you apply them in clinical?

7. What is conflict resolution? How can conflict be prevented?

CRITICAL THINKING ACTIVITIES

1. For a week, keep a log of your critical communications. Note who was involved in the communication, the context or situation in which it occurred, the time of day and day of the week, the message, the effectiveness of the communication, and what could have been done to improve communication. Compare four communication examples from your log. Identify examples of team coordination and collaboration.

2. Make a list of what you want to improve in your communication. What strategies might you use to improve your communication?

3. Why do you think delegation might be easy or difficult for you as an individual?

4. Have you been a member of a team/group or in a work situation in which there was conflict? Describe the situation (does not have to be a clinical situation), the events that occurred, your role in the situation, and the resolution. How did you feel about the experience? Could something have been done to prevent the conflict? Were you satisfied with the resolution? If not, what could have improved it?

5. View the video on incivility in the workplace: http://www.youtube.com/watch?v=NujWmw8z7sg Then identify three things you learned from the video that you found helpful. Discuss in teams.

ELECTRONIC REFLECTION JOURNAL

Describe your opinion of incivility in the healthcare workplace. Have you observed it or experienced it? What was your reaction?

CASE STUDIES

Case 1

A 70-year-old man in very good health experiences a syncopal episode after standing unsupported for 20 minutes. His pulse was 46 and color ashen with circumoral cyanosis. Paramedics were called, and he was taken to the nearest emergency department. After extensive tests and 3 weeks of home monitoring, it was determined that the patient needed a pacemaker. Following the pacemaker insertion, it was determined that his cholesterol was elevated, and he was started on medication. The patient stated that he had been put on statins once before by his primary care physician and was not able to tolerate them. This time, the medication was to be closely monitored.

One month following his pacemaker insertion and the start of this medication, the patient saw his primary care physician. The physician went over his lab tests, for which samples were drawn before the visit. When the patient asked about his cholesterol, he was told that no lipid levels had been measured. When the patient further asked about the report on his pacemaker surgery, the physician replied that he had no report.

This case presents a lack of care coordination, a lack of effective communication among team members, and potential for error, resulting in patient safety and quality-of-care issues.

Case Questions

1. What could have been done to prevent the confusion that this patient experienced?
2. Where and when might errors have occurred?
3. How does this case reflect the need for interprofessional teamwork?
4. Have you or a family member experienced similar situations when receiving health care? What happened? Now that you know more about teamwork and quality care, what is your perspective of your experience?

Case 2

Examine the important topic of care coordination at the AHRQ website: https://www.ahrq .gov/professionals/prevention-chronic-care/improve/coordination/index.html. Content and presentations on the topic are provided on the site. You are preparing a presentation for your unit's next staff meeting.

Case Questions

Outline your presentation using the information from the website and information for this chapter.

1. What are some examples of effective care coordination you have seen in your clinical experiences that you might include in your presentation?
2. What are examples from your clinical experiences when you thought care coordination should have been used that you might include in your presentation?

CASE STUDIES (CONTINUED)

Working Backward to Develop a Case

Write a brief paragraph that describes a case related to the following questions.

1. Why do we need to work together?

2. We work in teams all the time as nurses. You need to work in interprofessional teams, so what do we need to do to accomplish this?

3. What are the 3 Cs we need to address?

REFERENCES

American Association of Critical Care Nurses. (2005). AACN standards for establishing and sustaining healthy work environments: A journey to excellence. Retrieved from http://www.aacn.org/wd/hwe/content/hwehome.pcms?menu=hwe

American Nurses Association. (1997). *Position statement: Registered nurse utilization of unlicensed assistive personnel.* Washington, DC: Author.

American Nurses Association. (2014). Bullying andworkplace violence. Retrieved from http:www.nursingworld.org/Bullying-Workplace-Violence

American Nurses Association. (2015a). *Nursing: Scope and standards of practice.* Silver Spring, MD: Author.

American Nurses Association. (2015b). *Code of ethics for nurses with interpretive statements.* Silver Spring, MD: Author.

American Nurses Association. (2015c). *Position statement: Incivility, bullying, and workplace violence.* Silver Spring, MD: Author.

American Nurses Association & National Council of State Boards of Nursing. (2006). Joint statement on delegation. Retrieved from https://www.ncsbn.org/Delegation_joint_statement_NCSBN-ANA.pdf

Anthony, M., & Vidal, K. (2010). Mindful communication: A novel approach to improving delegation and increasing patient safety. *Online Journal of Issues in Nursing, 15*(2). Retrieved from http://nursingworld.org/MainMenuCategories/ANAMarketplace/ANAPeriodicals/OJIN/TableofContents/Vol152010/No2May2010/Mindful-Communication-and-Delegation.html

Baggs, J., Schmitt, M., Mushlin, L., Mitchell, P., Eldredge, D., Oaks, d., & Hutson, A. (1999). Association between nurse–physician collaboration and patient outcomes in three intensive care units. *Critical Care Medicine, 27,* 1991–1998.

Barnsteiner, J., Disch, J., Hall, L., Mayer, D., & Moore, S. (2007). Promoting interprofessional education. *Nursing Outlook, 55,* 144–150.

Burke, M., Boal, J., & Mitchell, R. (2004). Communicating for better care: Improving nurse–physician communication. *American Journal of Nursing, 104*(12), 40–47.

Curry, L., Spatz, E., Cherlin, E., Thompson, J., Berg, D., Ting, H., Decker, C., . . . Bradley, E. (2011). What distinguishes top-performing hospitals in acute myocardial infarction mortality rates? *Annals of Internal Medicine, 154,* 384–390.

Dartmouth College. (2010). Clinical microsystems. Retrieved from http://dms.dartmouth.edu/cms/

Dixon, J. (2008). The American Association of Critical Care Nurses standards for establishing and sustaining healthy work environments: Off the printed page and into practice. *Critical Care Nursing Clinical North America, 20*(4), 393–401.

Fabre, J. (2005). *Smart nursing.* New York, NY: Springer.

Fairchild, D., Hogan, J., Smith, R., Portnow, M., & Bates, D. (2002). Survey of primary care physicians and home care clinicians. *Journal of General Internal Medicine, 17,* 243–261.

Gawande, A. (2009). *The checklist manifesto: How to get things right.* New York, NY: Metropolitan Books.

Gessler, R., Rosenstein, A., & Ferron, L. (2012). How to handle disruptive physician behaviors. Find out the best way to respond if you're the target. *American Nurse Today, 7*(11), 8–10.

Gum, L., Prideaux, D., Sweet, L., & Greenhill, J. (2012). From the nurses' station to the health team hub: How can design promote interprofessional collaboration? *Journal of Professional Care, 26*, 21–27.

Hagenow, N. (2003). Why not person-centered care? The challenges of implementation. *Nursing Administration Quarterly, 27*(3), 203–207.

Heller, R. (1999). *Learning to lead.* New York, NY: DK Publishing.

Higgins, L. (1999). Nurses' perceptions of collaborative nurse–physician transfer decision making as a predictor of patient outcomes in a medical intensive care unit. *Journal of Advanced Nursing, 29*, 1434–1443.

Institute for Health Improvement. (2011a). SBAR. Retrieved from http://www.ihi.org/resources/Pages/Tools /SBARTechniqueforCommunicationASituational BriefingModel.aspx

Institute for Health Improvement. (2011b). PDSA cycle. Retrieved from http://www.ihi.org/resources/Pages /Tools/PlanDoStudyActWorksheet.aspx

Institute of Medicine. (2001). *Crossing the quality chasm.* Washington, DC: The National Academies Press.

Institute of Medicine. (2003). *Health professions education: A bridge to quality.* Washington, DC: The National Academies Press.

Interprofessional Education Collaborative Expert Panel. (2011). *Core competencies for interprofessional collaborative practice: 2016 update.* Washington, DC: Author. Retrieved from http://www.aacn.nche.edu /education-resources/ipecreport.pdf

Interprofessional Education Collaborative Expert Panel. (2016). *Core competencies for interprofessional collaborative practice: 2016 update.* Washington, DC: Author. Retrieved from https://ipecollaborative.org/uploads /IPEC-2016-Updated-Core-Competencies-Report _final_release_.PDF

Joint Commission, The. (2008). Sentinel event alert: Behaviors that undermine a culture of safety. Retrieved from http://www.jointcommission.org/sentinel_event_alert _issue_40_behaviors_that_undermine_a_culture_of_safety

Joint Commission, The. (2013). Sentinel event data: Root causes by event type 2004–2012. Retrieved from http://www.jointcommission.org/sentinel _event.aspx

Kupperschmidt, B., Kientz, E., Ward, J., & Reinholz, B. (2010, January). A healthy work environment: It begins with you. *Online Journal of Issues in Nursing, 15*(1). Retrieved from http://www.nursingworld.org/Main MenuCategories/ANAMarketplace/ANAPeriodicals /OJIN/TableofContents/Vol152010/No1Jan2010 /A-Healthy-Work-Environment-and-You.html

Lamb, G. (2013). Care coordination, quality, and nursing. In G. Lamb (Ed.), *Care coordination: The game changer.*

How nursing is revolutionizing quality care (pp. 1–10). Silver Spring, MD: American Nurses Association.

Lewis, P., & Malecha, A. (2011). The impact of workplace incivility on the work environment, manager, skill, and productivity. *Journal of Nursing Administration, 41*(1), 41–47.

Lower, J. (2007, September). Creating a culture of civility in the workplace. *American Nurse Today*, 49–51.

Luparell, S. (2008, April–May). Incivility in nursing education: Let's put an end to it. *NSNA Imprint*, 42–46.

McCallin, A. (2001). Interdisciplinary practice—a matter of teamwork: An integrated review. *Journal of Clinical Nursing, 10*, 419–428.

Maxfield, D., Grenny, J., McMillan, R., Patterson, K., & Switzler, A. (2005). Silence kills: The seven crucial conversations in healthcare. Retrieved from http://www.silenttreatmentstudy.com/silencekills /SilenceKills.pdf

Michalopoulos, A., & Michalopoulos, H. (2006). Management's possible benefits from teamwork and the nursing process. *Nurse Leader, 4*(3), 52–55.

Milgram, L., Spector, A., & Treger, M. (1999). *Managing smart.* Houston, TX: Gulf Publishing.

Nair, D., Fitzpatrick, J., McNulty, R., Click, E., & Glembocki, M. (2012). Frequency of nurse–physician collaborative behaviors in an acute care hospital. *Journal of Interprofessional Care, 26*(2), 115–120.

Nelson, E. C., Godfrey, M. M., Batalden, P. B., Berry, S. A., Bothe, A. E., McKinley, K. E., . . . Wasson, J. H. (2008). Clinical microsystems, Part 1: The building blocks of health systems. *Joint Commission Journal on Quality and Patient Safety, 34*(7), 367–378.

O'Keeffe, M., & Saver, C. (2014). *Communication, collaboration, and you.* Silver Spring, MD: American Nurses Association.

Rosenstein, A. (2002). Original research: Nurse–physician relationships: Impact on nurse satisfaction and retention. *American Journal of Nursing, 102*(6), 26–34.

Rosenstein, A., & O'Daniel, M. (2005). Disruptive and clinical behavior outcomes. *American Journal of Nursing, 105*(1), 54–63.

Singer, S., Molina, G., Zhonghe, L., Jiang, W., Nurudeen, S., Kite, J., . . . Berry, W. (2016). Relationship between operating room teamwork, contextual factors, and safety checklist performance. *Journal of American College of Surgeons, 233*(4), 568–580.

Thomas, E., Sexton, J., & Helmreich, R. (2003). Discrepant attitudes about teamwork among critical care nurses and physicians. *Critical Care Medicine, 31*, 956–959.

Trossman, S. (2014, November 21). Toward civility. *The American Nurse.* Retrieved from http://www .theamericannurse.org/index.php/2014/02/27/toward -civility/

U.S. Department of Health and Human Services. (2013). 2013 annual progress report to Congress: National strategy for quality improvement in health care. Retrieved from http://www.ahrq.gov/workingforquality/nqs/nqs2013annlrpt.htm

U.S. Department of Health and Human Services, Agency for Healthcare Research and Quality. (2014a). TeamSTEPPS® fundamentals course: Module 1. Introduction. Retrieved from http://www.ahrq.gov/professionals/education/curriculum-tools/teamstepps/instructor/fundamentals/module1/sintrol.html

U.S. Department of Health and Human Services, Agency for Healthcare Research and Quality. (2014b). Care coordination. Retrieved from http://www.ahrq.gov/professionals/prevention-chronic-care/improve/coordination/index.html

U.S. Department of Health and Human Services, Agency for Healthcare Research and Quality. (2016). Pocket guide: TeamSTEPPS®: Strategies and tools to enhance performance and patient safety. Retrieved from https://www.ahrq.gov/teamstepps/instructor/index.html

U.S. Department of Health and Human Services, Agency for Healthcare Research and Quality. (2017). TeamSTEPPS®. Retrieved from https://www.ahrq.gov/teamstepps/index.html

U.S. Department of Health and Human Services, Agency for Healthcare Research and Quality, Patient Safety Network. (2016). Learning through debriefing. Retrieved from https://psnet.ahrq.gov/primers/primer/36

Weinberg, D., Miner, D., & Rivlin, L. (2009). "It depends": Medical residents' perspectives on working with nurses. *American Journal of Nursing, 109*(7), 34–43.

Weinstock, M. (2010). Team-based care. *Hospital Health Network, 84*(3), 6, 28.

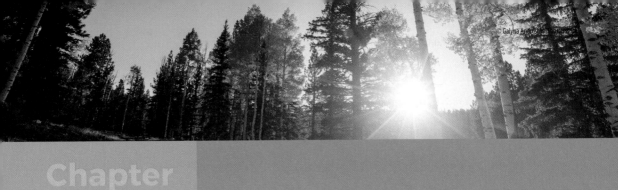

Chapter 11

Employ Evidence-Based Practice

CHAPTER OBJECTIVES

At the conclusion of this chapter, the learner will be able to:

- Discuss the core competency: Employ evidence-based practice.
- Discuss the relevance of nursing research.
- Discuss the relevance of evidence-based practice and its process.
- Compare and contrast evidence-based practice and evidence-based management.
- Discuss the need to improve implementation of evidence-based practice.
- Describe tools used to ensure use of evidence-based practice.

- Compare and contrast evidence-based practice, research, and quality improvement.
- Discuss importance of evidence-based practice for the nursing profession.
- Examine the impact that evidence-based practice has had over the last decade on nursing practice and management, nursing education, government initiatives, and nursing students.
- Discuss the role of student application of evidence-based practice.

CHAPTER OUTLINE

- Introduction
- The Core Competency: Employ Evidence-Based Practice
- Nursing Research
  - Historical Background
  - National Institute of Nursing Research
  - The Research Process
  - Types of Research Design
  - Research Funding
  - Ethics and Legal Issues
  - Barriers to and Facilitators of Research
  - Other Influential Organizations: Impact on Research

- Evidence-Based Practice
  - Definitions
  - Types of EBP Literature
  - Searching for EBP Literature: Evidence
  - The Roles of Staff Nurses Related to Systematic Reviews
- Evidence-Based Management
- Improving EBP Implementation
- Tools to Ensure a Higher Level of Use of EBP
  - Policies and Procedures Based on EBP
  - Clinical Guidelines Based on EBP
- Confusion: Difference in Research, EBP, and Quality Improvement

- Importance of EBP to the Nursing Profession
- Impact of Evidence-Based Practice over the Last Decade
  - Nursing Practice and Management
  - Nursing Education
  - Government Initiatives: Research and EBP
- Applying EBP as a Student

- Chapter Highlights
- Engaging in the Content
  - Discussion Questions
  - Critical Thinking Activities
  - Electronic Reflection Journal
  - Case Studies
  - Working Backward to Develop a Case
- References

KEY TERMS

Applied research
Basic research
Continuous quality
   improvement (CQI)
Evidence-based
   management (EBM)
Evidence-based practice
   (EBP)
Experimental study
Hypothesis

Institutional review board
Outcomes research
PICOT (patient-intervention–
   comparison–outcome–
   time)
Qualitative study
Quality improvement (QI)
Quantitative study
Randomized controlled trial
   (RCT)

Research
Research analysis
Research design
Research problem
   statement
Research proposal
Research purpose
Research question
Systematic review
Translational research

Introduction

This chapter focuses on the third healthcare professions core competency, the need for all healthcare professionals, including nurses, to use evidence-based practice (EBP). Evidence-based management (EBM) is also critical for effective healthcare delivery in all settings. The content provided in this chapter explores this core competency. Because research is an important component in understanding and using EBP and is a part of nursing content in nursing education programs, a brief introduction to nursing research is offered as well. EBP and EBM and their impact on nursing care and the nursing profession are described.

The Competency: Employ
Evidence-Based Practice

The Institute of Medicine (IOM, 2003) definition of **EBP** is to "integrate best research with clinical expertise and patient values for optimum care, and participate in learning and research activities to the extent feasible" (p. 4). EBP is connected to providing patient-centered care and improving quality care. Teams need to use EBP and EBM in making decisions and to ensure the most effective patient-centered care. Nurse managers and other nursing leaders also need to actively apply EBM. There is too long a time lag between conclusions of studies and then, if the results are significant, applying them in care delivery. Clearly, there is a great need to get research results to the patient sooner. Increasing use of evidence can improve the quality of care and avoid underuse, misuse, and overuse of care (Chassin, 1998). To the nurse, this means the ability to access the evidence, know what the evidence is and apply it, as appropriate for need, at the point of care. Using EBP affects comparison of alternatives and interventions such as prevention, diagnostic tests, or therapy; and, in some cases, leads to the decision that no intervention is the best choice. **Figure 11-1** illustrates the key elements related to this core competency.

In 2011, the IOM published additional information about the relevance of EBP to health care: "We seek the development of a learning health system that is designed to generate and apply the best evidence for the collaborative healthcare choices of each patient and provider; to drive the process of discovery as a natural outgrowth of patient care, and to ensure innovation, quality, safety, and value in health care. Our vision is for a healthcare system that draws on the best evidence to provide the care most appropriate to each patient, emphasizes prevention and health promotion, delivers the most value, adds to learning throughout the delivery of care, and leads to improvements in the nation's health. By the year 2020, 90 percent of clinical decisions will be supported by accurate, timely, and up-to-date clinical information, and will reflect the best available evidence. We feel that this presents a tangible focus for progress toward our vision, that Americans ought to expect at least this level of performance, that it should be feasible with existing resources and emerging tools, and that measures can be developed to track and stimulate progress" (IOM, 2011a, p. xi). This is a clear mandate to support EBP as a critical component of all healthcare delivery, regardless of healthcare provider or setting.

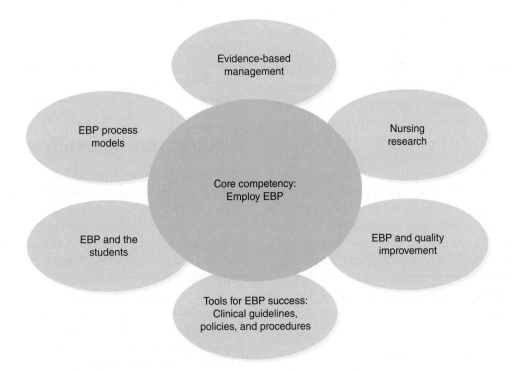

Figure 11-1 Employ EBP: Key Elements

Research results that can make a difference in health care in general, and in nursing in particular, need to be implemented in nursing practice. EBP is the major initiative used to increase the use of best practice or evidence in making clinical decisions. It is important to note that EBP includes more than just research results (IOM, 2003). Best practice clinical decisions also require healthcare provider expertise and patient assessment, as well as inclusion of the patient's perspective (patient preferences and values). It is easy to confuse research utilization and EBP. Research utilization usually involves using knowledge gained from one study, with limited regard to provider expertise, patient assessment, and patient preferences and values. EBP, by comparison, is a much more organized approach to getting research into practice—tailored to individual patient needs and should be based on evidence from more than one study.

A critical question is: How much evidence from research is actually applied? Research done for research's sake, without ever influencing clinical research or making it into practice, has limited value. There are growing efforts to change this by increasing EBP content—not just research content—in all levels of nursing education, undergraduate through graduate. Efforts are also being made to improve staff education about EBP so that nurses in practice can gain and maintain essential competencies to increase EBP in clinical settings. In this chapter, it is important to recognize that research cannot be discussed without considering EBP; research and EBP should be interconnected. As part of this relationship, science must be accessible. EBP provides methods for making science more accessible to the practitioner who does not have a lot of time to pore over research study reports to determine what works and what does not work and compare one study with another in detail.

Stop and Consider #1

EBP is an important competency due to its affect on quality health care.

Nursing Research

The first step in using EBP effectively is to understand research. **Research** is a systematic investigation that includes research development, testing, and evaluation. It is designed to develop or contribute to generalizable knowledge. One of the major sources of best evidence for practice comes from research results. Nursing is considered a science discipline in that much of the knowledge base for nursing practice includes theoretical and evidence-based knowledge (ANA, 2015a).

Two major types of research approaches are: basic and applied. **Basic research** is designed to broaden the base of knowledge, rather than solve an immediate problem, and is typically done in a laboratory setting. Results from basic research may be used to develop **applied research**, which is designed to find a solution to a practical problem. It is often referred to as clinical research and is usually carried out in a non-laboratory setting. Nurses typically are more involved in applied research, although some nurses are involved in basic research. **Outcomes research** is a newer approach. This type of research focuses on determining the effectiveness of healthcare services and patient outcomes.

Historical Background

How has the nursing profession developed nursing research (American Nurses Association [ANA], 2015a)? Florence Nightingale did have some interested in clinical research. Although Nightingale used the data she collected to measure some patient outcomes and improve care, the nursing community really did not pay much attention to research early in its history.

When nurses began to earn advanced degrees, this trend resulted in some studies about nurses and nursing education, but research was still not an important part of nursing. In the 1920s and 1930s, a few very early studies focused more on nursing care. Some of these studies were published in the *American Journal of Nursing*, making them the first studies to be published in a nursing journal, although the conduct of nursing studies was not common. It took time for more studies to be done, and time to develop nursing researchers.

In the 1950s, greater interest in nursing research emerged, and the journal *Nursing Research* was launched. In the 1970s and 1980s, more nurses conducted studies and more nurses obtained graduate degrees (including doctoral degrees); thus, nursing researchers were more qualified. Master's programs in nursing typically required courses on research and completion of an extensive master's thesis based on a study conducted by the student; however, this was eliminated as the PhD in nursing became available. Nursing theorists were very active in the 1960s and 1970s, adding to the scholarly work, as discussed in other chapters.

Nursing organizations in the United States and internationally support nursing research and have described their views of research; for example, the International Council of Nurses (ICN, 2010) is "committed to supporting nursing research as a powerful tool for generating new knowledge and evidence to underpin nursing practice. Nursing has an obligation to society to provide care that is continually researched and evaluated. Nurses working singly or in multidisciplinary research teams can offer new insights and unique perspectives to the research process. Nursing research provides opportunities for linkages between those involved in the research process, practicing nurses, other health professionals, policy makers, and the public. With the rapid advances in knowledge and technology, nursing research serves as a framework for organizing facts and evidence into a coherent and usable format. A research network provides a vehicle for continual exchange of knowledge and experience." This effort allows for greater global sharing of research information and expertise. The American Association of Colleges of Nursing (AACN, 2006) statement on research includes the following principles: "Nursing researchers bring a holistic perspective to studying individuals, families, and communities; their research takes a biobehavioral, interdisciplinary (interprofessional), and translational approach to science. The priorities for nursing research reflect nursing's commitment to the promotion of health and healthy lifestyles, the advancement of quality and excellence in health care, and the critical importance of basing professional nursing practice on research."

The AACN position statement also identifies major research focus areas. The first area, clinical research, includes interventions that might be used, from acute to chronic care experiences across the entire life span; health promotion and preventive care to end-of-life care; and care for individuals, families, and communities in diverse settings. The second area is health systems and outcomes research, which focuses on identifying ways that the organization and delivery of health care influence quality, cost, and the experience of patients and their families. The third focus is on nursing education—research that explores more effective and efficient educational processes and new teaching–learning practices to incorporate technology in the learning process, intergenerational learning differences and their impact on education, and the development of methods to improve lifelong learning and commitment to leadership.

National Institute of Nursing Research

The National Institute of Nursing Research (NINR), established in 1985, is part of the National Institutes of Health (NIH). It is important that nursing have a presence in the most prestigious national research system in the United States. As discussed in other chapters about scholarly work, the NINR conducts research that has an impact for the nursing profession and also allocates funding for nursing studies that may be conducted in other institutions such as universities and clinical organizations. Interprofessional research is also encouraged and funded by the NINR, which describes how nursing research develops knowledge for the following purposes (2014):

- Build the scientific foundation for clinical practice.
- Prevent disease and disability.
- Manage and eliminate symptoms caused by illness.
- Enhance end-of-life and palliative care.

The NINR is physically located at the NIH campus in Rockville, Maryland. When funded research is conducted at the NINR campus, it is referred to as an intramural or internal study. Grants are also awarded for outside, or extramural, studies that are conducted at the researcher's home institution or in collaboration with several institutions. The NINR's current strategic plan identifies its goals to invest in research focusing on the following areas (NINR, 2016):

- Enhance health promotion and disease prevention.
- Improve quality of life by managing symptoms of acute and chronic illness.

- Improve palliative and end-of-life care.
- Enhance innovation in science and practice.
- Develop the next generation of nurse scientists.

In comparing the ICN and AACN statements with the NINR purposes and strategic plan goals, there are clear similarities, and thus, these organizations provide a more consistent statement about nursing research and the profession's overarching view of research.

The Research Process

The research process is similar to the nursing process; it is a problem-solving method. **Exhibit 11-1** describes the steps of the quantitative experimental research process. The specific plan for conducting the study is the research design and methods. In the proposal, the researcher describes *what will be done*, and in the research report or published article, poster, or presentation after the study is completed, the researcher describes what *was* done.

First, the researcher develops a plan or proposal for the study. This written document describes recent

---

Exhibit 11-1 Steps in the Quantitative Experimental Research Process

I.   Description of problem statement, including background and significance

II. Identification of research question(s) and hypothesis

III. Identification of the purpose(s) of the study: Explain how the findings might be used

IV. Review of literature: Summary of critical literature (theoretical and research literature) that applies to the study.

V.   Theoretical framework: Theories and conceptual models organize research findings into a broader conceptual context and include conceptual and operational definitions of the variables (independent and dependent) in the framework. (This step is not done for all studies.)

VI. Ethical considerations: Description of informed consent for participants/subjects and the institution review board process

VII. Research design and methods
  A. Research design
    1. Identify the research design. Is the study a quantitative study or a qualitative study? Identify the specific sub-design (for example, experimental, quasi-experimental, and descriptive).
    2. Provide an adequate rationale for choosing the research design.
    3. Identify independent and dependent variables (if required for the study design).

Exhibit 11-1 *(continued)*

B. Sample and sample selection
   1. Describe the sample population.
   2. Provide sample criteria (inclusion and exclusion criteria).
   3. Describe sample size using power analysis.
   4. Describe how participants/subjects who meet the criteria will be selected as study subjects: sampling method.
   5. If applicable, describe how groups or treatments/interventions will be assigned in the sample.
C. Setting
   1. Briefly describe the setting for the study.
   2. Describe how access to the study setting will be obtained.
D. Measurement and instrumentation
   1. Discuss the origin and type of measurement instruments.
   2. Describe why the instrument(s) is (are) appropriate to study the problem (that is, why the instrument can produce data that to answer the study question).
   3. If an instrument is developed for the study, describe how it will be developed and how it will be tested for reliability/validity; pilot-test it before using it in the study.
   4. Describe the reliability and validity of the instrument (if used). Evaluate and report relevant reliability and validity data from previous research or a pilot conducted for the study.
E. Data collection
   1. Describe the data collection process and procedures chronologically and clearly enough to allow for replication (describe them in sufficient detail so that a stranger could use this procedure and collect the data as intended).
   2. Identify who will collect the data, and describe the training required. Provide data collection forms as needed.
   3. Discuss control features for study procedures.
F. Data analysis (This step is completed after the previous steps are completed, but the proposal plan needs to describe the data analysis plan that *will* be used.)
   1. Describe specific data analysis plan for each hypothesis or study question. Identify appropriate statistical tests and the rationale for their use in analyzing each study question or hypothesis and participant demographic data. Include the level of measurement of each variable and selected level of significance. (This proposal is a plan for the study, as data are not analyzed until after collected and then included in the final report.)
   2. Specify and justify the level of significance (that is, 0.05, 0.01) for statistical results and findings.
G. Limitations
   1. Ensure that limitations are clearly identified and appropriate.
VIII. Development of budget for the study

Details about analysis of results and conclusions are not included in the proposal, but rather in the final report when the study is complete.

relevant literature on the problem area, describes the research topic or problem, and defines the processes or steps that will be followed to answer the research question(s). The **research proposal** is used to plan the research and also may be used to apply for research funding. It is the critical document used to obtain approval for a study and institutional review board (IRB). The proposal is written in the future tense because the research has not yet been done.

There must be an assessment to identify and describe the problem, formulating the **research problem statement**. The researcher does this assessment using the researcher's individual expertise, reviewing the literature, and possibly interviewing other experts. The review of literature and any other sources is included in the research proposal and in the subsequent research report of results. The researcher (or researchers) primarily examines previous studies by reading their published reports of results to consider relevance to the researcher's proposed study.

The researcher then identifies the study question(s) and hypothesis(ses). The **research question** is concise, developed before the research is conducted and stated in the research proposal. The **hypothesis** is the formal statement of the expected relationship or relationships between two or more variables in a specified population, which is the sample. The hypothesis is stated before the research is conducted and included in the proposal. Some studies do not have hypotheses, such as qualitative studies in which the emphasis is on describing a situation or perception rather than on measuring the variable of interest. The question and hypothesis flow from the description of the research problem statement and the research question(s). The researcher also needs to consider the **research purpose**—describing the potential uses of the results.

In nursing research, particularly qualitative studies, the researcher may identify a theory or a conceptual model to organize the findings. The theory or model is described and related to the research question. For example, if a study was developed to investigate patient education about diabetes, Orem's theory on self-care might be used as the framework for the study. Nursing research studies that use a conceptual framework may or may not rely on a nursing theory, some may use a non-nursing theory. It is important that the framework represents the phenomenon of interest and guides the research question and the measurement of the variable(s). For example, if the nurse is studying blood pressure in a premature infant, the study would most likely use a scientific, physiologically based framework to support factors that influence blood pressure. This all sets the stage for the actual research, which requires that problem assessment and identification are clear. These steps are similar to the assessment and nursing diagnosis phases in the nursing process.

The **research design** and methods are complex. They include the details related to type of study (research approach and design), the sample and the means by which the sample is selected, the setting for the study, measurement and data collection instruments, the data collection process (what exactly will be done to collect the data), data analysis, and a description of potential limitations. The plan should be clear and detailed. This information, or the plan, is called a proposal until the research is conducted. The study is conducted after funding is received. Most research requires funding, and some studies are very expensive to conduct. This step could be compared to implementing a care plan.

The last part of the research process is the **research analysis** and description of the results and conclusions. The proposal describes how the data will be analyzed, but the actual analysis of data cannot occur until the study has been conducted. What did the analysis of data demonstrate, and what are the implications of the data? The researcher needs to consider the proposal—what was planned, how the study was implemented, and the plan for data analysis—so that the outcomes are identified, just as would be done in the nursing process. This can be compared to the evaluation that determines whether patient outcome goals were met based on the nursing process or care plan.

Types of Research Design

The research design describes the plan for the study in detail and explains how the study will be conducted. Research study designs are categorized into two broad categories: quantitative or qualitative. In **quantitative studies**, the research question focuses on how many or how much; in **qualitative studies**, the research question focuses on feelings or experiences. Not all quantitative research studies are **experimental studies**. To be experimental, a study must meet three criteria:

- *Manipulation of intervention:* The researcher administers an intervention to the participants/subjects (sample). This intervention represents the independent variable(s). The researcher wants to identify the effect of the independent variable on the dependent variable or determine if the independent variable causes the dependent variable(s).
- *Control:* The researcher controls some of the experimental situation and uses a control group from the sample, which does not experience the intervention (independent variable). Total control is not usually possible, but efforts must be made to have as much control of the situation as possible. This is easier to do in a laboratory setting as compared to applied or clinical research where there are many factors, many of them unknown, that affect the patient or the sample.
- *Randomization:* The researcher assigns participants/subjects in the sample to the experimental and to the control group using systematic methods, ideally randomization.

Data collection in a quantitative study is highly structured. Examples of data collection methods include structured interviews; collection of biophysiological data, such as blood pressure, blood, urine, and other physiological parameters; questionnaires or surveys; rating scales; structured observation; and many other methods. In quantitative studies, data analysis involves the use of statistics.

Data collection in qualitative studies is less structured than in a quantitative study. A qualitative study might use focus groups, diaries, logs, observation, and open-ended interviews. Analysis of data does not rely on statistics or mathematical equations. The researcher is less detached and may interact actively with the participants/subjects to obtain the best data possible. In fact, the researcher is often considered the instrument of the qualitative research because of the researcher's involvement. Data are analyzed as the study progresses and may lead the researcher in a different direction or to collect additional data. However, data that are not covered in the informed consent cannot be collected without IRB approval for the change. The goal is to understand the issue deeply, not to intervene, and also to see results or compare groups.

Research Funding

Funding is a critical part of any research because it provides the resources to conduct the research, such as researcher salary, staff pay, space (office, lab) supplies, animal costs, and so on. Funding sources vary widely: universities, private donations, foundations and organizations, local and state governments, and the federal government. The federal government is the largest source of grant monies, but private sector organizations also fund research at high levels such as the specialty organizations (for example, American Cancer Society) and healthcare professional organizations. Funding sources determine the amount of the funding and length of time it is awarded. The research proposal includes a budget that should be realistic but also should consider the funding amounts the funding source(s) is providing. There are three approaches a researcher may take to obtain funding:

1. Identify a problem and develop a proposal. This proposal is sent to funding sources that might have an interest in the particular problem.
2. Develop a research proposal that specifically addresses a problem area that a funding source

has identified as a critical need area. This is called a request for proposals or request for applications, and in this case, the researcher must carefully follow all the requirements for the proposal.

3. Sometimes funding sources require the researcher to conduct a pilot study or have data that indicate greater need for research about a particular problem. Indeed, in many cases, having some data to support the research is critical to getting funding for a study.

Once the written proposal is completed and submitted, it is scrutinized to see whether it meets a set of very specific requirements. These requirements can vary from one funding source to another, and deadlines differ. The proposal then goes through the grant review process, which can take months. Typically, peer groups identified by the funding source review grant proposals.

It is extremely difficult to get funding. The federal government grants are highly competitive, and the major source of such funds is the NIH. Congress sets the NIH's budget. Nursing research is funded by similar sources, as is other healthcare research. Funds are also available to support training programs and service programs, which are typically not considered research studies—for example, for schools of nursing to develop a new nurse practitioner or doctor of nursing practice program, offer a nurse residency program, implement programs to increase student retention, or establish a nurse managed clinic. There are also grants for healthcare organizations to develop new services such as in public/community health. Funding for these types of projects and programs typically comes from the Health Resources and Services Administration, which is part of the U.S. Department of Health and Human Services (HHS), but other government sources may also offer these grant opportunities. These funds are not research grants, but rather program grants, but they still require a detailed proposal. Program grants are very important as they provide monies to try new practice or delivery approaches or changes

in healthcare professions education or education opportunities that would not otherwise be tried due to financial barriers.

Ethics and Legal Issues

When ethics and legal issues are considered in relation to research, the first concern is to protect the rights of human participants/subjects. A second area that the researcher considers is how best to balance benefits and risks/harm in the studies. Ethics and legal issues are discussed in other chapters, but here we focus on their implications for research. There are many studies in which participants might potentially be harmed. Research ethics emphasizes the need to be clear about participant/subject risks whenever possible. The third ethical and legal issue is informed consent, which is also important in healthcare service delivery. The last concern is institutional review—that is, review of the proposal to ensure that participant/subject rights are protected and the study is planned in an effective manner that meets the sponsoring organization's standards. This topic is discussed in text content focused on ethical and legal issues.

Today, because of past concern about research ethics and standards, there is greater control to prevent problems with research and ethics. An example demonstrating recognition of ethics is the ANA's *Code of ethics with interpretive statements*, which focuses on multiple rights related to clinical practice but also to research: Provision 3, "the nurse promotes, advocates for, and protects the rights, health, and safety of patients," and Provision 8, which notes that nurses in collaboration with "other health professionals and the public protects human rights, promotes health diplomacy, and reduces health disparities" (ANA, 2015b, pp. 9, 31).

After many major experiences of abuse in research, discussed in this text, efforts were instituted to prevent further problems. One of the strategies was the creation of the **institutional research board**. This committee reviews research before it is conducted to ensure that the study is conducted ethically. Any study that involves human subjects should obtain approval from their institution's IRB (for example, university, healthcare organization). IRBs are mandated to review all research that involves human subjects in institutions that receive federal funds. The purpose is to protect participants/subjects from unnecessary risk or from risks that outweigh potential benefits. Particularly vulnerable populations include the following groups:

- Neonates (newborns)
- Children
- Pregnant women and fetuses
- Persons with mental illness
- Persons with cognitive impairment
- Terminally ill persons
- Persons confined to institutions (for example, prisons, long-term care hospitals)

Examples of questions that might be considered by an IRB prior to approval of a proposed study include the following:

- Will the participant/subject be deceived, and if so, is it necessary for the integrity of the research?
- Does the participant/subject understand the purpose of the project and completely understand his or her role in the project and potential risk of harm and benefits? (informed consent process; who will conduct and what will the participant/subject be told)
- Are there obvious costs or hidden costs to people if they participate? Can they withdraw at any time? Are there any incentives such as cost of transportation?
- What are the benefits, if any, to the participant/subject?
- What are the risks, immediate and long term (if known), to the participant/subject?
- How will the researcher protect the participant's/subject's right to confidentiality?
- Whom should the participants/subjects contact with questions?
- What will be done with the results of the study?

Barriers to and Facilitators of Research

Research is not easy to accomplish. Barriers need to be turned into facilitators for research to be successful. Barriers could include any of these issues; suggested methods for removing the barrier are noted here:

- *Lack of funding:* Researchers need to plan for and obtain adequate funding; most research is costly to implement. As the research is conducted, the researcher needs to manage the budget.
- *Lack of sufficient time:* Good research takes planning and time to accomplish. The researcher needs blocks of time to work on a study, so this requires a schedule that makes sense for the researcher's required workload and other staff involved in the study. Some investigators are involved in research on a full-time basis.
- *Lack of research competencies:* Research expertise is developed over a period of years. Finding a mentor or mentors is important; working with researchers who have been successful can assist a novice researcher.
- *Lack of participants/subjects for the sample:* If the study includes participants/subjects, it is not always easy to find them in the number required or for the required circumstances. This takes time and creativity, and at all times, ethical principles must be considered. The researcher needs to be realistic when planning the study. Participants/subjects may also leave a study at any time, and this loss of sample size can result in a negative result for the study.
- *Inability to find the right setting:* Finding and securing a setting that agrees to participate in the study can be problematic because it requires contacts and communication. The setting also must consider how the study will impact its patients, staff, functioning, and so on.

- *Lack of statistical expertise:* Researchers should find a statistical expert to consult; researchers work in teams and need to work with different experts.

Other Influential Organizations: Impact on Research

The ANA identifies research as an important issue for professional nursing. "Nurses use research to provide evidence-based care that promotes quality health outcomes for individuals, families, communities and health care systems. Nurses also use research to shape health policy in direct care, within an organization, and at the local, state and federal levels. Nurses conduct research, use research in practice, and teach about research. The ANA supports nursing research with a variety of resources such as the Research Toolkit" (ANA, 2016). Its website offers research news, information about research needs, and resources, and the ANA research agenda focuses on (2016):

- The value of nursing contributions to safety, reliability, quality, and efficiency
- Factors that increase the impact of nurses on quality and efficiency
- Use of National Database of Nursing Quality Indicators to enhance patient safety, quality care, and efficiency
- Nurse workforce issues
- Population health issues

Stop and Consider #2

Nursing research needs to improve and expand.

Evidence-Based Practice

What is the purpose of EBP? The use of EBP in nursing leads to more effective decision making to guide the use of limited resources, control costs, and improve quality (Jennings & Loan, 2001). An EBP nursing review is not nursing research. This review involves identifying evidence to answer an EBP question.

How do you get from EBP to research? You might not. At the conclusion of an EBP review, reviewers might find that there is not sufficient evidence to answer the clinical question. The review is referred to as a systematic review. If an EBP review indicates that evidence is already available, there is no need to perform additional research. Thus, an EBP review does not mean that research is conducted or that it must be conducted. In most cases, however, sufficient nursing research is not available to settle most nursing questions. This means that research conducted by nurses prepared in research may be needed to fill the gap in the knowledge base, though most nurses would not conduct this research because they are not prepared to do so.

Definitions

"Decisions about the care of individual patients should be based on the conscientious, explicit, and judicious use of current best evidence. This means that individual clinical expertise should be integrated with the best information from scientifically based, systematic research and applied in light of the patient's values and circumstances" (IOM, 2008, p. 2). This does not mean that all patient care decisions are based on research evidence or only research evidence as there are other types of evidence. Other sources of knowledge or evidence exist, including the following (Melnyk & Fineout-Overholt, 2014):

- *Best research evidence.*
- *Clinical expertise:* The clinician's knowledge and experience or what the nurse, physician, and others on the healthcare team contribute to the care process.
- *Patient values and preferences/circumstances:* This represents the individual patient's own concerns, preferences, expectations, and social and financial resources that affect health and

health care. These factors can change over time and with each unique healthcare need and encounter.

- *Clinical data (assessment) and history:* A patient's assessment includes important evidence that should be considered in treatment decisions.

As nursing students soon discover when they search for nursing EBP literature, there is a problem in this field: The nursing and allied health professions are not as far along in implementing EBP as medicine. The amount of nursing research must increase—not just in quantity, but also in quality and relevance to nursing practice. Also, nursing health interventions are not captured effectively in medical records, which affects the quantity and quality of nursing data that might be found in these records, if this is the an important source for data (IOM, 2003). Examples of nursing data include those related to patient pain, dehydration, skin breakdown, lifestyle change, patient knowledge deficiencies, and nonadherence with treatment. Furthermore, nursing interventions often are evaluated in descriptive or qualitative studies rather than in quantitative studies. Quantitative studies are ranked higher than qualitative studies when evaluating or ranking EBP evidence from research studies, but they are still considered sources of evidence.

The **PICOT (patient–intervention–comparison–outcome–time)** or EBP question should be part of every search for evidence to improve practice. The goal is to ask a searchable and answerable question to identify the best evidence to answer the question. The acronym stands for the patient/population, intervention, comparison, outcome, and time (Melnyk & Stillwater, 2010). EBP questions must be specific—describing each of the elements so that the search for evidence will reach the best conclusions.

How is the PICOT question used? The following describes the process (Melnyk & Stillwater, 2010):

1. Identify a burning clinical issue or question.
2. Collect the best evidence relevant to the question.
3. Critically appraise that evidence before it is used.

4. Integrate the evidence with the other parts of EBP: patient preferences and values, your clinical expertise, assessment information about the patient and the patient's history.
5. Evaluate the practice decision or change.

Types of EBP Literature

EBP literature is different from typical clinical literature and research literature (that is, published articles about studies). The key component of EBP literature is a systematic review. A **systematic review** is a "the consolidation of research evidence that incorporates a critical assessment and evaluation of the research (not simply a summary) and addresses a focused clinical question using methods designed to reduce the likelihood of bias" (DiCenso, Guyatt, & Ciliska, 2005, p. 570). The key characteristic of systematic reviews that identifies their value is their critique of multiple studies related to the same research question to determine best evidence available. There are several types of systematic reviews, but all types (1) include clear criteria for conducting the review process and (2) review not only of research reports, but also may review data from large databases and include published articles that are opinion or essay with the goal of finding as much available evidence as possible that meet the question and related criteria (Brown, 2009). During the assessment process, when evidence is reviewed, a standard hierarchy or rating system is used.

The increasing interest in EBP and need to better understand implications for healthcare delivery led to the publication of in-depth analysis of research issues and EBP. Some of these reports are briefly described here:

- *Knowing what works in health care: a roadmap for the nation* (IOM, 2008): This report emphasizes the need to use EBP and to identify diagnostic, treatment, and prevention services based on what works effectively. Cost must also be considered in clinical decisions, and it impacts quality care. Critical factors that need to be considered are constraining healthcare costs, reducing geographic variation in the use of healthcare services, improving quality, empowering healthcare consumers, and making healthcare coverage decisions.

- *Clinical practice guidelines we can trust* (IOM, 2011b): This report discusses the importance of developing effective clinical guidelines based on best evidence and then applying those guidelines when appropriate. The guidelines should be based on systematic reviews, developed by knowledgeable multidisciplinary experts, consider important patient subgroups and patient preferences, provide clear explanations of the logical relationships between alternative care options and health outcomes, and revise as needed.
- *Finding what works in health care: standards for systematic reviews* (IOM, 2011c): This report focuses on research and EBP and emphasizes the importance of systematic reviews. Standards to ensure quality care should be based on systematic reviews that include assessment of individual studies and synthesis of the evidence. This information should then be shared through publication so that it can be applied in healthcare delivery.

Searching for EBP Literature: Evidence

The first step in finding evidence is to look for a systematic review that addresses the identified PICOT question. If these reviews cannot be found, published articles describing randomized controlled trials/studies should be sought. **Randomized controlled trials (RCTs)** are often referred to as the gold standard in research design. They involve a true experiment; there is control over variables, randomization of the sample, use of a control group and an experimental group, and manipulation of an intervention or interventions

(independent variable). The results of an RCT provide the strongest support for a cause-and-effect relationship. Not all studies meet these criteria.

Two important EBP literature databases are the Cochrane Database of Systematic Reviews and the Joanna Briggs Institute EBP Database. A third source is the Agency for Healthcare Research and Quality (AHRQ) and its collection of evidence-based national clinical guidelines (NCGs). A brief description of each of these databases follows:

- *The Cochrane Database of Systematic Reviews:* This center develops, maintains, and updates systematic reviews of healthcare interventions to allow practitioners to make informed decisions. It is located in London.
- *Joanna Briggs Institute EBP Database:* This organization represents an international collaboration among nursing and allied health centers. It is located in Australia. Its main purpose is to train professionals to conduct systematic reviews.
- *NCGs:* This source is U.S. government based, through the AHRQ, although the guidelines come from many different sources. Guidelines are discussed within other sections of this chapter.

Sigma Theta Tau International, the nursing honor society, is also active in supporting and developing EBP through its online publication, *Online Journal of Knowledge Synthesis for Nursing*. This journal provides full-text systematic reviews to guide nursing practice. It is available by subscription. University libraries may have access via a university subscription, so students may be able to access the journal through their university library.

The Roles of Staff Nurses Related to Systematic Reviews

Nurses may be involved in developing systematic reviews by reviewing studies based on specific criteria, but this is not common for most nurses. Reviewing studies using systematic review procedures takes special expertise and in-depth knowledge of statistics, so this would not be something every nurse could do. It should not be an expectation that staff nurses will do these reviews. The staff nurse's most important role is that of consumer: applying knowledge from systematic reviews. Using the PICOT method to guide them, nurses search for the systematic reviews through databases (for example, Cochrane, Joanna Briggs, Clinical Guideline Clearinghouse, and other professional literature review). After evidence is found, nurses examine the validity of the evidence, its relevance, and its applicability to the EBP question and may then apply the evidence in their practice.

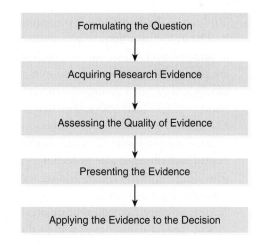

Figure 11-2 The EBM Process

Data from Kovner, A., Fine, D., & D'Aquila, R. (2009). *Evidence-based management in healthcare*. Chicago, IL: Health Administration Press.

Stop and Consider #3

EBP depends on more than just research evidence.

Evidence-Based
Management

Most nurse managers and non-nurse managers, such as someone on a committee making decisions that relate to management of services, do not typically use evidence from research to actively assist in making management decisions. Many use the professional literature, which does not always describe research, but rather provides more content and descriptions of practice. Included in one of the American Organization of Nurse Executives' (2017) goals is facilitation and support of research and development to advance nursing administrative practice and quality patient care. **EBM** is "systematic application of the best available evidence to the evaluation of managerial strategies for improving the performance of health services organizations" (Kovner & Rundall, 2009, p. 56). The definitions for EBM and EBP are not that different. More research that focuses on nursing

management and leadership is needed. The results of these studies may then be considered evidence and incorporated into leadership and management decisions. **Figure 11-2** describes the EBM process.

Stop and Consider #4

Nurses need to apply more EBM.

Improving EBP
Implementation

It has not been easy to incorporate EBP into practice. Some healthcare organizations have been more successful than others. Over time, greater use of EBP will occur, but some barriers still need to be overcome by most organizations:

- *Lack of knowledge about EBP and its value:* EBP has been added to nursing curricula in the last 5 to 10 years, so many practicing nurses have limited knowledge of EBP.

This gap in the knowledge base requires healthcare organizations to play catch-up to improve staff knowledge of EBP. There are now greater numbers of resources for faculty and students through the increased number of EBP textbooks and inclusion of EBP content in research textbooks.

- *Limited time in practice settings:* Staff are rushed and often just able to keep up with providing required care, so adding more responsibilities is difficult.
- *Nursing shortage:* Some healthcare organizations may have insufficient staff to allow nurses time to consider EBP effectively.
- *Greater need to emphasize both knowledge and practical approaches:* This barrier applies to both nursing education and practice settings.
- *Concern that EBP represents a cookbook approach to care:* EBP may be considered a cookbook approach if it is used without assessment and clinical reasoning and judgment. Every patient must be viewed as an individual (patient-centered care).
- *Lack of knowledge about EBP resources:* To make evidence available and usable, more information is needed regarding searching for resources, accessing resources, and analyzing resources.
- *Lack of resources to find information:* For example, staff may not have easy access to the Internet, access to appropriate databases, and library support.
- *Limited recognition by employers regarding the value of EBP:* Nurses are not given time to find EBP evidence and then apply it—even though the healthcare organizations says they want care to be evidence-based.

The recommendation is that EBP needs to be used more effectively; healthcare professionals should have these abilities to (IOM, 2003, pp. 57–58):

- Know where and how to find the best possible sources of evidence.
- Formulate clear clinical questions.

- Search for the relevant answers to the questions from the best possible sources of evidence, including those that evaluate or appraise the evidence for its validity and usefulness with respect to a particular patient or population.
- Determine when and how to integrate these new findings into practice.

Nursing services within a healthcare organization (or any type of healthcare organization) need to plan carefully so that staff have knowledge of EBP and time to ensure staff can effectively apply EBP and evaluate the outcomes. The first step is staff preparation. Some staff members are not ready to engage in EBP. Given that most staff did not graduate from nursing education programs within the last few years (the average age of nurses is older than 45 years), staff may not have had EBP content in their nursing programs or limited content. This is a major hurdle for healthcare organizations. In an effort to remedy potential staff knowledge deficit, many healthcare organizations have integrated EBP content into their staff education programs. EBP is now standard content in pre-licensure and graduate nursing programs, which is reducing the problem of staff that might have limited knowledge of EBP. **Table 11-1** describes strategies individual nurses and healthcare organizations may use to overcome barriers to EBP.

Stop and Consider #5
There are many barriers to effective EBP.

Tools to Ensure a Higher
Level of Use of EBP

EBP evidence should be incorporated into standards of care that guide nursing practice and education. This can reduce practice variation and provide greater consistency based on evidence to improve quality and safety (Newhouse, 2006, 2007). In practice, two

Table 11-1 Strategies to Overcome Barriers to Adopting EBP

Barrier	Strategy
Lack of time	Devote 15 minutes a day to reading evidence related to a clinical problem.
	Sign up for emails that offer summaries of research studies in your area of interest.
	Use a team approach when considering policy changes to distribute the workload among members.
	Bookmark websites having clinical guidelines to promote faster retrieval of information.
	Evaluate available technologies (that is, personal digital assistant) to create time-saving systems that allow quick and convenient retrieval of information at the bedside.
	Negotiate release time from patient care duties to collect, read, and share information about relevant clinical problems.
	Search for established clinical guidelines because they provide synthesis of existing research.
Lack of value placed on research in practice	Make a list of reasons healthcare providers should value research, and use this list as a springboard for discussions with colleagues.
	Invite nurse researchers to share why they are passionate about their work.
	When disagreements arise about a policy or protocol, find an article that supports your position and share it with others.
	When selecting a work environment, ask about the organizational commitment to EBP.
	Link measurement of quality indicators to EBP.
	Participate in EBP activities to demonstrate professionalism that can be rewarded through promotions or merit raises.
	Provide recognition during National Nurses Week for individuals involved in EBP [and EBM] projects.
Lack of knowledge about EBP and research	Take a course or attend a continuing education offering on EBP.
	Invite a faculty member to a unit meeting to discuss EBP.
	Consult with advanced practice nurses.
	Attend conferences where clinical research is presented, and talk with presenters about their studies.
	Volunteer to serve on committees that set policies and protocols.
	Create a mentoring program to bring novice and experienced nurses together.
Lack of technological skills to find evidence	Consult with a librarian about how to access databases and retrieve articles.
	Learn to bookmark important websites that are sources of clinical guidelines.
	Commit to acquiring computer skills.

(Continues)

Table 11-1 (*continued*)

Barrier	Strategy
Lack of resources to access evidence	Write a proposal for funds to support access to online databases and journals. Collaborate with a nursing program for access to resources. Investigate funding possibilities from others (that is, pharmaceutical companies, grants).
Lack of ability to read research	Organize a journal club where nurses meet regularly to discuss the evidence about a specific clinical problem. Write down questions about an article, and ask an advanced practice nurse to read the article and assist in answering the questions. Clarify unfamiliar terms by looking them up in a dictionary or research textbook. Use one familiar critique format when reading research. Identify clinical problems and share them with nurse researchers. Participate in ongoing unit-based studies. Subscribe to journals that provide uncomplicated explanations of research studies.
Resistance to change	Listen to people's concerns about change. When considering an EBP project, select one that interests the staff, has a high priority, is likely to be successful, and has baseline data. Mobilize talented individuals to act as change agents. Create a means to reward individuals who provide leadership during change.
Lack of organizational support for EBP	Link organizational priorities with EBP to reduce cost and increase efficiency. Recruit administrators who value EBP. Form coalitions with other healthcare providers to increase the base of support for EBP. Use EBP to meet accreditation standards or gain recognition (that is, Magnet recognition).

Reproduced from Schmidt, N., & Brown, J. (2015). *Evidence-based practice for nurses: Appraisal and applications of research.* Burlington, MA: Jones & Bartlett Learning.

major tools are commonly used to ensure a higher level use of EBP: (1) healthcare organization policies and procedures and (2) clinical guidelines.

Policies and Procedures Based on EBP

Much of the care in healthcare organizations is defined by policies and procedures, which are important guides for care within healthcare settings. Organizations develop these written guides to inform staff about expectations related to care and management. Policies and procedures are not new to health care, and in reviewing resources such as research results and systematic reviews, this may lead to revision of policies and procedures or development of new policies and procedures. What is the evidence to support a policy or procedure? The difficulty in nursing is there may not yet be evidence such as from research, but policies and procedures should state the research evidence used (if it exists) to support the content. Many healthcare organizations are now trying to improve their policies and procedures by reviewing them from an EBP perspective. Unfortunately, this is a time-consuming process.

Clinical Guidelines Based on EBP

An evidence-based guideline is one of the strongest sources for EBP, along with systematic reviews. Clinical guidelines are described as follows (U.S. Department of Health and Human Services [HHS] & Agency for Healthcare Research and Quality [AHRQ], 2016): "A guideline that provides a purposeful and clear evaluation of the effectiveness of therapeutic modalities. Effectiveness is defined as a measure of the benefit resulting from an intervention for a given health problem under average conditions of use. This form of evaluation considers both the efficacy of an intervention and its acceptance by those to whom it is offered. It answers the question: Does the practice do more harm than good to people to whom it is offered?" Expert panels or professional organizations develop clinical practice guidelines, and these guidelines should be evidence based. An important source for guidelines is the National Guideline Clearinghouse, which is sponsored by the AHRQ providing a commonly used searchable database of guidelines that are used to improve patient outcomes.

Stop and Consider #6
Using clinical guidelines may better ensure effective EBP.

Confusion: Difference
in Research, EBP, and Quality Improvement

Research, EBP, and quality improvement (QI) are not the same, but they are interrelated. Although QI is not discussed in detail in this chapter, it is important to clarify the differences in these three terms and processes for the purposes of this discussion. *Research* is systematic investigation of a problem, question, issue, or topic that uses a specific scientific process to gain new knowledge. Results from studies can be used as evidence to support clinical decisions, although not all research concerns clinical problems and related decisions or has an impact on quality care. An example of research that is clinically focused and would have an impact on quality is a nurse who questions the best method for preventing patient falls in a long-term care facility and wants to consider new interventions. This nurse might develop a research study to gather data to examine how two different groups of patients respond to a new intervention to prevent falls. In doing so, the nurse would follow the research process described elsewhere in this chapter.

By comparison, *EBP* focuses on systematic review and appraisal of evidence, including not only research results, but also the patient's assessment and history data, the clinician's expertise, and the patient's preferences and values. In this case, the same nurse who wondered about factors related to falls might take a different approach, the EBP approach. The nurse would pose a PICOT question, such as "Which factors influence patient falls in a long-term care facility?" The nurse would look for systematic reviews to answer this question and would use systematic reviews, if found, to guide practice; doing so would impact quality care.

QI, which now focuses more on **continuous quality improvement** (CQI), is the process that aims to ensure patients receive the best care when they need it and outcomes are met on an ongoing basis (Finkelman, 2018). CQI is "a structured organizational process for involving personnel in planning and executing a continuous flow of improvements to provide quality healthcare that meets or exceeds expectation" (Sollecito & Johnson, 2013, p. 4). Healthcare organizations are involved in CQI on a daily basis as the healthcare organization staff tries to understand outcomes and improve them. In the same example noted with falls, a CQI project might include monthly collection of HCO data related to the number of falls and specific information about the falls (that is, factors related to the falls). The HCO would examine the seriousness of the problem by using root-cause analysis and might then institute a change in practice or management, such as requiring identification of patients at risk for falls in medical records and putting labels in the patient areas. The HCO would then track data to see if there is any change in the number of falls for at-risk patients—what are the outcomes of using these interventions, though many factors could impact the outcomes since this is not an experimental study with controls.

- Will the evidence help me provide quality care?
- Were all clinically relevant outcomes considered?
- Are the benefits worth the potential harm and costs?

Changing how care is delivered is a major undertaking because there are always barriers to change. It takes an organized approach to implement EBP in a healthcare delivery system. Reimbursement for services—medical and nursing—is increasingly based on whether the guidelines for care are evidence-based. As the financial incentive to implement EBP grows, so will integration of EBP. **Exhibit 11-2** describes role criteria that support EBP functions for the staff nurse, nurse manager, advanced practice registered nurse, and nurse executive.

Stop and Consider #7
Research, EBP, and QI are different but related.

Stop and Consider #8
Every nurse is responsible for using EBP.

Importance of EBP
to the Nursing Profession

As noted in a number of expert reports, EBP can improve care. Nursing care should be supported by evidence, but it is not uncommon for nursing care to be provided in a manner that is best described as "we have always done it this way." This type of approach may not always lead to quality care that best meets patient outcomes, and it may not be the most cost-effective approach. "Evidence-based practice is a problem-solving approach to making clinical, educational, and administrative decisions that combines the best available scientific evidence with the best practical evidence" (Newhouse, 2006, p. 337). In this process, EBP increases nurses' clinical knowledge; this in turn, leads to greater freedom to act, increasing nurses' autonomy and feeling of empowerment. The following are the critical questions for each nurse to ask (Kramer & Schmalenberg, 2005, p. 278):

Impact of Evidence-Based
Practice over the Last Decade

Since the publication of the *Quality Chasm* reports, covering the last decade, and the publication of *The future of nursing* report (IOM, 2010), there have been many changes in the delivery of care by nurses. Notably, EBP has influenced many of these changes in nursing practice, nursing models and frameworks, education, and nursing research. The following content discusses some of the impact on nursing.

Nursing Practice and Management

It was recognized early on that integrating EBP in the healthcare delivery system, nurses as individual care providers, microsystem and system leaders, and policy makers at all levels of government would have to implement EBP. The Magnet Recognition Program® includes EBP as one of its

Exhibit 11-2 Sample EBP Performance Criteria for Nursing Roles

Staff Nurse

- Questions current practices.
- Participates in implementing changes in practice based on evidence.
- Participates as a member of an EBP project team.
- Reads evidence related to the nurse's practice.
- Participates in QI initiatives.
- Suggests resolutions for clinical issues based on evidence.

Nurse Manager

- Creates a microsystem that fosters critical thinking.
- Challenges staff to seek out evidence to resolve clinical issues and improve care.
- Role-models EBP.
- Uses evidence to guide operations and management decisions.
- Uses performance criteria about EBP in evaluation of staff.

Advanced Practice Registered Nurse

- Serves as a coach and mentor in EBP.
- Facilitates locating evidence.
- Synthesizes evidence for practice.

- Uses evidence to write/modify practice standards.
- Role models use of evidence in practice.
- Facilitates system changes to support use of EBPs.

Nurse Executive

- Ensures the governance reflects EBP if initiated in councils and committees.
- Assigns accountability for EBP.
- Ensures explicit articulation of organizational and department commitment to EBP.
- Modifies the mission and vision to include EBP language.
- Provides resources to support EBP by direct care providers.
- Articulates the value of EBP to the chief executive officer and governing board.
- Role-models EBP in administrative decision making.
- Hires and retains nurse managers and advanced practice nurses with knowledge and skills in EBP.
- Provides a learning environment for EBP.
- Uses evidence in leadership decisions.

Reproduced from Schmidt, N., & Brown, J. (2015). *Evidence-based practice for nurses: Appraisal and applications of research.* Burlington, MA: Jones & Bartlett Learning. Modified from Titler, M. (2014). Developing an evidence-based practice. In G. LoBiondo-Wood & J. Haber (Eds.), *Nursing research: Methods and critical appraisal for evidence-based practice* (8th ed., pp. 418–440). St Louis, MO: Mosby Elsevier.

recognition elements—a factor that has encouraged an increasing number of healthcare organizations to adopt nursing EBP and actively pursue staff knowledge of EBP so that EBP can be effectively implemented. Evidence has also been used more extensively to support new practice initiatives such as TeamSTEPPS®. However, even when a program is based on evidence and is well developed, it is not easy to implement and sustain an EBP program. Much more is needed to improve practice and use

evidence to do so. Both of the programs noted here are discussed in other chapters.

Nursing Education

EBP is included in the five healthcare professions core competencies, which in turn provides more support for the call to include EBP in nursing education (IOM, 2003). Nursing education accreditation standards also now include EBP. To prepare students in these core competencies, schools of nursing EBP content is provided at both the undergraduate and graduate levels. Healthcare organizations also include more content on EBP in their staff education. Professional literature, textbooks, and journals are available to support nursing EBP preparation.

Government Initiatives Supporting Research and EBP

There is increasing recognition that a critical need exists for evidence to support strategies employed to improve care. Examples of two initiatives that have been developed to meet this need are the Clinical and Translational Science Awards (CTSA) and the Patient-Centered Outcomes Research Institute (PCORI). The CTSA's goal is to decrease the time taken to move research into practice; as a consequence, this initiative has driven translational research. **Translational research** had been described in two ways: (1) the application of discoveries generated in the laboratory and in preclinical studies to the development of trials and studies in humans and (2) research aimed at enhancing the adoption of best practices in the community. Determining comparative effectiveness of prevention and treatment strategies, for example, is part of translational science (National Institutes of Health, 2010). PCORI (2014) focuses on research that addresses patient-centered outcomes. The federal government also supports comparative effectiveness research and provides resources so that state-of-the-science information is available (HHS & AHRQ, 2017).

Applying EBP
as a Student

Nursing curricula are including more content on EBP for both undergraduate and graduate students. The location of this content in the curriculum can vary from school to school, but typically it is associated with nursing research content and then emphasized throughout the curriculum. This content is not something that should be presented in isolation from other nursing content and clinical experiences. Instead, students need to actively pursue understanding of EBP and use of evidence in their practice. When you are assigned or select patients for clinical experiences, part of the preparation should be to search for current research evidence found in professional literature and then incorporate this evidence in the care plan and practice. This search should extend beyond the patient diagnosis to nursing problems. Students typically use certain types of EBP data—for example, patient values and preferences, patient history, and assessment data—but they also need to include research evidence and often do not consider their own clinical expertise level as evidence for practice.

The more you examine and use EBP, the more it will become an integral part of your practice as a student, as well as your practice after graduation. Merely completing a few assignments on EBP or taking an exam on EBP will not cause you to develop the core competency to use EBP. Instead, you need to make a commitment to practice at the best possible level; to get there takes practice, and that practice should include EBP.

Stop and Consider #9
EBP is now part of nursing education and practice and several important government programs.

Stop and Consider #10
You need to use EBP as a student.

CHAPTER HIGHLIGHTS

- EBP as a core competency is connected to providing patient-centered care, QI, and interprofessional teams.
- Application of EBP has increased because of the recognition of the large translation gap between bench (scientific) research and its impact (that is, its use in practice).
- Research is a systematic investigation of a specific problem.
- The relationship between research and EBP centers on the fact that the best evidence comes from research findings.
- Basic research is designed to broaden the base of knowledge rather than to solve an immediate problem.
- Applied research is designed to find a solution to a practical problem.
- Nursing research is inextricably linked to the profession's mandate to protect the public and promote the best possible patient outcomes.
- The NINR was established in 1985, providing nursing with representation at the NIH.
- The research process, like the nursing process, is based on problem solving.
- Research can be either quantitative or qualitative design; some studies include both. In quantitative studies, the research question(s) focus on how many or how much; in the qualitative design, the research question(s) focus on feelings or experiences.
- IRBs focus on participant/subject rights. The IRB is charged with the responsibility of ensuring that a research participant/subject's rights are protected and that the study is planned in an effective manner that meets scientific standards, particularly theory and informed consent.
- EBP uses evidence from research results, patient assessment and other sources, clinical expertise, and information about patient preferences and values.
- The key component of EBP literature is systematic reviews.
- The involvement of staff nurses in the EBP process is critical to its eventual integration in a healthcare organization's culture of care delivery.
- EBM is critical for effective management of care in all types of settings.
- Research, EBP, and QI are not the same. Research focuses on the scientific method to deduce answers to questions; EBP focuses on the use of supporting data to support interventions; and QI focuses on a system or process to measure and systematically examine quality of care at a macro (or system) level or a micro (or patient) level.
- Nursing education has begun to shift from pure research content with additive information on EBP to a focus on EBP while teaching how research underlies much of EBP.
- Government initiatives such as PCORI support research and EBP.
- Students need to apply EBP in their clinical experiences.

ENGAGING IN THE CONTENT

Discussion Questions

1. What does the core competency "employ evidence-based practice" mean?
2. What is the research process?
3. How does research relate to EBP?
4. What is a systematic review? How do systematic reviews relate to EBP? What is their value to practice?
5. Why is EBP important to nursing practice?
6. What are the barriers to implementing EBP, and how might some of them be overcome?
7. Why is EBM important to healthcare delivery?
8. Which factors would you consider when implementing EBP in a nursing unit?

CRITICAL THINKING ACTIVITIES

1. In an EBP review, you begin by describing the clinical problem or scenario. At the University of Washington's website (http://libguides.hsl.washington.edu/content.php?pid=231619&sid=1931590), you will find examples of clinical problems and scenarios. The PICOT method is used to clearly define a specific clinical problem. This site shows you how to move from the clinical problem/scenario to a clinical question using a PICOT question. How would you summarize this process?

2. Write a PICOT question. After you have written your PICOT question, compare it with questions developed by other students (this can be done in a small group). Ask members of the group to identify the *P, I, C, O,* and *T* in your question, and do the same with the other questions. Select one PICOT question and see if the group can find a systematic review dealing with it. If you cannot find a systematic review, then discuss what this means. Identify PICOT questions for your clinical patients.

3. Visit the NINR website and review the current strategic plan (https://www.ninr.nih.gov/aboutninr/ninr-mission-and-strategic-plan). What examples are given on the site to demonstrate how nursing research is making a difference? Do any of these examples surprise you (nursing involvement, type of study, results)? What is your own school doing in the area of nursing research?

4. Visit the National Institute of Health ethics program website (http://ethics.od.nih.gov/default.htm). Review one of the posted topics. Why did you select this topic? Summarize what you have learned from this site.

5. If you are interested in learning more about the Tuskegee study as an example of need for research ethics, visit The National Academics online ethics center (https://www.cdc.gov/tuskegee/timeline.htm). What happened in this study? What were the ethical issues that should have been considered? Does your school have an IRB office? If so, visit its website and review the informed consent forms and Health Insurance Portability and Accountability Act forms.

ELECTRONIC REFLECTION

Consider how you might improve your practice first as a student and then as a nurse. Develop the steps you will take to work to improve, and then track your results annually.

CASE STUDIES

Case 1

Health professionals noticed that ventilator-dependent adults often developed pneumonia. They started questioning what might be going on. They reviewed the literature and found that there was little evidence to support this phenomenon, although a few studies had addressed the topic. Subsequently, more and more institutions examined ventilator-associated pneumonia (VAP). Based on these reviews, guidelines or best practices were developed to decrease the incidence of VAP in adults. Now, research and EBP studies examine VAP as a measure of quality of care, consider costs associated with VAP versus preventive costs, and use VAP as a benchmarking tool for quality care and patient safety (Ruffell & Adamcova, 2008; Uckay, Ahmed, Sax, & Pittet, 2008).

Case Questions

1. Can you find one published article describing a single study and also a systematic review focusing on VAP and related care issues? If so, what evidence does it provide? How is a single study different from a systematic review?
2. Can you find a clinical guideline on VAP? What evidence is provided?
3. What care approach is used in a clinical setting in which you have practicum? How does it relate to what you have learned from the systematic review and/or clinical guideline?

Case 2

You have just taken a new position in a cardiac care unit. A month after you start the job, you have a question about a procedure and the rationale for its use. You go to your staff mentor, and she tells you to just follow the procedure as written, as it makes work easier. This is not what you expected.

Case Questions

1. What might be your response to your mentor?
2. How might this interaction affect your view of your mentor?
3. At your next monthly meeting with the nurse manager, what might you say about this issue?
4. What does this tell you about EBP on the unit?
5. What might be improved in this unit's practice?

Working Backward to Develop a Case

Write a brief paragraph that describes a case related to the following questions.

1. What do we need to do to increase use of EBP?
2. Why is this important to us? We are all very busy.
3. Why is the documentation of EBP something we should consider?

REFERENCES

American Association of Colleges of Nursing. (2006). *AACN position statement on nursing research*. Washington, DC: Author.

American Nurses Association. (2015a). *Scope and standards of practice*. Silver Spring, MD: Author. Appendix: *Code of ethics with interpretive statements*.

American Nurses Association. (2015b). *Code of ethics with interpretive statements*. Silver Spring, MD: Author.

American Nurses Association. (2016). *Nursing research*. Retrieved from http://www.nursingworld.org /EspeciallyForYou/Nurse-Researchers

American Organization of Nurse Executives. (2017). *American organization of nurse executives*. Retrieved from http:// www.aone.org/about/overview.shtml

Brown, S. (2009). *Evidence-based nursing*. Burlington, MA: Jones & Bartlett Learning.

Chassin, M. (1998). Is healthcare ready for Six Sigma quality? *Milbank Quarterly, 76*, 565–591.

DiCenso, A., Guyatt, G., & Ciliska, D. (2005). *Evidence-based nursing: A guide to clinical practice*. St. Louis, MO: Elsevier Mosby.

Finkelman, A. (2018). *Quality improvement: A guide for integration in nursing*. Burlington, MA: Jones & Bartlett Learning.

Institute of Medicine. (2003). *Health professions education: A bridge to quality*. Washington, DC: The National Academies Press.

Institute of Medicine. (2008). *Knowing what works in health care: A roadmap for the nation*. Washington, DC: The National Academies Press.

Institute of Medicine. (2010). *The future of nursing: Leading change, advancing health*. Washington, DC: The National Academies Press.

Institute of Medicine. (2011a). *Clinical data as the basic staple for health learning: Workshop summary*. Washington, DC: The National Academies Press.

Institute of Medicine. (2011b). *Clinical guidelines we can trust*. Washington, DC: The National Academies Press.

Institute of Medicine. (2011c). *Finding what works: Standards for systematic reviews*. Washington, DC: The National Academies Press.

International Council of Nurses. (2010). *Nursing research network*. Retrieved from http://www.icn.ch/networks/icn-networks/

Jennings, B., & Loan, L. (2001). Misconceptions among nurses about EBP. *Journal of Nursing Scholarship, 33*, 121–127.

Kovner, A., & Rundall, T. (2009). Evidence-based management reconsidered. In A. Kovner, D. Fine, & R. D'Aquila (Eds.), *Evidence-based management in health care* (pp. 53–78). Chicago, IL: Health Administration Press.

Kramer, M., & Schmalenberg, C. (2005). Best quality patient care: A historical perspective on Magnet hospitals. *Nursing Administration Quarterly, 29*, 275–287.

Melnyk, B., & Fineout-Overholt, E. (2014). *Evidence-based practice in nursing and healthcare*. Philadelphia, PA: Lippincott Williams & Wilkins.

Melnyk, B., & Stillwater, S. (2010). Asking compelling, clinical questions. In B. Melynik & E. Fineout-Overholt (Eds.), *Evidence-based practice in nursing and healthcare* (pp. 25–39). Philadelphia, PA: Lippincott Williams & Wilkins.

National Institute of Nursing Research. (2016, September). *The NINR strategic plan: Advancing science, improving lives*. Retrieved from https://www.ninr.nih.gov/sites /www.ninr.nih.gov/files/NINR_StratPlan2016 _reduced.pdf

National Institute of Nursing Research. (2014). *What is nursing research?* Retrieved from http://www.ninr.nih.gov/

National Institutes of Health. (2010). *Institutional clinical and translational science award (US4)*. Retrieved from http://grants.nih.gov/grants/guide/rfa-files/RFA-RM -10-001 .html#SectionI

Newhouse, R. (2006). Examining the support for evidence-based nursing practice. *Journal of Nursing Administration, 36*, 337–340.

Newhouse, R. (2007). Diffusing confusion among evidence-based practice, quality improvement, and research. *Journal of Nursing Administration, 37*(10), 432–435.

Patient-Centered Outcomes Research Institute. (2014). *About us*. Retrieved from http://www.pcori.org/about -us/landing/

Ruffell, A., & Adamcova, L. (2008). Ventilator-associated pneumonia: Prevention is better than care. *Nursing Critical Care, 13*(1), 44–53.

Sollecito, W., & Johnson, J. (2013). The global evolution of continuous quality improvement: From Japanese manufacturing to global health services. In W. Sollecito & J. Johnson (Eds.) *McLaughlin and Kaluzny's continuous quality improvement in healthcare* (4th ed., pp. 1–48). Burlington, MA: Jones & Bartlett Learning.

Uckay, I., Ahmed, Q., Sax, H., & Pittet, D. (2008). Ventilator-associated pneumonia as a quality indicator for patient safety? *Clinical Infectious Diseases, 46*(4), 557–563.

U.S. Department of Health and Human Services, & Agency for Healthcare Research and Quality. (2016, July 16). *National guideline clearinghouse: Glossary*. Retrieved from https://www.guideline.gov/help-and-about /summaries/glossary

U.S. Department of Health and Human Services, & Agency for Healthcare Research and Quality. (2017). *What is comparative effectiveness research?* Retrieved from http://effectivehealthcare.ahrq.gov/index.cfm /what-is-comparative-effectiveness-research1/

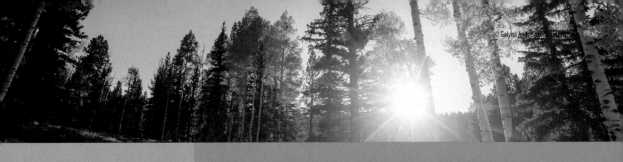

© Galyna Andrushko/Shutterstock.

Chapter 12

Apply Quality Improvement

CHAPTER OBJECTIVES

At the conclusion of this chapter, the learner will be able to:

- Discuss the relevance of the core competency: Apply quality improvement.
- Describe the current status of healthcare quality.
- Explain the need for a blame-free culture of safety and critical concerns of healthcare safety.
- Discuss the integration of quality improvement in healthcare delivery.
- Describe examples of safety initiatives.
- Examine the National Quality Strategy.

- Explain two new major federal initiatives to improve care and control costs: hospital-acquired conditions and 30-day unplanned readmissions.
- Examine examples of high-risk healthcare activities.
- Describe examples of tools and methods used to monitor and improve health care.
- Describe quality improvement measurement and analysis.
- Discuss the roles of nurses and nursing as a profession in improving health care.

CHAPTER OUTLINE

- Introduction
- The Competency: Apply Quality Improvement
- Quality Health Care
- To Err Is Human: Impact on Safety
- Crossing the Quality Chasm: *Impact on Quality Care*
- Envisioning the National Healthcare Quality Report: Need for Monitoring
  - Defining Quality Health Care
- Safety in Health Care
  - Critical Safety Terms

- A Culture of Safety and a Blame-Free Work Environment
- Staff Safety
- Quality Improvement
- Examples of Safety Initiatives
  - The Joint Commission
  - Healthcare Report Cards
- National Quality Strategy
- Federal Initiatives to Improve Care: Hospital-Acquired Conditions and 30-Day Unplanned Readmissions

- Examples of High-Risk Healthcare Activities
  - Medication Administration
  - Care Transitions and Handoffs
  - Failure to Rescue
  - Alarm/Alert Fatigue
  - Missed Nursing Care
- Tools and Methods to Monitor and Improve Healthcare Delivery
  - Utilization Review/Management
  - Benchmarking
  - Assessment of Access to Healthcare Services
  - Medication Reconciliation
  - Standardized Communication Methods
  - Rounds
- Incident Reports
- Sentinel Events
- Measurement and Analysis
  - Data Collection
  - Analysis
- Patient Outcomes and Nursing Care: Do We Make a Difference in Quality Improvement?
- Chapter Highlights
- Engaging in the Content
  - Discussion Questions
  - Critical Thinking Activities
  - Electronic Reflection Journal
  - Case Studies
  - Working Backward to Develop a Case
- References

KEY TERMS

Accreditation	Hospital-acquired complication (HAC)	Quality improvement (QI)
Adverse event	Incident report	Rapid response team (RRT)
Alarm or alert fatigue	Indicator	Root-cause analysis (RCA)
Benchmarking	The Joint Commission	Rounds
Blame-free environment	Measure	Safe care
Care transition	Medication error	Safety
Continuous quality improvement (CQI)	Medication reconciliation	Sentinel event
Culture of safety	Missed nursing care	STEEEP®
Effective care	Misuse	Structure
Efficient care	National Quality Strategy (NQS)	Surveillance
Equitable care	Near miss	Timely care
Error	Outcomes	Transforming Care at the Bedside (TCAB)
Failure to rescue	Overuse	Triple Aim
Healthcare quality	Patient-centered care	Underuse
Healthcare report card	Process	Utilization review/management (UR/UM)

Introduction

This chapter discusses the fourth healthcare core competency: Apply quality improvement (QI). The content includes information about the key quality and associated safety reports (*Quality Chasm* series) and their recommendations. The role of accreditation of healthcare organizations (HCOs) is also related to the need to improve care. Nurses and nursing as a profession assume major roles in ensuring that care is safe and outcomes are reached, resulting in quality care. **Appendix A** is an important resource for this content, providing additional content and terminology to assist in greater understanding of quality health care.

The Competency: Apply
Quality Improvement

The fourth healthcare profession core competency is to apply QI. The description of this core competency follows: "Identify errors and hazards in care; understand and implement basic safety design principles, such as standardization and simplification; continually understand and measure quality of care in terms of structure, process, and outcomes in relation to patient and community needs; and design and test interventions to change processes and systems of care, with the objective of improving quality" (Institute of Medicine [IOM], 2003, p. 4). **Figure 12-1** identifies the key elements of this competency.

Current data indicate that there are serious problems with health care in the United States—its safety, its quality, and waste and inefficiency. In 2014, the U.S. Congressional Subcommittee on Primary Health and Aging held a meeting to examine healthcare errors: "Preventable medical errors in hospitals are the third leading cause of death in the United States, a Senate panel was told today. Only heart disease and cancer kill more Americans . . . Medical harm is a major cause of suffering, disability, and death—as well as a huge financial cost to our nation," Senator Bernie Sanders commented (I-Vt.). The press release went on to state, "each year as many as 440,000 people die due to a preventable medical error in hospitals. Compared with other nations, the United States is about average. In addition to deaths and injuries, medical errors also cost billions of dollars. One study conducted in 2011 put the figure at $17 billion a year. Counting indirect costs like lost productivity due to missed workdays, medical errors may cost nearly $1 trillion each year. . ." (U.S. Congress, Subcommittee on Primary Health and Aging, 2014). Experts comment on healthcare quality by noting recent studies supporting the comments to congress—if we identified errors as a disease, then when tracking death rates per disease errors would be the third leading cause of death in the U.S. (Makary, 2016). This is a strong statement, and it should drive us to greater efforts to improve. The picture is not all bleak as there has been improvement since the report, *To err is human*, but there has not been enough. The examples provided in this chapter content and in **Exhibit 12-1** indicate major problems still exist 18 years after the publication of *To err is human* (IOM, 1999).

Stop and Consider #1
Every nurse is expected to meet the QI competency.

Quality Health Care

Since the late 1990s, there has been considerable growing examination of healthcare quality. The Institute of Medicine (IOM), now known as the Academy of Medicine, is a leader in this effort, consulting with experts, collecting and analyzing data, and publishing reports with recommendations on a variety of topics related to healthcare quality. Its series of reports is often referred to as the *Quality Chasm* reports.

To Err Is Human: *Impact on Safety*

The first report in the *Quality Chasm* series was *To err is human: Building a safer health system*

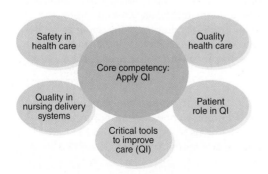

Figure 12-1 Apply QIs: Key Elements

Exhibit 12-1 Examples of Quality Care Issues

The following represent several examples of problems that have occurred in last few years in healthcare organizations that have had a serious impact on patients and their health outcomes. Some have been resolved, and some are ongoing.

National Institutes of Health Clinical Center

The NIH Clinical Center has long been thought of as an exemplar healthcare setting that offers care for unique problems and clinical trials for research studies; however, in 2016, there was significant criticism of the center and its care. Leadership at the center disputed the claims of poor quality (Kaiser, 2016). The report identifies several recommendations for improvement: (1) Fortify a culture and practice of safety and quality; (2) strengthen leadership for clinical quality, oversight, and compliance; and (3) address sterile processing of all injectables and the specifics of the sentinel event that set this review in operation (NIH, ACD, 2016).

Veterans Health Administration

In 2014, there was extensive reporting of abuse with the Veterans Health Administration focused on patients put on wait lists for long periods of time or never seen. This in itself is poor care, but added to this were changes made in documentation indicating that there were not problems with getting appointments. This is fraud and unethical and has been investigated by the Inspector General for the VA. In 2016, problems continued in some VA medical centers—for example, the Inspector General investigating care and misconduct (Krause, 2016). Other problems have been identified in other VA medical centers, such as environment concerns in the operating rooms and fraud and cover-ups with nurses' involvement (Rebelo & Santora, 2016).

A Nurse as a Whistleblower

A nurse in an academic health center sues the health center for covering up infections and then limiting use of standard checking of equipment routinely used in procedures to ensure sterility (Beckers Hospital Review, 2016). If equipment is not checked then, data collected would not identify problems and performance would appear to be better than it might be. The nurse asked that this not be done and an external audit be conducted. This was rejected. The nurse is suing under the whistleblower law, which allows a person to report and file a lawsuit. Employers cannot retaliate for this type of employee action.

Lost Newborn Body

An academic medical center loses the body of a newborn after death during delivery. This is an unusual situation and is a sentinel event. There are procedures and policies that should be applied when a death occurs in a healthcare organization, including care of the body. This did not happen in this case when a woman delivered twins; one was stillborn and the second lived an hour (CBS News, 2015; Fieldstadt, 2015). The hospital even searched the city dump but did not find the body (Butts, 2015).

Whistleblower: Visiting Nurse Service Fraud

At one of the largest nonprofit home healthcare agencies in the United States, a senior manager filed a whistleblower lawsuit for fraud that resulted in hundreds of millions of dollars taken from Medicare and Medicaid. The fraud included falsified and improper billings. This resulted in many patients receiving a fifth or less of their prescribed care. Patients were not told about changes in the service level nor were physicians notified. An example of fraud was a nurse who claimed to have made 20 patient visits for 9 patients in one day. Other nurses made similar claims of visits that could not have been made in the timeframe identified.

Exhibit 12-1 (continued)

Sources:

Beckers Hospital Review (2016). *UC health nurse sues health system for covering up scope-related outbreak*. Retrieved from http://www.beckershospitalreview.com/quality/uc-health-nurse-sues-health-system-for-covering-up-scope-related-outbreak.html; Bernstein, N. (2016, September 24). *Whistleblower suit accuses visiting nurse service of fraud*. Retrieved from http://www.nytimes.com/2016/09/24/nyregion/whistle-blower-suit-accuees-visiting-nurse-service-of-fraud.html; Butts, R. (2015, September 29). *Search of landfill fails to find newborn*. Retrieved from http://www.usatoday.com/story/news/nation/2015/09/29/newborn-boy-body-landfill/73017012/; CBS News (2015, September 29). *Cincinnati hospital apologizes for lost remains of baby*. Retrieved from http://www.cbsnews.com/news/university-of-cincinnati-medical-center-apologizes-for-lost-remains-of-baby/; Fieldstadt, E. (2015). *Body of newborn baby goes miss at University of Cincinnati Medical Center*. Retrieved from http://www.nbcnews.com/news/us-news/body-newborn-baby-goes-missing-university-cincinnati-medical-center-n435696; Kaiser, J. (2016, June 3). *NIH in uproar over report slamming clinical center, leadership shake up*. Retrieved from http://www.sciencemag.org/news/2016/06/nih-uproar-over-report-slamming-clinical-center-leadership-shakeup; Krause, B. (February 15, 2016). *Cincinnati VA at center of misconduct investigation*. Retrieved from http://www.disabledveterans.org/2016/02/15/cincinnati-va-at-center-of-misconduct-investigation/; National Institutes of Health (NIH), & Advisory Committee to the Director (ACD). (2016). *Reducing risk and promoting patient safety for NIH intramural clinical research. Final report*. Retrieved from https://acd.od.nih.gov/Red_Team_final_report_4262016.pdf; Rubelo, K., & Santora, M. (2016, September 19). *Deaths, fraud allegation, and an inquiry into a Long Island VA hospital*. Retrieved from https://www.nytimes.com/2016/09/20/nyregion/inquiry-into-northport-va-hospital-long-island.html?_r=1

(IOM, 1999). This report explored the status of safety in the U.S. healthcare delivery system. The results were dramatic, with data indicating serious safety problems in hospitals. This examination did not include other types of healthcare settings, such as ambulatory care, home care, long-term care, and many other types of sites. More research was needed to provide data about the quality of care and safety in these settings. A recent example of such research is the report published by the Agency for Health Research and Quality (AHRQ): *AHRQ health information technology, ambulatory safety and quality. Findings and lessons from the AHRQ ambulatory safety and quality program*. This report describes studies about ambulatory care, but the report notes that more information is needed to support strong conclusions (U.S. Department of Health and Human Services [HHS] & Agency for Healthcare Research and Quality [AHRQ], 2013b). As is discussed in this chapter, effective understanding or quality requires clear data that are useful for monitoring and measuring healthcare outcomes.

Some of the data from the initial *Quality Chasm* report that disturbed the public and healthcare providers included the following and set the stage for the drive to improve care (IOM, 1999, pp. 1–2):

- When data from one study were extrapolated, the result suggested that at least 44,000 Americans die each year as a result of a medication error. Another study indicated the number of deaths from this cause could be as high as 98,000 (American Hospital Association, 1999).

- More people die in a given year as a result of medical errors than from motor vehicle accidents (43,458), breast cancer (42,297), or acquired immunodeficiency syndrome (AIDS) (16,516) (U.S. Department of Health and Human Services, Centers for Disease Control and Prevention, & National Center for Health Statistics, 1998).
- Healthcare delivery costs represent over more than half of total healthcare national costs, which includes lost income, lost household production, disability and the actual healthcare delivery costs (Thomas et al., 1999).

The data described here are no longer current but are important in understanding the significance of this report. Later in this chapter, HCO accreditation is discussed in detail; however, it is important to note here that accreditation, focusing on evaluating the quality of care in HCOs, has long been a driving force in health care. It is clear from *To err is human* that this has not been enough to improve care at the level needed.

The media took note of *To err is human* and its recommendations, and soon worrisome stories appeared on the evening news and in newspapers; special in-depth news reports asked, "How safe are you when you go in for health care?" Consumers began to ask questions. Healthcare errors experienced by patients and errors reported in the media reduce the public's trust in the healthcare system. The result is that patients and families now question their care more. Some patients now want a family member or friend with them when they are in the hospital, not just for support but also to act as a protector from errors. When a patient experiences an error, the patient's trust level drops, and this has an impact on how the patient approaches future care. There is a positive side to this situation: More patients are demanding to be informed about their care and, therefore, are becoming more involved in the care process.

The first important issue when trying to do something to prevent errors and improve care is to recognize there is not a specific single answer to this problem. Changing the status of quality care requires multiple planned strategies in practice and management and an increase in QI education in professional healthcare programs such as nursing education and staff training.

Crossing the Quality Chasm: *Impact on Quality Care*

Crossing the quality chasm (IOM, 2001a) is the report that followed *To err is human* (IOM, 1999) in the *Quality Chasm* series. This report's major message is that the U.S. healthcare system is in need of fundamental improvement. Although the healthcare delivery system has undergone many changes—such as the development of new drugs, medical technology, and informatics that have improved care and care options—more needs to be done. The 2001 report provides valuable information to help nurses better understand quality issues in the healthcare system; however, if this information is not applied to improve care, it serves little purpose. The report identifies six aims or goals for improvement. These aims state that care should have the following characteristics: safe, timely, effective, efficient, equitable, and patient-centered care (**STEEEP**®) (IOM, 2001a, pp. 5–6). This care ensures that patients receive the care they need, when they need, in the most cost-effective manner and that efforts are made to prevent problems that might occur due to the care such as an error. As noted in other *Quality Chasm* reports, care must also recognize diversity and ensure that disparities are limited. The critical element that connects all of this is the care is focused on the patient with the patient participating in the care process. All of the healthcare professions' core competencies relate to STEEEP, and these aims are now considered to be critical elements for all healthcare delivery (IOM, 2003).

The *Quality Chasm* series is unique in that each report does not stand alone, but rather expands on previous reports in the series. This interconnectedness makes it important that readers understand the general information in each report, the ways in which the reports relate to one another, and the recommendations and joint implications for nursing and health care. For example, STEEEP is related to all of the reports and now is a central feature in HCO QI programs and in national QI initiatives to better ensure continuous quality improvement (CQI).

To ensure an improved healthcare system meets the six aims identified in the *Crossing the quality chasm* report, new rules for the 21st century were developed to guide care delivery describing a vision of health care, though we are not there yet. The rules are included here with additional comments about their relationship to nursing (IOM, 2001a, p. 67).

1. *Care based on continuous healing relationships. Patients should receive care whenever they need it—access is critical.* Health needs are not static, and care must change to meet the needs. Consider these factors and examples: the nurse–patient relationship, continuum of care, collaboration and coordination, HCO services and systems, diversity, interprofessional teams, communication, and nursing standards.

2. *Customization based on patient needs and values.* This rule relates directly to patient-centered care. Patient needs and values also constitute one of the sources of evidence for evidence-based practice (EBP). Consider these factors and examples: nursing care and planning, interprofessional teams, patient-centered care, collaboration and coordination, diversity, patient rights, and patient education, all of which relate to nursing standards and to the nursing code of ethics.

3. *The patient as the source of control.* Patients need information to make decisions about their own care—this is essential to patient-centered care. Healthcare systems and professionals need to share information with patients and bring patients into the decision-making process. Consider these factors and examples: plan of care, interprofessional care, informed consent provides patient information to the decision maker, privacy and confidentiality, patient education, patient rights and professional ethics, and informatics.

4. *Shared knowledge and the free flow of information.* Patients need access to their medical information, and clinicians also need access. This rule relates to all the core competencies, and particularly to the fifth competency—applying informatics. Consider these factors and examples: informatics, interprofessional teams, sharing information in the nursing care process, patient-centered care, privacy and confidentiality, patient education, computerized documentation, professional ethics, and standards.

5. *Evidence-based decision making.* Patients need care that is based on the best possible evidence available. Care should not vary illogically from clinician to clinician or from place to place. Consider these factors and examples: patient-centered care, nursing research and other areas of research, research informed consent, and plan of care.

6. *Safety as a system property.* Patients need to be safe from harm that may occur within the healthcare system. There needs to be more attention placed on system errors rather than just individual errors. Consider these factors and examples: patient-centered care, CQI, nursing care provided in a safe manner, inclusion of safety in the plan of care, patient safety and errors, staff safety, culture of safety, and reimbursement (for example, Medicare rules limit reimbursement if a patient experiences a fall).

7. *The need for transparency.* The healthcare system should make information available to patients and their families that allow them to make informed decisions when selecting a health plan, hospital, or clinical practice or when choosing among alternative treatments. This should include information that describes the system's performance on quality, EBP, and patient satisfaction. Consider these factors and examples: interprofessional teams, informatics, privacy and confidentiality, informed consent, research, patient education, report cards, ethics and standards, and national reports on quality and disparity.

8. *Anticipation of needs.* Healthcare providers and the health system should not just react to events that may occur with patients, but should anticipate patient needs and provide care needed. Consider these factors and examples: assessment, interprofessional teams, nursing care process, plan of care, collaboration and coordination, HCO services, patient satisfaction, diversity, outcomes.

9. *Continuous decrease in waste.* Resources should not be wasted—including patient time. Consider these factors and examples: use of resources for care delivery, costs of care, access to care and services, staff communication, and issues of misuse, overuse, and underuse.

10. *Cooperation among clinicians.* Collaboration and communication are critical among healthcare professionals and systems (interprofessional teamwork). Consider these factors and examples: interprofessional team, plan of care requires team collaboration and coordination.

These rules provide a vision of what healthcare delivery should be *if* we are to ensure quality care for all. They provide nurses with a guide in developing improvement initiatives and strategies.

Envisioning the National Healthcare Quality Report: *Need for Monitoring*

Envisioning the national healthcare quality report (IOM, 2001b) is the follow-up report to the *Crossing the quality chasm* (IOM, 2001a). Up until this time, the United States did not have a structured method to monitor and measure healthcare quality. This report addresses this problem and describes a framework for collecting annual national data about healthcare quality and focusing on how the U.S. healthcare delivery system performs in providing personal health care. The Agency for Healthcare Research and Quality (AHRQ) is mandated to collect data using this framework and then publish an annual report describing current status of U.S.

healthcare quality, which is made available on the Internet. This report should "serve as a yardstick or the barometer by which to gauge progress in improving the performance of the healthcare delivery system in consistently providing high-quality care" (IOM, 2001b, p. 2). Elsewhere in this chapter, healthcare report cards are discussed. An annual national report card does not replace the need for individual HCOs to monitor their own quality. The information from the national annual report card can be used by HCOs in comparing their QI data with national data and developing services. Healthcare professionals (providers), insurers, and health policy makers may use the information to better understand current healthcare quality and consider strategies to improve. Nurse educators should use this information in planning curricula and teaching–learning strategies to ensure that students are prepared to practice effectively based on current needs.

Because the quality report and the national disparities report were interrelated, in 2010 they were merged into one report, the National Quality and Disparities Report (QDR) (HHS & AHRQ, 2010). This report is designed to meet the following needs: use measurement based on best methods; identify issues that improve or act as barriers to quality care; collect data about care quality; educate the public, healthcare professionals, organizations, and so on, about quality care; assist policy makers in improving care; identify key benchmarks; compare U.S. health care with other countries; continue to improve measurement so that data are available and useful; examine healthcare issues that might affect quality of care; and report data and results. The annual report tracks outcomes for the priority areas of care and the adjusted priorities based on annual results.

We now have more than 10 years of data from these monitoring reports, and the reports influence decisions made about health policy and QI. Because it takes time to collect and analyze data, the published reports are typically 2 years behind the current year.

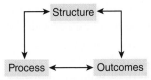

Figure 12-2 Three Elements of Quality

The monitoring methods used to collect and analyze the data are reviewed periodically to ensure their usefulness and quality of the data, and changes have been made as needed. The current National Healthcare QDR can be accessed at the AHRQ's website.

Defining Quality Health Care

There is no universal definition of **healthcare quality**—a fact that has made it difficult to assess quality. For this discussion, the following definition will be used in this chapter and is applied in other chapters: "degree to which health services for individuals and populations increase the likelihood of desired health outcomes and are consistent with current professional knowledge" (IOM, 1990, p. 4). Quality is a complex concept, and who is defining it can make a difference; for example, a nurse, a physician, and a patient may all have different definitions of quality.

This definition of quality includes three elements, which usually are included in the discussion of quality care and monitoring care and described in **Figure 12-2** (Donabedian, 1980):

1. **Structure**: The environment in which services are provided; inputs into the system, such as patients, staff, and environments.
2. **Process**: The manner in which services are provided; the interactions between clinicians and patients.
3. **Outcomes**: The results of services; evidence about changes in patients' health status in relation to patient and community needs.

Stop and Consider #2
It is not easy to define quality health care.

Safety in Health Care

Safety is a critical component of quality care. It is important to recognize the relationship of safety and quality because it is easy to assume that safety is something different from quality care rather than to view it as an integral component of QI. An effective HCO QI program monitors all aspects of quality so safety for patients and staff would be included. There is no question that healthcare providers, including nurses, have long been concerned about providing safe care for their patients. If one interviewed healthcare providers, they would say that they want to keep their patients safe. This belief was somewhat shattered when the U.S. Congress and President's Clinton's Advisory on Consumer and Quality in the Healthcare Industry requested that the IOM initiate an examination of healthcare safety and make recommendations based on its findings. Here we explore the topic of safety in healthcare quality: what it is and what can be done to better ensure safe care for all. As will be discussed, this examination expanded to something more than a focus on healthcare safety.

Critical Safety Terms

Through the IOM's emphasis on healthcare quality, this organization expanded knowledge about safety and errors, in part by undertaking identification and definition of key terms. This development of a common terminology is an important step in addressing the issue. To effectively collect and analyze data nationally requires a shared terminology. **Appendix A** provides a summary of definitions for some critical terms. The following terms are part of this effort, and they have relevance to nurses who need to be directly involved in initiatives to improve care in HCOs, at the individual healthcare professional level, and in health policy (Chassin & Galvin, 1998; IOM, 1999).

- **Safety**: Freedom from accidental injury. *Example*: The patient leaves the hospital after surgery and a 3-day stay with no complications with expected outcomes reached.

- **Error**: The failure of a planned action to be completed as intended or the use of the wrong plan to achieve an aim. Errors are directly related to outcomes. There are two general types of errors: error of planning and error of execution. Errors harm the patient, and some, not all, errors may be preventable. *Example*: The patient is given the wrong medication.

- **Adverse event**: An injury resulting from a medical intervention; in other words, an injury that is not a result of the patient's underlying condition. Not all adverse events are caused by errors, and not all are preventable. It requires greater examination and analysis to determine the possible relationship between an error and an adverse event. When an adverse event is the result of an error, it is considered a preventable adverse event. *Example*: A patient is given the wrong medication and experiences a seizure. If the patient does not have a seizure disorder, this is more likely an adverse event, but much more needs to be known about the cause(s). How did the error that led to the adverse event happen? The following factors are expected to increase the risk of medication adverse events in the future: development of new medications, discovery of new uses for older medications, aging of the U.S. population, and greater use of medications for disease prevention (U.S. Department of Health and Human Services [HHS] & Centers for Disease Control and Prevention [CDC], 2012).

- **Misuse**: Avoidable complications that prevent patients from receiving the full potential benefit of a service. *Example*: The patient receives a medication that is not prescribed and that conflicts with the patient's allergies; the patient experiences anaphylaxis.

- **Overuse**: Potential for harm from the provision of a service exceeds the possible benefit. *Example*: An elderly patient is on multiple medications, and the patient's multiple healthcare providers do not know the medications that have been prescribed by different healthcare providers.

- **Underuse**: Failure to provide a service that would have produced a favorable outcome for the patient. *Example*: The patient is not able to get a specialty service needed for cancer because of distance from resources, or the patient's insurer will not cover a medication for arthritis that could make the patient more mobile.

- **Near miss**: Recognition that an event occurred that might have led to an adverse event. This does not mean an error occurred, but that it almost occurred. It is important to understand these errors because they provide valuable information for preventing future actual errors. *Example*: The surgical team is preparing for surgery to repair a patient's knee. The right knee is prepped, but soon after, the team checks the records and goes through a safety check list prior to beginning surgery, the call-out, and check-back, to ensure that the correct knee is exposed—only to find out that it is the left knee that requires surgery. The team stops and replans the surgery. If there is no consideration of why this error almost happened, then the team cannot learn from it and hopefully prevent future errors. One model for understanding near misses and prevention of an error is the Endhoven model (van der Schaaf, 1992), which was adapted by nursing to identify three sources of errors Henneman and Gawlinski (2004, p. 196):

1. *Technical failure (system error)*: Physical items such as software, equipment, or other materials are not designed correctly, are working incorrectly, or are not available when needed.

2. *Organizational failure (system error)*: Such errors relate to complex factors that affect

how work is carried out in the healthcare setting, such as staff orientation, staff expertise, protocols, policies and procedures, clinical pathways, management priorities, budget, and organizational culture.

3. *Human failure:* This failure results from behaviors related to skills, rules, and knowledge. Safety mechanisms should include reliable system defenses and the availability of adequate human recovery. Human intervention such as from nurses can prevent adverse outcomes even when high-risk incidents develop into error incidents.

- **Sentinel event**: This type of event has a serious negative patient outcome (unexpected death, serious physical or psychological injury, or serious risk). *Example*: A patient commits suicide while in the hospital for treatment of diabetes.

If the examination of healthcare quality had concluded with the *To err is human* report, the major impact of the report and its recommendations would most likely have been diluted (IOM, 1999). This, however, did not happen. In 2004, due to recognition that much more needed to be known about the quality of health care, follow-up reports were published. The approach of the *Quality Chasm* series has been (1) to describe a problem using data and expert knowledge, (2) identify recommendations to respond to the problem(s), and (3) identify monitoring methods and possible interventions or solutions. *Patient safety: Achieving a new standard for care* (IOM, 2004a) focuses on the need to establish a national information infrastructure and the need for data standards. These elements help healthcare providers and payers improve monitoring outcomes. Having a common language/terminology to use in discussions about safety and errors is critical in meeting the goal to develop a national information infrastructure to support monitoring of care. It also addresses the fifth healthcare professions core competency, which focuses on informatics. This is

another example that illustrates how the reports, data, recommendations, and methods to monitor change are all interconnected. They are clearly interwoven with the need to develop core competencies so that healthcare providers can meet the need to improve care. As discussed later and in other chapters, there are now major initiatives that respond to the concerns noted in the *Quality Chasm* reports.

A Culture of Safety and a Blame-Free Work Environment

The typical HCO approach to errors in health care has been to identify the staff member who made the error, supported by requiring staff to complete incident reports that describe errors. This type of approach is punitive in nature and has not been effective in reducing errors, as noted in the 1999 report (IOM). It has not been effective because most errors are not made by an individual, but rather are complex and most likely system errors. When an error occurs, the question should not be "Who is at fault?" but rather "Why did our defenses fail?" (Reason, 2000). Communication, collaboration, and coordination (interprofessional teamwork); staffing levels and expertise; staff knowledge; patient acuity level; equipment; delivery processes; the role of the patient in care; and many other factors affect actions taken or not taken in health care. The healthcare system has focused on the blame game and not on designing and using structured methods to find out more about all the factors related to an error. Staff members need to feel comfortable—not fearful—in reporting errors. The goal now should be a **blame-free environment** or a **culture of safety** in which staff can practice and openly discuss potential errors or near misses and actual errors. If staff members worry about implications such as impact on their position or performance, they may not report an error. This can have serious consequences for patients and prevent the system from improving. This type of fear may also prevent staff from communicating near misses, from which much can be learned about potential errors. In the past, if a nurse made a medication error, the nurse might have been routinely required to take a medication review course and an exam on medication administration with no consideration of analyzing the causes of the error. The following are examples of questions that are important to consider for this situation in a culture of safety, demonstrating the complexity of an error:

- What are the key questions we should consider?
- Was the prescription transcribed correctly?
- Was the order not the best choice for the patient and patient's problem?
- Was an error made in what the physician intended to order or what the team agreed would be the best approach?
- Was the correct medication sent by pharmacy? Correct dose? Correct method of administration? Correct time?
- Did the error involve placing a patient medication in the wrong patient medication box?
- Was there an equipment malfunction (for example, intravenous equipment, monitoring equipment)? Was there a computer error?
- What were the distractions and interruptions when the medication was prepared and administered?
- Were monitoring guidelines followed (for example, vital signs checked)? If data indicated certain actions should be taken, were they taken? If not, why?

Did the nurse check the patient's identification correctly? To accomplish the goal to move to a culture of safety, there must be (1) greater understanding of its essential elements, (2) a decrease in barriers to creating the culture, (3) development and implementation of strategies to create the safety culture, and (4) evaluation of outcomes (IOM, 2004a). Hospitals and other HCOs are moving toward cultures of safety, but it will take time and effort to change staff and administration attitudes and behaviors.

It is particularly important to have effective HCO leadership to guide and support the development of a culture of safety (Anderson, 2006). Trust is important in this type of culture—staff must trust management and vice versa. A topic that comes up often from all types of healthcare professionals is concern about revealing errors and near misses. This is based on past experiences. Moving away from blame means that staff members must trust that they will not be automatically blamed or punished for errors that are out of their individual control. Another aspect of this issue is related to individual staff expectations; nurses feel that they should not make mistakes, that the care they provide should be perfect. This is not a reality-based perspective. Errors will inevitably be made that are caused by many factors. Improvement is, of course, critical, but to think that errors will never be made is not realistic. There is no doubt that the number of errors needs to decrease. Moreover, there is no doubt that what has been done to address errors has not yet been fully effective. To be truly effective, disclosure must be present with maximum transparency. Ensuring transparency and involving patients are the most difficult aspects of ensuring a culture of safety (Anderson, 2006). "A fundamental principle of the systems approach to error reduction is the recognition that all humans make mistakes and that errors are to be expected, even in the best organizations" (Reason, 2000, p. 768).

It is important to note that a no-blame culture of patient safety does not mean a lack of individual accountability (Wachter & Pronovost, 2009). There is greater emphasis on the recognition of the impact of the system on errors, but nurses and other healthcare providers still have accountability for their own practice. When an individual fails to adhere to a safety standard that one would be expected to know and apply, and there are no system issues for this failure, then an individual staff member may be accountable for the error. Reporting is an important component of professional accountability. This means healthcare professionals recognize the importance of QI and are committed to active participation in the QI process.

Despite all of these reports, data, and initiatives to improve care and respond to errors—for example, with checklists to ensure that the correct side or body part is operated on in surgery—major problems persist. The Joint Commission reports that wrong site, wrong patient, and wrong procedure continue to be major problems, representing the most frequently reported sentinel event—for example 1,196 events reported for first 9 months of 2015 (Joint Commission, 2015). Such errors are increasing, not decreasing. For example, consider what happened with a patient who was scheduled to have cardiac bypass surgery. When a nurse asks the patient to sign the consent form, it listed a different procedure. The patient, who was a physician, pointed out the error and refused to sign. A half-an-hour later, another nurse brought the patient another consent form to sign, but it was also incorrect. The third consent form was correct and signed by the patient. This should never happen. What if the patient had not noticed or did not have the background to understand that the surgical procedure described was not what was agreed upon between the physician and the patient? This experience also took staff time and increased stress for the patient and family just prior to surgery. Patient trust in staff was significantly reduced, and as the patient left the hospital, he said, "What has happened to nurses? I have worked with them for years, but their practice has gone downhill. I could have been killed in there." This same patient experienced several critical near misses with intravenous medications that could have led to cardiac arrest if the patient had not noticed the errors and told the nurse to stop giving the medication immediately; an error that was repeated the next day. It highlights the fact that much more needs to be done to improve care and that changing the culture is much more complicated than thought.

It is important to recognize that some HCOs continue to have blame cultures, and more attention should be given to the personal reaction of staff involved in errors, particularly errors that lead to the death of a patient. How much debriefing occurs, and are staff blamed and in what way? In 2011, a neonatal nurse with 24 years' experience was involved in medication error that led to the death of an 8-month-old baby, though at the time it was not clear the error was the actual cause of the death. Immediately after the incident, the nurse was escorted from the hospital, put on administrative leave, and then fired several weeks later. Seven months later, the nurse committed suicide. The hospital in which this event occurred had been following a "just culture" approach for more than 3 years, but this example does not demonstrate this type of culture (Aleccia, 2011). Does this incident send a message not to mention mistakes? How effective was the organization's "just culture"? How can employers help staff so that staff do not become secondary victims if they cannot cope with the result of an error? Emotional distress after an event is not uncommon for staff. In a survey of 3,000 physicians in the United States and Canada, 92% reported experiencing an adverse event, and of those physicians, 81% reported some job-related stress associated with the adverse event (U.S. Department of Health and Human Services [HHS], Agency for Healthcare Research and Quality [AHRQ], & Patient Safety network [PSNet], 2016a). Recovery requires time, but it is critical that HCOs maintain an environment of support and offer the provider assistance. Getting support from peers is also important, as is having a break from work responsibilities immediately after the adverse event and having some time to talk about the event in an environment that is not threatening.

The establishment and maintenance of an effective culture of safety requires leadership. This is so critical that The Joint Commission published a sentinel event alert entitled: The essential role of leadership in developing a safety culture (2017a). It recognizes that when leaders in HCOs do not create an effective culture of safety, this results in adverse events. The sentinel alert notes that leadership is needed for effective support of event reporting and to provide feedback to staff and others who are reporting safety concerns, promote an environment in which staff who report events are not intimidated, use the

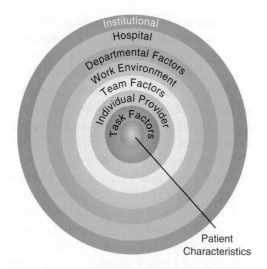

Patient
Characteristics

Figure 12-3 System-Level Factors That Affect Safety

Reproduced from Agency for Healthcare Research and Quality. (2015, June). *Collaborative unit-based safety program (CUSP) toolkit. Understand the science of safety: Presentation slides.* Retrieved from http://www.ahrq .gov/professionals/education/curriculum-tools/cusptoolkit /index.html

reporting data to improve, and alert management to staff burnout. This type of leader supports a just culture, a reporting culture, and a learning culture at all levels of the organization.

It is important for students who are involved in a near miss or an error to discuss the experience openly with faculty and ask for support. Faculty need to provide support to students when these situations occur or get qualified persons to assist the student. If this is not done, it reinforces a blame culture—schools of nursing need to establish cultures of safety or just cultures (Penn, 2014). As we move toward a system view of errors, factors described **Figure 12-3** support a culture of safety.

Staff Safety

To err is human focused on patient safety, not staff safety, but the report did state that "creating a safe environment for patients will go a long way in addressing issues of worker safety as well" (IOM, 1999, p. 20). This lack of information about staff

safety in this report does not mean staff safety is not important—it is very important. Another report, *Keeping patients safe: Transforming the work environment of nurses* (IOM, 2004b), includes content related to staff safety, particularly nurses. Nursing staff is not immune to workplace injuries. The Occupational Safety and Health Administration (OSHA) is the federal agency that is responsible for monitoring safe workplaces and provides guidance and resources to ensure workplace safety. The American Nurses Association (ANA) is a strong advocate for safety for nurses in all types of healthcare settings. Its position statements on staff safety provide guidelines for healthy work environments. Examples of some of the position statements are available at the ANA website, such as *Personnel policies and HIV in the workplace, HIV infection and nursing students, HIV testing,* and others. Some of the key safety issues for nursing staff other than those mentioned are highlighted here. These statements can be accessed via the ANA website.

- *Needlesticks:* Hospital-based healthcare workers experience approximately 385,000 needlesticks and other sharps injuries annually, with 5.6 million at risk for exposure (HHS & CDC, 2015; U.S. Department of Labor & Occupational Safety and Health Administration, 2016). These exposures can lead to hepatitis B, hepatitis C, and human immunodeficiency virus, the virus that causes AIDS. At least 1,000 healthcare workers are estimated to contract serious infections annually from needlestick and sharps injuries. Registered nurses (RNs) working at the bedside experience the majority of these exposures. More than 80% of needlestick injuries can be prevented with the use of safer needle devices, but HCOs must provide them—and nurses need to demand that they are available.

- *Infections:* As noted, healthcare workers are often exposed to communicable diseases via needlesticks. Other examples of infections staff may be exposed to include tuberculosis,

Staphylococcus, cytomegalovirus, influenza, and bacteria. Influenza spread has been linked to suboptimal vaccination levels of healthcare workers (Polygreen et al., 2008). Bacterial infections have sometimes been linked to glove contamination (Diaz et al. 2008). A recent infectious disease is the Ebola virus that spread from Africa and also the Zika virus, transmitted by mosquitos but not contagious in the work environment, unless the nurse is working in an area where the infected mosquitos exist. Both of these situations are examples of the global impact of infectious diseases today; people travel globally, and healthcare providers go to assist other countries in providing health care for emergencies and on a routine basis.

- *Ergonomic safety:* Nurses experience a significant number of work-related back injuries and other musculoskeletal disorders. Because of these injuries, nurses may transfer to other units or other healthcare settings, and sometimes they may leave nursing. Typical injuries are to the neck, shoulder, and back. Nursing practice requires a lot of patient handling, and factors such as the patient's weight, height, body shape, age, dependency, and medical status are important to consider as ergonomic issues. There has been an increase in weight in the U.S. adult population in general, and this has increased the risk of injury. The physical setting also is a factor in increasing risk. There should be enough space to provide care and when moving the patient. Nurses should consider the types of equipment available to assist with moving patients, request assistance, and discuss their work needs with management, noting the importance of these factors to quality care and staff and patient safety. The ANA's "Handle with Care" campaign addresses work-related musculoskeletal disorders (Castro, 2004). Its goal is to develop and implement a proactive, multifaceted plan to promote the issue of

safe patient handling and the prevention of musculoskeletal disorders among nurses in the United States. Through a variety of activities, the campaign seeks to advocate, educate, and facilitate change from traditional practices of manual patient handling to emerging technology-oriented methods. Nursing education and staff education needs to include content and experiences to facilitate the use of the most effective handling methods. In addition, more emphasis should be placed on assistive patient handling equipment and devices. Students need to learn how to use this equipment, too. In 2013, the ANA expanded its initiative on safe patient handling by publishing *Patient handling and mobility: Interprofessional national standards*, in collaboration with an interprofessional group to establish safe environments for nurses and patients (ANA, 2013).

Standard 1. Establish a culture of safety.

Standard 2. Implement and sustain a safe patient handling and mobility (SPHM) program.

Standard 3. Incorporate ergonomic design principles to provide a safe environment of care.

Standard 4. Select, install, and maintain SPHM technology.

Standard 5. Establish a system for education, training and maintaining competence.

Standard 6. Integrate patient-centered SPHM assessment, plan of care, and use of SPHM technology.

Standard 7. Include SPHM in reasonable accommodation and post-injury return to work.

Standard 8. Establish a comprehensive evaluation system.

- *Violence:* Violence may not be a typical staff safety concern that a student would first think of when asked about safety in the healthcare workplace, but it may be a problem. There is greater risk for violence in emergency departments, psychiatric/substance abuse departments, and long-term care facilities; however, such incidents may occur anywhere. Patients and families may not be able to control their anger appropriately. The nurse may also be in a situation in which violence that is not directly related to the nurse or health care occurs, such as providing home care in a community in which there is often violence. Staff members need training so that they can prevent violence when possible—particularly training on how to identify signs of escalation and how to de-escalate a situation when possible. They need to know how to protect themselves when violence cannot be prevented. In areas such as psychiatry, this training is more common. Signs of escalation include a sudden change in behavior, clenched jaws or fists, threats, pacing, increased movement, shouting, use of profanity, increased respirations, and staring or pointing. These signs do not mean that the person will become violent, but rather that the nurse should be more aware of the person's behavior and communication to determine if the person is escalating. Protecting oneself is very important: The nurse may decide it is safer to leave the room stay near the door or keep the door open, but not appear to be blocking the door; ask other staff to be present; or call for security assistance. It is also important when any weapon is noted in patient belongings to secure the weapon and call for professional assistance such as the HCO's security and the police. HCOs should have a policy and procedure describing expected staff response to this type of situation. This information should also include requirements for police who are carrying weapons (for example, when entering a mental health unit they must remove their guns). Additional content on workplace violence is discussed in other content in this text.

- *Chemical exposure:* OSHA offers information on preventing workplace injuries caused by exposure to chemicals, which is something nurses may encounter during the course of their work. The Environmental Working Group and Healthcare Without Harm, in collaboration with the ANA and the Environmental Health Education Center of the University of Maryland's School of Nursing and supported by numerous state and specialty nursing organizations, conducted an online survey of workplace exposures and disease conditions among 1,500 nurses. This comprehensive survey indicated that participating nurses who were exposed frequently to sterilizing chemicals, housekeeping cleaners, residue from drug preparation, radiation, and other hazardous substances reported increased rates of asthma, miscarriage, and certain cancers and an increase in birth defects (in particular, musculoskeletal defects) in their children. There are limited workplace safety standards for the hundreds of hazardous substances to which nurses are exposed on the job (Environmental Working Group, 2007). Other reviews of nurses' workplace safety identifies concerns such as anesthetic gases, hand and skin disinfection, latex (for example, gloves), medications such as antiretroviral medications and chemotherapeutic agents, mercury-containing devices, personal care products, and sterilization and disinfectant agents such as ethylene oxide and glutaraldehyde. The ANA continues to monitor risks for nurses (Trossman, 2017). Nurses need to be aware of past and current data that indicate specific potential problems in order to protect themselves and their colleagues from exposure and prevent injuries and health problems. In addition, nurses need to be alert to developing symptoms of allergies to drugs and products, which can directly affect their health and practice.

Stop and Consider #3
Safety is a component of quality health care.

Quality Improvement

Healthcare QI focuses on the healthcare system. The system is fragmented and in need of improvement. Plsek defines a system as "the coming together of parts, interconnections, and purpose. While systems can be broken down into parts, which are interesting in and of themselves, the real power lies in the way the parts come together and are interconnected to fulfill some purpose. The healthcare system in the United States consists of various parts (e.g., clinics, hospitals, pharmacies, laboratories) that are interconnected (via flows of patients and information) to fulfill a purpose (e.g., maintaining and improving health)" (2001, p. 309). This does not mean that meeting individual patient needs and individual patient care improvement are not important. Each patient's care is part of the overall emphasis on healthcare improvement and is integrated in the system. Ultimately, the goal is that each patient's outcomes will be met.

The Institute for Healthcare Improvement (IHI) suggests that new designs can and must be developed to simultaneously accomplish three critical objectives—that is, the **Triple Aim**, which is now integrated in most efforts, both by HCOs and in health policy, to improve care on a continuous basis (CQI). The aims are (Institute for Healthcare Improvement [IHI], 2007):

1. Improve the health of the population.
2. Enhance the patient experience of care (including quality, access, and reliability).
3. Reduce, or at least control, the per capita cost of care.

You will observe and may be involved in issues of quality care as a student and as a nurse in practice. Entering the healthcare system and the nursing profession, you may have doubts that QI is an important topic, particularly if you have found the health system to be effective for you and your family. In this case, this might demonstrate that the healthcare system or HCO in which you received care had an effective QI program that you might not know about. There are, however, serious problems that have been reported routinely in major reports, by the government, and by consumers. The content in this chapter is critical for you as a nurse who must engage in efforts to improve care on a daily basis for your individual patients and the healthcare system.

QI needs to be viewed as a continuous process so it is often referred to as **CQI**. When QI is discussed, there are several perspectives to consider. The first and most critical is your individual practice, the practice of all healthcare professionals. What you do as a nurse has a direct impact on patient outcomes and quality. This chapter and other content in this text guide you in understanding your responsibilities and need to engage in CQI. There is no end point to QI, so it is continuous or referred to as CQI. There are two other perspectives that affect individual healthcare professionals and in total the quality of healthcare. One of the perspectives is the HCO QI program that is designed to support the HCO's efforts to maintain and improve care quality. The second view is the health policy perspective—QI initiatives from the local, state, and national levels. All of these perspectives should be in sync to provide effective health care for patients, families, and communities.

Implementing **QI** "requires that health professionals be clear about what they are trying to accomplish, what changes they can make that will result in an improvement, and how they will know that the improvement occurred" (IOM, 2003, p. 59). Healthcare complexity is mentioned many times as a barrier to understanding quality and improving healthcare delivery. Its consumers are very diverse in their needs, diagnoses, ethnic and cultural backgrounds, and overall health status, including genetic background, socioeconomic factors, patient preferences for health care, community differences, and healthcare coverage/reimbursement. Health care cannot be viewed in the same manner as other businesses (such as the automobile industry) that might manufacture or sell one product or a series of highly related products. Healthcare products/services vary based on the medical problem and the patient; the setting; the expertise of clinical staff; the desires of the patient; treatment options; patient prognosis; the expertise of the healthcare providers and HCOs; health policy and legislation; and advances in science, medical technology, and health informatics technology (HIT). In specialty areas such as obstetrics, psychiatry, emergency care, intensive care, home care, and long-term care, there is great variation within services—in their interventions, roles of the patient and family, patient education needs, prognosis and outcomes, and so on. It is expensive to develop and maintain effective QI programs, but The Joint Commission requires such programs for all its accredited organizations. QI programs should guide HCOs to improve care (Finkelman, 2018).

Because of the complex nature of quality, developing an HCO QI program that addresses monitoring and improving healthcare quality is in and of itself a complex process. HCOs typically have a department with staff that focus on CQI. This requires a budget for these efforts, and the program must plan, implement its plans, monitor, measure quality, and then identify interventions and solutions to maintain quality or improve quality. Effective appraisal of the scientific facts suggests that health care can be improved by closing the wide gaps between prevailing practices and the best-known approaches to care and by developing new forms of care. This requires planning and careful evaluation of results. One model for improvement focuses on three key questions (Berwick & Nolan, 1998, p. 209):

1. What is the HCO trying to accomplish?

2. How will the HCO know whether a change is an improvement?

3. What change can the HCO try that it believes will result in improvement?

For an HCO to have an effective QI program, nurses and other health professionals need to be knowledgeable and competent in a number of areas (IOM, 2003). All aspects of the healthcare environment are important to consider such as patients and staff and their interactions; patient and healthcare outcomes; and changes in science, technology, and needs of individuals and communities. HCOs need to consider and compare factors with other HCOs and similar healthcare systems to determine best current practices and then develop and apply interventions to improve care. This all requires an understanding of quality issues—errors, risks, human factors—that affect quality care for patients and staff safety, monitoring, and measurement. Surrounding all of this is the need to integrate interprofessional teamwork in CQI and also in care practice. **Figure 12-4** illustrates the importance of quality in the healthcare system, emphasizing critical thinking and teams focused on safe, effective, and efficient care delivery.

Stop and Consider #4
QI is a continuous process.

Examples of Safety Initiatives

A number of important safety initiatives have been stimulated by the *Quality Chasm* series. The IHI, for example, was established in 1991. It describes itself as "a reliable source of energy, knowledge, and support for a never-ending campaign to improve healthcare worldwide. The IHI helps accelerate change in healthcare by cultivating promising concepts for improving patient care and turning those ideas into action" (IHI, 2014). The IHI also focuses on STEEEP. The 5 Million Lives campaign is one example of an IHI safety initiative. This voluntary global initiative sought to protect patients from 5 million

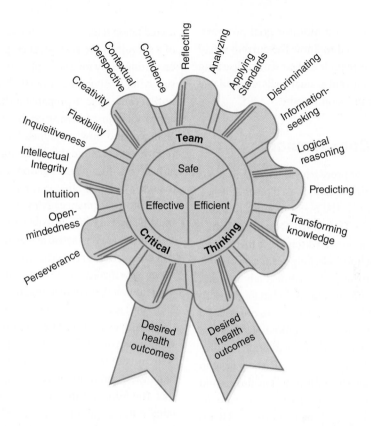

Figure 12-4 Medallion of Quality Health Care through Critical Thinking

Reproduced from Rubenfeld, M., & Scheffer, B. (2015). *Critical thinking tactics for nurses.* Burlington, MA: Jones & Bartlett Learning.

incidents of medical harm over 2 years (December 2006–December 2008). This initiative led the IHI to further develop its resources to improve healthcare quality, such as an improvement map designed to help hospitals deal with the multiple requirements they face and to focus on high-leverage changes to transform health care (IHI, 2011).

Another initiative, a collaborative effort between the IHI and the Robert Wood Johnson Foundation, focuses mostly on nursing—**Transforming Care at the Bedside (TCAB)**. TCAB is a "unique innovation initiative that aims to create, test, and implement changes that will dramatically improve care on medical/surgical units, and improve staff satisfaction as well" (IHI, 2017). This program

guides pilot studies to improve care, and QI studies are developed at the point-of-care by staff in practice, which offers many opportunities for improvement.

The Joint Commission's annual safety goals, which were first introduced in 2003, is a safety initiative that has an impact on many HCOs. Each year, The Joint Commission identifies safety goals that should be the focus of every Joint Commission–accredited HCO. These goals are based on the critical, current safety concerns based on data The Joint Commission collects and analyzes from its accredited HCOs, as well as other sources of information about healthcare safety. Their surveyors also emphasize the safety goals during accreditation visits. HCOs typically provide staff education related to the goals and monitor goal progress. Nursing students need to know the current safety goals and integrate them into their clinical learning experiences. The current annual goals are available on The Joint Commission website.

The Joint Commission

Accreditation is the process by which organizations are evaluated on their quality, based on established minimum standards. The major organization that accredits HCOs is **The Joint Commission**, a nonprofit organization accrediting more than 20,500 HCOs, including hospitals, long-term care organizations, home care agencies, clinical laboratories, ambulatory care organizations, behavioral health organizations, and healthcare networks or managed care organizations. It has accredited HCOs since 1951, and over that time, the accreditation requirements and process have changed. Participating in a Joint Commission survey is time consuming and costly, but it is necessary for HCOs. For example, nursing education programs need to use HCOs with current Joint Commission accreditation for student practicum/clinical experiences. As The Joint Commission has changed, its emphasis on quality care has also changed. CQI is now the major focus of the accreditation process, which includes safety.

Nurses serve on the Joint Commission Nursing Advisory Council, which advises its parent organization about nursing concerns and care issues related to quality. Nurses who work in HCOs eventually experience a Joint Commission survey. After initial accreditation is received, The Joint Commission makes a visit to the HCO every 3 years to complete its intensive survey for accreditation renewal, and it may even make unscheduled visits. For the scheduled visits, the HCO is given a date and has 9–12 months to prepare for the visit. Preparing for the visit involves gathering information and data for The Joint Commission, educating staff about the standards, conducting mock surveys to prepare staff, and so on. The HCO should meet the expected accreditation standards at all times, not just at the time of a survey. In the past, great emphasis was placed on getting ready for The Joint Commission visit and surviving it; afterward, the HCO was less vigilant until it came time to prepare for the next visit. This approach of just focusing on the survey eventually changed, and now accredited HCOs must submit reports on certain data to The Joint Commission annually, with a plan of action for areas noted in the self-assessment that may require improvement (periodic performance review); in addition, HCOs must be prepared for possible unscheduled visits.

Nurses are very active in preparing for the survey and during the survey visit. The Joint Commission survey now involves more direct care staff in the visits by including them in meetings to discuss care in the HCO and asking individual staff questions during the survey visit. If students are present during the visit, surveyors may ask them questions. The goal is to find out if patients are achieving the expected outcomes, and if not, why. Examples of outcomes that The Joint Commission assesses include mortality rates, length of stay, sentinel events, adverse incidents, complications, readmission rates, patient/family satisfaction, referrals to specialists, patient adherence to discharge plans or treatment plans, achievement of safety goals, prevention adherence services (for example, mammograms, Pap smears, immunizations), and more.

The Joint Commission standards have been developed, evaluated, and revised over the years to meet the changing needs of healthcare delivery. These standards form the framework for accreditation. The accreditation of hospitals focuses on a number of areas and issues, for example (The Joint Commission, 2017b, 2017c):

- Environment of care
- Emergency medicine
- Human resources
- Infection prevention and control
- Information management
- Leadership
- Life safety

- Medication management
- Medical staff
- National patient safety goals
- Nursing
- Provision of care, treatment, and services
- Performance improvement
- Record of care, treatment, and services
- Rights and responsibilities of the individual
- Transplant safety

Because The Joint Commission accredits a broad range of HCOs, there are differences in the minimum standards and in how the various healthcare settings might monitor care and outcomes. Consider home care agencies: These agencies may use other national evaluation approaches that are not related to or led by The Joint Commission. The home care outcome-based approach to QI, known as the Outcome and Assessment Information Set (OASIS), was developed in the 1990s by the U.S. Department of Health and Human Services. It offers a database for collecting and organizing home care data so that outcomes can be analyzed (U.S. Department of Health and Human Services [HHS] & Centers for Medicare and Medicaid Services [CMS], 2012). This database focuses on a group of data elements that represent core items of a comprehensive assessment of home care patients. The key question is: Did the patient benefit from the home care services? In this type of system, home care agencies from all over the country input their QI data. The OASIS is managed through the CMS and offers a national view of home healthcare quality.

Healthcare Report Cards

Healthcare report cards provide specific performance data about an HCO at specific intervals, with a focus on quality. The report can be used by the HCO to compare its outcomes with report cards published by other similar HCOs or with a large state or national database (benchmarking). This information can be helpful in improving care in the HCO by identifying what the HCO is doing well and what needs improvement as compared with

other similar HCOs. Some of these report cards are now accessible on the Internet and can also be used by consumers (patients, families). Nurses use them when searching for new jobs to obtain evaluation data about a specific HCO. In some cases, insurers use healthcare report cards to assess an HCO and compare it with similar HCOs. The goal is to examine performance based on clearly defined criteria.

Examples of other changes in QI focus on sharing information with patients and rewards for QI performance. Today, public reporting is more common, so report cards may be made public. This sharing of predetermined quality and efficiency measures with performance data informs patients and stakeholders about provider performance (Dunton, Gonnerman, Montalvo, & Shumann, 2011).

Value-based purchasing is also used today. Value-based purchasing is a payment system that provides financial rewards for performance. Such a system, in addition to public reporting, may incentivize providers to improve outcomes. There is, however, a risk that pay-for-performance may act as an incentive to "cut corners," to take steps to ensure data "looks positive" when it is not. An example is found in **Exhibit 12-1** describing how the Veteran's Administration medical system changed records that provided data on appointments and wait times in order to improve performance.

In 1994, the ANA began an investigation of the impact of workforce restructuring and redesign on the safety and quality of patient care in acute care settings. This investigation led to the development of a nursing report card in 1998, the National Database of Nursing Quality Indicators® (NDNQI®) (ANA, 2014). This occurred around the time that the *Quality Chasm* series began to address healthcare quality. The ANA wanted to "explore the nature and strength of the linkages between nursing care and patient outcomes by identifying nursing quality indicators" (Pollard, Mitra, & Mendelson, 1996, p. 1). This initiative also provides a framework for educating nurses, consumers, and policy makers to evaluate the contributions of nursing within the acute care setting by tracking the quality of nursing care provided in such settings. The NDNQI made it clear that data on nursing and outcomes were lacking—that is, the methods of HCO used to collect data at that time were not nursing specific. Patients come into the acute care setting primarily because they need around-the-clock care, which is the focus of nursing care, and yet data on this care were lacking.

The NDNQI was initially managed by the University of Kansas School of Nursing, under contract to ANA; it is now part of Press Ganey, a company that offers HCOs services to evaluate quality and patient satisfaction (Press Ganey, 2014, 2017). As of early 2017, there were more than 2,000 hospitals participating in this database. Ninety-five percent of Magnet® recognized facilities participate in NDNQI. This initiative "provides each nurse the opportunity to review the evidence, evaluate their practice, and determine what improvements can be made" (Montalvo & Dunton, 2007, p. 3). The participating institutions submit their nursing-sensitive indicator data to the electronic database, which allows for the collection of a large amount of data for evaluation and for research. The NDNQI database indicators focus on the characteristics of the nursing workforce, nursing processes, and patient outcomes. To assist with more effective comparisons, reports are provided to hospitals with information about patient population, unit type, and hospital bed size. The result is the nursing profession's quality report card. With the exception of Magnet hospitals, participation in the NDNQI process is voluntary; therefore, only participating HCOs are reflected in the data.

Some of the nursing-sensitive indicators are now included in other public reporting such as data collected by the National Quality Forum (NQF), but there needs to be more representation of nursing-sensitive indicators in public reporting on the status of healthcare quality (Dunton et al. 2011). The NQF is an important national quality initiative, and one with which the NDNQI collaborates. The

NQF Strategic Plan for 2016–2019 focuses on four purposes (2017a):

1. Accelerate development of needed measures.
2. Reduce, select, and endorse measures.
3. Drive measure implementation of prioritized measures.
4. Facilitate feedback on what works and what does not work.

The NQF examines some of the critical care issues that need to be considered to meet these purposes. Currently, the NQF endorses about 300 measures, which are used in more than 20 federal public reporting, pay-for-performance programs; state programs; and the private sector, but it does not develop measures (NQF, 2017b). The NQF also identifies areas where more measures are needed to reduce gaps and attempts to ensure measures are effective.

The National QDR, discussed earlier in the chapter, also serves as another report card. It now represents the major national annual report on the status of care in the United States.

Stop and Consider #5
Healthcare accreditation supports QI, but it cannot ensure it.

National Quality Strategy

A provision in the Affordable Care Act of 2010 requires the HHS to develop the **National Quality Strategy (NQS)**. The AHRQ led the development of the strategy and now administers the NQS. An evidence-based approach along with a collaborative effort was used, including feedback from more than 300 stakeholders representing the federal government, especially the HHS; the states; the private sector; and multi-stakeholder groups such as healthcare professional organizations (Finkelman, 2018). The NQS is a groundbreaking initiative supporting national measurement and QI at multiple levels: community, practice settings, and individual physicians (HHS, 2011). As the strategy was developed, a critical problem was noted. There were too many measures and no control or evaluation of measures, causing measurement redundancies and overlap that may negatively affect the value of results.

The NQS priorities are patient safety, person-centered care, care coordination, effective treatment, healthy living, and care affordability and, as noted, are also monitored as part of the annual QDR and correlate with other initiatives such as *Healthy People 2020*. The NQS establishes priorities, and this information about outcomes related to the priorities is then included in the annual NQS report to Congress (HHS, 2015; HHS & AHRQ, 2015b). Thus, data for the NQS annual report originates from multiple HCOs and government agencies.

Patient-centered care is a core factor in the NQS, supporting earlier work emphasizing patient-centered care. The major purpose of the NQS is to provide a national approach to measure quality and ensure higher quality care for all, which correlates with the Triple Aim and STEEEP. The NQS recommends that all HCOs adopt the Triple Aim and STEEEP, and many are meeting this recommendation.

More systematic measurement methods are needed to effectively assess quality and maintain CQI. The NQS now provides a framework for better development and coordination across the HHS to establish core sets of measures to improve measurement for multiple populations and healthcare services. It is clear we need to have better control and coordination of measurement—confusion does not support effective CQI. The six strategy priorities are (HHS & AHRQ, 2015b):

- Making care safer by reducing harm caused in the delivery of care
- Ensuring that each person and family is engaged as partners in their care
- Promoting effective communication and coordination of care

- Promoting the most effective prevention and treatment practices for leading causes of mortality
- Working with communities to promote wide use of best practice to enable healthy living
- Making quality care more affordable for individuals, families, employers, and government by developing and spreading new healthcare delivery models

Figure 12-5 provides an overview describing how NQS works. It is important to consider the entire healthcare delivery system rather than just focus on the hospital setting. For example, there are an estimated 1 billion ambulatory care visits per year and 35 million hospital admissions, and 1 in 10 patients develop a healthcare-acquired condition (National Patient Safety Foundation, 2015). The plan applies to all types of healthcare settings and is intended to address the entire continuum of care.

It is recommended that other healthcare programs, private and public, adopt the NQS; however, it is not required—though more healthcare programs and quality initiatives do correlate with the NQS. The AHRQ provides tools and resources to support implementation of the NQS (HHS & AHRQ, 2015). The NQS annual reports to Congress are posted on the AHRQ website. The 2015 congressional report states "across the nation the National Strategy for Quality Improvement in Health Care (NQS) brings together federal agencies, healthcare payers, purchasers, providers, consumers, and other partners in pursuit of improved health and health care for all Americans. The NQS serves as a framework for aligning stakeholders across private and public sectors at the federal, state, and local levels" (U.S. Department of Health and Human Services [HHS], 2015).

Stop and Consider #6

The NQS should be integrated into our view of nursing practice to ensure QI.

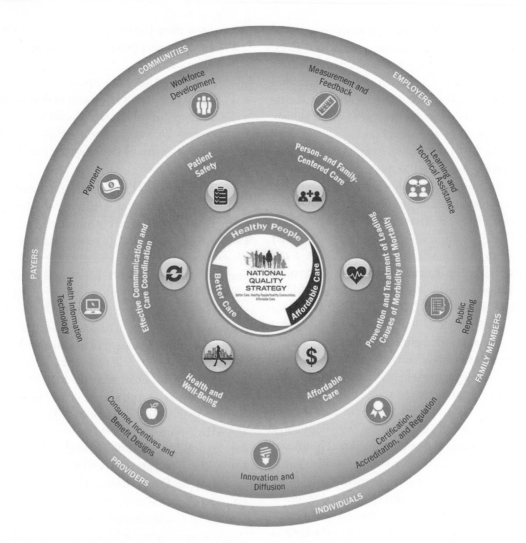

Figure 12-5 NQS: How It Works

Reproduced from Agency for Healthcare Quality and Research. (2015, July). *National Quality Strategy: Overview (PowerPoint presentation).* Retrieved from http://www.ahrq.gov/workingforquality/toolkit.htm

Federal Initiatives to
Improve Care: Hospital-Acquired Conditions and 30-Day Unplanned Readmissions

In an effort to improve care and reduce costs in 2007–2008, the Centers for Medicare and Medicaid Services (CMS) introduced a major change in its reimbursement policy. It will no longer pay for care for complications that occur in the hospital that could have been prevented, now referred to as **hospital-acquired complications (HACs)**. Examples of types of complications that are no longer covered include falls, hospital-acquired decubiti, performing the wrong procedure, and administering the wrong blood type. This policy has major implications: Who will now pay for the care for HACs?

Ultimately, the HCO may hold the bill and have to cover the costs. HCOs are limited in what they can charge a Medicare patient personally. This issue is complex and serious, but the major message from the CMS and other insurers is that when errors are made, there are costs involved, and performance is associated with cost. For many reasons, HCOs have problems maintaining a stable budget, and this change in reimbursement practice has a major impact on the financial status of hospitals. This CMS decision has a potential major impact on HCO finances. For example, suppose a patient who is covered by Medicare falls in the hospital and incurs an injury. Treatment for that injury may not be charged to Medicare and may not be charged to the patient. The hospital must provide care but will receive no payment for doing so. It is uncertain how hospitals will respond to this change long-term though they are developing methods to prevent HACs, some more successful than others.

In addition, in 2011, Medicaid issued its list of HACs that might occur in hospitals. In July 2012, Medicaid implemented a policy of not paying for these HACs if they occurred in hospitalized patients covered by Medicaid. Examples of some of these events, similar to Medicare's list, are blood incompatibility, falls and trauma, hypoglycemic coma, and surgery on the wrong patient or wrong body part (Galewitz, 2011). The list of HACs for Medicare and Medicaid may change over time based on data related to common complications and errors, and the CMS website maintains an updated list of HACs. In early 2008, some of the major insurers came out in support of this approach, announcing zero tolerance for HACs and identifying their own list of such events. Hospitals are now required to be aware of all HACs regardless of insurer, and as noted here, they do not all include the same HACs on their lists. Nurses can make a difference in preventing HACs, and they need to be involved in determining interventions to prevent these conditions or other "never" events, as they are sometimes called. To be more involved, nurses need to understand HACs

and why they are important. The targets for HACs are (1) high volume and cost; (2) identified as a complication, comorbidity, or major complication as connected with CMS diagnosis-related groups; and (3) reasonably preventable using evidence-based guidelines (HHS & CMS, 2016, p. 3). In the past, the CMS identified problems that are now called HACs as care quality problems (such as for air embolism, pressure ulcers, catheter-associated urinary tract infection, foreign object retained after surgery, and others), and they were not associated with limited reimbursement for care and thus were covered. Now the attention turns to evidence-based guidelines to improve care focused on the HACs and need for HCOs to provide care that will prevent these problems.

For each HAC, several associated EBP guidelines are available that should be used to prevent these problems. This emphasizes the importance of EBP and need for CQI. The CMS's goal is to stimulate hospitals to improve care—to decrease preventable hospital-acquired conditions—and this has begun to happen. A second goal is to decrease care costs. Asking HCOs to improve care did not seem to work, so the CMS turned to incentivizing by limiting payment if care performance was not at the expected level. In spring 2014, the HHS announced: "New preliminary data show an overall 9% decrease in hospital-acquired conditions nationally during 2011 and 2012. National reductions in adverse drug events, falls, infections, and other forms of hospital-induced harm are estimated to have prevented nearly 15,000 deaths in hospitals, avoided 560,000 patient injuries, and [avoided] approximately $4 billion in health spending over the same period. Hospital readmissions fall by 8% for Medicare beneficiaries. In 2010 there were 145 HACs per 1,000 discharges and in 2012 132 HACs per 1,000 discharges" (HHS, 2014). Data from the 2015 National Scorecard on Rates of Hospital-Acquired Conditions "shows that about 125,000 fewer patients died and more than $28 billion in health care costs were saved from 2010 through 2015 due to a 21 percent drop in hospital-acquired conditions (HACs). In total, hospital patients experienced more than 3 million fewer HACs from 2010 through 2015. HACs include adverse drug events, catheter-associated urinary tract infections, central line associated bloodstream infections, pressure ulcers and surgical site infections, among others" (HHS & AHRQ, 2016). The current data indicate significant improvement. This improvement supports partnerships to improve care and structured initiatives to monitor and respond to problems, and it may demonstrate that we do need to motivate healthcare providers to improve performance by including a financial incentive.

Along with the development of the initiative to reduce HACs, unplanned readmissions for any cause to an acute care hospital within 30 days of discharge have come under CMS scrutiny to improve care and reduce costs. This initiative now requires that hospitals do the following (HHS & AHRQ, 2014a, p. 5):

- *Analyze the root causes of readmissions:* Understand patterns and trends for the HCO and the local community for comparison; understand the patient's perspective, for example, effectiveness of communication and coordination. Data should be tracked routinely.
- *Inventory and align the current readmission reduction efforts to meet the needs of the HCO's targeted patients:* This should be an in depth inventory; the AHRQ guide provides several tools (Hospital Inventory, Cross-Continuum Team Inventory, and Conditions of Participation Checklist) so that the HCO can understand what it currently does to prevent and/or respond to the problem to better plan changes.
- *Examine the extent to which the current readmission reduction efforts meet the needs of the HCO targeted patients:* Combine previous information about methods HCOs may use.
- *Improve hospital-based processes to better target and serve targeted patients' needs:* With the

above information, set aims and objectives and then identify strategies that will be part of the program. Examples of strategies are use of checklists, arrange for post-discharge follow-up, flag discharge more than 30-days in chart, develop transitional plans, engage the patient and when appropriate the family with the patient's permission, and identify high-risk patients.

- *Expand and strengthen cross-setting partnerships:* Implement strategies to increase collaboration with cross-setting partners.
- *Provide enhanced services to patients at high-risk of readmission:* Implement strategies for high-risk patients.

Nurses are directly involved in this problem because discharge planning and patient education are critical elements in preparing patients for discharge and establishing an effective post-discharge trajectory so that patients do not need to be readmitted within 30 days of discharge. Teach-back, asking patients to repeat information they have learned, is used by many nurses to better ensure that patients and families understand the information they need post-discharge (Peter, Robinson, & Jordan, 2015). Patients and families should also be involved in discharge planning to ensure that the plan would work post-discharge for the patient and the environment in which the patient will be living. Consideration needs to be given to support services that might be required such as home health care, follow-up phone calls and other communication with healthcare providers, and support for caregivers. We cannot control all aspects of the patient's life and condition, but we need to do as much as we can to ensure their success post-discharge.

Stop and Consider #7

The CMS decided that care was not improving for its beneficiaries, so it began to incentivize improvement with threat of loss of payment for services.

Examples of High-Risk
Healthcare Activities

As has been stated, we cannot eliminate all errors and healthcare quality concerns; however, we can reduce them—and we need to do this much more. There are some healthcare activities (for example, nursing interventions, procedures, treatment) that are of higher risk for errors and quality problems than others. The Joint Commission's annual safety goals identify high-risk concerns in health care—and the goals change annually. There are factors that increase risk, and these should guide us in developing plans to reduce risk. We know that poor communication is a critical factor to consider. Today, with increasing use of and development of technology—both for communication and use in in treatment methods—we have opportunity for positive outcomes, but this also increases risk (Finkelman, 2018). We also know that staff need to be competent, and this requires not only

improvement in academic professional education, but also lifelong learning. **Figure 12-6** provides an overview of the five drivers of clinical quality and safety. This description highlights risk areas, or factors that may affect risk, and the same factors can be used to guide decisions and interventions to reduce risk and improve care. This section discusses several examples of high-risk healthcare activities for nurses.

Medication Administration

Medication administration via any route or for any medication is a high-risk treatment intervention. A **medication error** is a "preventable event that may cause or led to inappropriate medication use or patient harm while the medication in control of the healthcare professional, patient, or consumer" (U.S. Department of Health and Human Services & Food and Drug Administration, 2015). The medication use process includes documenting, dispensing, administering, and monitoring.

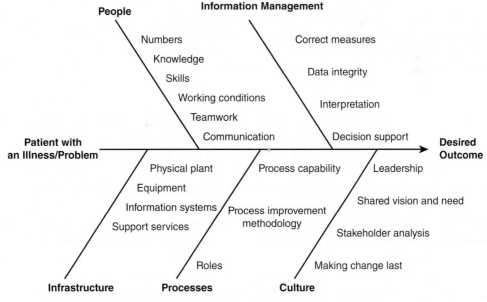

Figure 12-6 Five Drivers of Clinical Quality and Patient Safety

Table 12-1 Common Sources of Medication Error

Ambiguous orders	Incorrect drug selected
Drug device use	Incorrect patient
Environmental stress	Insufficient drug information
Errors in communication/ miscommunication of drug orders	Insufficient information about other drugs patient is on (therapeutic duplication)
Error-prone abbreviation	Insufficient laboratory information
Illegible handwriting	Known allergy
Improper dose	Limited patient education
Incomplete orders	Limited staff education
Incomplete/insufficient monitoring	Look-alike or sound-alike drugs
Incomplete patient information/patient information unavailable	Poor communication

Reproduced from Youngberg, B. (2013). *Patient safety handbook* (2nd ed.). Burlington, MA: Jones & Bartlett Learning.

Common sources of medication errors are identified in **Table 12-1**. Students and staff must apply methods to reduce medication errors. Some of these methods include the following: know and respond when high-alert medications are administered (drugs that are of higher risk for patient harm); report and analyze near misses; ask for help when needed; avoid distractions and interruptions during the medication administration procedure; if in doubt, ask for help (for example, other nurses, pharmacist, physician); double check and verify; listen to the patient and family when they question something; do not use workarounds; be alert to allergies; apply sterile technique when required; follow policies and procedures; document in a timely manner; do not document medications you have not administered; provide appropriate patient education about medications; and routinely apply the five rights of medication administration.

Much time is spent in nursing education on medication administration. Such content and learning activities focus on the five rights of medication administration, which emphasize safe medication administration: right patient, right medication, right dose, right time, and right route. The goal in applying the five rights is to reduce errors; however, they also are the common areas for errors and when nurses need to be alert. Other rights have been identified that are not included in the long-recognized five rights: right documentation, right to refuse medication, and right to evaluation and monitoring (Anderson and Townsend, 2010). Another right that is suggested is to identify the right indication or reason for using the medication (Walton, 2014). An example of how these rights impact care and QI, which relates to HIT, is administering the medication at the right time or time ordered. This has been a potential problem for some time, particularly as more HCOs use electronic medical records and bar codes. A common accepted policy that was supported by the CMS was that medications should be administered within 30 minutes of the ordered time. The Institute for Safe Medication Practice (ISMP, 2011) expressed concern about what happens when nurses cannot meet this standard. The typical response is to use workarounds or shortcuts because nurses do not want this to be considered an error. The ISMP conducted a survey of 17,500 nurses. The majority of the nurses believed that trying to meet the 30-minute deadline leads to problems and errors. With electronic methods (medical records and use of bar codes), more data are now available regarding the actual times medications are administered, and this has led to negative views, with late administration being considered an error. This viewpoint does not consider that most nurses are capable of making commonsense clinical decisions and are aware of medications for which administration time is a critical element and the need to consider individual patient status issues. This example demonstrates how analysis of a quality problem may lead to change and improvement, but it also demonstrates that many factors and many stakeholders may be involved.

Care Transitions and Handoffs

Care transition is a time of change for the patient, family, and staff. It occurs when a patient's care is transferred from one staff member to another, one unit to another, one HCO to another, and from an HCO to the patient's home—it also occurs between students and staff and vice versa. Communication is the key issue: the key cause of problems if it is ineffective and the key strategy to improve handoffs when it is effective. There are also other factors that interfere with effective handoffs, such as stressful work environment, staffing levels, interruptions, problems with sharing digital information (as discussed in chapter on informatics), HIT equipment problems, leadership and management concerns, lack of staff preparation and understanding of the transition process, multitasking, and ineffective teamwork (Finkelman, 2018). It is important for staff to ask questions and expect to receive required information so that the patient's care can continue as needed and in a safe manner. Use of standardized communication methods can help reduce problems and are discussed later in this chapter.

Failure to Rescue

Failure to rescue is a time of potential critical risk for patients; it is a time when staff miss something about the patient's condition and then do not intervene as needed. There are many reasons this may occur such as inadequate staffing levels, staff competency and ineffective use of critical thinking and clinical reasoning/clinical judgment, ineffective response to alarms or alerts or malfunction of alarm equipment, distractions and emergencies, lack of routine monitoring such as rounds and other methods/surveillance, and ineffective communication from one staff to another (for example, during handoffs). A common method used to reduce failure to rescue is use of **rapid response teams (RRTs)**. These teams of experts in care of the critically ill respond to a call to the bedside to assess the patient and determine best treatment, which may mean transferring the patient to intensive care. A systematic review of studies on the use of RRTs indicates that 20% of the patients in the sample seen by the RRT had experienced an adverse event, and 80% of these events were preventable (Amaral et al., 2015). Most of the events were not reported through the expected reporting system. The recommendation from the review is that calling for RRT assistance should be a trigger to investigate if an adverse event occurred.

Alarm/Alert Fatigue

With the growing use of technology, there is recognition that technology provides many advantages and improves care, but also may lead to more problems. **Alarm or alert fatigue** occurs when staff do not respond or are slow to respond to an alarm from a device such as a cardiac monitor, bedside physiological monitor, infusion pump, or ventilator. Why does this happen when the alarms are supposed to direct us to immediate assessment and response? In some cases, on a single unit such as an intensive care unit there can be several hundred alarms per patient in a day. If you multiply this number by the number of patients on a unit, it is easy to see how these alarms can, over time, stress staff; added to this is the problem that between 85% and 99% of the alarms are false, requiring no clinical intervention (Finkelman, 2018; Joint Commission, 2013). When there are many alarms for multiple patients, the risk of a poor response increases. This problem has increased so much that The Joint Commission issued a sentinel event alert for medical device alarm safety in hospitals (Joint Commission, 2013), and in 2016, improving response to alarms was included in The Joint Commission's annual safety goals.

Missed Nursing Care

Missed nursing care is considered to be an issue that nurses need to attend to more in their practice and in their CQI responsibilities. It is a type of error of omission, representing "needed nursing care that is delayed, partially completed, or not completed at all" (HHS, AHRQ, & PSNet, 2016b). Due to the increased concern about this type of error—which has a negative impact on care coordination, implementation of care, and patient outcomes, thus increasing risk that the patient will not get care required or other errors may occur—the AHRQ has developed a patient safety primer on missed nursing care (HHS, AHRQ, & PSNet, 2016b). In a systematic review of 42 studies, 55% to 98% of the nurses in the samples reported that they had missed one or more items required for assessment; most of this occurred during the last shift (Jones, Hamilton, & Murry, 2015). This review also noted that missed nursing care is associated with decreased patient satisfaction and higher rates of adverse events. The major predictors of missed nursing care are staffing levels, the work environment, and teamwork. This is then where nursing should focus its strategies to prevent missed nursing care. When nurses feel time pressure and competing demands during a shift, there is increased risk that something that should be done is not done or not done completely. We know that efforts to develop a positive work environment

with effective teams and team members who help one another plus a culture of safety with an emphasis on CQI support nurses to work more effectively and improve patient care. Nurses also need to work in environments in which work needs are met, not just appropriate staffing levels, but also access to clinical supplies, equipment, medications, and HIT. Having these resources reduces missed nursing care—care cannot get done if the nurse does not have the resources to provide the care.

Stop and Consider #8
There are many care situations that are times of high risk for errors.

Tools and Methods
to Monitor and Improve Healthcare Delivery

Other chapters include content about some of the methods used by HCOs to monitor and improve healthcare delivery. Some of these are related to nursing professional issues such as standards of care; HCO policies and procedures; clinical pathways and protocols; licensure and credentialing to better ensure competency for practice; application of evidence-based care; interprofessional teams and teamwork; HCO risk management focused on possible legal concerns, which also affect quality care; and healthcare regulation and legislation. In this section, we discuss other, more specific CQI tools and methods used by HCOs. Nurses are involved in the use of these tools and methods. This discussion does not include all possible tools and methods. **Appendix A** augments this content.

Utilization Review/ Management

Utilization review/management (UR/UM) is the process of evaluating the necessity, appropriateness, and efficiency of healthcare services for specific patients or patient populations. HCOs use utilization review data in a number of ways—for example, to determine access and usage of services, if a service is no longer needed, whether or not a new service is needed, and to review the relationship of data to patient outcomes. Data are primarily obtained from medical records to determine necessity, appropriateness, and timeliness of healthcare services. Utilization review data are connected to financial concerns for the HCO and its budget (for example, whether the HCO is serving enough patients to meet its budget, types of procedures and their reimbursement, and so on). Utilization review is administered by the HCO administration, although nurses may participate as data collectors and in the analysis process. Nurses should participate in decisions about changes that might be made in clinical services. The QI program may use some of the UR data.

Benchmarking

Many hospitals and other types of HCOs use benchmarking. **Benchmarking** is the process of comparing performance to an external standard. It can help staff members and management understand how their performance compares to other HCOs, and this may then motivate them to engage in improvement. "Benchmarking can stimulate healthy competition, as well as help members of a practice reflect more effectively on their own performance" (HHS & AHRQ, 2013a).

One popular benchmarking approach is Six Sigma. This rigorous and systematic methodology utilizes information (management by facts) and statistical analysis to measure and improve an HCO's operational performance, practices, and systems by identifying and preventing defects in processes. The goal is to anticipate and exceed stakeholder expectations and increase effectiveness. (Six Sigma, 2017).

Assessment of Access to Healthcare Services

Access to healthcare services is important to monitor and improve as part of the QI process. Communities are concerned about whether their citizens have access to care. The *Healthy People 2020* initiative considers access to be a critical issue across the United States for all types of healthcare needs (HHS, 2017). The QDR also monitors access to care. When a patient does not have access, the patient's health status is at risk, and further complications may occur.

Medication Reconciliation

Patients often take many medications, and a key concern is how these medications interact with one another. **Medication reconciliation** is "creating the most accurate list possible of all medications a patient is taking, including drug name, dosage, frequency, and route, and comparing that list against the physician's admission, transfer, and/or discharge orders with the goal of providing correct medications to the patient at all transition points within the hospital (could be throughout continuum of care)" (Ketchum, Grass, & Padwojski, 2005, pp. 78–79). Responsibility for completing the medication reconciliation procedure needs to be clarified in a policy and procedure. Use of routine tracking is important. HCOs should have a standardized form on which to record the information. If the patient takes a lot of medications and cannot remember all the information, medication reconciliation can take time to complete and may be inaccurate. The Joint Commission now requires that its accredited HCOs use medication reconciliation routinely. If problems arise in reconciling medications, then errors can result in omitted medications, incorrect dosage, incorrect route, incorrect timing, use of the same medications that are different formulations, use of drugs that do not interact effectively with one another, and failure to discontinue contraindicated medications (Rozich et al. 2004).

Standardized Communication Methods

HCOs are now using more standardized communication methods. This is mostly due to the recognition that errors are often associated with ineffective communication. There are many methods now used or incorporated with other methods to address QI problems. An example of the latter is that during handoffs, HCOs may require that specific information be shared. Staff members are trained in using the structured script to provide critical information and thus make sure this information is not forgotten. In a study of standardized communication used during handoffs, recurrent types of content covered in various standardized methods are identified as introduction, patient/administrative data/necessary patient information, danger or risk(s), background/history, situation/story/framework, follow-up care needs, awareness of error risk to prevent errors, dialogue, questions, ownership/custody, document, and thank you (Nasarwanji, Badir, & Gurses, 2016, p. 241). Two standardized communication methods discussed here are SBAR and checklists.

The SBAR, or situation–background–assessment–recommendation, is discussed in more detail in content about teams, but it is important to recognize that this method is part of CQI. It is used to prevent QI problems by ensuring clear communication during times when important information is required. It is easy to get off track in communication, but during communication from one healthcare provider to another, such as a nurse calling a physician about a patient, it is important to stay on track. The SBAR and other similar methods help to focus the conversation.

Checklists are also discussed in content about teams. They have become a common tool used to guide staff during certain aspects of care with the goal of ensuring that critical steps are taken. Teams provide a collective vigilance to identify potential risk of errors or to quickly identify when an error has occurred, shifting from individual accountability and thus providing a better chance to catch a new miss (potential error) (Jeffs, Lingard, Berta, & Baker,

2012). Checklists support team vigilance. The most common area of use is in surgery—prior to surgery and/or after surgery. When checklists are used, any staff member may interrupt and question—for example, a step was missed or something was done that should not have been done according to the checklist. This method may be used in many situations, but the HCO should have clear checklists that staff understand. Staff need to be involved in the development of checklists, provide feedback for improvement, and use the checklists as a checklist that is not used is then not effective. Use of checklists not only acts as a method to prevent QI problems, but may also provide QI data.

Rounds

Rounds have been used in healthcare for a long time. The types of rounds, however, have changed over time. **Rounds** provide opportunity to gain information through observation and communication. They may be used by an individual staff member checking on his or her patients or by teams, which may be profession specific (such as a nursing team or physicians/residents/medical students) or interprofessional. All units should use some form of interprofessional rounds to ensure consistent assessment, clearer communication, and planning for patient care. Rounds do not always focus on the patient directly. There may be administrative rounds when the nurse manager goes through the unit and is focused on many issues such as safety, cleanliness, and work environment and may also observe patient care in process or talk to patients and families. Safety rounds may be used when certain staff—often managers, but also clinical staff—go through the unit focusing on risks for staff and patient safety. Clinical rounds focus on the patient and should be patient centered—with patient engagement. This may seem strange, but it is important. In the past, rounds were often done around the patient with little effort made to include the patient. It is also important to recognize that rounds disturb the patients—patients' rest and quiet, concerns about privacy, and concerns that others may be making decisions in which they have no input or limited input. Rounds may be routine or unscheduled, such as the nurse decides to check on assigned patients. Routine rounds happen at scheduled times, specific staff are involved, and the purpose is clear. Documentation may be part of rounds, either during the rounds, which is typical, or immediately after rounds. QI concerns may be identified during rounds. If so, they require follow-up. HCOs should have policies and procedures about rounds and also about how they relate to the QI program.

Incident Reports

Incident reports have long been used by HCOs as a method for staff to report errors or problems with care. HCOs have policies and procedures to guide staff in the use of incident reports. This is an HCO standardized form that is completed by staff involved in an event. The HCO identifies the types of events that require reporting. These forms are used by the QI program to track events such as infections, medication errors, treatment and procedure errors, patient complaints, falls, security issues, harm to staff, sentinel events, and regulatory compliance (U.S. Department of Health and Human Services [HHS] & Office of the Inspector General [OIG], 2012). Management, including nursing management, review the reports to provide up-to-date information on QI and to assist in identifying situations that require an immediate response. Incident reports have been used in blame cultures to identify staff involved and then take steps to resolve problems focused on staff actions and the staff member—often leading to punitive responses. Over time, this has had a negative impact on staff completion of reports, which is not helpful because valuable information is lost (HHS & OIG, 2012). There is more effort now in cultures of safety to reduce this focus—to view incident reports as a source of data to be used in HCO QI efforts to assess care processes from a system perspective.

Sentinel Events

As described earlier, **sentinel events** are "unexpected events that happen to patients resulting in major negative outcomes, such as unexpected death or critical physical or psychological complications that can lead to major alteration in the patient's health" (Finkelman, 2018, p. 221). These are events that require immediate response—for example, a suicide in the hospital, wrong-site surgery, or a life-threatening post-operative complication. Staff responsible for QI must analyze the event (use root-cause analysis [RCA], discussed in the next section) and collaborate with other staff to respond. The Joint Commission publishes sentinel event alerts on its website based on information it receives from its accredited HCOs. This information is provided so that others can be alert to potential risks. Not all errors are sentinel events, and HCOs need to determine if the event is to be classified as sentinel. Often, sentinel events are unique or happen rarely but response is required, including steps to prevent reoccurrence.

Stop and Consider #9
There are many methods and tools used to prevent or resolve quality care concerns.

Measurement and Analysis

Measures/indicators provide performance data to better understand actual practice, identify problems, and assist in best practice changes for improvement by identifying topics that will be monitored to determine performance and expected outcomes. A **measure** is a "standard used as a basis for comparison, a reference point against which other things can be evaluated" (HHS & AHRQ, 2014b). **Indicators** are aggregate measures for broader application. Data provide information about potential quality concerns and areas that need more examination and also help to track changes over time. Why is this done? "We cannot really measure 'quality care' per se so we use measures as an 'indicator' of quality—although they are not a direct measure of quality care" (HHS & AHRQ, 2004). "Measuring a health system's inputs, processes, and outcomes is a proactive, systematic approach to practice-level decisions for patient care and the delivery systems that support it. Data management also includes ongoing measurement and monitoring. It enables an organization's CQI team to identify and implement opportunities for improvements of its current care delivery systems and to monitor progress as changes are applied. Managing data also helps a CQI team to understand how outcomes are achieved, such as, improved patient satisfaction with care, staff satisfaction with working in the organization, or an organization's costs and revenues associated with patient care" (U.S. Department Health and Human Services & Health Resources and Services Administration, 2011a, 2011b). It is important to recognize that once something is identified as a measure, this puts that situation or action in the list of important activities—it draws attention to the issue and typically means staff will pay more attention to the issue, and more resources may be directed at interventions to prevent or resolve a problem. This may or may not be a positive result—for example, if the measure is not that important, something that is more important is ignored. "Nurses function as the gatekeepers of health care, and nursing systems serve as important leverage points" (VanFosson, Jones, & Yoder, 2016, p. 126).

Measurement must be planned, evaluated, and revised as needed. The HCO QI program is responsible for the measurement plan and then its implementation. "It is critical that an HCO's QI program and plans identify clear steps to be taken to ensure that the CQI activities have direction. This direction is provided by overall goals, which typically are fairly universal and often focus on the six aims (STEEEP®); however, more specific direction is required. Measures/indicators provide this direction to assist in reaching the overarching goals" (Finkelman, 2018, pp. 329–330).

Data Collection

The HCO QI program collects data to monitor and assess its QI status. There are many sources of data. Some of the sources are designed specifically to collect QI data. Other sources, such as the electronic medical record, are used primarily for other purposes and then may also be used as a source of CQI data. The purpose of this record is documentation of patient care for clinical purposes—sharing information; documenting what will be done and what was done; records of testing, procedures, and medication administration; monitoring, such as vital signs; and so on. This, however, is also valuable data for CQI. When using data from methods that were not primarily designed for CQI data collection, there is some risk that the data will not be what is needed; data may be missing or not understood; and data may be difficult to retrieve. The QI program must plan carefully what data will be collected and the best source for the data.

The focus above is on HCO data collection; however, CQI data are also collected for broader purposes. The government collects data, as has been discussed in this text for *Healthy People 2020*, the QDR, NQS, CMS programs, and many other initiatives. The NDNQI® is an example of a health profession database that requires data collection. The Joint Commission and the Magnet Recognition Program® also collect data from HCOs that are accredited or recognized by these organizations. Data collection and measurement has become a complex process and, at times, is confusing with multiple measures and indicators.

Analysis

Analysis of data or review of performance is a complex process conducted by an HCO's QI program. The goal is better understanding of the data. The data may be analyzed from a broad perspective, such as all data about medication errors; from a more focused perspective, such as intensive care unit medication errors or the HCO's intravenous medication errors; may compare data using benchmarking, for example, comparisons with other, similar HCOs or comparing clinical units within the HCO; and the analysis may be focused on specific incidents using RCA to understand an incident or event.

RCA is now used by most HCOs, particularly hospitals. It is an error analysis system that recognizes system factors are more important than individuals when an error occurs. The RCA process includes the following steps (Finkelman, 2018; U.S. Department of Health and Human Services, Agency for Research and Healthcare Quality, & Health Information Technology, 2013):

1. Select the team to complete the RCA. The team should include experts related to the event. For example, if the error occurred in surgery, team members should include representatives from the surgical staff from the operating room, anesthesiology, other relevant healthcare professionals such as surgeons and nurses, laboratory technicians, radiologist, infusion team, pharmacy, infection control (depending on the error), and management. Staff educators may also participate.
2. As the team analyzes the situation and error, it creates a flow chart to describe the situation.
3. The team then examines the flow chart for areas of failure.
4. The team uses CQI tools to consider data collected and possible root causes.
5. The team redesigns the process for improvement (if required) based on the analysis results.
6. The HCO implements the changes, ideally first through a pilot, and then spread to other areas as appropriate for the improvement strategy/intervention.

Key questions the RCA team asks during RCA are:

- What happened?
- Who was involved?
- When did it happen?
- Where did it happen?
- What is the severity of the actual or potential harm?
- What is the likelihood of reoccurrence?
- What are the consequences?

The team analyzing the problem or error usually uses brainstorming, flow charts, and cause-effect diagrams to clearly describe the problem and factors related to it. Typical contributing factors are categorized as (Finkelman, 2018, p. 363):

- *Environmental factors* (for example, work environment, staff safety, safety culture-type, ethical-legal concerns)

- *Organizational factors* (for example, staffing levels/mix, staff availability and roles, support staff, clear policies, administrative support, effective leadership, access to equipment and supplies, documentation, use of rounds and other communication methods, attitudes toward patients and families/patient-centered care)
- *Staff/team* (for example, supervision of staff, communication, team membership, quality of teamwork, team leadership and functioning, availability of expertise)
- *Individual staff factors* (for example, level of knowledge, competency, and experience, fatigue, stress, expectations, position description, staff safety)
- *Task factors* (for example, clear protocols and/ or guidelines, use of checklists, lab tests and other procedures, description of tasks, policies)
- *Patient factors* (for example, stress, communication, accessible patient information, diversity factors, comorbidities, status on admission, past history, 30-day unplanned readmission, discharge plans)

Work in healthcare environments is complex, and many factors affect how staff perform (Roth, Wieck, Fountain, & Hass, 2015). Common human factors that affect staff performance, and thus quality care, are fatigue and sleep problems, stress, hunger, illness, unfamiliarity with a task, inexperience, shortage of time, inadequate checking, interruptions, noise, poor procedures to follow, unwillingness or inability to ask for help, and language and culture factors (Finkelman, 2018). These factors can be used to develop strategies to improve care by preventing these factors or reducing them.

The analysis must lead to clear views of issues so that it can be used to plan for interventions to prevent problems or to solve problems. Gap analysis may be part of the process—identification of where you want to be and comparison with current status. Staff members need to be informed about the analysis and results. If they are not informed, it is very difficult to engage them in QI. Nurses should be involved in all phases of analysis.

Patient Outcomes
and Nursing Care: Do We Make a Difference in Quality Improvement?

Keeping Patients Safe: Transforming the Work Environment of Nurses (IOM, 2004b) is an early *Quality Chasm* report that focuses on acute care or care provided in the hospital setting; however, it is relevant here because much of the content can also be applied to nursing in other types of settings and even to current nursing practice. This report also has a different focus from the later report *The Future of Nursing, Leading Change, Advancing Health* (IOM, 2010). The earlier report states, "When we are hospitalized, in a nursing home, or managing a chronic condition in our own homes—at some of our most vulnerable moments—nurses are the healthcare providers we are most likely to encounter, spend the greatest amount of time with, and be dependent upon for our recovery" (IOM, 2004b, p. ix). The report emphasizes designs for a work environment in which nurses can provide safer, higher quality patient care. The content discusses changes in nursing shortage and staffing, healthcare errors, patient safety risk factors, central role of the nurse in patient safety, and work environment threats to patient safety. In discussing errors, the focus moves away from a punitive, blaming environment and emphasizes the need to view errors more from a system perspective, supporting the major message from *To Err Is Human* (IOM, 1999). Some of the factors that influence errors from a system perspective are highlighted in this report, including equipment failures, inadequate staff training, lack of clear supervision and direction, and inadequate staffing levels—these have not become major issues in QI programs. The central message in the report is that we need to transform the healthcare work environment, an ongoing need. This critical report identifies six major concerns for direct care in nursing (IOM, 2004b):

1. *Monitoring patient status or surveillance:* This is different from assessment. **Surveillance** is defined as "purposeful and ongoing acquisition, interpretation, and synthesis of patient data for clinical decision-making" (McCloskey & Bulechek, 2000, p. 629). If surveillance is not effective, the result may be termed failure to rescue—missing an opportunity to prevent complications.

2. *Physiologic therapy:* This is the most common visible intervention performed by nurses.

3. *Helping patients compensate for loss of function:* Teamwork is important to accomplish this—for example, nursing, physical therapy, medicine, and so on.

4. *Providing emotional support,* which is critical for patients and their families.

5. *Education for patients and families:* This has become more difficult to accomplish due to work conditions, staffing levels, patient acuity, and shorter lengths of stay.

6. *Integration and coordination of care:* Patients' needs are complex, and care is complex, often resulting in multiple forms of care provided by multiple providers.

This report recommends (1) adopting transformational leadership and evidence-based management, (2) maximizing the capability of the workforce, (3) understanding work processes so that they can be improved, and (4) creating and sustaining cultures of safety (IOM, 2004b). Nursing leadership must be very active throughout the HCO. Nurse leaders must represent staff, support the need for effective change, facilitate input from direct care nursing staff, and expand communication and collaboration. Leadership is a reoccurring theme throughout this text. The HCO needs to support ongoing staff learning—for example, through effective orientation for an appropriate length of time, ongoing training; nurse residency programs, funding support for nurses to return to school to complete higher degrees, establishing partnerships with schools of nursing, providing opportunities for interprofessional educational experiences, and so on. All this requires resources that management must ensure are available—for example, adequate staffing is critical. All HCOs struggle with the challenges of how best to fill positions and retain staff. Excessive documentation can lead to less time for patients, which can affect safety and quality. There is need for computerized documentation with decision-making support, which many HCOs have today. Work design is discussed in depth in the *Keeping Patients Safe* report (IOM, 2004b); physical space and design—for example, lighting, size of the unit, and the ability to get to equipment easily and quickly—and how these may affect safety are also addressed (IOM, 1999). *The Future of Nursing* report also emphasizes nursing leadership and the need for nurses to be leaders in HCOs and in CQI (IOM, 2010).

Woven throughout all of the recommendations is the need for EBP and the need to base decisions on evidence. "As nurses are the largest component of the healthcare workforce and are also strongly involved in the commission, detection, and prevention of errors and adverse events, they and their work environment are critical elements of stronger patient safety defenses" (IOM, 2004b, p. 31).

Based on what is known about QI and its importance, it is natural to assume that nurses are very active in QI and have assumed leadership in improving care, but this is not necessarily the case, particularly with new nurses. When a 2008 survey on this topic was sent to nurses who graduated between 2004 and 2005, 436 responded (a rate of 69.4%). According to the researchers, "Overall, 159 (38.6%) of new nurses thought that they were 'poorly' or 'very poorly' prepared about or had 'never heard of' QI. Their perceptions of preparation varied widely by the specific topic. Baccalaureate (BSN) graduates reported significantly higher levels of preparation than associate degree (ADN) graduates in EBP; assessing gaps in practice, teamwork, and collaboration; and many of the research-type skills such as data

collection, analysis, measurement and measuring resulting changes" (Kovner, Brewer, Yingrengreung, & Fairchild, 2010, p. 29). The authors of this study indicate that more needs to be done in nursing education on this critical content to help students see the connection between QI concepts and practice.

Subsequently, a second study was done that compared the 2004–2005 graduates with graduates from 2007–2008 (539 RNs who worked in 15 states). Not much difference was apparent in their responses, indicating little had changed in nursing education to better prepare new nurses for QI (Djukic, Kovner, Brewer, & Bernstein, 2013). Although more hospitals are providing staff education for new graduates, hospitals in general need to collaborate more with schools of nursing so that nursing graduates are better prepared and then require less staff education, which is costly for the hospitals.

A 2015 publication discusses education gaps and solutions for early-career, front-line nurse managers' education and participation in QI (Djukic, Kovner, Brewer, Fatehi, & Jun, 2015). These are key concerns if we want care to improve. We need leaders at all levels in QI, but unit managers have a major impact on QI and in increasing staff nurse engagement—but are these managers prepared for this need? A sample of 42 early-career, front-line nurse managers was part of study to examine this issue. The results indicate that about 30% of the sample thought they were very prepared based on 12 QI indicators. Did they indicate that the sample was engaged in specific clinical efforts to improve care on their unit more than once a month? Thirty-five percent noted that they had been involved in this manner. More than 50% indicated that they received good organizational support for QI efforts, with 30% receiving reward for their QI contributions. This study then demonstrates that some nurse managers are prepared and participate, though the sample for the study was small.

Nurses need to participate actively in the NQS although historically nurses have provided weak QI leadership. Means by which nurses can participate include the National Priorities Partnership, Measures Application Partnership, and the NDNQI (Kennedy,

Murphy, & Roberts, 2013). Nurses need to actively engage in the national quality agenda.

The American Association of Critical-Care Nurses conducted a study to examine calculated decisions of nurses to not speak up when nurses have knowledge of errors (Maxwell, Grenny, Lavandero, & Groah, 2011). One aspect of the study examined the use of four common survey safety tools (universal protocol checklist, World Health Organization checklist, SBAR when used with a handoff protocol, and drug-interaction warning systems). In the study, the nurses were asked how often they had been in situations where one of these tools was effective, warning them of a problem that might have been missed and harmed a patient if a tool had not been used. The results indicated that 85% (2,020) of the nurses said they had been in this situation at least once, and 29% (693) said they were in this situation at least a few times a month. This would indicate that these tools do make a difference and lead to improved care.

Other data from the same study, however, were not so positive. Maxwell and colleagues (2011) also examined the effectiveness of these safety tools, which may be undercut by "undiscussables" as noted in their sample: 58% (1,403) of the nurses said they had been in situations where it was either unsafe to speak up or they were unable to get others to listen. Seventeen percent (409 of the 1,403) said they were in this situation at least a few times a month. This type of data attests to the complexity of QI. Understanding data requires consideration of the problems; the challenges in identifying, monitoring, and measuring the problems; and the influence of human factors. Findings reported in this "Silent Treatment" study show that only a small minority of nonsupervisory nurses spoke up when they had a concern related to dangerous shortcuts, incompetence, or disrespect. Only 9% spoke up in all three of these situations, and only 14% spoke up in two of the three. "The goal is to connect to people's existing values to stimulate their passion for keeping patients safe. The most effective way to make this connection is through sharing personal experiences. The least effective way is to resort

to verbal persuasion: data dumps, lectures, sermons, and rants" (Maxwell et al. 2011, p. 10). Thus, it is important to get staff to share stories of near misses, patient injuries, or examples of when they discuss error prevention and harm to a patient. Staff can relate more to stories, and they will remember them.

Nurses also must be engaged in error recovery. We know that not all errors can be prevented, though we are making efforts to reduce errors. Error recovery "includes identifying, interrupting, and correcting medical errors in a timely fashion" (Gaffney, Hatcher, & Milligan, 2016, p. 906). This nursing role is invisible for the most part when a near miss occurs. Gaffney et al. systematic review of studies on error recovery notes that nurses typically used strategies to identify, interrupt, and correct errors that included knowledge of the patient and the patient's problems, knowledge of the environment, and awareness of the plan of care. Nurses gain this knowledge, which may affect error recovery, through collection of data, surveillance, communicating with others (team), continuity of care, asking questions and sharing information. "When these strategies were not effective, being physically present was key in verbally interrupting or creating delays to correct potential errors" (2016, p. 914). Development of clinical judgment comes with experience, and this assists in error recovery.

Other ways that more nurses can participate in the quality agenda is through development and implementation of standards; involvement in shared governance and decision making about QI; serving on QI committees in HCOs and for professional organizations; engaging in health policy development at the local, state, and national levels; undertaking research and using evidence to improve practice; and engaging in active discussions with colleagues and other healthcare professions about QI. There is need for change in the healthcare system, and the following is critical: "The 21st century healthcare system envisioned by the committee—providing care that is evidence based, patient centered, and systems oriented—also implies new roles and responsibilities for patients and their families, who must become more aware, more participative, and more demanding in a care system that should be meeting their needs. And all involved must be united by the overarching purpose of reducing the burden of illness, injury, and disability in our nation" (IOM, 2001a, p. 20). **Figure 12-7** describes a framework of nursing care performance illustrating how nursing care intersects with QI.

Stop and Consider #11

Every nurse must engage in QI every day.

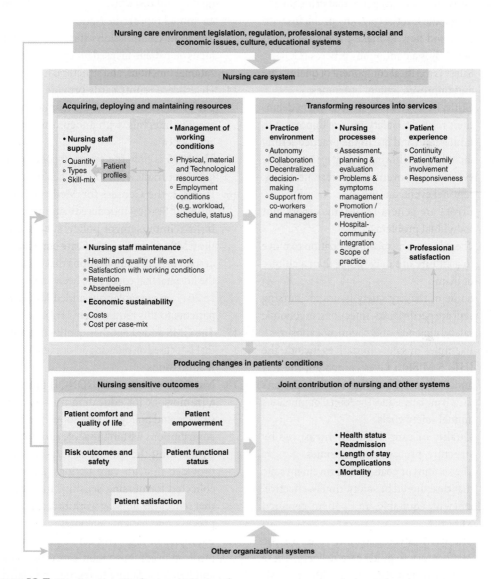

Figure 12-7 Nursing Care Performance Network

CHAPTER HIGHLIGHTS

1. The IOM published a number of critical reports related to quality health care in the United States—the *Quality Chasm* series.

2. QI is aimed at processes that critically examine the level of care, any problems with care, and how to make patient outcomes better. It is a continuous process (CQI).

3. Safety is a critical component of quality care and improved patient outcomes.

4. Critical terms that require consistent definitions related to safety and are important to understand and use in the practice setting include the following: safety, error, adverse event, misuse, overuse, underuse, near miss, sentinel event, and RCA.

5. Errors are generally systems errors, not individual problems.

6. There is a strong recommendation to move to a culture of safety rather than a culture of blame.

7. Some of the key safety issues for nursing staff are needlesticks, infections, ergonomic safety, violence, and chemical exposures.

8. Examples of safety initiatives include the IHI's 5 Million Lives campaign, the IHI and Robert Wood Johnson Foundation's TCAB initiative, and The Joint Commission's annual safety goals.

9. Quality of care is usually measured by structure, process, and outcomes.

10. The six aims or goals for improvement state that care should be safety, timely, effective, efficient, equitable, and patient-centered STEEEP.

11. The IOM developed new rules for the 21st century to guide care delivery. These rules provide a vision for healthcare quality and are directly related to the six aims and to the healthcare professions core competencies.

12. The United States now collects national quality and disparities data and publishes an annual report: the National QDR.

13. The Joint Commission's standards for QI focus on patient-focused functions, organizational functions, and structural functions.

14. Healthcare report cards provide specific performance data about an organization at specific intervals, with a focus on quality and safety.

15. The NQS is now the major improvement guide for framework for U.S. health care.

16. In 2007, the Centers for Medicare and Medicaid Services introduced a major change in its reimbursement policy, stating that the CMS will not pay Medicare benefits for certain patient complications that occur in the hospital that could have been prevented. In 2011, new regulations added Medicaid patients to this requirement (HACs).

17. The CMS added another quality initiative that is focused on reducing 30-day unplanned readmissions.

18. Nursing's report card (NDNQI) provides a framework for educating nurses, consumers, and policy makers about nursing's contributions within the acute care setting by tracking the quality of nursing care provided in acute care settings. Data are collected for nursing-sensitive indicators that reflect the nursing workforce, nursing process, and patient outcomes.

19. Examples of high-risk care activities are medication administration, care transitions and handoffs, failure to rescue, and alarm /alert fatigue.

(Continues)

CHAPTER HIGHLIGHTS (CONTINUED)

20. Examples of methods used to measure and monitor safety and quality include utilization review, benchmarking, assessment of access to care, medication reconciliation, standardized communication, rounds, incident reports, and sentinel reports.

21. *Keeping Patients Safe* (IOM, 2004b) recommended the following: (1) adopting transformational leadership and evidence-based management, (2) maximizing the capability of the workforce, (3) understanding work processes so that they can be improved, and (4) creating and sustaining cultures of safety.

22. *The Future of Nursing* (IOM, 2010) emphasizes nursing leadership and need for nursing engagement in QI.

23. Much more needs to be done to prepare nurses for CQI and to assume leadership in CQI.

ENGAGING IN THE CONTENT

Discussion Questions

1. How do the six aims (STEEEP) to improve quality relate to the rules for the 21st century (IOM) and the healthcare professions core competencies (IOM)?

2. Describe the culture of safety. How does this compare to the blame culture?

3. What is accreditation? Who is the major provider of accreditation for HCOs?

4. Discuss the definition of *quality*.

5. Describe four examples of tools and methods used to improve care.

CRITICAL THINKING ACTIVITIES

1. Divide up into teams, with each team taking one of the rules for the 21st century. Develop a defense for this rule and share with the other teams.

2. Visit the National Healthcare QDRs website to review the current reports on healthcare quality and disparities (https://www.ahrq.gov/research /findings/nhqrdr/index.html). After reviewing data on the dimensions of quality, what have you learned? Select one of the areas monitored and summarize key issues. Share this with others who have reviewed different clinical conditions.

3. In student teams, examine the website for the Toolkit for Using the AHRQ Quality Indicators (https://www.ahrq.gov/professionals /systems/hospital/qitoolkit/index.html). Each team should review the information and summarize the key points that they would

(Continues)

CRITICAL THINKING ACTIVITIES (CONTINUED)

use to explain the purpose of the toolkit and value to nursing practice.

4. Visit the OSHA Workplace Violence website, https://www.osha.gov/SLTC/healthcarefacilities /violence.html, to learn about this important staff safety problem and possible solutions. Review the guidelines for healthcare workplace violence. What solutions are recommended, and what is your opinion of the solutions?

5. Select one of the common quality care issues, such as hand washing, decubiti, and so on, and search for information about the topic and how care can be improved.

6. Select two of the online patient safety resources found at National Patient Safety Foundation website (http://www.npsf .org/?page=professionals). How might nurses use this resource?

ELECTRONIC REFLECTION JOURNAL

In your journal, describe an example of a QI problem that you have observed or were directly involved in while in clinical practice. Remember to follow the Health Insurance Portability and Accountability Act rules when recording your information.

CASE STUDIES

Case 1

A 21-year-old woman presented to the emergency department of an urban hospital with a history of systemic lupus. Her complaint was dehydration, dizziness, and feeling faint. The woman also had a recent history of being dehydrated, complicated by renal involvement from lupus and having to receive bolus fluids. She was on multiple medications, including steroids and methotrexate. An intravenous (IV) line was started, and blood was drawn for labs. The emergency department physician returned to report that the lab values were within normal limits, yet the young woman felt no better. She stated that she still felt dehydrated, her blood pressure felt low, and she normally received more IV fluids and a steroid injection when she felt this way. The physician indicated that he felt no need for this treatment, but when the patient insisted on more fluids, he agreed to continue them for a while and to give her an injection of steroids. The patient asked, "Do you want to give me anti-nausea medication first?" The physician stated that there was no indication. The patient told him that she was always nauseated following steroids and had sometimes vomited if no antiemetic were administered first. The physician argued but finally grew tired and walked away. The steroid injection was given, and nausea ensued. When the

CASE STUDIES (CONTINUED)

patient got home a few hours later, the patient called her rheumatologist and urologist (neither had been available when the illness occurred because of the late hour). They repeated her labs the next day, only to find that she was severely dehydrated, and many values, including renal panel, were outside normal limits.

Case Questions

1. What are the critical issues in this case description?
2. Consider the six aims (STEEEP) to better ensure quality care. How might they apply to this patient?
3. Is this patient-centered care? Why or why not?
4. If you were the nurse assigned to this patient in emergency department, what could you have done?

Case 2

A patient has been admitted to an ambulatory surgical unit for a hernia repair. He is a physician, and his wife is a nurse. After his surgery, his wife is taken to the post-anesthesia care unit (also known as recovery) to see her husband. The unit is configured with cubicles divided with curtains. In the patient area, there is the stretcher with the patient, monitors, and a computer with a stool in front of it. The patient is recovering from anesthesia but can communicate. The nurse is "glued to" the computer, rarely looking at the patient when speaking to him. The patient has a history of atrial fibrillation and takes a number of cardiac medications. The nurse says that he is going to put a medication into the IV; he indicates the medication name, and begins to do so. At the same time, the patient becomes alert and says, "No." Just at that time, the curtain opens and the anesthesiology resident says loudly, "Stop that order." Both physicians knew (the patient and the resident, although the resident should not have made the order) that there was a contraindication for mixing certain drugs.

A few hours later, the patient is getting ready for discharge in the ambulatory surgical unit, and his wife is present. During the admission process, the nurse was also "glued to" computer when assessing the patient, rarely looking at the patient and more concerned with typing in information rather than assessment. At the time of discharge, the nurse comes in and reads through a list of discharge directions, strongly emphasizing that the patient should take all of his routine medications when he gets home. The patient says, "All of them?" (He is testing the nurse, as he knows the answer to this question.) The nurse says, "Yes." The patient says, "I don't think so. Aspirin should not be taken right after surgery, and I take it daily as routine medication." The nurse did not seem to understand what he said and did not respond.

In this situation, the doctor should not have written an order for all medications after discharge; however, in both incidents the nurse had responsibilities and provided ineffective, unsafe care that was stopped by the patient before a serious problem occurred. The patient and his wife left the hospital fed up with the quality of care. Both incidents were described in the patient satisfaction survey the patient received, but the patient never heard from the hospital. This was an academic health center with a medical school and nursing school attached to the university. The patient will not return to this hospital for surgery.

CASE STUDIES (CONTINUED)

Case Questions

In this example of a case that actually occurred, it is clear that physician errors led to near misses, but it is also clear that nursing actions led to near misses.

1. What is a "near miss"?
2. Describe each of the near misses and the roles of the physicians and the nurses in each incident.
3. Which system issues might have been involved?
4. What could have been done to prevent these near misses?
5. What do you think hospitals should do when patients describe incidents like these in patient satisfaction surveys?
6. What was the impact of technology in this case?

Working Backward to Develop a Case

Write a brief paragraph that describes a case related to the following questions.

1. Can you provide us with comparison data for the last 5 years?
2. Was the procedure followed as described and based on best evidence?
3. What role should staff nurses assume?

REFERENCES

Aleccia, J. (2011). Nurse's suicide highlights twin tragedies of medical errors. Retrieved from http://www.msnbc .msn .com/id/43529641/ns/health-health_care/# .Tm0By09A8j8

Amaral, A., McDonald, A., Coburn, N., Xiong, W., Shojana, K., Fowler, R., . . . Adhikari, N. (2015). Expanding the scope of critical care rapid response teams: A feasible approach to identify adverse events. A prospective observational cohort. *BMJ Quality and Safety, 24*(12). Retrieved from http://qualitysafety.bmj .com/content/24/12/764

American Hospital Association. (1999). *Hospital statistics.* Chicago, IL: Author.

American Nurses Association. (2013). *Safe patient handling and mobility: Interprofessional national standards across the care continuum.* Retrieved from http://www .nursingworld .org/handlewithcare

American Nurses Association. (2014). NDNQI®. Retrieved from http://www.nursingquality.org/#intro

Anderson, D. (2006). Creating a culture of safety: Leadership, teams, and tools. *Nurse Leader, 4*(5), 28–41.

Anderson, P., & Townsend, T. (2010). Medication errors: Don't let them happen to you. *American Nurse Today, 5*(3). Retrieved from http://www.americannursetoday. com/medication-errors-dont-let-them-happen-to-you/

Berwick, D., & Nolan, T. (1998). Physicians as leaders improving healthcare. *Annals of Internal Medicine, 128,* 289–292.

Castro, A. (2004). Handle with Care: The American Nurses Association's campaign to address work-related musculoskeletal disorders. *Online Journal of Issues in Nursing, 9*(3). Retrieved from http://www.nursingworld .org/MainMenuCategories/ANAMarketplace/ANA Periodicals/ OJIN/TableofContents/Volume92004 /No3Sept04/ HandleWithCare.aspx

Chassin, M., & Galvin, R. (1998). The urgent need to improve healthcare quality. *Journal of the American Medical Association, 280,* 1000–1005.

Diaz, M., Silkaitis, C., Malczynski, M., Noskin, G., Warren, J., & Zembower, T. (2008). Contamination of examination gloves in patient rooms and implications for transmission of antimicrobial-resistant microorganisms. *Infection Control and Hospital Epidemiology, 29*(1), 63–65.

Djukic, M., Kovner, C., Brewer, C., & Bernstein, I. (2013). Early career registered nurses' participation in hospital quality improvement *Journal of Nursing Care Quality, 39*(1), 198–207.

Djukic, M., Kovner, C., Brewer, C., Fatehi, F., & Jun, J. (2015). Educational gaps and solutions for early-career nurse managers' education and participation in quality improvement. *Journal of Nursing Administration, 45*(4), 206–211.

Donabedian, A. (1980). *Explorations in quality assessment and monitoring, Vol. I: The definition of quality and approaches to its assessment.* Ann Arbor, MI: Health Administration Press.

Dunton, N., Gonnerman, D., Montalvo, I., & Schumann, M. (2011). Incorporating nursing quality indicators in public reporting and value-based purchasing initiatives. *American Nurse Today, 6*(1), 14–17.

Environmental Working Group. (2007). Nurses' health and workplace exposures to hazardous substance. Retrieved from http://www.ewg.org/research/nurses-health

Finkelman, A. (2018). *Quality improvement. A guide for integration in nursing.* Burlington, MA: Jones & Bartlett Learning.

Gaffney, T., Hatcher, B., & Milligan, T. (2016). Nurses' role in medical error recover: An integrative review. *Journal of Clinical Nursing, 25*, 906–917.

Galewitz, P. (2011). Medicaid to stop paying for hospital mistakes. Retrieved from http://www.kaiserhealthnews.org

Henneman, E., & Gawlinski, A. (2004). A "near-miss" model for describing the nurse's role in the recovery of medical errors. *Journal of Professional Nursing, 20*(3), 196–201.

Institute for Healthcare Improvement. (2007). *Triple aim.* Retrieved from http://www.ihi.org/offerings/initiatives/tripleaim/Pages/default.aspx

Institute for Healthcare Improvement. (2011). *Five million lives campaign.* Retrieved from http://www.ihi.org/IHI/Programs/Campaign

Institute for Healthcare Improvement. (2014). *Institute for healthcare improvement.* Retrieved from http://www.ihi.org

Institute for Healthcare Improvement. (2017). *Transforming care at the bedside.* Retrieved from http://www.ihi.org/engage/initiatives/completed/tcab/pages/default.aspx

Institute for Safe Medication Practice. (2011). *Medication errors.* Retrieved from http://www.ismp.org/pressroom/PR20100909.pdf

Institute of Medicine. (1990). *Clinical practice guidelines: Directions for a new program.* Washington, DC: The National Academies Press.

Institute of Medicine. (1999). *To err is human: Building a safer health system.* Washington, DC: The National Academies Press.

Institute of Medicine. (2001a). *Crossing the quality chasm: A new health system for the 21st century.* Washington, DC: The National Academies Press.

Institute of Medicine. (2001b). *Envisioning the national healthcare quality report.* Washington, DC: The National Academies Press.

Institute of Medicine. (2003). *Health professions education: A bridge to quality.* Washington, DC: The National Academies Press.

Institute of Medicine. (2004a). *Patient safety: Achieving a new standard for care.* Washington, DC: The National Academies Press.

Institute of Medicine. (2004b). *Keeping patients safe: Transforming the work environment of nurses.* Washington, DC: The National Academies Press.

Institute of Medicine. (2010). *The future of nursing: Leading change, advancing health.* Washington, DC: The National Academies Press.

Jeffs, L., Lingard, L., Berta, W., & Baker, G. (2012). Catching and correcting near misses. The collective vigilance and individual accountability trade off. *Journal of Interprofessional Care, 26*, 121–126.

Joint Commission, The. (2013). *Sentinel event alert. Medical device alarm safety in hospitals.* Retrieved from http://www.jointcommission.org/sea_issue_50

Joint Commission, The. (2015). *Joint commission updates on sentinel event statistics.* Retrieved from https://www.ecri.org/components/HRCAlerts/Pages/HRCAlerts111815_Joint.aspx

Joint Commission, The. (2017a). *Sentinel event alert. The essential role of leadership in developing a safety culture.* Retrieved from https://www.jointcommission.org/issues/article.aspx?Article=s6ej6wvxeEkJWMY931rGSTZ2OaisY4Fzd5u3Y%2BzeeUU%3D

Joint Commission, The. (2017b). *Accreditation survey activity guide for healthcare organizations, 2017.* Retrieved from https://www.jointcommission.org/assets/1/18/2017_Organization_SAG.pdf

Joint Commission, The. (2017c). *Hospitals.* Retrieved from https://www.jointcommission.org/standards_information/hap_requirements.aspx

Jones, T., Mailton, P., & Murry, N. (2015). Unfinished nursing care, missed care, and implicitly rationed care: State of the science review. *International Journal of Nursing Studies, 52*, 1121–1137.

Kennedy, R., Murphy, J., & Roberts, D. (2013, September 30). An overview of the national quality strategy: Where do nurses fit? *Online Journal of Issues in Nursing, 18*(3). doi Retrieved from http://www.nursingworld.org/MainMenuCategories/ANAMarketplace/ANAPeriodicals/OJIN/TableofContents/Vol-18-2013/No3-Sept-2013/National-Quality-Strategy.html

Ketchum, K., Grass, C., & Padwojski, A. (2005). Medication reconciliation. *American Journal of Nursing, 105*(11), 78–85.

Kovner, C., Brewer, C., Yingrengreung, S., & Fairchild, S. (2010). New nurses' views of quality improvement education. New nurses views on quality improvement education. *Joint Commission on Journal on Quality and Patient Safety, 36*(1), 29–35.

Makary, M. (2016, May 3). Medical error—the third leading cause of death in the U.S. *British Medical Journal.* Retrieved from http://www.bmj.com/content/353/bmj.i2139

Maxwell, D., Grenny, J., Lavandero, R., & Groah, L. (2011). *The silent treatment: Why safety tools and checklists aren't enough to save lives.* VitalSmarts, AORN, & AACN. Retrieved from http://www.aacn.org

McCloskey, J., & Bulechek, G. (2000). *Nursing interventions classification (NIC).* St. Louis, MO: Mosby.

Montalvo, I., & Dunton, N. (2007). *Transforming nursing data into quality care: Profiles of quality improvement in U.S. healthcare facilities.* Silver Spring, MD: American Nurses Association.

Nasarwanji, M., Badir, A., & Gurses, A. (2016). Standardizing handoff communication. Content analysis of 27 handoff mnemonics. *Journal of Nursing Care Quality,* July/September, 238–244.

National Patient Safety Foundation. (2015). *Free from harm.* Retrieved from www.npsf.org/free-from-harm

National Quality Forum. (2017a). *NQF strategic plan 2016–2019.* Retrieved from http://www.qualityforum.org/NQF_Strategic_Direction_2016-2019.aspx

National Quality Forum. (2017b). *Work in quality measurement.* Retrieved from http://www.qualityforum.org/about_nqf/work_in_quality_measurement/

Penn, C. (2014). Integrating just culture into nursing student error policy. *Journal of Nursing Education, 53*(9), S107–S109.

Peter, D., Robinson, P., & Jordan, M. (2015). Reducing readmissions using teach-back. Enhancing patient and family education. *Journal of Nursing Administration, 45*(1), 35–42.

Plsek, P. (2001). Redesigning healthcare with insights from the science of complex adaptive systems. In Institute of Medicine, *Crossing the quality chasm* (pp. 309–322). Washington, DC: National Academies Press.

Pollard, P., Mitra, K., & Mendelson, D. (1996). *Nursing report card for acute care.* Washington, DC: American Nurses Publishing.

Polygreen, P., Chen, Y., Beekmann, S., Srinivasan, A., Neill, M., Gay, T., & Cavanaugh, J. (2008). Elements of influenza vaccination programs that predict higher vaccination rates: Results of an emerging infections network survey. *Clinical Infectious Diseases, 46*(1), 14–19.

Press Ganey. (2014). *Press Ganey acquires national database of nursing quality indicators.* Retrieved from http://pressganey.com/pressRoom/2014/06/10/press-ganey-acquires-national-database-of-nursing-quality-indicators-%28ndnqi-%29

Press Ganey. (2017). *Nursing Quality (NDNQI®).* Retrieved from http://www.pressganey.com/solutions/clinical-quality/nursing-quality

Reason, J. (2000). Human error: Models and management. *British Medical Journal, 320*(7237), 768–770.

Roth, C., Wieck, K., Fountain, R., & Haas, B. (2015). Hospital nurses' perceptions of human factors contributing to nursing errors. *Journal of Nursing Administration, 45*(5), 263–269.

Rozich, J., Howard, R., Justeson, J., Macken, P., Lindsay, M., & Resar, R. (2004). Standardization as a mechanism to improve safety in healthcare. *Joint Commission Journal Quality and Safety, 30*(1), 5–14.

Six Sigma. (2017). *What is six sigma?* Retrieved from http://www.isixsigma.com/new-to-six-sigma/getting-started/what-six-sigma/

Thomas, E., Studdert, D., Newhouse, J., Zbar, B., Howard, K., Williams, E., & Brennan, T. (1999). Costs of medical injuries in Utah and Colorado. *Inquiry, 36,* 255–264.

Trossman, S. (2017, January 17). Hazardous conditions. Study links miscarriages and working with certain drugs. Retrieved from http://www.theamericannurse.org/2012/04/02/hazardous-conditions/

U.S. Congress, Subcommittee on Primary Health and Aging. (2014, July 17). *Medical mistakes are 3rd leading cause of death in U.S.* Retrieved from http://www.sanders.senate .gov/newsroom/press-releases/medical-mistakes-are-3rd-leading-cause-of-death-in-us

U.S. Department of Health and Human Services. (2014). *Press release: New HHS data show quality improvements saved 15,000 lives and $4 billion in health spending.* Retrieved from https://www.hhs.gov/about/news/2014/05/07/new-hhs-data-show-quality-improvements-saved-15000-lives-and-4-billion-in-health-spending.html

U.S. Department of Health and Human Services (HHS). (2015, December 1). *National patient safety efforts save 87,000 lives and nearly $20 billion in costs.* Retrieved from https://www.hhs.gov/about/news/2015/12/01/national-patient-safety-efforts-save-lives-and-costs.html#

U.S. Department of Health and Human Services. (2017). *Healthy people 2020.* Retrieved from https://www.healthypeople.gov/

U.S. Department of Health and Human Services, & Agency for Healthcare Research and Quality. (2004, July). *General questions about the AHRQ QIs. AHRQ quality indicators.* Retrieved from www.qualityindicators.ahrq.gov/FAQs_Support/default.aspx

U.S. Department of Health and Human Services, & Agency for Healthcare Research and Quality. (2010). *National healthcare quality and disparities reports.* Retrieved from http://www.ahrq.gov/qual/qrdr10.htm

U.S. Department of Health and Human Services. (2011, March 11). *Press release: National quality strategy will promote better health, quality care for Americans.* Retrieved from https://wayback.archiveit.org/3926/20140108162236/http://www.hhs.gov/news/press/2011pres/03/20110321a.html

U.S. Department of Health and Human Serviced, & Agency for Health Research and Quality. (2013a). *Practice facilitation handbook.* Chapter 7: Measuring and benchmarking clinical performance. Retrieved from https://www.ahrq.gov/professionals/prevention-chronic-care/improve/system/pfhandbook/mod7.html

U.S. Department of Health and Human Serviced, & Agency for Health Research and Quality. (2013b). *AHRQ health information technology, ambulatory safety and quality. Findings and lessons from the AHRQ ambulatory safety and quality program.* Retrieved from http://healthit.ahrq.gov/sites/default/files/docs/page/alternate-findings-and-lessons-from-the-ahrq-ambulatory-safety-and-quality-program.pdf

U.S. Department of Health and Human Services, & Agency for Healthcare Research and Quality (AHRQ). (2014a, August). *Hospital guide to reducing Medicaid readmissions.* Publication No. 14-0050-EF. Retrieved from http://www.ahrq.gov/professionals/systems/hospital/medicaidreadmitguide/index.

U.S. Department of Health and Human Services, & Agency for Healthcare Research and Quality. (2014b, October). *AHRQ Quality Indicators™ Toolkit for hospitals: Fact sheet.* Retrieved from http://www.ahrq.gov/research/findings/factsheets/quality/qifactsheet/index.htmlU.S. Department of Health and Human Services (HHS). (2015a). *National strategy for quality improvement in health care 2015 annual progress report to Congress.* Retrieved from http://www.ahrq.gov/news/nqs.htmlU.S. Department of Health and Human Services (HHS). Agency for Healthcare Research and Quality (AHRQ). (2015b, June). *National healthcare quality and disparities report: Chartbook on care affordability.* Retrieved from http://www.ahrq.gov/research/findings/nhqrdr/2014chartbooks/careafford/careafford-care.html

U.S. Department of Health and Human Services, & Agency for Healthcare Research and Quality. (2016). *National scorecard on rates of hospital-acquired conditions 2010 to 2015: Interim data from national efforts to make health care safer.* Content last reviewed December 2016. Retrieved from http://www.ahrq.gov/professionals/quality-patient-safety/pfp/2015-interim.html

U.S. Department of Health and Human Services, & Agency for Research and Healthcare Quality, & Health Information Technology. (2013, May). *Root cause analysis.* Retrieved from https://healthit.ahrq.gov/health-it-tools-and-resources/workflow-assessment-health-it-toolkit/all-workflow-tools/root-cause-analysis

U.S. Department of Health and Human Services, Agency for Healthcare Research and Quality, & Patient Safety network. (2016a). *Support for clinicians involved in errors and adverse events (second victims).* Retrieved from https://psnet.ahrq.gov/primers/primer/30

U.S. Department of Health and Human Services, Agency for Healthcare Research and Quality, & Patient Safety network. (2016b). *Missed nursing care.* Retrieved from https://psnet.ahrq.gov/primers/primer/29/missed-nursing-care

U.S. Department of Health and Human Services, & Centers for Disease Control and Prevention. National Center for Health Statistics. (1998). Births and deaths: Preliminary data for 1998. *National Vital Statistics Report, 47*(25), 6.

U.S. Department of Health and Human Services, Centers for Disease Control and Prevention, & (2012). *Medication safety basics.* Retrieved from https://www.cdc.gov/medicationsafety/basics.html

U.S. Department of Health and Human Services, & Centers for Disease Control and Prevention. (2015). *Sharps safety in healthcare settings.* Retrieved from https://www.cdc.gov/sharpssafety/

U.S. Department of Health and Human Services, & Centers for Medicare and Medicaid. (2012). *Outcome and assessment information set.* Retrieved from https://www.cms.gov/Medicare/Quality-Initiatives-Patient-Assessment-Instruments/OASIS/index.html

U.S. Department of Health and Human Services, & Centers for Medicare and Medicaid Services. (2016, April 28). *Evidence-based guidelines for selected hospital-acquired conditions.* Final report. Retrieved from https://www.cms.gov/Medicare/Medicare-Fee-for-Service-Payment/HospitalAcqCond/Downloads/2016-HAC-Report.pdf

U.S. Department of Health and Human Services, & Food and Drug Administration. (2015). *Medication errors.* Retrieved from http://www.fda.gov/Drugs/DrugSafety/MedicationErrors/default.htm

U.S. Department Health and Human Services, & Health Resources and Services Administration. (April 2011a). *Performance management and measurement.* Retrieved from http://www.hrsa.gov/quality/toolbox/508pdfs/performancemanagementandmeasurement.pdf

U.S. Department Health and Human Services, & Health Resources and Services Administration. (April 2011b). *Managing data for performance improvement.* Retrieved from http://www.hrsa.gov/quality/toolbox/methodology/performanceimprovement/index.html

U.S. Department of Health and Human Services, & Office of the Inspector General. (2012). *Hospital incident reporting systems do not capture most patient harm.* Retrieved from https://oig.hhs.gov/oei/reports/oei-06-09-00091.pdf

U.S. Department of Labor, & Occupational Safety and Health Administration. (2016). *Needlestick/sharps injuries.* Retrieved from https://www.osha.gov/SLTC/etools/hospital/hazards/sharps/sharps.html

van der Schaaf, T. (1992). *Near miss reporting in the chemical process industry* (Unpublished doctoral dissertation). Eindhoven University of Technology, Eindhoven, Netherlands.

VanFosson, C., Jones, T., & Yoder, L. (2016). Unfinished nursing care: An important performance measure for nursing care systems. *Nursing Outlook, 64*, 124–136.

Wachter, R., & Pronovost, P. (2009). Balancing "no blame" with accountability in patient safety. *New England Journal of Medicine, 361*(14), 1401–1406.

Walton, B. (2014). Are you prepared to prevent medication errors? *Ohio Nurse,* (March), 10–15.

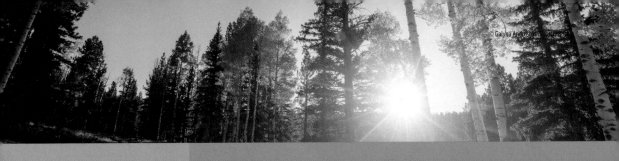
© Galyna Andrushko/Shutterstock

Chapter 13

Utilize Informatics

CHAPTER OBJECTIVES

At the conclusion of this chapter, the learner will be able to:

- Discuss the core competency: Utilize informatics.
- Discuss the relevance of the two recent federal reports on health information technology.
- Describe health informatics and its relationship to nursing.
- Explain the purpose of documentation and key issues related to informatics and documentation.
- Explain the importance of meaningful use.
- Critique the need for standardized terminologies in healthcare delivery.

- Explain systems and terminologies as they relate to health informatics.
- Examine informatics types and methods used in healthcare delivery.
- Describe new and expanding future approaches for applying informatics and technology in health care.
- Explain the importance of HIPAA.
- Compare and contrast high-touch care with high-tech care.
- Discuss the need for nursing leadership in health informatics technology.

- Clinical Decision Support Systems
- Tablets and Smartphones
- Computer-Based Reminder Systems
- Access to Patient Records at the Point of Care
- Internet Prescriptions
- Nurse Call Systems
- Voice Mail and Texting
- Telephone for Advice and Other Services
- Internet or Virtual Appointments
- Online Support Groups for Patients and Families
- The Future of Health Informatics and Medical Technology
  - Nanotechnology
  - Wearable Computing

- Telehealth and Remote Telemetry Monitoring
- Robotics
- Genetics and Genomics
- Medical Devices
- HIPAA: Ensuring Confidentiality
- High-Touch Care versus High-Tech Care
- Nursing Leadership in Health Informatics
- Chapter Highlights
- Engaging in the Content
  - Discussion Questions
  - Critical Thinking Activities
  - Electronic Reflection Journal
  - Case Studies
  - Working Backward to Develop a Case
- References

KEY TERMS

Clinical data repository
Clinical decision support systems
Clinical information system
Clinical provider order-entry system (CPOES)
Coding system
Computer literacy
Dashboard
Data
Data analysis software
Data bank
Data mining
Database

Electronic medical/health record (EMR/EHR)
Email list
E-measurement
Encryption
Health Insurance Portability and Accountability Act of 1996 (HIPAA)
Informatics
Information
Information (cognition) overload
Information literacy
Interoperability

Knowledge
Meaningful use
Minimum data set
Nomenclature
Nursing informatics (NI)
Personal health record (PHR)
Scorecard
Security protections
Software
Standardized terminology
Telehealth
Telenursing
Wisdom

Introduction

This chapter concludes the section that focuses on the healthcare profession core competencies with a discussion of the fifth core competency: utilize informatics. Informatics technology (IT) is an important topic in all areas of life today; with the explosion of technology, there are many opportunities for communication and sharing of knowledge. The impact of health informatics technology (HIT) on nursing care is explored here. Other issues that need to be addressed are documentation; confidentiality and privacy of information; and technology and informatics methods used in practice, education, and research. This chapter also includes content about biomedical equipment or medical devices, an expanding area in

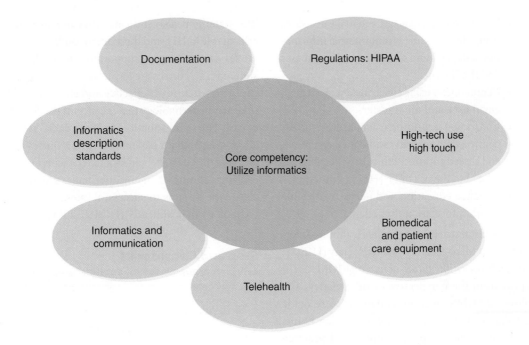

Figure 13-1 Utilize Informatics: Key Elements

healthcare technology that affects nurses and nursing care. Some of this equipment also uses IT. Nurses today cannot avoid technology, whether it is used in communication, care provision, or monitoring the quality of care. The chapter concludes with a discussion about the potential conflict between high-touch care versus high-tech care and the need for nursing leadership in health informatics—important issues for nurses to consider. **Figure 13-1** identifies key elements in this competency.

The Core Competency:
Utilize Informatics

The fifth healthcare profession core competency is "communicate, manage knowledge, mitigate error, and support decision making using information technology" (Institute of Medicine [IOM], 2003, p. 4). **Informatics** entails more than just understanding what is HIT and its clinical implications.

It also includes how that technology is used to prevent errors and improve care, particularly in the measurement of care. From the initial use of computers to share information, to management of financial records, to the current use of informatics with more emphasis on patient care, there has been a major move toward HIT application in health care. Some examples are greater use of informatics to find evidence to implement evidence-based practice (EBP); use of informatics in research; greater consumer access to information via the Internet; and more specific clinical applications, such as reminder and decision systems, telehealth, online prescribing, and use of email for provider–provider communication and patient–provider communication. The *Quality Chasm* report on healthcare professions core competencies concludes that every healthcare professional should meet the following informatics competencies (IOM, 2003, p. 63):

- Employ word processing, presentation, and data analysis software.

- Search, retrieve, manage, and make decisions using electronic data from internal information databases and external online databases and the Internet.
- Communicate using email, instant messaging, email lists, and file transfers.
- Understand security protections such as access control, data security, and data encryption, and directly address ethical and legal issues related to the use of IT [HIT] in practice.
- Enhance education and access to reliable health information for patients.

A position statement from the Healthcare Information and Management Systems Society (HIMSS, 2011) addresses *The future of nursing* (IOM, 2010) report from the perspective of informatics. The following HIMSS recommendations were made and align with *The Future* report on the key points of nursing leadership, education, and practice (HIMSS, 2011):

- Partner with nurse executives to lead technology changes that advance health and the delivery of health care.
- Support the development of informatics departments.
- Foster the evolution of the chief nursing informatics (NI) officer role.
- Transform nursing education to include informatics competencies and demonstrable behaviors at all levels of academic preparation.
- Promote the continuing education of all levels of nursing, particularly in the areas of electronic health records (EHRs) and HIT.
- Ensure that data, information, knowledge, and wisdom form the basis of 21st-century nursing practice by incorporating informatics competencies into practice standards in all healthcare settings.
- Facilitate the collection and analysis of interprofessional healthcare workforce data by ensuring data collected from existing IT systems.

The statement also indicates that nurses play a critical role in HIT and there are expanded roles for nurses—there is strong support for nursing leadership in HIT. "Nurses are key leaders in developing the infrastructure for effective and efficient health information technology that transforms the delivery of care. Nurse informaticists play a crucial role in advocating both for patients and fellow nurses who are often the key stakeholders and recipients of these evolving solutions. Nursing informatics professionals are the liaisons to successful interactions with technology in healthcare" (HIMSS, 2011).

Stop and Consider #1

Every nurse applies the informatics competency.

The Federal Health
Informatics Reports

The federal government increased its involvement in HIT, particularly through the U.S. Department of Health and Human Services (HHS), Office of the National Coordinator for Health Information Technology (ONC). This office published *Health information technology: Patient safety action & surveillance plan*, which identifies advantages for greater use of the electronic medical record (EMR), a key HIT example found in healthcare organizations (HCOs) (HHS & ONC, 2013, pp. 5–6):

- Increase clinicians' awareness of potential medication errors and adverse interactions.
- Improvement of the availability and timeliness of information to support treatment decisions, care coordination, and care planning.
- Make it easier for clinicians to report safety issues and hazards.
- Give patients the opportunity to more efficiently provide input on data accuracy than what paper records would allow.

These continue to be advantages in linking EMRs to quality improvement. The increased use of electronic records was initially driven and still is driven by important federal legislation, the Health Information Technology for Economic and Clinical Health Act of 2009, known as HITECH. All of this set the stage for greater federal involvement in HIT.

In 2015, the HHS published a report, *Connecting health and care for the nation: A shared nationwide interoperability roadmap, draft version 1.0.* The purpose of this extensive report is to describe a roadmap supporting **interoperability** or "the ability of a system to exchange electronic health information with and use electronic health information from other systems without special effort on the part of the user" (HHS & ONC, 2015a, p. 18). This is a critical element in making HIT more accessible and sharing information across systems and providers. A second report describes the federal health IT strategic plan for 2015–2020. **Figure 13-2** describes the framework for this strategic plan, including the vision, mission, and four goals. The key issue is access to information when needed by people. **Figure 13-3** highlights the vision that guides the strategic plan, focusing on high-quality care, lower costs, a healthier population, and engaged individuals—thus providing patient-centered care. This is a good example of how HIT is not just about computers and software. There needs to be a relationship between the technology and care delivery—needs and outcomes. Important principles should be followed when HIT plans are developed (HHS & ONC, 2015b, pp. 20–21).

- Build upon the existing health IT infrastructure.
- Recognize that one size does not fit all.
- Empower individuals giving them more access to information.
- Leverage the market—greater need now for seamless flow of electronic clinical health information.
- Simplify.
- Maintain modularity and provide flexibility to the system as change will be ongoing.
- Consider the current environment and support multiple levels of advancement.
- Focus on value.

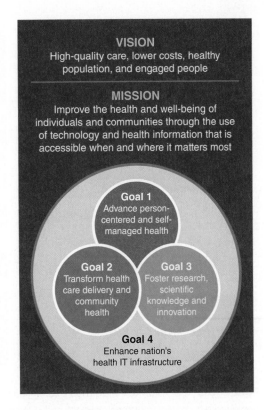

Figure 13-2 Federal Health IT Strategic Plan: Vision, Mission, and Goals

Reproduced from U.S. Department of Health and Human Services. The Office of National Coordinator for Health Information Technology. (2015). *Federal health IT strategic plan.* 2015–2020. p. 6. Retrieved from https://www.healthit.gov/sites/default/files/9-5-federalhealthitstratplan final_0.pdf

- Protect privacy and security in all aspects of interoperability.
- Include scalability and universal access.

These two reports—the strategic plan and follow-up initiatives—demonstrate the importance of HIT and the need for better standards and consistency, as well as the important role of the federal government through the work done by HHS and its agencies.

Undoubtedly, there has been major expansion in the use of HIT. The HHS through the ONC must now report annually to Congress on the status of HIT. The 2016 report indicated that prior to 2009, most

High-Quality Care

❖ Individuals care is patient centered, accessible, and safe, and interventions address behavioral, social, and environmental determinants of health (*National Quality Strategy*)

❖ Individuals benefit from improvement and innovation, and new knowledge is captured as part of care experience (*Health and Medicine Division of the National Academies of Sciences, Engineering, and Medicine*)

Lower Costs

❖ Individuals, families, employers, and governments benefit from more affordable quality care through new delivery models (*National Quality Strategy*)

Healthier Population

❖ Individuals, families, clinicians, and communities focus on prevention and wellness (*National Prevention Strategy*)

Engaged Individuals

❖ Individuals are active in managing their health and partnering in their health care (*ONC Person at the Center*)

Figure 13-3 The Vision to Guide the Federal Health IT Strategic Plan 2015–2020

Reproduced from U.S. Department of Health and Human Services. The Office of National Coordinator for Health Information Technology. (2015). *Federal health IT strategic plan. 2015–2020*. p. 13. Retrieved from https://www.healthit .gov/sites/default/files/9-5-federalhealthitstratplanfinal_0.pdf

HCOs—including hospitals, physician practices, clinics, and so on—used paper documentation. Sharing was done using fax machines. Indicating major improvement, the ONC notes that seven years later, 78% of physician practices and 96% of hospitals use a certified electronic medical/health record (EMR/EHR; HHS & ONC, 2016a, 2016b). Now there is more emphasis placed on creating a better seamless and secure system that considers interoperability.

Stop and Consider #2

The federal government is very involved in ensuring effective health information technology.

Informatics

Informatics is complex, and the fact that it is changing daily makes it even more difficult to keep current with this field. Healthcare delivery has been strongly influenced by the changes in informatics, but what is informatics? "Technology is revolutionizing the way that healthcare is delivered with a steady infusion of new solutions into clinical environments. At the same time, outside of healthcare, both clinicians and consumers are learning to incorporate technological solutions into their daily lives with tools like high-speed data networks, smart phones, handheld devices, and various forms of patient engagement in social media exchanges. Bringing these types of technologies into the healthcare marketplace will transform the time and place for how care is provided. Having individuals who understand the unique complexities of healthcare practices along with how to best develop technological tools that positively affect safe patient care is essential. Nurses integrating informatics solutions into clinical encounters are critical for the transition to an automated healthcare environment that promotes the continuum of care across time and place, in addition to wellness and health maintenance activities" (HIMSS, 2011).

Some nurses may hold health informatics positions, as discussed later in this chapter, but all nurses use HIT in their positions—it is not an area that only concerns a specific nursing specialty. HIT is now a critical element throughout the healthcare delivery system. "It is a foundational tool to change the healthcare industry; however, it is not an instant fix. Rather, it is one tool in the arsenal of health reform. Health IT impacts quality by providing users the unique ability and opportunity to truly capture and derive the benefits from data. This allows users to translate seemingly independent pieces of data into meaningful conclusions that, if applied and implemented correctly, can improve the health of individuals and populations; lower costs; and help tailor healthcare to individual patient needs. Health IT can be implemented and employed in such a way as to support the National Quality Strategy and help achieve the 3-part aim of better care, better health, and lower cost" (Kennedy, Murphy, & Roberts, 2013).

Description and Definitions

Informatics has opened doors to many innovative methods of communication with patients and among providers, individuals, and HCOs of all types, some of them discussed in this chapter. HIT often saves time but can also lead to information overload. With these changes comes greater risk of inappropriate access to information through hacking and other means. Informatics is also used to evaluate HCO and individual healthcare provider performance. The use of HIT has a major impact on quality improvement (Finkelman, 2018). Today, it is much easier to collect, store, and analyze large amounts of data that, in the past, were collected by hand. Insurers rely heavily on informatics as they provide insurance coverage, manage data, and analyze performance, which has a direct impact on whether care is covered for reimbursement. Informatics allows governments at all levels—local, state, national, and international—to collect and use data for policy decision making and evaluation.

Informatics has its own language and is a highly specialized area. Nurses do not have to be informatics experts, but they do need to understand the basics. Some common IT terms that most people know are *Internet* and *e-mail*. Other terms that nurses should know are highlighted here (Glassman & Rosenfeld, 2015; American Nurses Association [ANA], 2008):

- **Clinical data repository:** This is a physical or logical compendium of patient data pertaining to health; an information warehouse used to store data longitudinally, in multiple forms (text, voice, images, and so on).
- **Clinical decision support systems:** These systems are computer applications designed to facilitate human decision making. Decision support systems are typically rule based, using a knowledge base with a set of rules to analyze data and information to reach recommendations.
- **Clinical information system:** This is an information system that supports the acquisition, storage, manipulation, and distribution of clinical information throughout an HCO, with a focus on electronic communication, using HIT applied at the point of clinical care. Typical clinical information system components include **EMRs/EHRs**, clinical data repositories, decision support programs (such as application of clinical guidelines and checking drug interaction), handheld devices for collecting data and viewing reference material, imaging modalities, and

communication tools such as electronic messaging systems.

- **Coding system:** This is a set of agreed-upon symbols (frequently numeric or alphanumeric) associated with a concept representation or terms to allow exchange of meaning. Examples are the SYNTEGRITY Perioperative Nursing Data Set (PNDS) and the Clinical Care Classification System.
- **Computer literacy:** Specific knowledge and skills are required to use basic computer applications and computer technology.
- **Data:** These are discrete entities described objectively without interpretation.
- **Dashboard:** A method to provide a quick view of data using key elements of concern.
- **Data analysis software:** Computer software used to analyze data; used in health care to meet regulatory requirements, performance assessment and quality improvement, accreditation, and research.
- **Data bank:** A method used to store a large amount of information; may include several databases.
- **Database:** A collection of interrelated data organized according to a scheme to serve one or more applications with data stored so that several programs can use the data without concern for data structures or organization. An example is the National Database of Nursing Quality Indicators, discussed in other content in this text.
- **Data mining:** This is a method used to locate and identify unknown patterns and relationships within data.
- **Email list:** A list of email addresses can be used to send an email to many addresses simultaneously.
- **Encryption:** A method used to change information into a code, usually for security reasons so as to limit access to that information.
- **Information:** This represents data that have been interpreted, organized, or structured.

- **Information literacy:** This is the ability to recognize when information is needed and then to locate, evaluate, and effectively use that information.
- **Minimum data set:** This describes the minimum categories of data with uniform definitions and categories; concerns a specific aspect or dimension of the healthcare system that meets the basic needs of multiple data users.
- **Nomenclature:** This is a system of designations (terms) that is elaborated on according to preestablished rules. Examples include Systematized Nomenclature of Medicine—Clinical Terms International and International Classification for Nursing Practice.
- **Scorecard:** This is a metric method used by management to assess and track performance, typically related to the HCO's agenda (or unit, service, department); it can focus on clinical, financial, and other indicators. Another term that may be used is *report card*.
- **Security protections** (access control, data security, and data encryption): Methods used to ensure that information is not read or taken by unauthorized persons.

The role of HIT in e-measurement and quality care has become increasingly more important in recent years (Dykes & Collins, 2013). **E-measurement** is the secondary use of electronic data to populate standardized performance measures (National Quality Forum [NQF], 2017). The NQF is engaged in ensuring effective e-measures are available so that data can be used for clinical documentation and reused to measure patient outcomes that are clear and consistent. This endeavor, which is very complex, remains far from complete at this time.

A current problem in our everyday lives and in our professional lives is **information (cognitive) overload**, which is an "interpretation that people make in response to breakdowns, interruptions, interruptions of ongoing projects, or imbalances between demand and capacity" (Weick, 2009, p. 76). We are so overwhelmed with information that we may experience it as a barrier in using the information and, in some cases, it may interfere with our decision making and work that must be done. Interruptions, attention issues, and not having enough time can also influence information overload, making it a greater problem. The bottom line is this problem can lead to other problems (Sitterding, 2015). We are attached to our devices personally and now more and more in our work in health care. Managing the use of devices and information is a critical requirement for success. Information and accessibility to information has a positive impact on quality care; however, we are learning that this can also have a negative impact, which may prevent us from reaching outcomes—we have too much information or we cannot manage the information effectively.

Nursing Standards: Scope and Standards of Nursing Informatics

NI is a specialty that integrates nursing science, computer science, and information science to manage and communicate data, information, knowledge, and wisdom in nursing practice. NI supports consumers, patients, nurses, and other providers in their decision making in all roles and settings. This support is accomplished through the use of information structures, information processes, and HIT. The goal of NI is to "improve the health of populations, communities, families, and individuals by optimizing information management and communication" (ANA, 2008, p. 1).

Undergraduate nursing programs may include HIT in the curriculum, sometimes as a course on informatics, but not all programs include this content. This omission from nursing education programs is a problem because of the greater emphasis on informatics as a healthcare professions core competency. Some schools of nursing offer master's degrees in NI.

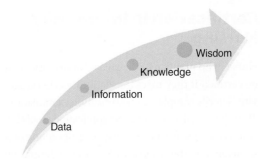

Figure 13-4 From Data to Wisdom

Data alone are not useful—understanding the data and then using this **knowledge** is what is important. This view is important to include in discussions with students. The steps in moving from data to **wisdom** can be described as data naming, collecting, and organizing, following this pattern: (1) information—organizing and interpreting; (2) knowledge—interpreting, integrating, and understanding; and (3) wisdom—understanding, applying, and applying with compassion. **Figure 13-4** illustrates this process. Nelson and Joos define *wisdom* as "the appropriate use of knowledge to manage and solve human problems. It is knowing when and how to apply knowledge to deal with complex problems or specific human needs" (1989, p. 6). Knowledge and wisdom are related: "While knowledge focuses on what is known, wisdom focuses on the appropriate application of that knowledge. For example, a knowledge base may include several options for managing an anxious family, while wisdom would help decide which option is most appropriate for a specific family" (ANA, 2008, p. 5). Data are important to the delivery of nursing care, but without effective analysis, it is not useful to us. In hospitals, data can be used to evaluate outcomes, identify problems for a specific group of patients, and assist in making plans for change to improve care. In the community, aggregated data are often collected to better understand the health issues in a population or community and to formulate a plan of action.

Certification in Informatics Nursing

Nurses who practice in the area of informatics can be certified if they meet the eligibility criteria and satisfactorily complete the certification examination. The following list identifies the application eligibility criteria required for the informatics certification exam sponsored by the American Nurses Credentialing Center (ANCC). The nurse must (ANCC, 2016):

- Hold a current, active registered nurse license in a state or territory of the United States or the professional, legally recognized equivalent in another country.
- Have practiced the equivalent of 2 years full-time as a registered nurse.
- Hold a bachelor's or higher degree in nursing or a baccalaureate degree in relevant field.
- Have completed 30 hours of continuing education in informatics within the last 3 years
- Meet one of the following practice hour requirements:
    a. The nurse must have practiced a minimum of 2,000 hours in informatics nursing within the last 3 years.
    b. The nurse must have practiced a minimum of 1,000 hours in informatics nursing in the last 3 years and must have completed a minimum of 12 semester hours of academic credit in informatics courses that are a part of a graduate-level informatics nursing program.
    c. The nurse must have completed a graduate program in NI containing a minimum of 200 hours of faculty-supervised practicum in informatics.*

These are not simple eligibility criteria; they take time to meet. They also provide a good overview of the need for expertise in this area.

The informatics nurse is involved in activities that focus on the methods and technologies of information handling in nursing, such as the development, support, and evaluation of applications, tools, processes, and structures that help nurses to manage data in direct care of patients as well as in nursing education and research. Informatics nurses can be involved in a variety of information systems, including theory formulation, design, development, marketing, selection, testing, implementation, training, maintenance, and evaluation. They may hold positions in HCOs, such as in clinical practice, management, or education; serve as an HIT consultant; and hold positions that support research. It is clear that a nurse who wants to function in this specialty area must have excellent computer skills, understand practice needs for information, and know how best to apply HIT to nursing practice. The nurse must also be able to work collaboratively in interprofessional teams and demonstrate leadership. By advocating for the needs of the practicing nurse, the informatics nurse represents all nurses in practice—clinical, education, and research—as applies to the specific situation.

Informatics: Impact on Care

Effective use of informatics can lead to safe, quality care. Application of informatics, however, does not guarantee perfection. It is commonly thought that work processes will be better if using IT; however, potential glitches need to be considered so that problems will be prevented. Examples include the following: clear expectations for staff HIT use and outcomes, ease of use, staff time for HIT training, quality of HIT training, staff time required to use HIT, monitoring of errors and methods used to address problems, accessibility to HIT such as access to a computer or device that supports the task, acceptance of HIT by staff, methods used to introduce HIT changes and communication of these changes, HIT tech support, and so on. Introducing and maintaining HIT requires careful planning with input from staff that will use HIT.

Nurses need to assume an active role in the development of HIT for patient care and not wait to be asked to participate. When an HCO is choosing

---

*© American Nurses Credentialing Center (ANCC) 2016. Reprinted with permission.

an EMR system, nurses need to be involved to ensure that the system meets nursing care documentation requirements and that relevant data can be collected to assist nurses in providing and improving care. Nurses may serve in key HIT roles to guide development and implementation. Nurses may also serve as resources in identifying needs and testing systems to ensure that the systems are nurse–user friendly. Many nurses who provide feedback about systems do not have special HIT training; they review the system to determine if it is user friendly for nurses who have limited informatics knowledge and help to determine if the system meets documentation needs and standards. All nurses need to be skilled in managing and communicating information, but most nurses are primarily concerned with the content of that information and getting it when they need it.

In today's dynamic healthcare environment, coordination of care is very important. One of the barriers to seamless coordination is the lack of interoperable computerized records with hospitals and also office-based physicians (Bodenheimer, 2008). Interoperability is receiving more attention on the national level, as discussed earlier in this chapter. A problem that is not yet fully solved is the need to share information from one system to another, which is a limitation that needs to be resolved for better coordination of care. For example, it should be possible to share current information among healthcare providers in private practice, clinics, and hospitals when it is needed. All of this requires greater use of standardized definitions related to data and measurement to ensure objectivity and reliability of data, allow for comparisons, consistently track data over time, and increase opportunity to provide/observe empirical evidence of outcomes (Glassman & Rosenfeld, 2015).

Innovative methods to improve coordination that focus on informatics have been developed. One method is to use electronic referral (e-referral.) This approach allows a healthcare provider to send an email to another provider, such as a specialist, with information about the patient and ask for consultation. In many situations, such communication eliminates the need to see the patient. The specialist reviews information such as lab reports, surgical reports, and so on, and the specialist can share opinion and treatment recommendations with the other healthcare provider. It is critical that reimbursement be provided for this type of service, or it will not be used. Health Insurance Portability and Accountability Act of 1996 (HIPAA) requirements must also be considered, with all parties working together to ensure patient privacy. Timely information flow from the hospital to post-hospital care should improve patient coordination. Not having this is a major drawback; even though the technology to improve it is available, it is not freely used.

Implications for Nursing Education and Nursing Research

Informatics is important not only for practice, but also for nursing education and nursing research. Today, there is greater use of IT in nursing education than was the case in the past. The increased use of online courses throughout the nursing curriculum, at both the undergraduate and graduate levels, has revolutionized nursing education. This has led to the need for faculty to consider use of more interactive learning methods. Moreover, as students use more technology in their personal lives, they expect correspondingly greater use of IT in education. Such tools as tablets and smartphones and Internet tools and apps such as Facebook, Instagram, and Twitter provide instant information and can be very interactive. These methods can also be used to increase student–faculty communication and have the potential to provide different means of student–faculty supervision in the clinical area. This is particularly true in areas such as public/community health when students visit multiple sites and faculty move from site to site to spend time with students. Informatics also affects simulation experiences for students, allowing faculty to create complex learning scenarios that use the computer and computerized equipment and, in many cases, provide opportunity for students to use an EMR system in a simulated environment.

Nursing research uses informatics in data collection and analysis; it saves time and improves the quality of data collection and analysis. Researchers have greater access to tools that can make their work easier and organize and save data for later use. It is then easier to analyze the data to determine research results. Nurse researchers and their staff do some of this work, and specialists such as statisticians may assist in using technology.

Stop and Consider #3

Health informatics is now integrated in practice, management, education, and research.

Documentation

Over time, clinical documentation has increased in terms of its relevance to nurses and to other healthcare professionals, thus increasing its impact on patient care and patient outcomes. Today it is expected that documentation should be accurate and accessible to those who need and should have access given confidentiality and privacy law requirements, as has been the case for a long time. Many different staff document in the medical record. Documentation must describe nursing practice, which should be evidence based. Both nurse managers and nurses involved in direct care are accountable for ensuring that documentation meets the expected standards. Nurse educators in academic and HCO settings are also involved in ensuring effective documentation. Documentation meets many needs, such as clear communication for the team and others who need the information to provide care and meet legal and ethical, accreditation, documentation, and reimbursement and budget requirements. We now place greater emphasis on documentation as a source for quality improvement and research data.

The format and content of nursing documentation have also changed. It is a professional responsibility to document planning, actual care provided, and outcomes. Care coordination and continuity are supported by documentation. With many different staff caring for patients around the clock and use of interprofessional teams, it is critical that a clear communication mechanism exists, and the key mechanism is documentation. Verbal communication is important, but a written document must be available. Staff can refer to such documentation when other care providers are not available. Through documentation, outcomes and evaluation of patient care are made clear.

The medical record is a legal document, and as such, rules must be followed when creating and amending it. Once documentation has been created, changes to it must be accompanied by a note indicating who made the change(s) and when (date and time), following HCO policy and procedure. Only certain staff may document; they must note the date and time on the documentation and include their name and credentials. If there are questions about care or a legal action, such as a malpractice suit, the medical record is the most important source of evidence. Consequently, medical records must be saved. A nurse can say that he or she provided certain care, but if it is not documented, then it is as if that care did not occur.

The following provides a list of the advantages of using EMRs (U.S. Department of Health and Human Services [HHS] & HealthIT.gov, 2015):

- Quick access to patient information from multiple locations to assist in providing coordinated, efficient care
- Decision support, clinical alerts, reminders, and medical information
- Performance-improving tools, real-time quality reporting
- Legible, complete documentation that facilitates accurate coding and billing
- Interfaces with labs and other sources of information

- Safer, more reliable prescribing
- Reduction in errors when multiple caregivers are involved in the care—care coordination
- Improvement of care transitions (handoffs) between settings
- Up-to-date information for emergency care—care coordination

The summary of the following guidelines should also be considered in documentation (Iyer & Camp, 1999):

- Do not include opinion, but only objective information in documentation. The nurse does not make subjective comments (for example, comments about the patient being uncooperative, lazy, or impolite). Nurses document only what they have done and objective data. A nurse does not document another staff member's actions. Supervision of care, however, can be documented.
- Write neatly and legibly. Many HCOs now use computerized documentation, although not all HCOs have moved to an EMR system. If a computerized system is used, typos (typographical errors) may be a problem. Other issues may arise in electronic systems that use a checklist for a particular section of the EMR but do not allow for narrative notes. Nurses and others may be frustrated when they cannot add a narrative note.
- Use of copy and paste feature in an EMR/EHR increases risk of errors, particularly perpetuating an error (Yadav et al., 2016).
- Use correct spelling, grammar, and medical terminology.
- Use authorized abbreviations. Using unapproved abbreviations increases the risk of errors.
- Use graphic records to record specified patient data, such as vital signs and medication administration.
- Record the patient's name on every page (for hard-copy medical records); this should be part of the EMR.
- Follow HCO policies and procedures about verbal and telephone orders.

- Transcribe orders carefully; double-check and ask questions if an order is not clear. In computerized systems, orders do not need to be transcribed; however, this does not mean that there is no risk of an error. All orders need careful review, and if they are not clear, they may require follow-up.
- Document omitted care.
- Document medications and outcomes.
- Document patient noncompliance/nonadherence and the reason(s) for it.
- Document allergies, and use this information to prevent errors and complications.
- Document sites of injections and other procedures.
- Record all required information about intravenous therapy and blood administration.
- Report abnormal laboratory results.
- Document as soon as possible after care is delivered. If documentation is done late, note this in the record. The nurse should not leave blank areas to come back to for later documentation.
- When quoting, use quotation marks and note the person who made the statement.
- When documentation is corrected because of a mistake, follow the HCO policies regarding corrections as per a hard-copy record or electronic record. Medical records are never rewritten or destroyed by staff.
- Document patient status change.
- When contacting the physician, document the time, date, name of physician, reason for the call, content, physician response, and steps taken after the call. This note should not include subjective analysis of the response such as the physician's attitude.

The Joint Commission does not provide details as to what must be in a medical record (the term used by The Joint Commission for this document is *record of care/treatment and services*), but it does provide some guidelines that are required for accreditation as follows with additional comments (Clark, 2011; Joint Commission, 2011, 2016):

- The minimum content that should be included is the patient's name, address, date of birth, name of any legally authorized representative, assessment, diagnosis, clinician notes and actions, signatures and countersignatures as required, dates, details of procedures performed, laboratory reports, medications administered, and treatment plans. Other data may be included.
- The record should be clear and understandable.
- The record provides a system of communication and in doing so is a source of data for quality improvement monitoring.
- Storage of documents must be secure and reasonable. For example, security requirements need to identify who has access to records and prevent casual viewing by non-staff. All Medicare storage rules must be followed. Today, with increased risk of problems with computer systems or hacking, HCOs need a policies and procedures to assist staff when there may be problems with the EMR and access.
- HIPAA requirements must be followed—ensuring patient privacy and confidentiality. HCOs should have policies and procedures that support HIPAA and staff must adhere to them.
- Use acceptable abbreviations identified by the HCO.

These guidelines apply to hospital medical records. The content is somewhat different for medical records in other types of settings, such as ambulatory care, long-term care, and home care, although some information and guidelines are the same. It is important for all HCOs to have clear documentation policies and procedures and ensure that staff are aware of them and follow them. When changes occur, staff must be informed so that the new requirements will be met.

Stop and Consider #4

Documentation is a critical communication method for the care team.

Meaningful Use

Meaningful use focuses on use of certified EHR technology for the following purposes (HHS & HealthIT.gov, 2014):

- Improve quality, safety, efficiency, and reduce health disparities.
- Engage patients and family.
- Improve care coordination, and population and public health.
- Maintain privacy and security of patient health information.

The American Recovery and Reinvestment Act of 2009 specifies the following three components of *meaningful use* (HHS & CMS, 2014):

- Use of certified EHR in a meaningful manner (for example, e-prescribing)
- Use of certified EHR technology for electronic exchange of health information to improve quality of health care
- Use of certified EHR technology to submit clinical quality measures and other such measures selected by the Secretary of HHS

Meaningful use identifies specific objectives that eligible professionals and hospitals must achieve to qualify for Centers for Medicare and Medicaid Services (CMS) reimbursement. Given that most hospitals receive CMS reimbursement, most hospitals have a strong incentive to follow these requirements. Nurses are also required to consider meaningful use, particularly if they are in leadership positions where decisions about HIT are made. Ultimately, it is hoped that meaningful use compliance will result in the following benefits:

- Better clinical outcomes
- Improved population health outcomes

- Increased transparency and efficiency
- Empowered individuals
- More robust research data on health systems

All of the meaningful use purposes are in line with the *Quality Chasm* reports on quality and are associated with continuous quality improvement.

Stop and Consider #5
Meaningful use relates to nursing practice.

Standardized Terminology

Health care has expanded in multiple directions and includes the services of many different healthcare providers. Ensuring effective communication among these myriad providers is not always easy. Certainly, there are issues regarding willingness to communicate, lack of time to communicate, and so on, but a critical problem is the lack of a common professional language/terminology. For those entering healthcare profession, such as nursing students, this is probably a surprising comment. Each healthcare professional area has its own terminology. There are some common medical terms, but each profession has specific terminology that is often not known or understood by other healthcare professionals. "Creating a common language is no small task. Developing and adhering to distinct profession-specific terms may be a manifestation of professionals' desire to preserve identity, status or control" (IOM, 2003, p. 123). This problem affects all the core competencies and the ability to develop educational experiences that meet the competencies across healthcare professions, such as nursing, medicine, pharmacy, and allied health. The issue of shared terminology is even more important in HIT because informatics is dependent on language, requiring a shared terminology. We now recognize its effect on practice and interprofessional teams. A **standardized terminology** is a collection of terms with definitions for use in information systems, databases. This enables comparisons to be made because the same term is used to denote the same condition, and it is necessary for effective documentation in EMRs/EHRs.

It is recognized that we need a common language across health professions supporting the five core healthcare professions competencies. Accomplishing this requires that healthcare professionals are willing to actively work together to achieve this goal. The HHS has been tasked with meeting this goal, though it is a difficult goal to reach—getting different healthcare professionals to accept a universal terminology. This will require compromises and has yet to be fully accomplished. The ANA notes that: "The data element sets and terminologies are foundational to standardization of nursing documentation and verbal communication that will lead to a reduction in errors and an increase in the quality and continuity of care. It is through standardization of nurse documentation and communication of a patient's care that the many nurses caring for a patient develop a shared understanding of that care" (2006). These statements are an example of why developing and accepting a universal language is difficult but necessary, but they also illustrate how it is easy to approach this from silos—focused on individual healthcare professions. Such statements are nursing focused, but all healthcare professions need to address this issue using interprofessional collaboration.

Determining how best to move from a specific profession approach to a collaborative approach to solve this problem is the challenge. The Library of Medicine (NLM), serving as the coordinating body for clinical terminology standards within HHS, offers products and services for HCOs and healthcare professionals that support interoperability and the unambiguous exchange of health data (National Institutes of Health [NIH] & U.S. National Library of Medicine [NLM], 2016a). The website for NLM provides a current overview of activities focused on standardized terminologies.

Systems and
Terminologies

Informatics is not as simple as email and the Internet. Informatics in general and HIT include many database systems, terms, and other factors that make this a complex area. The following provides examples illustrating the complexity of HIT:

Systematic Collection of Nursing Care Data or Data Element Sets

- *Nursing Minimum Data Set:* This data set describes patient problems across healthcare settings, different populations, geographic areas, and time. It provides clinical data to assist in identifying nursing diagnoses, nursing interventions, and nursing-sensitive patient outcomes. In addition, the Nursing Minimum Data Set is useful in assessing resources used in the provision of nursing care. The goal is to link data between HCOs and providers. Data can also be used for research and healthcare policy.
- *Nursing Management Minimum Data Set:* This data set focuses on nursing administrative data elements in all types of settings.

Interface Terminologies

- *Clinical Care Classification:* The clinical classifications software for the *International classification of diseases*, 10th revision, Clinical Modification (ICD-10-CM), is a diagnosis and procedure categorization scheme that can be used in many types of projects to analyze data on diagnoses and procedures. The software is based on ICD-10-CM, a uniform and standardized coding system. ICD-10-CM includes more than 13,600

diagnosis codes and 3,700 procedure codes (U.S. Department of Health and Human Services, Centers for Disease Control and Prevention, & National Institute for Occupational Safety and Health, 2016).

- *Nursing Intervention Classification and Nursing Outcome Classification:* The North American Nursing Diagnosis Association (NANDA) focuses on nursing diagnoses, Nursing Intervention Classification (NIC) on nursing interventions, and Nursing Outcome Classification (NOC) on nursing outcomes (NANDA, 2017; University of Iowa, Center for Nursing Classification and Effectiveness, 2017).
- *Omaha System:* The Omaha System is a comprehensive, standardized taxonomy designed to improve practice, documentation, and information management. It includes three components: the problem classification scheme, the intervention scheme, and the problem rating scale for outcomes. When the three components are used together, the Omaha System offers a way to link clinical data to demographic, financial, administrative, and staffing data (Omaha System, 2011). The Omaha System is used in home health care, community health, and public health services.
- *PNDS:* The PNDS is a standardized nursing vocabulary that addresses the perioperative patient experience from preadmission until discharge, including nursing diagnoses, interventions, and outcomes. This set was developed by a specialty organization, the Association of periOperative Registered Nurses (2017) and recognized by the ANA as a data set useful for perioperative nursing practice. This standardized system is now called SYNTEGRITY PNDS. It is an IT tool that can be personalized by HCOs to meet individual organization needs. The framework supports electronic documentation, patient quality and EBP, a common language/

terminology, and a method to collect and compare data. It connects nursing diagnoses, care implementation, and assessment to measure outcomes.

Examples of Multiprofessional Terminologies

- *Logical Observation Identifiers Names and Codes:* This clinical terminology classification is used for laboratory test orders and results. It is a system designated for use in U.S. federal government systems for the electronic exchange of clinical health information (NIH & NLM, 2008). This system can be used to collect data about assessments and outcomes for nursing and other healthcare services.
- *Current Procedural Terminology:* This code is used for reimbursement (American Medical Association, 2016).
- *Systematized Nomenclature of Medicine— Clinical Terms:* This comprehensive clinical terminology is one of several standards approved for use in U.S. federal government systems for the electronic exchange of clinical health information (NIH & NLM, 2016b). The system is applicable to nursing and other healthcare services and focuses on diagnoses, interventions, and outcomes.

With the increased use of technology for documentation, nursing has been more concerned about two issues (Schwiran & Thede, 2011):

- How to differentiate nursing's contributions to patient care from those of medicine
- How to incorporate descriptions of nursing care into the health record in a manner that is commensurate with its importance to patients' welfare

This requires systems that can meet these needs; therefore, nurses need to engage in HIT so that nursing can be better represented in decisions about EMRs.

In a study conducted by Schwiran and Thede (2011), the researchers examined nurses' knowledge of and experience with standardized nursing technologies. The results indicate that most nurses do not have much knowledge of or experience with standardized nursing technologies, such as the NIC, NOC, and NANDA. They may have used these technologies in their nursing education, but not in practice after graduation. Given the increasing use of informatics in healthcare settings, such a lack of knowledge and experience may hamper nurses' ability to participate actively in HIT development and evaluation and better ensure that nursing practice is supported.

Stop and Consider #7

Nursing is more involved in approaches to develop and improve health information technology.

Informatics: Types
and Methods

For informatics to be effective, three concerns must be addressed. First, the HCO must have effective and easily accessible HIT support services. Staff must be able to pick up the telephone and get this support. Failure of the information system has major implications for patient care and increases staff stress, so backup systems are critical. The second critical concern is staff training. This requires resources: financial resources, trainers, and time. Time is needed for staff to attend training, and there must be recognition that it takes time for staff to learn how to use a system—and during this time, there is an impact on care and work processes. Incorporation of informatics with any of the methods described next (and others that are not included here) requires a major change in care delivery. Change is stressful for staff, and it needs to be planned, representing the third concern. Trying to implement too many changes at one time may increase staff stress, affect the success of using more informatics in the future, decrease staff motivation to participate, and increase the risk of errors that might affect patient outcomes. Change is discussed in several chapters in this text.

It is not difficult to find nurses who will complain about a hospital's attempt to increase the use of informatics, particularly if it has been badly planned. Often, in these complaints, staff members note that the system selected was not effective and they had no part in the decision and implementation process. Equipment and **software** is very costly, and decisions regarding them are critical—getting an ineffective system or bad fit for what is needed only increases costs and management and staff stress. Time must be taken to evaluate equipment and software to make sure they meet the needs and demands of the organization and users such as nurses. Examples of current activities in this area are automated dispensing of medications and bar coding; computerized monitoring of adverse events; the use of EMRs/EHRs, provider order-entry systems, clinical decision support systems, use of devices such as tablets and smartphones, computer-based and reminder systems; access to patient records at the point of care; prescribing via the Internet; using nurse call systems, voice mail, and the telephone for advice and other services; use of Internet or virtual appointments; and online support groups for patients and families. These methods are discussed in this section.

It is important to note that there is now a serious risk with the use of electronic methods for documentation and communication today. Hacking has become more common with IT in general, and there have been incidents of hacking health records. Why would this be done? One reason is health records often include personal identification information that might be used for illegal purposes, such as to obtain addresses, telephone, email addresses, credit card information, and social security numbers (McCain, 2014; Pagliery, 2014; Peterson, 2015). Another experience that some HCOs have had is hacking data or control of data and then the hacker(s) demand a ransom for the HCO to regain access to the system (Conn, 2014). This can happen to small or large HCOs. All of this emphasizes that the data we have are important—valuable—not only to us and to our patients, but also to others who may not have the same goals. We must be careful and use appropriate passwords and procedures to protect data. We see an increasing use of emails as a method to communicate with patients—sharing important personal information. Is this wise? Patients are often asked and encouraged to provide their email—but it is their choice to make, and in all cases, it should be their decision. We need to take care with what we put in emails or what we ask patients to send in an email, for example, social security numbers should never be sent in an email. When we keep data for healthcare, we have ethical and legal responsibilities to ensure the information is accurate and safe.

Automated Dispensing of Medications and Bar Coding

Pharmacies in all types of HCOs are using or moving toward expanding use of automatic medication dispensing systems with bar coding. These systems select the medication based on the order and prepare it in single doses for the patient. The bar code is on the packaged dose. This code can then be compared with the bar code on the patient's identification band using a handheld device. This type of system can decrease errors, and it supports all five rights of medication administration, as discussed in other content in this text. Bar coding can also be used to collect data about prescribed and administered drugs. Data then may be used for monitoring quality improvement and for research. Bar coding systems are expensive to install and maintain, but they can make a difference in reducing errors and can reduce time required for all medication administration steps.

Computerized Monitoring of Adverse Events

Computerized systems that monitor adverse events assist in identifying and monitoring adverse events. Developing and using a database of these events facilitates analysis of data and the development of interventions to decrease adverse events. A major problem with data collection, such as for adverse events, is not using structured collection—overdoing collection and ending up with data that are not needed or not in a format that could be used. Careful planning is required to identify information or data needed and how it will be accessed and used to prevent this from occurring.

Electronic Medical/Health Records

EMRs/EHRs are slowly replacing the written medical record for an individual patient while the patient receives care within a specific healthcare system. A second type of electronic documentation system is the **personal health record (PHR)**. The PHR is less common than the EMR, but the goal is for it to become standard in the future. The PHR is a computer-based health record for which data are collected over the long term—for a lifetime. With the patient's permission, the healthcare provider can access this record easily to obtain information. To reach this point, there must be agreement on a minimum data set—uniform definitions of data (that is, standardized language/terminology) that would enable all healthcare providers to understand and use the information. There is still much to be done to make this a reality in every HCO, including clinics and medical offices, but the technology is already available.

The EMR/EHR is a record of the patient's history and assessment, orders, laboratory results, description of medical tests and procedures, and documentation of care provided and outcomes. Current requirements for electronic records referred to as the Common Clinical Data Set guides EMR content. The following are the minimum requirements identified by the HHS (HHS & ONC, 2015a):

- Patient name
- Sex
- Date of birth
- Race
- Ethnicity
- Preferred language
- Smoking status
- Problems
- Medications
- Medication allergies
- Vital signs
- Care plan field(s), including goals and instructions
- Procedures
- Care team members
- Immunizations
- Unique device identifier(s) for the patient's implantable device(s)
- Notes/narrative

Care plans are included. It should be easy to input, search, and review information, and it should be possible to print reports. Electronic data can be stored over the long term, which is harder to do with written records. Written records require significant storage space, and they may not be easy to find once archived. In addition, written records can be less readable over time. The hard-copy record is not always easy to access when it is needed in a hospital unit. If one person is using the record, others cannot use it. With the EMR, this is not a problem as long as staff can access the computerized record system. EMR systems do require security and backup systems to ensure that data are not lost in the event of a power outage, natural disaster, or other event that may make access difficult.

Electronic documentation has many advantages such as timeliness of care. Staff can document as care is provided or soon after, providing a system for all members of the team to view the care process when needed. Documentation may take place at the unit workstation, at a hallway computer station, at the bedside in the hospital, or in an examining room in a clinic. Bedside systems are better because they are easy to access when the nurse or other healthcare professional needs information, and point-of-care documentation is enhanced. This all improves documentation and communication. Other advantages are legibility; greater access to records for multiple users; increase in efficiency and effectiveness in the work environment; less opportunity to change records inappropriately; inclusion of safety elements, such as alerts for allergies or incompatible drug orders, and reminders to do certain tasks or add certain information to the record; ability to print records when need; and more accurate and accessible data for reimbursement, budget, and quality improvement.

It is important to recognize that when HCOs change to electronic documentation or make changes in a current electronic system, this is a time of great disruption in clinical practice and workflow processes, typically with negative staff responses to the change process and/or the change itself (Ford, Silvera, Kazley, Diana, & Huerta, 2016). A study conducted by Barnett, Mehrotra, Jena, and Newhouse (2016) also refer to the disruption in work processes during transition to electronic records, particularly noting the negative impact on patient outcomes. In this study of 17 hospitals transitioning to electronic methods, the hospitals demonstrated more problems with adverse patient outcomes than hospitals that were not transitioning to electronic records. All of this affects the culture of safety. HCOs and their providers must have time to adjust to the change and to recognize the benefits and, during change, be alert to prevent errors.

Clinical Provider Order-Entry System

A **clinical provider order-entry system (CPOES)** may be included in an EMR, although it may also be a stand-alone system. The healthcare provider inputs orders into this system rather than using a hard-copy record. This is an expensive system to implement. One clear advantage of the CPOES is legibility; written orders are often very difficult to read because handwriting varies, and this may cause errors. It also takes time to transcribe written

physician/provider orders into a form in which the orders can be used. During this process, the risk of transcription errors increases. Typing orders into a computer can also lead to typos, but this is less of a problem than errors with handwritten orders. A systematic review of 34 studies on CPOES used identified key areas of the EMR and its CPOES that may be associated with CPOES errors: computer screen display, drop-down menus and auto-population, wording, default settings, nonintuitive or inflexible ordering, repeat prescriptions and automated processes, users' work processes, and clinical decision support systems (Brown et al., 2016). The studies reviewed identified examples of how an EMR and its CPOES might have weaknesses in these areas—such as incomplete medication lists that led to prescription error, misinterpretation of text, and lack of flexibility in the CPOES so the staff member uses a workaround—increasing the risk of an error. Drop-down menus need to include safeguards to prevent selection errors. Another study examined alerts of automated identification of antibiotic overdoses and adverse drug events via a CPOES (Kirkendall et al., 2016). This study highlights alert fatigue, which is discussed in this text. If providers get a number of alerts, there is increased chance they will override the alert because of too many alerts—viewing them as irritants to getting work done. Alert systems need to be carefully reviewed and revised to reduce alerts that are not critical.

Clinical decision support systems can be included with the CPOES. The Brown and colleagues systematic review concludes that development of better clinical decision support systems may reduce errors and improve workflow (2016). Combining the CPOES with the decision support system enhances the provider order-entry system and can lead to improved care and a decrease in errors as noted in the Brown study.

CPOES is not only a clinical tool to assist in providing effective care, but it also offers a source of information about quality improvement—data that may be used by the QI program. Analysis of medication order voiding provides critical information for why providers who write the orders void them or why the system voids them (Kannampallil et. al., 2017). Kannampallil and colleagues examined 6 years of CPOES data, looking at void and not void orders and reasons for the voiding. In the sample, 0.49% of the all orders were voided, with most voiding due to medication ordering errors. The use of a voiding provides the HCO with an easy method for self-reporting of near-miss medication ordering errors, and the data should be used to assess the current status within the HCO and develop strategies to reduce need for voiding orders.

Clinical Decision Support Systems

Clinical decision support systems have led to major changes in healthcare delivery. These systems provide immediate information that can influence clinical decisions. Some of the systems actually intervene when an error is about to be made. For example, when an order for a medication is put in a patient's EMR, the computerized system might indicate the patient is allergic to that medication by immediately sending an alert, stopping the order. The nurse can also get alerts for a variety of potential problems such as the patient at risk for falls or decubiti.

In the past, nurses depended on textbooks or journals that the unit or hospital library might have available to find information, and such searches were often not done effectively. Easy electronic access to current information eliminates many problems related to obtaining information when needed. This, too, can improve the quality of care. EBP relies heavily on access to EBP literature, which is most easily accessible via the Internet and databases. As is true for all electronic methods, healthcare professional critical thinking, as well as clinical reasoning and judgment, must still be applied. Errors can still be made with technology. When HIT is used, staff may go on "automatic pilot," assuming the electronic

system will catch all potential errors, which is not always the case.

More research is needed to fully understand the impact of clinical decision support systems on patient outcomes. Romano and Stafford's (2011) study indicated that there was no consistent association between such systems and the quality of care in an investigation that included 3 billion patient visits. Only one of 20 indicators—diet counseling for high-risk adults—demonstrated significantly better performance when clinical decision support systems were utilized. In contrast, earlier studies had shown that use of the clinical decision support systems improved outcomes. A critique of the 2011 study questions whether the results were influenced by the following factors: (1) Clinical decision support system rules may have been different in the systems studied; (2) the study focused on medication management, whereas earlier studies were broader; and (3) the study looked at the outcome of a single visit rather than the cumulative effect. More research is needed to understand use of this method and better determine the effectiveness of using clinical decision support systems, which is a complex research area.

Tablets and Smartphones

Tablet computers are very popular with the general public and also in the workplace. Most mobile telephones now have Internet capability, such as access to the Internet and storage of information. These phones give users quick access to information, Internet, email, and text messaging, and of course, telephone service. Such handheld devices can hold a significant amount of information, serve as a calendar, keep contact information, monitor tasks, and so on, and are an effective method for transmission of information.

Nurses who use tablets and/or smartphones carry information with them and can look up side effects of a medication or any other type of medical information necessary as they provide care. In some cases, the nurse can access EMRs to get to patient information through the tablet. Some textbooks can now be uploaded into tablets, such as pharmacology and clinical laboratory resources. This is useful information for the nurse to have available—it is accessible in seconds at the point of care. Nurses working outside a structured setting, such as in public/community health or in home care, may also find this type of system useful for support information and documentation needs (patient information, visit data, and so on); however, they must be very careful to maintain HIPAA regulations. Tablets are used in public/community health to collect data such as health assessments; data are stored locally on the tablet and then uploaded to a secure cloud server (that is, a server that is encrypted to protect personal health information) when the user is back in network/wireless range. Any time such technology is used, the data must be protected to keep information secure and confidential. It is not only the concern about security of information, but also the devices, which can be lost and should be used with security codes. HCOs should have clear policies and procedures for actions staff should take if a device is lost or a person(s) who should not have access to the information gains access to the device. If the healthcare provider is using these devices for oral communication in any location, he or she must be careful to ensure privacy.

Computer-Based Reminder Systems

Computer-based reminder systems are used to communicate with patients via email or text messages to remind them of appointments and screenings and to discuss other health issues. In the future, these methods will most likely take the place of telephone calls to remind patients of appointments. Any reminder system must also maintain HIPAA regulations. For example, the healthcare provider must ensure that only authorized parties have access to the computer and email data. More narrowly

defined, only the patient should have access to the information unless the patient wants the information shared. An example of concern about privacy is using a patient's work email or work mobile phone. Employers have the right to view employee emails and phones, and thus private health information may be shared if the employer does view employee information and devices.

Access to Patient Records at the Point of Care

Many hospitals are moving toward providing access to the patient records either in the patient's room or in the hallway via computers. In the future, more nurses will carry small laptops or tablets that allow access to the EMR when needed for work requirements. This reduces time spent returning to the workstation to get information and allows for more timely documentation—it can be completed as soon as care is provided. This reduces errors and improves quality because all care providers know when care has been provided in a timely manner. Point-of-care access decreases the chance that details may be forgotten, documented incorrectly, or not documented at all. In addition, it saves nurses time and eliminates the need to delay documentation. For example, if they do not have this type of immediate access, nurses may document at certain times during the shift such as midmorning or near the end of a shift, requiring them to find a block of time to complete documentation without interruptions. This is an approach that can lead to errors, incomplete data in the record if the nurse forgets information, and situations in which other providers need current patient information that has not yet been documented.

Internet Prescriptions

There has been rapid growth in consumer access to prescribed medications via the Internet. The medications are then mailed to the patient. The consumer must be careful and check the legitimacy of the source to prevent errors.

Nurse Call Systems

Nurse call systems are a form of informatics that is very important in communication within a healthcare system. They allow for improved and efficient communication and are a great improvement on the old method of yelling out for a staff member or a unit speaker system calling for staff. Many types of nurse call systems exist, such as pagers, light signals, buzzers, methods that allow patients to talk directly to nurses through an easily accessible direct audio system, smartphones, miniature label microphones, and locator badges. The goal is to get a message to the right person as soon as possible while maintaining privacy and confidentiality. Doing so can improve care, improve patient satisfaction, reduce errors, and make staff more efficient, thus preventing the unnecessary work of trying to obtain and share information.

Voice Mail and Texting

Computer-based messaging systems are found in all healthcare settings today so that staff and others can leave and receive voice and text messages; for example, staff and patients can use these systems, often reducing the need for callbacks. Complicated systems may annoy consumers, however, and there is an impersonal quality to this form of communication, though it is part of everyday life today. One has to be very careful about leaving voice mails and even text messages. Clearly, others may listen to or view messages, and this may lead to a HIPAA violation.

Telephone for Advice and Other Services

Mostly, insurers use patient advice systems, although some HCOs and providers provide these services as well. In such systems, staff determine the caller's problem or questions and provide advice. Typically,

insurers develop standard protocols or clinical pathways that the nurses use to respond to common questions, but nurses must still use professional judgment when providing advice. This type of service should not become "cookbook" care in which there is no consideration of assessment and individual patient needs. Assessment is the key to successful telephone nursing because it enables providers to identify the caller's problems and interventions required that may or may not be found in the guidelines. Some physician offices have telephone advice services that are manned by a physician in the practice or by a nurse. Pediatric practices are the most common type of practice using this system. Patient advice systems via telephone require clear documentation policies and guidelines that include content related to who called, when, and for what reason; the required assessment data; problem(s); and recommended interventions—as well as any follow-up taken, such as a return call by the service to check on the patient. Telephone advice systems are typically used to answer questions, remind patients of appointments or follow-up needs, and check in on how a patient is doing.

Many hospitals now use the telephone to begin the admission process for patients with scheduled admissions, procedures, and testing. Patients are called before the scheduled date, asked questions related to required information, and told what to expect and any required preparation. Pretesting may also be scheduled prior to hospital admission. This saves the hospital time, is more cost-effective, and may be more convenient for the patient. This method can also identify problems that may affect patient care so that they can be addressed early on.

Internet or Virtual Appointments

The Internet may be used as a means for increasing accessibility to physicians, advanced practice registered nurses, or other healthcare professionals or making appointments. The Internet is used today to obtain advice from health professionals. Portable family histories can be maintained in this fashion and passed on to a new primary care provider. Patients and families who have limited resources—financial, transportation, or insurance—can more easily receive medical advice in this format if they have Internet access. It also keeps some patients from missing work or taking a child or other family member to an appointment. Some virtual methods allow the patient and the healthcare provider to see each other, which may provide more effective communication between the patient and provider. Many of these sites link to cellular devices to send an alert of high importance to whoever is on call for virtual hours. These types of services have increased, providing quick connection with health professionals to get answers to questions, provide patient monitoring data, and/or make decisions about next steps such as an appointment or to go in for emergency services. Mental health services may also be provided in this format.

Online Support Groups for Patients and Families

Online support groups can focus on any problem or disease. Patients and their families may use chat rooms, email, and websites for information sharing. Consumers gain information, education about their health and health needs, and support from others with similar problems. A healthcare provider may or may not be involved. Privacy issues must be discussed with participants, along with the risk of lack of privacy. Blogging has also become very popular and can be done by anyone with some basic technology information. This can make information from consumers more available to other consumers; however, as is true with any information available on the Internet, the accuracy of that information is important. Blogging can lend support and let consumers know they are not alone with their problems.

Many of these methods use the Internet. It can be an excellent source for all types of information,

including health and medical information. When the Internet is used as a source of health information, it is important to evaluate the websites because they are not all of the same quality. A nurse needs to consider the following factors when evaluating a website:

- *The source or sponsor of the website:* The government, academic institutions, healthcare professional organizations, and HCOs sponsor the most reliable websites.
- *Current status of the information:* When was it posted or revised?
- *Accessibility of the information on the site:* Can one find what one needs?
- *References provided for content when appropriate:* Sources should be cited, and data should be current.

As is true with all methods such as the ones discussed in this section, patient confidentiality must be maintained. Notably, the risk of confidentiality problems increases with use of technology. There are many ways that privacy can be violated, such as viewing data, overhearing conversations, and obtaining actual documents. It is the responsibility of healthcare providers, HCOs, insurers, and consumers (patients, families) to consider privacy a critical issue whenever technology is used and to ensure as much as possible that information is safe—available only to those who need the information and for whom the patient wants the information shared.

Stop and Consider #8

During a single shift, a nurse will interact and use multiple types and methods of informatics.

The Future of Health
Informatics and Medical Technology

The future will continue to bring about expansion in the use of technology, informatics, and medical devices. This expansion is already in process. Cutting-edge technology is sometimes hard to believe, and some of these changes are discussed below.

Nanotechnology

Nanotechnology—microscopic technology on the order of one billionth of a meter—will likely affect the diagnosis and treatment of many diseases and conditions (Gordon, Lutz, Boninger, & Cooper, 2007). Some of the pending technologies are highlighted here:

- Sensing patients' internal drug levels with miniature medical diagnostic tools that circulate in the bloodstreams
- Chemotherapy delivered directly to a tumor site, reducing systemic side effects
- New monitoring devices for the home: a talking pill bottle that lets patients push a button to hear prescription information, bathroom counters that announce whether it is safe to mix two medications, a shower with built-in scales to calculate body mass index, measuring devices in the bathroom to track urine frequency and output and upload these data to a system or care manager, noninvasive blood glucose monitors to eliminate sticks, and sensors to compute blood sugar levels using a multi-wavelength reflective dispersion photometer

Wearable Computing

A computer can be worn, much as eyeglasses or clothing is worn, and interactions with the user are based on the context of the situation (ANA, 2008). Wearable fitness tools are now popular. With heads-up displays, embedded sensors in fabrics, unobtrusive input devices, personal wireless local area networks, and a host of other context sensing and communication tools, wearable computers can act as intelligent assistants or data collection and analysis devices. Many of these devices are available now using smart fabrics. Such wearable

computer and remote monitoring systems may depend on the user's activity so that the technology becomes transparent. Sensors and devices can gather data during the patient's daily routine, providing healthcare providers or researchers with periodic or continuous data on the person's health while he or she is at work, at school, exercising, or sleeping, rather than the current snapshot captured during a typical hospital or clinic visit. A few applications for wearable computing devices include sudden infant death syndrome monitoring for infants, ambulatory cardiac and respiratory monitoring, monitoring of ventilation during exercise, monitoring the activity level of post-stroke patients, monitoring patterns of breathing in asthma, assessment of stress in individuals, arrhythmia detection and control of selected cardiac conditions, and daily activity monitors (Ootex Specialty Narrow Fabrics, 2017).

Telehealth and Remote Telemetry Monitoring

Remote telemetry monitoring technology informs staff when a patient's condition has changed. The patient is placed on a monitor, and signals are sent to staff through a page system, which today may not even be within an HCO but, rather, an external alert to a healthcare provider. Staff may be informed, for example, of the patient's identity, heart rate, and readout of rhythm without being right next to the patient; status of labor contractions, and other monitoring needs.

Telehealth, or telemedicine, is the use of telecommunications equipment and communication networks for transferring healthcare information between participants at different locations, applying telecommunication and computer technologies to the broad spectrum of public health and medicine. This technology offers opportunities to provide care when face-to-face interaction is impossible (such as in home care, school-based care, and rural areas) and can be used in a variety of settings and situations as long as the equipment is available.

Two-way interactive video is the most effective telehealth method. **Telenursing** refers to the use of telecommunications technology used to provide nursing care. This may be done with audio and/or visual—it is a virtual method of care.

Issues that arise with telehealth include the cost of equipment and its use; training for staff and for patients if they need to actively use the equipment; limited or no insurance coverage for telehealth services; the need for clear policies, procedures, and protocols; privacy and confidentiality of information; and regulatory issues (for example, a nurse who is located and licensed in one state providing telenursing for a patient in another state where the nurse is not licensed).

A systematic review of 58 studies on telehealth concluded that "the most consistent benefit has been reported when telehealth is used for communication and counseling or remote monitoring in chronic conditions such as cardiovascular and respiratory disease, with improvements in outcomes such as mortality, quality of life, and reductions in hospital admissions as well as for psychotherapy as part of behavioral health" (U.S. Department of Health and Human Services & Agency for Healthcare Quality and Research, 2016, pp. vi–vii). The report discusses the need for research about expanding implementation of telehealth and elimination of barriers to use areas such as consultation in maternal and child health, use for triage in urgent care, and new delivery models. Future applications will arise, and nurses need to consider how this might be used more in nursing practice. Telehealth also has implications for international health care because it provides a method for connecting expertise to patients who may need care that is not accessible in their home country—for example, during disasters.

Robotics

Robots have been used for many years to deliver supplies to patient care areas, and its use has expanded. Robotics enables remote surgeries and virtual reality surgical procedures. Hand-assist devices help patients regain strength after a stroke (Science Daily, 2016). Robots may provide a remote presence to allow physicians to virtually examine patients by manipulating remote cameras (Thomas, 2015). They are also used for microscopic, minimally invasive surgical procedures. For example, the da Vinci surgical system helps surgeons perform such procedures as mitral valve repairs, hysterectomies, and prostate surgeries (Intuitive Surgical, 2017). This type of surgery has increased, decreasing some of the past surgical risks, decreasing the need for long hospital stays, and supporting more rapid overall recovery. In the future, robots may also be used in direct patient care—for instance, to help lift obese patients.

Genetics and Genomics

The use of genomics has expanded as knowledge about genetics has become more accessible, as discussed in other content in this text. *Healthy People 2020* added a goal related to this expanding area: "improve health and prevent harm through valid and useful genomic tools in clinical and public health practices (*Healthy People 2020*, 2016). Genetic data, especially once data are integrated into EMR/EHR/PHR, are expected to advance customized patient care and medications targeted to individual responses to medications—precision medicine is recognized as a critical aspect of future health care. This is leading to more precise customization of treatment and medication based on the patient's unique DNA profile and how the patient responded to medications and other interventions in the past. This will dramatically change how patients are managed for specific diseases and conditions and will extend into the prevention of some diseases. The inherent complexity of customized patient care will demand computerized clinical decision support that reflects individual needs and health history. Predictive disease models based on patients' DNA profiles are emerging as clinicians better understand DNA mapping. These advances have implications for a new model of care and for informatics and nursing care. Nurses' participation in the development of genomic HIT solutions is important. Nurses are beginning to collaborate more with bioengineers and informatics experts to develop new products, participate in research using these products, and help to develop implementation and evaluation plans to use with these products. More than ever, patients will need to be partners in this development as part of patient-centered care.

Medical Devices

Development of medical devices has improved medical care. Some of these devices assist with diagnosis and others with treatment, rehabilitation, and ongoing health maintenance. Nurses use medical equipment everyday, some of which is associated with informatics. The HCO is responsible for ensuring that the equipment functions effectively and responding when questions are asked about its use or repair is required. Nurses also have responsibilities for reporting problems to appropriate persons in the organization. As use of medical devices has expanded, so has adverse events associated with devices. One concern is incident reporting is not yet clear on reporting of medical device concerns, resulting in underreporting of these incidents (Polisena, Gagliardi, Urbach, Clifford, & Fiander, 2015). The U.S. Food and Drug Administration (FDA) Med-Watch adverse event reporting program focuses on reporting medical device concerns, noting examples of medical devices that should be reported when adverse events occur. The following is a list of examples (Simone, Brumbaugh, & Ricketts, 2014; U.S. Department of Health and Human Services & Food and Drug Administration, 2017): electric beds such as electric shock or patient entrapment, patient lifts resulting in falls, peritoneal dialysis machines (for example, increased intraperitoneal pressure), foley catheters (for example, infections, breakage), and so on. The FDA provides updated information on medical device problems on its website.

Stop and Consider #9
The nursing profession needs to be up-to-date with changes in technology because many will affect nursing practice.

HIPAA: Ensuring
Confidentiality

The **HIPAA** has had a major impact on healthcare delivery systems and healthcare communication. Privacy and confidentiality have long been problematic issues in health care. Because HIPAA focuses on the issue of information and confidentiality, it applies to HIT. The law also requires data security and electronic transaction standards. With the growth of information sharing, it became increasingly evident that existing means of transactions and systems were not ensuring privacy and confidentiality—key elements that had long been part of the healthcare delivery system.

Privacy is the right of a person to have personal information kept private. As discussed in this text, this relates to professional ethics and also has legal implications. Privacy restrictions even apply to all family members, unless the adult patient specifically communicates that it is acceptable for family members to be given information. This cannot be assumed. HIPAA requires that only necessary information be shared among providers, including insurers. Patients may also access their medical records.

Health information cannot be openly shared by healthcare providers—for example, discussing patient information in public places, calling a patient's work or home and leaving a message that reveals information about health or health services, and so on—must not be done. Carrying documents outside an HCO with patient identifier information is prohibited; this constraint has implications for students who may take notes or have written assignments that include this information. How information is carried such as in tablets, laptops, or smartphones is also of concern. For example, taking pictures on smartphones in clinical settings is a privacy violation. Many institutions have implemented strict policies about taking patient photos, even if they are de-identified. As a nurse, you should make sure you know your employer's policies on smartphone and email use in a clinical setting and follow them.

Development of new technology has been moving so fast that critical prior issues have not always been addressed effectively. The 1996 law, however, requires that staff know the key elements of HIPAA and apply them. As a result, HCOs and healthcare profession schools, such as nursing programs, are required to provide information and training about HIPAA. Patients are informed about HIPAA when they enter the health system; they are given written information and asked to sign documents to indicate that they have been informed. Ensuring that the requirements are met must be incorporated into HIT. It is easy for patients and staff to report HIPAA violations to HHS via its website. Violations are examined, and the provider may have to pay a fee for not following HIPAA regulations.

Stop and Consider #10

There is high risk of problems with privacy and confidentiality when using HIT.

High-Touch Care versus
High-Tech Care

High-touch care is why most people become nurses, but nursing is much more than this today. This chapter describes the growing influence of technology on all segments of health care. This influence will not decrease, but rather increase in the future. Nurses need to understand and know how to use technology that is applied to their practice areas. They need to be involved in the development of

this technology when possible, and they must be involved in the implementation of the technology. But there are concerns. When we "talk" through machines, do we lose information and the personal relationship? How can this be prevented so that we are not disconnected from our patients? How can we ensure that the information we are getting is correct and complete? Are people able to communicate fully through some of these other means? It is clear that over time, the public has become increasingly comfortable with informatics, which they are using more and more in their everyday lives, but when it comes to their health care, they may want more personal communication. As nursing increasingly adopts informatics, nurses need to keep in mind the potential for isolation and the continuing need for effective patient communication throughout the care process. Nurses, also, must not forget the need for touch and face-to-face communication. When a nurse uses a computer or some type of handheld device while asking the patient questions and does not look at the patient, this does not engage the patient in the process.

The future will include many more new uses of technology; change is ongoing. For example, the e-intensive care unit (eICU) is used to monitor patients from afar to improve patient outcomes (Rouse, 2017). In this example, a system is attached to four hospitals in Iowa and their ICUs. This system allows intensivists at a remote monitoring center to view patients' vital statistics, electrocardiograms, ventilators, and X-ray and lab results. The eICU includes two-way conference video capability so that patients and staff can interact when required. This type of system has advantages; for example, experts can be located in one place and then consult with multiple locations and staff that may not have the required experts. This is particularly useful in providing expert medical care for residents in rural and remote areas. There is no reason that this type of system is limited to physician consultation because nurses use it, too. For example, a nurse clinical specialist might view patient data and consult on patient care with nurses in an ICU in an external location from where the nurse specialist is located. There is potential for increased access to information and expertise. The other side of this innovation coin is the effect on the touch side of care when the provider is not actually in the room with the patient. It is not clear how this might affect care because these types of systems are very new.

Stop and Consider #11

A computer can stand in the way of relating to patients.

Nursing Leadership
in Health Informatics

We are currently at a critical junction for nurses and the informatics competency, with all nurses called upon to assume more leadership in the expansion of informatics in health care. This call to action corresponds to the recommendations in *The future of nursing* report (IOM, 2010). Ongoing implementation of the Affordable Care Act of 2010 led to further changes in healthcare delivery and more dependence on informatics, and nurse informaticists should be part of the structure that develops and implements greater use of informatics (HIMSS, 2011).

The report titled *Health IT and patient safety: Building safer systems for better care* (IOM, 2012) makes a strong statement that HIT is not something separated from care delivery or the providers of care. "We are at a unique time in health care. Technology—which has the potential to improve quality and safety of care as well as reduce costs—is rapidly evolving, changing the way we deliver health care. At the same time, health care reform is reshaping the health care landscape" (IOM, 2012, p. ix). This report highlights patient and family concerns about safety and shared responsibility. These same themes have also been emphasized throughout this text.

Stop and Consider #12

With the expansion of health informatics in all sectors of health care nurses need to be leaders by participating in this expansion and providing feedback.

CHAPTER HIGHLIGHTS

1. The fifth healthcare profession core competency is to utilize informatics.
2. The federal government published two reports on HIT, indicating increasing interest in this topic; the reports include a federal strategic HIT plan.
3. Health informatics is more than just looking at IT; it also involves understanding how that technology is used in providing care, preventing errors and improving care, research, and more.
4. Health informatics is used to evaluate the performance of HCOs and individual healthcare providers and has a major impact on quality improvement. Today, it is much easier to collect, store, and analyze large amounts of data than were collected by hand in the past.
5. Insurers rely heavily on informatics to provide insurance coverage, manage data, and analyze performance, which has a

(Continues)

CHAPTER HIGHLIGHTS (CONTINUED)

direct impact on whether care is covered for reimbursement.

6. Informatics provides opportunities for government at all levels—local, state, national, and international—to collect data and use them for policy decision making and evaluation.

7. A clinical information system is a method of data storage that is generally used at the point of care. It includes such elements as clinical guidelines, patient information, and pharmacopeias to check for drug interactions.

8. Computer literacy requires knowledge of basic computer technology.

9. Standardized language is a collection of terms with definitions for use in informational systems databases. Standardized language is necessary for documentation in EHRs.

10. NI is a nursing specialty that integrates nursing science, computer science, and information science to manage and communicate data, information, knowledge, and wisdom in nursing practice. This specialty has its own sets of standards, scope of practice, and national certification.

11. Informatics can directly affect care by providing data in a retrievable form for the purpose of assisting with clinical decision making. However, the data are only as reliable as the information entered in the computer.

12. In today's HCOs, documentation is often implemented in an electronic format.

13. Standardized terminology assists in promoting clearer communication across disciplines.

14. Interface terminologies include, but are not limited to, the Clinical Care Classification, the International Classification of Nursing Practice, NANDA, NIC, NOC, the Omaha System, and the SYNTEGRITY PNDS.

15. Multidisciplinary terminologies include, but are not limited to, the Logical Observation Identifiers Names and Codes and the Systematized Nomenclature of Medicine—Clinical Terms.

16. Examples of use of informatics in healthcare delivery include the automated dispensing of medications and bar coding for identification; computerized monitoring of adverse events; use of EMRs, provider order-entry systems, and clinical decision support systems; use of tablets and smartphones; access to patient records at the point of care; and Internet prescriptions, nurse call systems, voice mail, telephone for advice and other services, online support groups for patients, and Internet or virtual appointments.

17. HIPAA requires that patient data are kept secure and private.

18. Current and future uses of HIT and technology include such methods as telehealth, robotics, genomics, and others.

19. Technology may have an impact on the patient–provider relationship—leading to a conflict between high-tech and high touch-care.

20. As health informatics expands, nursing must be proactive in increasing its role in informatics and assume more leadership to improve health care through better informatics.

ENGAGING IN THE CONTENT

Discussion Questions

1. Explain how the core competency "utilize informatics" relates to the other four core competencies.
2. What is informatics? Why is it important in health care and nursing?
3. Describe the certification requirements for the role of the informatics nurse.
4. Describe four examples of healthcare informatics and implications for nursing.
5. Why is documentation important?
6. Explain how the EMR and PHR can increase quality of care and decrease errors. Provide examples.
7. Discuss issues related to confidentiality and informatics.

CRITICAL THINKING ACTIVITIES

1. Divide into teams. Identify an HCO (hospital or other type) in your local community and try to find out how it uses informatics and applies meaningful use. You can focus on the entire organization or select a department or a unit. Are there any future plans to increase the use of informatics? Teams should then compare and contrast their information.
2. In a team, develop six questions to ask a nurse who works in a hospital that uses an EMR. Each student on the team then interviews one registered nurse. After the interviews, combine your data and analyze the results.
3. Speak to a registered nurse who works in staff development/education in an HCO. Discuss the training that staff members receive for using informatics (for example, type of content, cost and time commitment, challenges). Share this information with classmates.
4. If you have used an EMR in clinical practice, what was it like for you? Did you get sufficient orientation? If not, what was missing? If you have not yet done this, interview a senior student and ask about the experience.
5. Which biomedical equipment have you used or seen used? How does the use of this equipment impact care?

ELECTRONIC REFLECTION JOURNAL

What is your opinion of the potential conflict between high-touch care and high-tech care? Describe some examples where you thought technology interfered with patient care, either for you or for something you observed. What could have been done to prevent this?

CASE STUDIES

Case 1

A 6-year-old has come to the attention of the child welfare department as a possible victim of sexual abuse. The child's school nurse reported the situation as required by law. The child lives in a very rural part of a western state. Rather than have the child travel a distance to experts, she was taken to the nearest clinic with sexual assault nurse examiners and a knowledgeable pediatrician skilled in sexual abuse examinations. At the time of the examination, pictures were taken of the child's body, including the genital area. These pictures were crucial if charges were to be filed. To ensure that an accurate diagnosis was made, local experts sought a second opinion because the results of the physical examination were not believed to be completely definitive. The experts for the second opinion were linked via the Internet and Internet videoconferencing equipment so that the two teams could talk and view de-identified (because the information was going across unsecure Internet channels) photos. Within 15 minutes, it was determined that the hymen was intact and no penetration had occurred. Other markers indicated that there was evidence of child abuse, but none that supported a claim of sexual assault. This case used an EMR, digitized photos, school records, and Internet consultation to arrive at a diagnosis that had both medical and legal implications.

Case Questions

1. Discuss the impact of the use of these methods in the case on the nurse–patient relationship and on patient confidentiality, including HIPAA requirements.
2. How else might this technology be used?
3. What is your opinion of the human, caring part of the care process in relation to this case description?

Case 2

The hospital where you work is assessing its EMR system, which has been in use for 1 year. You volunteered to be on the task force that is leading the review. The team meets to discuss critical issues that need to be addressed. Some of the issues are staff acceptance of the new system, errors, and information that is not easy to access in the EMR. The representative from the hospital finance team asks, "What about meaningful use?"

Case Questions

1. What is meaningful use?
2. Why is the team member's question important?
3. How might meaningful use affect what the task force does?

CASE STUDIES (CONTINUED)

Working Backward to Develop a Case

Write a brief paragraph that describes a case related to the following questions.

1. What should we tell them about our documentation concerns?
2. Why are we discussing quality improvement when we are talking about documentation?
3. The timeline—why do we need to consider it?

REFERENCES

American Medical Association. (2016). *CPT, standard edition*. Chicago, IL: Author.

American Nurses Association. (2006). *Nursing practice information infrastructure: Glossary*. Retrieved from http://www.nursingworld.org/npii/glossary.htm

American Nurses Association. (2008). *Nursing informatics: Scope and standards of practice*. Washington, DC: Author.

American Nurses Credentialing Center. (2016). *Informatics nurse certification*. Retrieved from http://www.nurse credentialing.org/InformaticsNursing

Association of periOperative Registered Nurses. (2017). *AORN syntegrity perioperative documentation solution*. Retrieved from http://www.aorn.org/aorn-org/syntegrity

Barnett, M., Mehrotra, A., Jena, A., & Newhouse, R. (2016). Adverse inpatient outcomes during the transition to a new electronic health record system: Observational study. *British Medical Journal*. Retrieved from http://www.bmj.com/content/354/bmj.i3835

Bodenheimer, T. (2008). Coordinating care: A perilous journey through the healthcare system. *New England Journal of Medicine, 358*, 1065–1071.

Brown, C., Mulcaster, H., Triffitt, K., Sittig, D., Ash, J., Reygate, K., . . . Slight, S. (2016). A systematic review of the types and causes of prescribing errors generated from using computerized provider order entry systems in primary and secondary care. *J Am Med Inform Assoc*. 2017 Mar 1;24(2):432–440

Clark, S. (2011). Medical record documentation makes top 10 non-compliance list for first half of 2010. *HIM Connection*. Retrieved from http://www.hcpro.com/CCP-258429-237/ Medical-record-documentation-makes-Joint-Commission- top-10-noncompliance-list-for-first-half-of-2010.html

Conn, J. (2014, December 17). *Patient data held for ransom at Illinois rural hospital*. Retrieved from http://www.modernhealthcare.com/article/20141217/NEWS/312179948

Dykes, P., & Collins, S. (2013). Building linkages between nursing care and improved patient outcomes: The role of health information technology. *Online Journal of Issues in Nursing, 18*(3). Retrieved from http://www.nursingworld.org/MainMenuCategories/ANAMarketplace/ANAPeriodicals/OJIN/TableofContents/Vol-18-2013/No3-Sept-2013/Nursing-Care-and-Improved-Outcomes.html

Finkelman, A. (2018). *Quality improvement: A guide for nursing integration*. Burlington, MA: Jones & Bartlett Learning.

Ford, E., Silvera, G., Kazley, A., Diana, M., & Huerta, T. (2016). Assessing the relationship between patient safety culture and EHR strategy. *International Journal of Health Care Quality Assurance, 29*(6), 614–627.

Glassman, K., & Rosenfeld, P. (2015). *Data makes a difference. The smart nurse's handbook for using data to improve care*. Silver Spring, MD: American Nurses Association.

Gordon, A., Lutz, G., Boninger, M., & Cooper, R. (2007). Introduction to nanotechnology: Potential applications in physical medicine and rehabilitation. *American Journal of Physical Medicine and Rehabilitation, 86*, 225–241.

Healthcare Information and Management Systems Society. (2011, June 17). *Position statement on transforming nursing practice through technology and informatics*. Retrieved from http://www.himss.org/ASP/index.asp

Healthy People 2020. (2016). *Genomics.* Retrieved from https://www.healthypeople.gov/2020/topics-objectives/topic/genomics

Institute of Medicine. (2003). *Health professions education.* Washington, DC: The National Academies Press.

Institute of Medicine. (2010). *The future of nursing: Leading change, advancing health.* Washington, DC: The National Academies Press.

Institute of Medicine. (2012). *Health IT and patient safety: Building safer systems for better care.* Washington, DC: The National Academies Press.

Intuitive Surgical. (2017). *da Vinci® surgery.* Retrieved from http://www.davincisurgery.com/

Iyer, P., & Camp, N. (1999). *Nursing documentation.* St. Louis, MO: Mosby.

Joint Commission, The. (2011). *Comprehensive accreditation manual for hospitals.* Chicago, IL: Author.

Joint Commission, The. (2016). Facts about the official "do not use" list of abbreviations. Retrieved from https://www.jointcommission.org/facts_about_do_not_use_list/

Kennedy, R., Murphy, J., & Roberts, D. (2013, September 30). An overview of the national quality strategy: Where do nurses fit? *Online Journal of Issues in Nursing, 18*(3). Retrieved from http://www.nursingworld.org/MainMenuCategories/ANAMarketplace/ANAPeriodicals/OJIN/TableofContents/Vol-18-2013/No3-Sept-2013/National-Quality-Strategy.html

Kannampallil, T., Abraham, J., Solotskaya, A., Phillip, S., Lambert, B., Schiff, G., . . . Glanter, W. (2017, February). Learning from errors: Analysis of medication order voiding in CPOE systems. *Journal of American Informatics Association.* Retrieved from https://academic.oup.com/jamia/article-abstract/doi/10.1093/jamia/ocw187/3038212/Learning-from-errors-analysis-of-medication-order?redirectedFrom=fulltext

Kirkendall, E., Kouril, M., Dexheimer, J., Courter, J., Hagedorn, P., Szczesniak, R., . . . Spooner, S. (2016). Automated identification of antibiotic overdoses and adverse drug events via analysis of prescribing alerts and medication administration records. *Journal of American Medical Informatics Association.* Retrieved from https://www.ncbi.nlm.nih.gov/pubmed/27507653

McCain, E. (2014). *Hackers target health data in new breach.* Retrieved from http://www.healthcareitnews.com/news/hackers-target-health-data-new-HIPAA-breach

NANDA International. (2017). *Home: NANDA.* Retrieved from http://www.nanda.org/

National Institutes of Health, & U.S. National Library of Medicine. (2008). *Logical observation identifiers names and codes.* Retrieved from http://www.nlm.nih.gov/research/umls/loinc_main.html

National Institutes of Health, & U.S. National Library of Medicine. (2016a). *NLM health standards executive summary for 2015.* Retrieved from https://www.nlm.nih.gov/healthit/executive-summaries/2015/index.html

National Institutes of Health, & U.S. National Library of Medicine. (2016b). *SNOMED CT.* Retrieved from https://www.nlm.nih.gov/healthit/snomedct/

National Quality Forum. (2017). *Submitting emeasures for NQF endorsement.* Retrieved from http://www.qualityforum.org/Electronic_Quality_Measures.aspx

Nelson, R., & Joos, I. (1989, Fall). On language in nursing; from data to wisdom. *PLN Vision, 6.*

Omaha System. (2016). *The Omaha system: Solving the clinical data-information puzzle.* Retrieved from http://www.omahasystem.org/

Ootex Specialty Narrow Fabrics. (2017). *Specialty narrow fabrics.* Retrieved from https://www.osnf.com/

Pagliery, J. (2014, August 18). *Hospital network hacked, 4.5 million records stolen.* Retrieved from http://money.cnn.com/2014/08/18/technology/security/hospital-chs-hack/index.html

Peterson, A. (2015, March 20). *2015 already the year of the healthcare hack—and it is only going to get worse.* Retrieved from https://www.washingtonpost.com/news/the-switch/wp/2015/03/20/2015-is-already-the-year-of-the-health-care-hack-and-its-only-going-to-get-worse/?utm_term=.fbdaf3770636

Polisena, J. Gagliardi, A., Urbach, D., Clifford, T., & Fiander, M. (2015). Factors that influence the recognition, reporting, and resolution of incidents related to medical devices and other healthcare technologies: A systematic review. *Systematic Review.* Retrieved from https://www.ncbi.nlm.nih.gov/pubmed/25875375

Romano, M., & Stafford, R. (2011). Electronic health records and clinical decision support systems: Impact on national ambulatory care quality. *Archives of Internal Medicine, 171,* 897–903.

Rouse, M. (2017). *Electronic intensive care unit (eICU).* Retrieved from http://searchhealthit.techtarget.com/definition/Electronic-Intensive-Care-Unit-eICU

Schwiran, P., & Thede, L. (2011). Informatics: The standardized nursing terminologies: A national survey of nurses' experiences and attitudes. *Online Journal of Issues in Nursing, 16*(2). Retrieved from http://nursingworld.org/MainMenuCategories/ANAMarketplace/ANAPeriodicals/OJIN/Columns/Informatics/Informatics-Participants-Perception-of-Comfort-in-the-Use.html

Science Daily. (2016). *Robotic brace aids stroke recovery.* Retrieved from https://www.sciencedaily.com/releases/2007/03/070321105223.htm

Simone, L., Brumbaugh, J., & Ricketts, C. (2014). Medical devices, the FDA, and the home healthcare clinician. *Home Healthcare Nurse, 32*(7), 402–408.

Sitterding, M. (2015). An overview of information overload. In M. Sitterding & M. Broome, (eds.) (2015). *Information overload. Framework, tips, and tools to manage in complex healthcare* environments. (pp. 1–9). Silver Spring, MD: American Nurses Association.

Thomas, L. (2015, November 15). *What is telemedicine?* Retrieved from http://www.news-medical.net/health/What-is-Telemedicine.aspx

University of Iowa, Center for Nursing Classification and Effectiveness. (2017). *Center for Nursing Classification and Effectiveness.* Retrieved from https://nursing.uiowa.edu/center-for-nursing-classification-and-clinical-effectiveness

U.S. Department of Health and Human Services, & Agency for Healthcare Quality and Research. (2016). *Telehealth: Mapping the evidence for patient outcomes from systematic reviews.* Technical Brief Number 26. AHRQ Publication No. 16-EHCO34-EF. Rockville, MD: AHRQ.

U.S. Department of Health and Human Services, Centers for Disease Control and Prevention, & National Institute for Occupational Safety and Health. (2016). *International classification of diseases (ICD-10).* Retrieved from https://wwwn.cdc.gov/eworld/Appendix/ICDCodes

U.S. Department of Health and Human Services, & Centers for Medicare and Medicaid Services. (2014). *Meaningful use.* Retrieved from http://www.cms.gov/Regulations-and-Guidance/Legislation/EHRIncentivePrograms/Meaningful_Use.html

U.S. Department of Health and Human Services, & Food and Drug Administration. (2017). *Medical device reporting.* Retrieved from https://www.fda.gov/medicaldevices/safety/reportaproblem/default.htm

U.S. Health and Human Services, & HealthIt.Gov. (2014). *Meaningful use definition and objectives.* Retrieved from http://www.healthit.gov/providers-professionals/meaningful-use-definition-objectives

U.S. Department of Health and Human Services, & HealthIT.gov. (2015). *What is an electronic medical record (EMR)?* Retrieved from http://www.healthit.gov/providers-professionals/electronic-medical-records-emr

U.S. Department of Health and Human Services, & The Office of National Coordinator for Health Information Technology. (2013). *Health information technology. Patient safety action & surveillance plan.* Retrieved from https://healthit.gov/sites/default/files/safetyplanhhspubliccomment.pdf

U.S. Department of Health and Human Services, & The Office of National Coordinator for Health Information Technology. (2015a). *Connecting health and care for the nation: A shared nationwide interoperability roadmap draft version 1.0.* Retrieved from https://www.healthit.gov/policy-researchers-implementers/interoperability

U.S. Department of Health and Human Services, & The Office of National Coordinator for Health Information Technology. (2015b). *Federal health IT strategic plan. 2015-2020.* Retrieved from https://www.healthit.gov/sites/default/files/9-5-federalhealthitstratplanfinal_0.pdf

U.S. Department of Health and Human Services, & The Office of National Coordinator for Health Information Technology. (2016a). *2016 report to congress on health IT progress.* Retrieved from https://www.healthit.gov/sites/default/files/2016_report_to_congress_on_healthit_progress.pdf

U.S. Department of Health and Human Services, & The office of National Coordinator for Health Information Technology. (2016b). *Adoption of electronic health record systems among non-federal acute care hospitals 2008-2015.* Data brief 35. Retrieved from https://www.healthit.gov/sites/default/files/briefs/2015_hospital_adoption_db_v17.pdf

Weick, K. (2009). *Making sense of the organization.* New York, NY: John Wiley & Sons.

Yadav, S., Kazanji, N., Narayan, K., Paudel, S., Falatko, J., Shoichet, S., . . . Barnes, M. (2016). Comparison of accuracy of physical examination findings in initial progress notes between paper charts and a newly implemented electronic health record. *Journal of American Medical Informatics Association, 24*(1), 140–144.

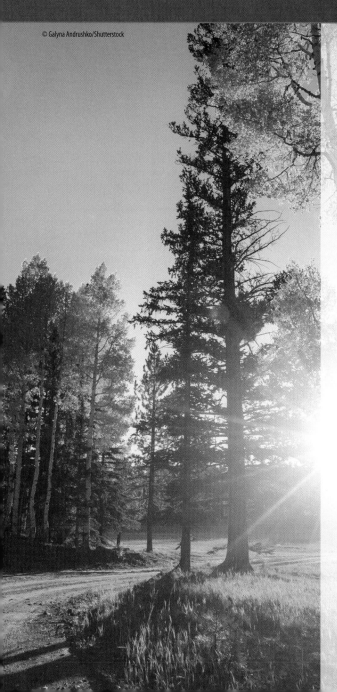

© Galyna Andrushko/Shutterstock

Section 4

The Practice of Nursing Today and in the Future

Section 4 concludes this text. It summarizes key concerns focusing on the future of nursing and the importance of nursing leadership. Change in the healthcare delivery system provides many opportunities for nursing, if nursing is ready for them.

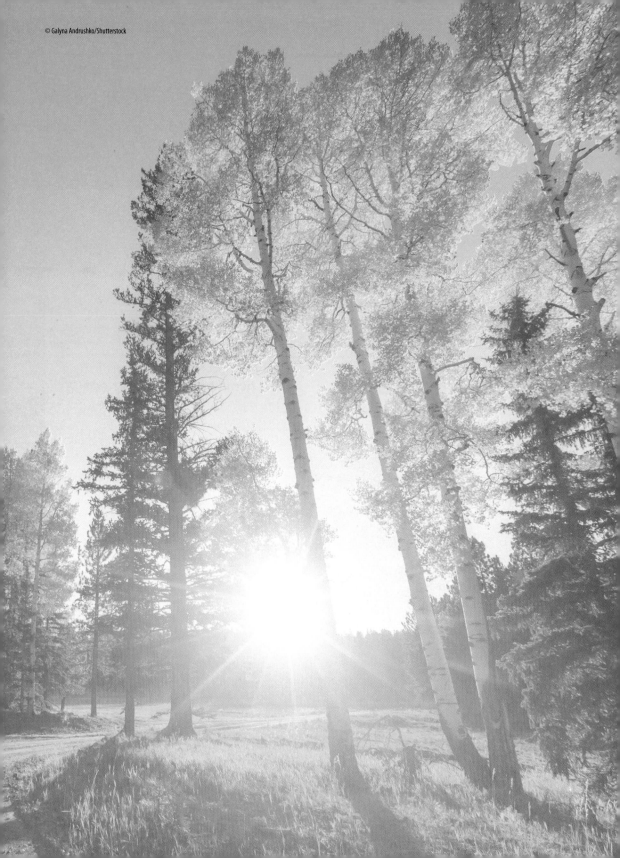

Chapter 14

The Future: Transformation of Nursing Practice through Leadership

CHAPTER OBJECTIVES

At the conclusion of this chapter, the learner will be able to:

- Discuss the relevance of leadership in nursing and management and the impact of shared governance.
- Examine the factors that influence nursing leadership and management.
- Examine the various healthcare settings, roles, and specialties for nurses and possible future changes in scope of practice.
- Critique examples of past and current professional practice models.
- Discuss the impact of legislation, regulation, and policy on nursing leadership and practice.
- Explain the importance of economic value to the nursing profession.

- Discuss the impact of the work environment on the nursing profession and the delivery of effective quality care.
- Explain why it is important for nurses to assume active leadership roles in quality improvement.
- Discuss how the Forces of Magnetism and the Magnet Recognition Program® are used to support effective, healthy nursing work environments and nursing leadership.
- Examine the future of nursing leadership to move the profession forward.

KEY TERMS

Accountability
Accreditation
Autonomy
Differentiated nursing practice
Forces of Magnetism

Leader
Leadership
Magnet Recognition Program®
Management
Manager

Peter Principle
Practice models
Responsibility
Shared governance
Transformational leadership

Introduction

This is the concluding chapter in this text, but in another sense, it is the beginning of your professional journey. Leadership is key to the success of the profession, so we end with discussion about leadership and tie together content found in this text. Content related to leadership is found throughout this text, such as in discussions about the development of the profession, nursing education, healthcare policy, legal and ethical issues, healthcare organizations (HCOs),

coordination and collaboration, communication, interprofessional teams, delegation, conflict resolution, evidence-based practice (EBP) and research, and the five healthcare core competencies. This discussion does not end with this text or in a course that introduces the critical elements of the nursing profession. Instead, this chapter marks a beginning because it highlights key concerns introduced elsewhere in the text, and the content focuses on the future of nursing and the need for greater leadership—both for the profession and for individual nurses. You are the future of nursing. This content also explores some of the emerging issues, trends, and initiatives important to the nursing profession and the need for greater nursing leadership. More changes are predicted for the future, but most are unknown.

Leadership and
Management in Nursing

Leadership is important for every nurse, whether the nurse is in a formal administrative/management position or not. Leadership characteristics and competencies are required to ensure that patients receive the care they need. These characteristics and competencies are also important in ensuring that the nursing profession is an active participant in the healthcare delivery system and in the development and implementation of healthcare policy. *The future of nursing* report supports this perspective by emphasizing the need for nurses to assume more leadership in health care, and to accomplish this, nurses need greater leadership competency (Institute of Medicine [IOM], 2010).

Leadership Models and Theories

A good place to begin to better understand leadership in nursing is with an overview of leadership models and theories, critical issues, and a comparison of **leadership** and **management**. Leadership and management are not the same, although effective managers need to demonstrate leadership. In general, earlier leadership models and theories emphasized control and getting the job done with little, if any, emphasis on creativity and innovation or staff participation in decision making. The following is a brief summary of some of the key models and theories to illustrate how they have changed over time.

- *Autocratic:* The formal leader (manager/ administrator) makes decisions for the staff;

the model assumes staff are not able and not interested in participating in decision making.
- *Bureaucratic:* The focus is on structure, rules, and policies, with decision making placed in the hands of the formal leader (manager/administrator). Staff members receive directions. This approach is related to the autocratic approach.
- *Laissez-faire:* The formal leader (manager/ administrator) turns over decision making to the staff; steps back from participation; and lets things happen with little, if any, direction. This can lead to problems because it often means the organization or process may be leaderless; it is a difficult balance to provide some leadership but to do so in the background.

These models and theories have long been used in health care. Indeed, some HCOs still use them or some adaptation of them. Nevertheless, these approaches are not effective in today's rapidly changing environment where staff want to participate more and seek recognition for their performance and expertise, but they still expect leaders to guide the overall process. Over time, new models and theories that built on one another were developed. Often, these changes began in other industries and then were adopted by HCOs. Some of these newer theories are highlighted here:

- *Deming's theory:* Effective organizations are dependent on group or team interaction.
- *Drucker's theory:* This theory, which is referred to as modern management, builds on Deming's recognition of the importance of staff team participation in the organization and yet also maintains the importance of individual autonomy.
- *Contingency theory:* Multiple variables affect situations, which in turn affect leader–member relationships, tasks, and position power.
- *Connective leadership theory:* The focus is on caring and connecting to others—individuals, groups, and organizations.

- *Emotional intelligence theory:* The focus is on leader–follower relationships, feelings, and self-awareness.
- *Chaos or quantum theory:* A more current theory, this model emphasizes interdependency, sensitivity to change, avoidance of predicting too far into the future, and accountability in the hands of those who do the work.
- *Knowledge management theory:* This theory turns attention to knowledge—the knowledge worker, knowledge-intense organizations, interprofessional collaboration, and accountability. It recognizes the importance of technology and information today. Although this is a new theory, it, too, has historical roots. For example, Drucker's theory used the term *knowledge worker* to describe a person who works with his or her hands and with theoretical knowledge. Knowledge workers are assets for HCOs—for example, nurses should focus on knowledge and application of knowledge rather than being overly concerned with staff titles and positions.

As changes were made in leadership models and theories in the last 20 years, there has been a movement toward greater staff participation, recognition of staff performance, staff and staff–manager relationships, and collaboration. This is very different from autocratic, bureaucratic, or even laissez-faire leadership approaches.

As a result of these changes, a newer leadership theory stands out today—a theory that has connections to the theories previously described. In early *Quality Chasm* reports, experts recommended that the best leadership style today for healthcare delivery is **transformational leadership** (IOM, 2003a). This approach emphasizes a positive work environment, recognition of the importance of change and using change effectively, rewarding staff for expertise and performance, and development of staff awareness of work processes so that they can engage in quality improvement (QI). Transformational leaders create vision and mission statements with the staff to guide the work of the organization. This leader is described as honest, energetic, loyal, confident, self-directed, flexible, and committed. Staff members are able to see these characteristics in a transformational leader and want to work for and with this leader. Some studies indicate that there is a connection between staff perceiving their nursing leaders as transformational leaders and staff perceptions of a positive work environment; there is less staff burnout and more staff engagement in the work environment and processes (Lewis & Cunningham, 2016). This type of study further supports the need for transformational leadership and also more nursing research to better understand this type of leadership.

Shared Governance: Empowering Nursing Staff

With the changing environment and changes in leadership and management models or theories, there is greater need to focus more on team efforts. This led to development and greater use of **shared governance** (shared decision making), which "can be viewed as a management philosophy, a professional practice model, and an accountability model that focuses on staff involvement in decision-making, particularly in decisions that affect their practice" (Finkelman, 2016, p. 115). Through shared governance, nurses in an organization can (Hess, 2004):

1. Control their professional practice.
2. Influence organizational resources that support practice.
3. Gain formal authority, which is granted by the organization.
4. Participate in decision making through committee structure.
5. Access information about the organization.
6. Set goals and negotiate conflict.

In this type of organization, nurses assume an active role in the management of the patient care services and thus have more control over their practice (Murray et al., 2016). Shared governance is a management model, emphasizing the need for nurses to share accountability and responsibility, and this typically leads to more staff commitment to the HCO. Nurses have the authority to make sure the right decisions are made about the work they do. **Accountability** means that the nurse accepts responsibility for outcomes or is answerable for what is done. **Responsibility** is to be "entrusted with a particular function" (Ritter-Teitel, 2002, p. 34). These aspects of management are connected to **autonomy**, or the right to make decisions and control actions. The best situation occurs when the nurse who provides care is also the staff member who works to resolve issues and ensure that patient outcomes are achieved at the point of care, limiting the number or layers of staff who must be involved. This approach is more effective in ensuring quality care than someone far above the direct care situation telling staff what they must do to improve. Shared governance is dependent on effective collaboration, communication, and teamwork and spreads departmental and organizational decision making over a large number of staff, providing for opportunities for more decentralized decision making. This approach, however, does not mean that managers can ignore their managerial and leadership responsibilities or that all decisions are made by the staff. If the process blocks decision making—for example, by taking too long to make a decision—then this model will not be effective. This approach means managers must do their jobs differently with inclusion of staff. Shared governance is not easy to develop, and sometimes it can become a barrier to delivery of efficient, high-quality care. It takes time to develop an effective shared governance structure and culture.

HCOs may vary in how they structure shared governance, but the principles are typically the same—as described here. For example, a hospital may have a nursing council with different nursing staff represented, and the council makes certain decisions for operation of nursing services with committees and task forces working on various aspects to ensure effective nursing care and meet staff work needs,

such as staffing, scheduling, education, salaries and benefits, promotion structure, and so on. Typically, hospitals that use a shared governance model find that staff members are more satisfied and turnover is lower. Staff like working in the organization. Not all hospitals use shared governance, and its implementation and effectiveness can vary widely.

Leadership versus Management

It is easy to confuse leadership and management. A **leader** can be a leader and not a manager, just as a manager can be a manager and not a leader. A leader provides overall guidance and supports staff engagement at all levels of the organization. A **manager** holds a formal management or administrative position and, in that position, focuses on four major functions: planning, organizing, leading, and controlling. Today, effective nurse managers need to be able to collaborate, communicate, coordinate, delegate, recognize importance of data and outcomes, manage resources (budget, staff, equipment, supplies, and so on), improve staff performance, build teams, and evaluate effectiveness and efficiency. In their position, they must actively support and apply EBP, evidence-based management (EBM), and QI. They use critical thinking and clinical reasoning and judgment, and they need to be flexible and able to adjust to change, using the planning process. This role has changed over time, particularly due to the changing healthcare environment and changes in leadership and management models. Currently, managers need more leadership and management competencies.

Someone who is described as a leader is viewed as such due to the person's ability to influence others; however, it does not necessarily mean that this person is in a formal management position. In contrast, managers have power because they hold a formal management position such as team leader, nurse manager, or chief nursing office. Ideally, all managers should also be leaders and viewed this way by their staff, but this does not always happen. Bennis and Goldsmith describe one viewpoint of the difference between leaders and managers (1997, p. 4): "There is a profound difference—a chasm—between leaders and managers. A good manager does things right. A leader does the right thing." A problem in organizations and in nursing is the **Peter Principle**, which occurs when someone is promoted beyond their leadership and management competencies required for a new position. This is a particular problem in nursing as it is not uncommon to promote a very competent clinical nurse to a management position and assume that this will lead to success. In many cases, it does not.

Major changes in healthcare delivery have led to the need for changes in leadership and in management. The following aspects of leadership have become more important, and they also have an impact on management (Porter-O'Grady, 1999, p. 40):

- Change focus from process to outcomes.
- Align role to the information infrastructure rather than to functional performance.
- Focus on team results rather than individual performance.
- Manage data complexes rather than individual events.
- Facilitate resources that then direct work.
- Transfer skill sets rather than make decisions for staff.
- Develop staff self-direction rather than giving direction.
- Focus on obtaining value rather than simply finding costs.
- Focus on consumer-driven structure rather than provider-based system.
- Construct horizontal relationships rather than maintain vertical control mechanisms.
- Facilitate equity-based partnerships rather than control individual behaviors.

Consideration of these factors provides greater opportunity to develop and implement transformational leadership; an effective nurse manager should demonstrate transformational leadership.

There are many myths about leadership that are important to address, and three of them are key for nursing leaders to consider as they develop their own leadership or develop other nurses for leadership (Goffee & Jones, 2000).

- *Everyone can be a leader.* This is not true. Everyone may have potential to be a leader; however, it is important to recognize that leadership competencies can and must be developed for a person to actually be a leader.
- *People who get to the top are leaders.* This is not true. There are many people in high-level administrative positions who would not be described as leaders; in some cases, they would not even be described as managers by their staff.
- *Leaders deliver business results.* This is not true. Leaders do not always meet expected outcomes; sometimes they are not effective managers.

HCOs need to work on developing leadership in nursing staff, and nurses need to work on developing their own leadership. Leaders do not just happen; they need education, guidance and support, mentoring, and so on.

Nursing Management Positions

Nurse managers today carry much more responsibility than in the past. The main purpose of management is to get the job done and make sure the job is done effectively. There are three common levels of management. The first level includes managers who work with staff daily to complete required work. The typical title at this level is nurse manager, though titles may vary by HCO. This person guides and supervises a unit's staff, both professional and nonprofessional, to ensure that quality patient care is delivered focused at the clinical unit level. The second level in an organization consists of middle managers who supervise multiple first-level managers. Such managers might include a nursing director who supervises all the unit nurse managers in the medical division or all the nurse managers in ambulatory care clinics and the emergency department. The upper level is the chief nursing officer. This nurse manager is responsible for the overall work of the nursing service and, in some cases, may be responsible for other services. Middle-level managers report to upper-level managers. Regardless of level, the manager must be able to perform management functions and ideally demonstrate leadership.

This description is the most common structure for nursing management in HCOs such as hospitals; however, there are variations from organization to organization. In addition, some staff may hold non-managerial positions, but they also need to be effective leaders and demonstrate some management functions such as planning. These individuals do not have supervisory responsibilities because they do not always direct staff, but they must influence staff. For example, a clinical nurse specialist (CNS), advanced practice registered nurse (APRN), clinical nurse leader (CNL), or nurse informaticist may hold this type of position.

Stop and Consider #1

Leadership and management are part of shared governance.

Factors that Influence
Leadership

Many factors influence the development of leadership competencies and the practice of effective leadership. Some of the factors are organization-based such as administrative support of effective leadership development, clear communication and processes, recognition and empowerment, and so on. Other factors are focused more on individuals who are leaders or aspire to improve and be leaders. Examples of factors are education (academic, staff education, continuing education [CE]), self-esteem, ability to communicate,

ability to ask for guidance, effective use of problem solving, ability to develop and communicate a vision, ability to engage others in the work process, and so on. The following sections include a discussion of some factors that should be considered in developing leadership at organizational and individual staff levels.

Generational Issues in Nursing: Impact on Image

Generational issues are important because multiple generations are part of the image of nursing and have an impact on nursing practice and management and, consequently, on leadership. When a person thinks of a nurse, which generation or age groups are considered? Most people probably do not realize that there is not one age group, but rather several represented in nursing. Today, nursing staff include representation from three active generations: (1) Baby Boomers, (2) Generation X, and (3) Generation Y. The so-called Traditional generation is no longer in practice, but it had a significant impact on the nursing profession and current practice. **Exhibit 14-1** identifies the time frames for these nursing generations.

Nurses in the four generations are different from one another. How does this affect the image of nursing? It means that the image of nursing is one of multiple age groups with different historical backgrounds and viewpoints. How nurses from each generation view nursing can be quite different, and their educational backgrounds vary a great deal, from nurses who entered nursing through diploma programs to nurses who entered through baccalaureate programs and on to graduate degrees. Some of these nurses have seen great changes in health care, and others see the current status as the way it has always been. Technology, for example, is frequently taken for granted by some nurses, whereas others are overwhelmed with technological advances. Some nurses have seen great changes in the roles of nurses, whereas other nurses now take the roles for granted—for example, the APRN role. If one asked a nurse in each generation for the nurse's view of nursing, the answers might be quite different—for example, how nurses practice, settings in which nurses practice, management responsibilities, and so on. If these nurses then tried to explain their views to the public, the perception of nursing would most likely consist of multiple images.

The situation of multiple generations in one profession provides opportunities to enhance the profession through the diversity of the age groups and their experiences, but it has also caused problems in the workplace. What are the characteristics of the various groups? How well do they mesh with the healthcare environment? How well do they work together? The following list summarizes some of the characteristics of each generation, including the traditional generation and its impact (American Hospital Association, 2002; Bertholf & Loveless, 2001; Finkelman, 2016; Gerke, 2001; Santos & Cox, 2002; Ulrich, 2001; Wieck, Prydun, & Walsh, 2002).

- *The Traditional (Silent or Mature) generation, born 1930–1940:* This generation is important because of its historical impact on nursing, but members of this group are no longer in practice. This group of nurses was hard working, loyal, and family focused, and they felt that duty to work was important. Many served in the military in World War II and the Korean War. This period occurred prior to the women's liberation movement. The characteristics of the traditional generation had a major impact

on how nursing services were organized and nurses' expectations of management. Some of this impact has been negative, such as the emphasis on bureaucratic structure, and it has been difficult to change in some HCOs.

- *Baby Boomers, born 1940–1964:* This generation, which is currently the largest in the work arena, is the group moving into the retirement process. This trend is predicted to lead to greater nursing shortage problems in the future. The Baby Boomer generation grew up in a time of major changes, including the women's liberation movement, the civil rights movement, and the Vietnam War. They had fewer professional opportunities than are available to nurses today because the typical career choices for women were either teaching or nursing. This began to change as the women's liberation movement grew, for example, opening up other opportunities, medicine, law, business, and so on. Within this generation, fewer men went into nursing, as was true of the previous generation. This group's characteristics include independence, acceptance of authority, loyalty to the employer, workaholic tendencies, and less experience with technology, although many in this group led the drive for adoption of more technology in nursing. This generation is often more materialistic and competitive and appreciates consensus leadership. It is a generation whose members chose a career and then stuck to it, even if they were not very happy with that choice.

- *Generation X (Gen-X), born 1965–1980:* The presence of Generation X, along with Generation Y, is growing in nursing. Members of this group are assuming more nursing leadership roles as the Baby Boomers retire. Gen-Xers are more accomplished in technology and very involved with computers and other advances in communication and information (social media), both in their personal lives and in healthcare delivery. They have experienced many changes in these areas in their lifetimes. These nurses want to be led, not managed, and they usually have not yet developed high levels of self-confidence and empowerment. What do they want in leaders? They look for leaders who are motivational, demonstrate positive communication, appreciate team players, and exhibit good people skills—leaders who are approachable and supportive. Baby Boomers, in contrast, would not look for these characteristics in a leader. Gen-Xers typically do not join organizations (which has implications for nursing organizations that need more members and active members), do not feel they must stay in the same job for a long time (which has implications for employers that experience staff turnover and related costs), and want a good balance between work and personal life (which means that they are less willing to bring work home). Compared with earlier generations of nurses, members of Generation X are more informal, pragmatic, technoliterate, independent, creative, intimidated by authority, and loyal to those they know; they also appreciate diversity. By contrast, the Baby Boomers with whom the Gen-Xers work often see things very differently. Baby Boomers

are more loyal to their employer, stay in the job longer, are more willing to work overtime (although they are not happy about it), and have greater long-term commitment. These differences may cause problems between the two generations, with Baby Boomers often occupying supervisory positions or senior faculty positions and Gen-Xers found in staff positions or beginning faculty positions, but moving into more leadership positions. It is a critical time of leadership transition in the profession.

- *Generation Y (Nexters, Millennials, Generation Next, Gen-Y), born 1980–present:* The Millennial generation is the newest generation in nursing, although second-career students and older students are also entering the profession who might be older and thus may represent an earlier generation. Key characteristics of this generation are optimism, civic duty, confidence, achievement, social ability, morality, and diversity. In work situations, they demonstrate collective action, optimism, tenacity, multitasking, and a high level of technology skill, and they are also more trusting of centralized authority than Generation X. Typically, they handle change better, take risks, and want to be challenged. This generation is connected to cell phones and personal tablets and use various social networking methods. They are tech savvy and expect to multitask. Sometimes, however, this makes it difficult for them to focus on one task.

In a profession that includes representatives from multiple generations, it is necessary to recognize that age diversity means variations in positive and negative characteristics among staff. Some will pull the profession backward if allowed, and some will push the profession forward. "In the workplace, differing work ethics, communication preferences, manners, and attitudes toward authority are key areas of conflict" (Siela, 2006, p. 47). This also has an impact on the nursing profession's image. As discussed here, nursing is not a profession that encompasses just one type of person or one age group, and people in different age groups are now entering nursing. We are long past the time when mostly 18-year-olds entered nursing education programs. As one generation moves toward retirement, the next generation will undoubtedly have a greater impact on the image of nursing. It is critical to avoid gender role stereotyping, and we need to increase the strength of nurses as one group of professionals, while still recognizing that these differences exist and appreciating how they might affect the profession.

Power and Empowerment

Power and empowerment are connected to the image of nursing and the ability to assume leadership. How one is viewed can affect whether the person is considered to have power—power to influence, to say what the profession is or is not, and to influence decision making. Nurses typically do not like to talk about power; they find it to be philosophically different from their view of nursing (Malone, 2001). This belief—that is, viewing power only in the negative—acts as a barrier to success as a healthcare professional and also affects teamwork, as discussed in other chapters. But what are power, powerlessness, and empowerment? They are critical elements influencing leadership.

To feel as if one is not listened to or not viewed positively can make a person feel powerless; this remains a longstanding problem for nurses. Many nurses believe that they cannot make an impact in clinical settings, and they are not listened to or sought out for their opinions. This powerlessness can result in nurses feeling like victims. The result may be resentment that is expressed as incivility, as discussed in other chapters in this text. This feeling of powerlessness can act against nurses when they do not actively address issues such as a negative image of nurses and when they allow others to describe

what a nurse is or make decisions for nurses. This failure to be proactive merely worsens their image and diminishes professional self-esteem; both reduce leadership.

What nurses want and need is power—to be able to influence decisions and have an impact on issues that matter. It is clear that power can be used constructively or destructively, but the concern here with the nursing profession is using power constructively. Power and influence are related. Power is about gaining control to reach a goal. There is more than one type of power, as described earlier in this text in content about teams and teamwork: informational, referent, expert, coercive, reward, and persuasive. The type of power a person possesses has an impact on how it can be used to reach goals or outcomes.

Empowerment is also an important issue for nurses today and is connected to leadership. Leaders who empower staff enable staff to act—a critical need in the nursing profession. Shared governance emphasizes empowerment. Basically, empowerment is more than just saying you can participate in decision making; staff need more than words. Empowerment is needed in day-to-day practice as nurses meet the needs of patients in hospitals, the community, and home settings. Empowerment also implies that some individuals may lose their power while others gain power. This can lead to conflict, which needs to be resolved so that it does not negatively affect the work environment and patient care.

Staff members who experience empowerment feel that they are respected and trusted to be active participants. This also helps them demonstrate a positive image to other healthcare team members, patients and their families, and the public. Nurses who do not feel empowered will not be effective in conveying a positive image because they will not be able to communicate that nurses are professionals with much to offer. Empowerment that is not clear to staff or not supported by management is just as problematic as lack of staff empowerment.

Empowered teams feel a responsibility for the team's performance and activities, which in turn can improve care and reduce errors.

Control over the nursing profession is a critical issue that is also related to the profession's image. Who should control the nursing profession, and who does? This is related to independence and autonomy—key characteristics of any profession. But a key question persists: *What should be the image of nursing?* As a profession, nursing does not appear to have a consensus about its image, given that the types of advertising and responses to these advertising initiatives vary. This topic is discussed in other chapters, and here it is mentioned again as one considers nursing leadership and what nurses need to do to become more effective leaders in a complex healthcare delivery system. Nursing needs to control the image and visibility of the profession, and in doing so, may exert more control over the solutions for the following four issues:

1. If nurses have a more realistic image, it is easier to support the types of services that nurses offer to the public.
2. If nurses have a more realistic image, it is easier to support an entry-level baccalaureate degree to provide the type of education needed.
3. If nurses have a more realistic image, it is easier to support the need for reimbursement for nursing services, which involves much more than patient hand holding.
4. If nurses have a more realistic image, it is easier to participate in the healthcare dialogue on the local, state, national, and international levels to influence policy.

Assertiveness

Earlier content in this text discussed assertiveness from the point of view of teams, but here we focus on nursing assertiveness and leadership. Assertiveness is demonstrated in a person's communication—direct and open with appropriate respect of others. When a person communicates in an assertive manner, verbal and nonverbal communication become congruent, making the message clearer. Assertive and aggressive communications are not the same. Assertive persons are better able to confront problems in a constructive manner and do not remain silent. The problems that the nursing profession has with its image have been influenced by nursing's silence caused by the inability to be assertive, but assertiveness is a critical leadership competency.

Smith (1975) identified some critical rules related to assertive behavior that can easily be applied to the difficulties that nursing experiences with its image and the need to increase its visibility and develop leadership. A summary of examples of these rules includes:

- Avoid over-apologizing.
- Avoid defensive, adverse reactions, such as aggression, temper tantrums, backbiting, revenge, slander, sarcasm, and threats.
- Use body language—such as eye contact, body posture, gestures, and facial expressions—that is appropriate to and that matches the verbal message.
- Accept manipulative criticism while maintaining responsibility for your decision.
- Repeat a negative reply calmly without justifying it.
- Be honest about feelings, needs, and ideas.
- Accept and/or acknowledge your faults calmly and without apology.

Katz identifies other examples of assertive behavior (2009, p. 267):

- Express feelings without being nasty or overbearing.
- Acknowledge emotions but remain open to discussion.
- Express self and give others the chance to express themselves equally.
- Use *I* statements to defuse arguments.
- Ask for and give reasons.

This information provides a guide to improve and maintain effective assertiveness.

Advocacy in Leadership

Advocacy is speaking on behalf of something important, and it is one of the major nursing roles. Other content discussed advocacy for patients, but now we turn to advocacy as applied to the nursing profession and the need for nursing leaders to advocate for staff. To do this successfully, nurses need to feel empowered and be assertive. All nurses represent nursing—acting as advocates in their daily work and in their personal lives. When someone asks a nurse, "What do you do?" the nurse's response is a form of advocacy for the profession. The goal is to provide a positive, informative, and accurate response.

Stop and Consider #2

Power and empowerment should be part of the image of nursing.

Scope of Practice:

A Profession of Multiple Settings, Positions, and Specialties

---

Healthcare delivery requires nurses with multiple competencies and specialties to fulfill many different roles in a variety of healthcare settings. Healthcare delivery is never static. For example, there is greater interest today in public/community health and thus more need for nurses to enter this area and hold a variety of positions. The following discussion considers some of the issues related to the variety of healthcare delivery settings and roles and implications for nursing leadership.

Multiple Settings and Positions

The practice of nursing takes place in multiple settings, thus offering multiple job possibilities for an individual nurse over the nurse's career span. Many nurses change their settings, positions, and specialties based on interest and jobs that they want to pursue during their career. Some examples of the many different nursing settings and positions are provided here, and some are discussed in other chapters.

- *Hospital-based or acute care nursing:* This is the area that most students think of first when considering nursing positions. It is what is most frequently illustrated in the media (films, television, and so on). Within this setting are multiple specialty opportunities and clinical/management/education/research positions.
- *Ambulatory care:* This is a growing area for nurses, and these venues are considered to be community-based settings. Many types of ambulatory care settings exist, such as clinics, private practice offices, ambulatory surgical centers (both freestanding and associated with hospitals), and diagnostic centers (both freestanding and associated with hospitals). There is greater expansion in this area today with more focus on public-/community-based care. Nurses hold clinical and management positions in ambulatory care facilities.
- *Public/community health:* This area, which is growing rapidly, is an important clinical site for nursing students, and within this setting are multiple opportunities. Examples include clinical/management/education positions in public/community health departments, clinics, school health facilities, tuberculosis control centers, immunization clinics, home health, substance abuse treatment, mental health, occupational health, and more. Nurses may also be involved in development and implementation of public policy at the local, state, and federal levels to improve health and healthcare quality.
- *Home care:* This setting is very broad, in that numerous home care agencies exist across the United States. Some are owned and managed by government agencies,

such as city health departments; others are owned and managed by other HCOs, such as a hospital or may be part of national healthcare corporations, for-profit HCOs, or not-for-profit HCOs. Nurses in this specialty practice in the patient's home. They may also hold management positions within the home care agency, and some nurses may even own home care agencies. We typically think only about nurses and home care aides as working in home care, but there are some physicians who make home visits (Wasik, 2016)—though this is not common. Could home medical care reduce healthcare costs? "Aging in place" is a new focus to help older adults stay in their homes as long as possible, but getting healthcare services acts a barrier for many older adults. With new technology, we can do much more in the home and communicate better with patients to monitor their status, as discussed in the chapter on informatics and technology. Physician home visits require more time due to travel and other factors, and one might question if this is the best use of resources—additional experience and data are needed to determine if expanding this approach is best. APRNs also may practice in the home setting, providing more expanded nursing services.

- *Hospice and palliative care:* This type of setting may be partnered with home care, or it may be a freestanding service. Hospice and palliative care can also be associated with an inpatient unit that is either part of a hospital system or a freestanding facility. Hospice care has a special mission: to include patients, families, and significant others in the dying process and make the patient as comfortable as possible while meeting the patient's wishes. Palliative care or comfort care is also used when a life-threatening condition is present that may or may not result in death. Many acute care hospitals now have palliative care teams that provide support to the patient, family, and the staff who care for these patients on a daily a basis.

- *Nurse-managed health clinics (NMHCs):* NMHCs have increased due to the increased healthcare insurance coverage provided through the Affordable Care Act of 2010 (ACA); if the ACA continues in the same form, then this increase will likely increase. These clinics are community-based, primary healthcare services that operate under the leadership of an APRN and focus on health education, health promotion, and disease prevention. The population targeted by NMHCs is usually the underserved. NMHCs are not-for-profit organizations and typically use a sliding scale for payments. They may be classified as Federally Qualified Health Centers (FQHCs) (Kovner & Walni, 2010). Since 2010, the number of FQHCs has grown. In 2012, the National Nurse-led Care Consortium, a nonprofit member association representing more than 200 NMHCs throughout the United States, was formed (2016). These clinics focus on delivering care at the neighborhood level, connecting social service delivery needs and resources, and partnering with the community to advance health equity.

- *Retail clinics:* A healthcare delivery growth area is retail clinics. These are clinics located in retail areas, such in a pharmacy, a large grocery store, or a mall. The goal is to provide easy access to the consumer. Most of these clinics use APRNs as their primary care provider. Sometimes a for-profit corporation owns them, and others may be owned by academic health centers . It was thought that these clinics would reduce emergency department visits for low-acuity conditions; however, a recent study indicates that this is not necessarily true—there is a slight decrease of emergency department visits for patients with private insurance (Martsolf et al., 2016).

The researchers attribute the latter result to the fact that most retail clinics are located in higher-income, suburban areas. These clinics may also serve as a source of referrals to a medical center. We need more data over time to understand the outcomes from this type of ambulatory care setting.

- *School nursing:* This setting is part of public/community health nursing. The focus is on the provision of healthcare services within schools. The role of the school nurse is changing dramatically. Some schools have very active clinics where nurses provide a broad range of healthcare services to students. Pediatric APRNs have become more involved in school clinics that provide more expanded services.
- *Occupational health:* This is a unique setting for nursing practice. Nurses who work in this area provide healthcare services in occupational or work settings. They provide emergency care; direct care, including assessment, screenings, and preventive care; and health and safety education, and they may work with employer management to ensure a safer work environment. They also initiate referrals for additional care. Some schools of nursing offer graduate degrees in this area.
- *Telehealth/telemedicine:* Nurses work in telehealth by monitoring patients, providing patient and family education, and directing care changes. Home health may also use this method; although it is still not common, it is considered a care service area that will increase.
- *Parish nursing:* Parish nursing takes place in a faith-based setting, such as a church or other religiously affiliated institution. The nurse is often a member of the faith-based institution. Healthcare services might include screenings and prevention, health education, and referral services for the members of the institution.
- *Office-based nursing:* Nurses work in physician practices. Some of the nursing staff may be APRNs, and some APRNs may have their

own practices. Depending on their level of education, these nurses provide assessment and direct services, assist the physician, monitor and follow-up with patients, and teach patients and families. APRNs provide more advanced nursing care in this setting.

- *Extended care and long-term care:* Many nurses work in this area. With the aging population increasing, nursing staff needs will increase. Positions may be located in residential or community-based centers. Nurses provide assessment, direct care, and support to patients and support and education to families.
- *Management positions:* Nurse managers are found in all HCOs. The key responsibilities of this functional position are staffing, recruitment, and retention of staff; planning, budgeting, and staffing; supervising; QI; supporting EBP; staff education; and ensuring overall functioning of the nurse manager's assigned unit, division, or department.
- *Nursing education (academic and staff education):* This is a functional position. Academic faculty teach in nursing education programs. Nurses may also hold positions in staff development or staff education within HCOs, focusing on staff orientation, ongoing staff education, and maintenance of continued competencies.
- *Nursing research:* Nurses are involved in research in HCOs, academic institutions, and in the public/community arena. They fill many research roles, including serving as the primary investigator designing and leading research studies, collecting data, and analyzing data. Some healthcare institutions refer to this role as a nurse scientist. Nurses are not just conducting nursing research; they are also responsible for helping other interprofessional team members conduct research. In addition, because research provides important evidence for EBP, they contribute to the expansion and use of EBP.

- *Informatics:* Nurses are active in the area of informatics as a specialty and as a part of their other responsibilities. A nurse might serve on the informatics committee or participate in planning for implementation of an electronic medical record; if the nurse has advanced informatics expertise, the nurse may lead or help with major organizational informatics planning, implementation, and evaluation. Additional content explaining this role and preparation is discussed in this text's content about health informatics technology (HIT). It is an important new role for nurses and HCOs.
- *Nurse entrepreneurship:* Nurses may serve as consultants or own a healthcare-related business. Some may be involved in developing new healthcare products or in technology development, including computer products. This is an area that most nursing students do not know much about because it is a less common role for nurses; however, it is likely that this area will expand in the future.
- *Nurse navigator:* This nurse helps a patient and family navigate the healthcare system. HCOs may use different titles for a nurse who fulfills these functions. The nurse may coordinate care among several professions or provide a bridge between transitional care settings. For example, the patient who has cancer and has been discharged home may require care coordination between the acute care facility and oncology and radiology services. The patient may also need home visits. The nurse navigator helps find services and coordinates the care. Some HCOs use case managers for this purpose, as do insurers.
- *Legal nurse consultant:* This nurse usually has completed additional coursework related to legal issues and health care, and the nurse may even be certified in this area. The legal nurse consultant works with attorneys and provides advice about health issues, reviews medical records and other documents, and assists with planning legal responses. Some nurse legal consultants are hired by HCOs to assist their attorneys and participate in risk management functions. Nurses may be expert witnesses providing expert testimony for cases. Some nurses are also attorneys and thus function in a dual role in the area of healthcare legal issues.

It is unknown what the future holds for new healthcare settings or new roles, but nursing history demonstrates that the likelihood of new roles emerging is high. In an interview with nursing leaders, Porter-O'Grady commented that mobility and portability would become very important in technotherapeutic interventions (Saver, 2006). Technology is extending into patients' lives, and the settings in which care is received will be less connected to hospitals. Others suggest that as patients demand more control as consumers, there will be more self-diagnostic tests (Saver, 2006). Examples might be apps that are used to monitor and identify medical problems or monitor diet or exercise. New roles for nurses, in turn, will emerge to support changes. For example, nurses will assume more active roles in positions concerned with healthcare quality, in pharmaceutical companies, as nurse practitioners in clinics located in retail stores, managing research and development departments associated with equipment or biomedical companies, working in or leading medical homes, and in counseling (Saver, 2006). All of this change is occurring now, with more expected in the future, and requires greater nursing leadership competency.

Nursing Specialties

Nursing specialties are part of the profession and expand professionalism. There are numerous general specialties in nursing, such as maternal–child (obstetrics)/women's health, neonatal, pediatrics, emergency, critical care, ambulatory care, public/community health, home health, hospice, surgical/perioperative, psychiatric/mental health/ behavioral health, nurse–midwifery, management, legal nurse consulting, nursing consulting, and many more. There are also subspecialties such as diabetic care, wound care, and renal dialysis. The most important reason specialties develop is to meet the need for focused practice experience and ensure that nurses receive the necessary education to provide specialized nursing. Nurses may also become interested in a type of patient or care setting and want to learn more about it, gain more experience, and work in that area. All specialty nursing is based on the core general nursing knowledge and competencies. The same specialty might be offered in multiple settings—for example, a certified nurse–midwife (CNM) might work in a hospital in labor and delivery, a private practice with obstetricians, a clinic, a freestanding delivery center, patients' homes, or a nurse's (APRN) private practice.

There are two ways to view a specialty. One view is based on the nurse who works in a specialty area and thus claims it as his or her specialty (for example, the nurse works in a behavioral health unit and is then considered a psychiatric nurse). A second view, combined with the first, is that the nurse has additional education and possibly certification in a specialty. For example, the psychiatric nurse may have a master's degree in psychiatric–mental health nursing and may be certified in this specialty. The key to truly functioning as a specialty nurse is making a commitment to gain additional education in the specialty. This also includes CE and may include certification.

There are many titles in nursing, but they all do not necessarily indicate a nurse's specialty. These titles are APRN, CNS, and CNL. The titles for CNM and certified registered nurse anesthetists (CRNA) make their specialties clear in their titles (midwifery and anesthesia, respectively). An APRN may focus on one or more multiple specialties, such as families, pediatric acute care, adult–gerontology primary care or acute care, pediatric primary care,

neonatal care, and psychiatric–mental health. A CNL does not typically focus on a specific clinical group in the CNL degree program; instead, this is a functional role that may be used in any type of specialty area. For example, a CNL may hold a position in a medical unit, a pediatric unit, or a women's health unit. The CNS title is also a broader term, but the CNS master's degree focuses on a specific clinical area—it is not a common title today, with increased use of APRNs and CNLs. Specialty education at the graduate level and certification support professionalism in nursing and help to ensure that nursing remains a profession. As discussed in education content, many of these positions are transitioning to an entry-level doctor of nursing practice (DNP) degree.

Nurse leaders must continually support staff and the need for professionalism within the work setting. They do this by recognizing education and degrees through differentiated practice, encouraging ongoing staff education (CE and academic), ensuring that standards are maintained, working to increase staff participation in decision making, helping staff who want to move into a management position accomplish this goal (for example, by directing staff to management-focused education to prepare for the role), and mentoring staff who want to pursue the management track. Nurse leaders also need to encourage staff to participate in professional organizations; publish in professional journals; attend professional conferences; submit abstracts for presentations; participate in EBP, QI, and research; and then recognize these staff accomplishments throughout the organization.

Advanced Practice
Registered Nurse: Changing Scope of Practice

There has been increasing development in the role of the APRN. "Nurses' role in primary care has recently received substantial scrutiny, as demand for primary care has increased and nurse practitioners have gained traction with the public. Evidence from many studies indicates that primary care services, such as wellness and prevention services, diagnosis and management of many common uncomplicated acute illnesses, and management of chronic diseases such as diabetes can be provided by nurse practitioners at least as safely and effectively as by physicians" (Fairman, Rowe, Hassmiller, & Shalala, 2010, p. 280).

The report *The future of nursing* recommends increased expansion of nurses' scope of practice in primary care focused on advanced practice (IOM, 2010). The critical factor that limits nurse practitioners' scope of practice is state-based regulations. The website for the Center to Champion Nursing in America provides resources about nursing and about nurse practitioners and their scope of practice. Data are provided describing how specific states regulate nurse practitioner practice.

Other changes are occurring due to legislation that are important to the APRN scope of practice. One example is the movement allowing APRNs to sign home health plans of care and certify Medicare patients for home health benefits. This change required legislation, and in 2013, bills were introduced in both the U.S. House of Representatives (H.R. 2504) and the Senate (S. 1332) Home Healthcare Planning Improvement Act, endorsed by the American Nurses Association (ANA) and others. This legislation would allow payment for home health services to Medicare beneficiaries when these services are delivered by (1) a nurse practitioner, (2) a CNS working in collaboration with a physician in accordance with state law, (3) a CNM, or (4) a physician assistant under a physician's supervision. This change would facilitate providing greater home care services to the rural and underserved areas. Because this is federal legislation, it must be passed by both the House and the Senate and signed by the president to become law; however, this legislation was referred to a committee in 2013 and now sits in committees waiting for committee

action to move forward, and most likely will not. This is an example of how legislation gets "frozen in committee," and this is not an uncommon result for proposed legislation. Sometimes the legislation is re-introduced in a different form. Legislation and nursing may be connected—for example, *The future of nursing* report highlights many new position opportunities for APRNs such as in community health centers, nurse-managed health centers, medical/health homes, and accountable care organizations—but most if not all of these would never exist without health policy changes or new health policy. Some of the ACA provisions support these new care settings, illustrating how important healthcare legislation may be to nursing and why it is important to monitor changes in legislation as they may mean changes for nursing; however, not all may be positive.

A number of barriers exist to expansion of the role of nurse practitioners in primary care, particularly state laws that limit scope of practice; reimbursement policies; and may increase professional tensions among nurse practitioners, physicians, and physician assistants. Policy solutions need to (1) remove unwarranted restrictions on scope of practice, (2) equalize payment and recognize nurse practitioners as eligible providers, (3) increase nurses' accountability, (4) expand nurse-managed centers, (5) address professional tensions and focus more on interprofessional teams, (6) fund education for the primary care workforce, and (7) fund research to examine outcomes (Naylor & Kurtzman, 2010, p. 898).

Stop and Consider #3

There are new nursing positions for not only APRNs, but for all nurses.

Professional Practice

Today, professional **practice models** are described as having an impact both on the nursing profession and on quality care. A model describes the view of professional nursing for a group or a HCO—it may be a verbal description, visual, or both. The American Nurses Credentialing Center defines a professional practice model as the "driving force of nursing care; a schematic description of a theory, phenomenon, or system that depicts how nurses practice, collaborate, communicate, and develop professionally to provide the highest-quality care for those served by the organization (e.g., patients, families communities)" (American Nurses Association [ANA] & American Nurses Credentialing Center [ANCC], 2013a, p. 74). Some HCOs are developing, or have developed, their own professional practice models, but all should include the description of its "mission, vision, and values; how the organization manages and governs; how the organization cares for its patients; how various professions relate to one another; and how the organization develops and recognizes employees" (Robert & Finlayson, 2015, p. 26). Elements of a successful professional practice model should support expected nursing profession standards, differentiated practice, shared governance, collaboration, leadership, EBP, teams, and ongoing staff education. All of these elements are important topics and discussed in this text.

Differentiated Nursing Practice

Differentiated nursing practice is part of developing a professional practice model. The subject of desired degree for entry into nursing practice continues to be an issue in the nursing profession. As discussed in content on education, a decision was made in 1965 to establish the baccalaureate in nursing (BSN) as the nursing entry-level degree. The emphasis on the BSN degree in hospitals as part of the **Magnet Recognition Program**® has made a difference. These HCOs usually have more registered nurses (RNs) with BSN degrees (59% compared to 34% in non-Magnet hospitals) (ANA & AACN, 2017). Studies (Aiken, Clarke, Sloane, Lake, & Cheney, 2008;

Blegen, Goode, Park, Vaughn, & Spetz, 2013; Friese, Lake, Aiken, Silber, & Sochalski, 2008; McHugh et al., 2012) indicate that there is a positive impact on patient care when more RNs have a BSN degree. We are seeing more students in BSN programs, and more nurses returning to complete a BSN degree.

Graduates from all types of nursing programs take the same licensure exam, and this complicates the differentiated practice. RN licensure is the same for all nursing graduates regardless of the type of degree earned, which complicates the understanding of differentiated practice. Boston defined **differentiated nursing practice** as "a philosophy that focuses on the structuring of roles and functions of nurses according to education, experience, and competence" (1990, p. 1). This does not mean that a graduate from one program is necessarily better than another because many individual factors determine effectiveness; rather, it indicates that graduates from each program enter practice having completed a curriculum associated with a level of education and related competencies.

Differentiated practice needs to be more evident in nursing and relates to professional practice models, which may identify required levels of education and competency. Many employers do not formally recognize a nurse's degree. It is rarely noted on employee identification badges, and if noted, the degree designation is difficult to read on small name badges. Patients, and many other staff, do not know about nursing degrees and roles—they group all nurses together into the RN group. Another issue is that salaries are often not based on the education level of the nurse, although they should be. Much needs to be done by the profession to address this area of concern, and this requires professional leadership.

Examples of Professional Practice Models

Why does an HCO need a professional practice model for nursing? The description of the Magnet forces and the Magnet model provide some reasons for the need: "Conceptual models provide an infrastructure that decreases variation among nurses, the interventions they will choose, and, ultimately, patient outcomes. Conceptual frameworks also differentiate forward thinking organizations from those where nursing has less of a voice" (Kerfoot et al., 2006, p. 20). These forward-thinking HCOs also tend to have a professional rather than technical view of nursing. A model offers nurses "a consistent way of framing the care they deliver to patients and their families" (Kerfoot et al., 2006, p. 21).

Examples of professional practice models are found in **Figures 14-1, 14-2, 14-3, 14-4**, and **14-5**. Some of these models are not used today, but it is important to understand their evolution; sometimes they are used again or are revised. Notably, the functional model is used less today, although total care may be used in critical care. Primary care was very popular in the 1980s, but it is less so now because it requires a greater number of RNs. However, some HCOs still use the primary care model, usually as an adaptation of the original model. The Forces of Magnetism for Magnet hospitals emphasizes the need for HCOs to implement a professional practice model. The Magnet Recognition Program, which is a nursing practice model, is discussed later in this chapter.

The American Association of Critical-Care Nurses' Synergy Model for Patient Care is an example of a current nursing model (Kerfoot et al., 2006). This model's core premise is closely related to the five healthcare professions core competencies, particularly patient-centered care, by describing

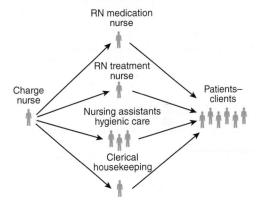

Figure 14-2 Functional Nursing Model

Reproduced from Hansten, R. I., & Jackson, M. (2004). *Clinical delegation skills: A handbook for professional practice.* Sudbury, MA: Jones & Bartlett Learning.

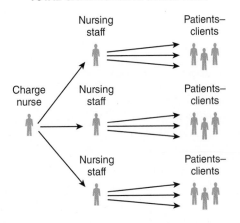

Figure 14-3 Total Patient Care Model

Reproduced from Hansten, R. I., & Jackson, M. (2004). *Clinical delegation skills: A handbook for professional practice.* Sudbury, MA: Jones & Bartlett Learning.

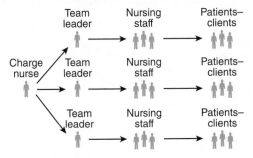

Figure 14-1 Team Nursing Model

Reproduced from Hansten, R. I., & Jackson, M. (2004). *Clinical delegation skills: A handbook for professional practice.* Sudbury, MA: Jones & Bartlett Learning.

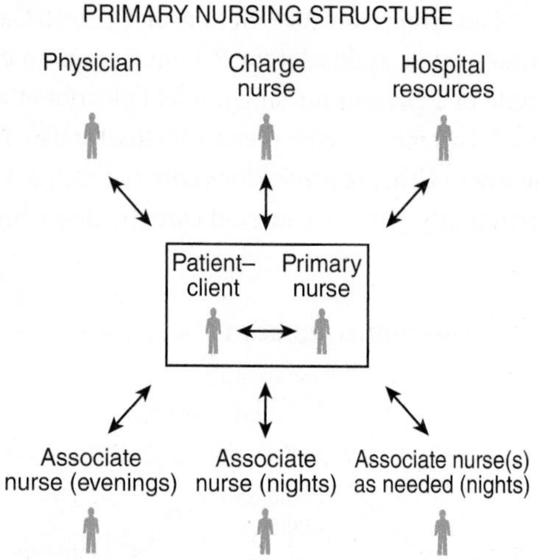

PRIMARY NURSING STRUCTURE

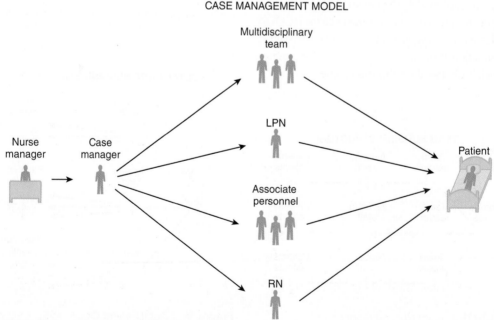

Figure 14-4 Primary Care Model

Reproduced from Hansten, R. I., & Jackson, M. (2004). *Clinical delegation skills: A handbook for professional practice*. Sudbury, MA: Jones & Bartlett Learning.

the needs of patients and families as the drivers of the characteristics and competencies of the nurse (American Association of Critical Care Nurses, 2017). The Synergy Model focuses on patient characteristics (resiliency, vulnerability, stability, complexity, resource availability, participation in care, participation in decision, and predictability) and nurse competencies (clinical judgment, advocacy, caring practices, collaboration, systems thinking, response to diversity, clinical inquiry, facilitation of learning, and clinical inquiry [innovator/evaluator]) (Harden & Kaplow, 2016). This model can be applied to all types of units, not just critical care.

Innovative new professional practice models have common elements (Kimball, Cherner, Joynt, & O'Neil, 2007). Specifically, they include an elevated RN role; greater focus on the patient; efforts

CASE MANAGEMENT MODEL

Figure 14-5 Case Management Model

Reproduced from Hansten, R. I., & Jackson, M. (2004). *Clinical delegation skills: A handbook for professional practice*. Sudbury, MA: Jones & Bartlett Learning.

to improve patient transitions and handoffs to decrease errors and make the patient more comfortable; leveraging of technology to enable care model design, such as electronic medical records, robots, bar coding, cell phone communication, and more; and greater emphasis on results or outcomes. The five healthcare professions core competencies also provide an effective start for a professional practice model (IOM, 2003b).

Stop and Consider #4

Differentiated practice has an impact on every nurse.

Impact of Legislation/

Regulation/Policy on Nursing Leadership and Practice

Legislation, regulations, and policies emphasize the need for nurses to work collaboratively with other stakeholders in shaping health policy through legislation and regulation. Nurses are involved and will continue to be involved at the local, state, national, and international levels. The current critical health policy issue is the Patient Protection and ACA. The increasing cost of health care, the increasing number of uninsured and underinsured individuals, and the growing aging population (along with concerns about the long-term ability of Medicare funds to cover all of their care) are all forces that helped to propel healthcare reform forward. The ACA, which focuses primarily on reimbursement/insurance, affects nurses and nursing care, and now the implementation phase requires active nursing participation to further develop this important policy. It will take time to evaluate the results of this initiative with regard to individual consumer satisfaction, access to care, quality of care, and of course, cost of care. These health policy issues have been and continue to be intense political battles,

particularly as changes are considered by the Trump administration. Changes that might be made due to change in administration are not known at this time but require nursing input as health policy is reviewed and revised or maintained. We need to recognize that even though the focus of ACA is on healthcare reimbursement, the legislation has had an impact on many areas of healthcare delivery; some may then be altered if ACA is repealed or changed.

Over the last decade, many agencies, through the establishment of state workforce centers, have examined the issue of the nursing supply and demand related to state legislation and regulation. State workforce centers focus on maintaining an adequate supply of qualified nurses within a state to meet healthcare needs (demand), providing analysis and strategies to address unmet needs (National Forum of State Nursing Workforce Centers, 2014). This initiative has been more successful on the state level than the federal/national level, though we need both perspectives to better prepare for supply and demand to meet staffing needs for all healthcare professionals. At the national level, a provision in the ACA established the National Health Care Workforce Commission. Its purposes are fivefold:

1. Serve as a resource for Congress, the president, and localities.
2. Coordinate activities of the Departments of Health and Human Services, Labor, Veterans Affairs, Homeland Security, and Education.
3. Develop and evaluate education and training activities.
4. Identify barriers to improved federal, state, and local coordination and recommend ways to address barriers.
5. Encourage innovation.

The commission was designed to include 15 members (each serving a 3-year term), and the commission as a whole to report to Congress. Membership must include no less than one representative from the following categories: healthcare workforce and health professions, employers, third-party payers, experts in healthcare services and health economics research, consumer representatives, labor unions, state or local workforce investment boards, and educational institutions. Although this commission was established and the Obama administration requested $3 million for the commission, this was not allocated; thus the commission has not been operational (Buerhaus & Retchin, 2013). This is described here as an example of how legislation might initiate a change, but if there is limited or no funding, the initiative can be blocked. With potential changes in ACA under the Trump administration, it is unclear if this ACA provision will ever be fully activated, though it is needed.

The American Academy of Nursing recently held a technology conference to examine work redesign and the use of technology as a means to transform nursing care. As this initiative evolved, a commission on the workforce was formed, led by representatives from both practice and education. It was quickly recognized that responses to nursing shortage problems must address the pipeline issue—that is, the faculty shortage, which in turn reflects on educational preparation of the workforce. A subcommittee addressing this issue included regulators from the National Council of Boards of Nursing, nursing education accreditation services such as from the National League for Nursing and the American Association of Colleges of Nursing, and officials from higher education and practice. The focus of this work is to identify barriers to increasing school of nursing enrollment and redesigning education at all levels. To make sweeping changes in this area, regulatory bodies also need to be included in the conversations to shape the new nursing educational models of the future. Quality of education to meet required competencies and differences in roles and responsibilities must also be considered. Work, such as done with this initiative, may then be used to support future legislation (state or federal) to address issues.

There is no doubt that quality care is a major issue addressed by healthcare legislation. Nurses need to be involved in these initiatives because they directly affect patient care every day in multiple settings. Healthcare legislation at the state level is also important to nurses. For example, many states are trying to pass legislation related to mandatory overtime and staff–patient ratios—and some states have already enacted these types of laws.

There is a nurses' caucus in Congress made up of nurses who serve in Congress. It serves as an important resource for nursing. More nurses are needed to run for office at the local, state, and national levels. Nurses who have an interest in politics and health policy have to plan for this activity, particularly if they want to run for office in the future. This requires a career plan with a time frame, mentoring, and experience in political activities.

Regulation is also an important issue today as change occurs both within the healthcare system and within nursing. One example is an initiative to change regulations related to APRNs, focusing on changes to allow APRNs to practice independently of physicians, when appropriate. Most states have not enacted such changes. There is often greater emphasis on the need for changes related to such issues as expansion of reimbursement for APRNs on the federal level. Reimbursement for APRNs represents a major change, and it will not be easy to accomplish.

Stop and Consider #5

To improve health care, we need more nursing leadership in health policy.

Economic Value
and the Nursing Profession

Salaries and benefits have long been a concern of nurses, which vary across the United States. Some nurses have unionized to get better salaries and benefits and to have more say in the decision-making process in the work setting. The nursing profession as a whole has yet to develop effective methods to determine their value in the reimbursement process and implications for HCO budgets, and it is important to solve this problem. How do nurses describe the value of nursing services? How do nurses identify costs of nursing services? Some efforts have been made to accomplish this, but there is much more to do. Within the fragmented healthcare system, nursing contributions are even more difficult to identify. Most HCOs' accounting systems are not able to capture or differentiate economic value provided by nurses (IOM, 2010).

APRNs have brought the issue of payment for nursing services to the forefront. Some examples of issues that have arisen relate to reimbursement. The Federal Employee Compensation Act—a law that provides healthcare services to federal employees who are injured on the job—has become important to APRNs. It is one of the last major federal healthcare programs to deny patient access to APRNs. APRNs are now covered medical providers in Medicare, Medicaid, Tri-Care, and some private insurance plans, and they serve as medical providers in the Veterans Administration, the U.S. Department of Defense, and the Indian Health Service. If they choose, most federal employees have access to APRNs through their federal employee health benefit plan.

Because greater emphasis has been placed on healthcare quality, there is now more focus on a pay-for-performance model—third-party payers and government determine payment for services based on performance or quality care (Saver, 2006). This change is exemplified by the Centers for Medicare and Medicaid Services' (CMS) and other insurers' refusal to pay for certain complications experienced by patients (hospital-acquired complications) or for 30-day post-discharge unplanned readmissions, as discussed in content on QI. In turn, this policy has an impact on nursing care and on budgetary decisions related to nursing. Because nurses are involved in most of the care associated with these complications and with discharge planning, nurses have an opportunity to exhibit leadership in these

areas and demonstrate that they can have a major impact on the quality of care and cost of care by developing effective interventions to assess risk and prevent these complications and prepare for more effective transitions to discharge.

Stop and Consider #6

We still do not have consistent and effective recognition of the economic value of nursing practice.

The Nursing Work
Environment

The nursing work environment is critical for quality care, patient satisfaction, staff satisfaction, recruitment and retention, HCO financial stability (for example, if an HCO has high staff turnover, the HCO will have higher expenses associated with recruitment and orientation), development of leadership and effective management, and effective use of interprofessional teams. This section discusses some issues relevant to healthy work environments.

The Work Environment and Leadership

Quality care is best provided in a healthy, functional work environment. Key issues are staff safety; communication; collaborative, positive work relationships; work design (space/facility); work processes; infrastructure that support staff participation in decision making; and an emphasis on positive work environments that support staff and reduce staff stress/burnout and high turnover rates and seek to develop staff. This requires an environment in which staff members respect one another and incivility is controlled, as discussed in other content in this text. Nurse managers need to develop and maintain a work environment that engages staff in work processes, decision making, and continuous quality improvement (CQI). Job resources, interpersonal relationships, job performance, and proactive work behavior are factors that influence the work environment (Warshawsky, Havens, & Knafl, 2012).

The future of nursing report highlights the unique needs of new graduates and recommends nurse residency programs as a means to increase retention of staff, guiding transition into the workplace and affecting the quality of care (IOM, 2010). The nursing profession is currently focusing much of its attention on APRNs; however, most nurses are not APRNs, but rather staff nurses who have complex staff needs and work in a complex environment. If these needs are not addressed, this omission will have a major negative impact on patient care—more significantly, it will affect quality as well as nursing practice. We need to know more about the problems, but more importantly, the nursing profession needs to actively address the problems for all nurses and not just focus on APRNs.

Workforce Issues and Effective Staffing

RNs represent a large number of healthcare professional healthcare providers in the United States: As of September 2016, there are a total of 3,880,565 RNs and 913,453 licensed practical nurses and licensed vocational nurses (LPN/LVNs) in the United States (National Council for State Boards of Nursing [NCSBN], 2016a). Of this number, 2,687,310 RNs and 695,610 LPN/LVNs were employed as of May 2015. Compared to 10 years ago, RN employment increased and LPN/LVN employment decreased. There are also now many more APRNs in a variety of healthcare roles and settings. "More than 250,000 APRNs are in the United States, categorized into four distinct roles: the certified nurse practitioner, the certified registered nurse anesthetist (CRNA), the certified nurse midwife (CNM), and the clinical nurse specialist. Certified nurse practitioners constitute nearly 70% of the total number of APRNs, with nurse practitioners reportedly numbered at

222,000 in 2014" (American Association of Nurse Practitioners, 2016). The CRNA accounts for approximately 20% of total APRNs (NCSBN, 2017, p. 4). Staffing in all types of healthcare settings has an impact on staff morale, staff retention, the budget, and quality care. Staffing is also a power issue—scheduling affects staff directly and their ability to engage in decision making. Fairness in patient assignments and staff scheduling has a positive impact on the manager–staff relationship (Cathro, 2013). All aspects of staffing are critical in the workplace environment. The fact that staffing needs are not static, even changing throughout the day, makes this a very complex workforce issue as noted in the following discussion.

We have a large number of RNs and will need more. Staffing is a critical concern in providing quality care, and multiple factors need to be considered: patient acuity and changes in status, staff expertise, mix of staff, supervision, budget, staff fatigue and stress, staff behaviors that may lead negativity such as incivility, physical environment, admissions and discharges, presence of students (any type of healthcare profession student), presence and quality of medical staff, access to resources such as a pharmacist, need and methods used to transport patients, use of electronic documentation, position descriptions, standards, policies and procedures, access to EBP resources, presence of family members or significant others, leadership within the HCO, budget, staff orientation and education, and more. These factors demonstrate that staffing is more than just the number of staff. There is increased interest from nursing leadership to better address these factors in the workplace. An example is staff fatigue from long hours and shift work. In 2016, the ANA held a webinar focused on helping nurse leaders deal with staff fatigue, emphasizing the need to implement evidence-based strategies to proactively address this problem—"to promote the health, safety, and wellness of registered nurses and ensure optimal patient outcomes" (ANA, 2016). The ANA also offers resources on nurse fatigue on its website.

A topic that has long caused concern for the nursing profession is potential and real nursing shortages (American Association of Colleges of Nursing [AACN], 2014). There have been periods of time when there were national shortages and regional shortages. In addition, individual HCOs may experience shortages, which may be due to budget cuts, recruitment problems, and poor HCO ratings, thus reducing applications for positions and/or leading to staff retention problems, and so on. A nursing shortage is expected as more nurses retire due to the number of nurses approaching retirement age. This is coupled with a growing need for more nurses with expansion of care services. According to the Bureau of Labor Statistics' employment projections for 2012–2022, released in December 2013, "Registered nursing (RN) is listed among the top occupations in terms of job growth through 2022. The RN workforce is expected to grow from 2.71 million in 2012 to 3.24 million in 2022, an increase of 526,800 or 19%. The Bureau also projects the need for 525,000 replacements nurses in the workforce bringing the total number of job openings for nurses due to growth and replacements to 1.05 million by 2022" (U.S. Department of Labor & Bureau of Labor Statistics, 2013).

Staffing and related workforce issues are directly related to nursing education. To meet demands, there must be sufficient graduates from nursing programs, and this means there must be sufficient qualified applicants in nursing program admission pools. A shortage of nursing faculty has led to nursing programs turning away qualified students, as discussed in other chapters. Efforts have been made to provide funding for graduate education to increase the faculty pool. We will also need more nurses who are competent to care for the growing aging population. This will require both pertinent clinical content and experiences with this population in nursing programs (pre-licensure and graduate levels) and staff education to increase staff competencies in this area.

The work environment is an important factor in recruiting and retaining nurses. The environment is high stress; however, some HCOs have more problems in this area leading to staff dissatisfaction, burnout, turnover, and a decrease in productivity. All of this may lead to a reputation of a poor place to work, and this drives employee applicants away. HCOs need to continually assess these issues and institute changes to reduce stress in the workplace, and staffing is one of these factors. "Ensuring adequate staffing levels has been shown to (ANA, 2014):

- Reduce medical and medication errors
- Decrease patient complications
- Decrease mortality
- Improve patient satisfaction
- Reduce nurse fatigue
- Decrease nurse burnout
- Improve nurse retention and job satisfaction"

Staff scheduling approaches should consider patient acuity; strategies for using unlicensed assistive personnel; staff skills and competencies (skill mix), education, and training required for specific settings; and effective use of delegation. Staffing levels are related to quality care and to meeting patient outcomes, as well as staff satisfaction and a healthy work environment. For example, a recent study reported that staffing in 71 acute care hospitals in two states indicated that work schedules are significantly related to patient mortality when staffing levels and characteristics were controlled (Trinkoff et al., 2011). This study relates to earlier work done led by Dr. Aiken about the impact of nurse staffing on patient mortality and quality care (Aiken, Clarke, Sloane, Sochalski, & Silber, 2002). "The safety of nurses from workplace-induced injuries and illnesses is important to nurses themselves as well as to the patients they serve. The presence of healthy and well-rested nurses is critical to providing vigilant monitoring, empathic patient care, and vigorous advocacy" (Trinkoff et al., 2008, p. 2473). The HCO needs to commit to developing and maintaining a culture of safety, and this must include staff safety issues. The level of staffing impacts staff safety—for example, if there are too few staff, this may lead to more staff stress and staff injuries—for example, when lifting patients without considering the most effective interventions and/or asking for help.

Appendix B provides some guidelines about staffing that are important for students to review to better understand staffing and scheduling. The guidelines also provide important information that should be considered when searching for first nursing positions—staffing should be an important topic in job interviews, and applicants need to be prepared with questions addressing this topic.

Interprofessional Teams and the Work Environment

Interprofessional teams are critical in today's healthcare workplace, as discussed throughout this text. One of the healthcare professions core competencies is the ability to use interprofessional teams effectively as teams have a major impact on the work environment. Despite this well-known need, an effective approach to preparing nursing students and other healthcare profession students to work on teams is still lacking. The assumption is these individual healthcare professionals will be able to work on teams after they graduate—but that outcome does not necessarily happen. Newhouse and Mills (2002, pp. 64–69) identified key points related to nurse–physician relationships that are important in the development of effective interprofessional teams:

- All teams are not created equal, but careful development of working relationships and clear goals can make all the difference.
- Successful teams are composed of competent team members with the necessary skills, abilities, and personalities to achieve the desired objectives.
- Teams composed of many professions/disciplines are able to expand the number and quality of actions to improve healthcare systems.

- Interprofessional teams work collaboratively to set and achieve goals directed toward innovative and effective care and efficient organizational systems.
- Nurses on the team represent the voice of nursing as a discipline responsible for the holistic care of patients.
- Positive relationships with physicians benefit the patient and enhance the work environment for nurses.
- Nurses must develop the skills to work collaboratively as professional members of the interprofessional team.

As has been discussed in this text, teams are a critical component of healthcare and interprofessional teams have become more important. Nurses, however, are also members of nursing teams. For both types of teams, team functioning is the same—the same teamwork principles apply. A study examined whether there was a relationship between nursing teamwork and the presence of nurse-sensitive outcomes (for example, pressure ulcers, falls, catheter-associated urinary tract infections) (Rahn, 2016). Rahn's study indicates there is a significant relationship, and improving teamwork can have a positive impact on reducing the occurrence of preventable adverse outcomes. Nursing needs to understand this in order to develop education (content and learning experience), leadership, and practice solutions to reduce adverse patient outcomes. This is a critical part of QI. Another factor that is important to consider with any type of team (nursing or interprofessional) is changing team membership, a problem for most healthcare teams. Leaders need to monitor this factor and its impact on team functioning. Lack of long-term team membership may be a problem as well as increasing the need for team orientation, which is not often a routine requirement. If a nurse leader can improve teamwork, this may have a direct impact on performance, improving care.

Improving the Work Environment

Nurses need to take the lead in HCOs to improve the work environment—by identifying concerns, helping to identify supporting data and analyzing the data, understanding retention of staff, assisting in the development of strategies to resolve problems, and tracking outcomes to improve the work environment and level of care. It has been noted that staff are using workarounds more, which increases risk of errors in a work environment. A *workaround* is an effort to get something done without following the expected process, standards, policy, or procedure. This situation means staff do not recognize or understand a potential risk for error so that it is difficult to correct and improve. Efforts to improve and develop an effective,

healthy work environment need to consider the five healthcare professions core competencies and critical elements in the work culture. **Exhibits 14-2** and **14-3** describe examples of improvement strategies.

The March 2014 issue of *Charting nursing's future*, a newsletter that was created following the publication of *The future of nursing* report, describes an emerging blueprint to transform the nurses' work environment that recommends providers, policy makers, and educators use the following strategies (Robert Wood Johnson Foundation, 2014, p. 8):

- Monitor nurse staffing and ensure that all healthcare settings are adequately staffed with appropriately educated, licensed, and certified personnel.
- Create institutional cultures that foster professionalism and curb disruptions.

Exhibit 14-2 Transition Policy and Strategies

Goal: Anticipate and prepare the nurse labor market for impending shortages, thereby reducing their duration and impact and lowering the economic and noneconomic costs to patients, nurses, and hospitals.

Strategies	Transition Policy
Demand strategies	<ul><li>Speed up development and adoption of technology and use nonprofessional nursing personnel more effectively</li><li>Remove barriers to efficiency and redesign the work content and organization of nursing care</li><li>Strengthen management decision making</li><li>Avoid regulating nurse staffing</li></ul>
Supply strategies	<ul><li>Accommodate an older RN workforce</li><li>Accelerate improvements in working conditions</li><li>Expand the capacity of nursing education programs</li><li>Continue to inform the public about opportunities in nursing</li></ul>
Wage strategies	<ul><li>Assist hospitals and other healthcare employers in financing needed RN wage increases</li><li>Avoid imposing controls on RN wages</li></ul>

Reproduced from Buerhaus, P. I., Staiger, D. O., & Auerbach, D. I. (2009). *The future of the nursing workforce in the United States: Data, trends, and implications.* Sudbury, MA: Jones & Bartlett Learning.

> ### Exhibit 14-3 Long-Run Policy and Strategies
>
> **Goal:** Expand employment of RNs in the long run by eliminating barriers that lead to an inadequate supply of RNs and by appropriately valuing the contributions of RNs.
>
> | Strategies | Long-Run Policy |
> |---|---|
> | Supply strategies | • Remove barriers to hiring foreign-educated RNs
• Remove stigmas and barriers facing men and Hispanics |
> | Demand strategies | • Reinforce development of pay-for-performance systems
• Increase the number of nursing-sensitive outcomes included in pay-for-performance systems |
>
> Reproduced from Buerhaus, P. I., Staiger, D. O., & Auerbach, D. I. (2009). *The future of the nursing workforce in the United States: Data, trends, and implications.* Sudbury, MA: Jones & Bartlett Learning.

- Harness nurse leadership at all levels of administration and governance.
- Educate the current and future workforce to work in teams and communicate better across the health professions.

All of these strategies relate directly to the healthcare professions core competencies discussed throughout this text.

Finding the Right Workplace for You

Students begin the process of finding the right work environment for themselves when their clinical courses begin. You begin to consciously or unconsciously assess each work environment you encounter by asking, "Would I want to work here?" In doing so, you also begin to integrate your ideas about nursing, "What is a nurse?" and "Is this profession right for me?" Socialization into the profession begins at this stage. By the time senior year arrives, you are actively beginning to consider positions after graduation. Along with your review of **Appendix B** to gain a better understanding of staffing, which is a critical issue to consider when assessing positions, review **Appendix C**, which provides tips related to finding the right workplace for you.

Stop and Consider #7

You need to be involved in improving the healthcare work environment.

Quality Improvement
and Nursing Leadership

There is no question that all nurses need to be more active in CQI. The American Organization of Nurse Executives supports nursing leadership in HCOs and describes key principles that need to be considered to guide the role of the nurse in future patient care delivery, including in CQI. This is described in **Figure 14-6**. Nurse managers and administrators need to be leaders in the HCO in setting QI direction and determining strategies to improve care at all levels and engaging nursing staff in the process. Some nurses should serve in key QI positions. At the health policy level, nurses should be active at the local, state, and federal levels in the development of QI health policy; they may assume many roles to provide leadership in the health policy-making process. Nursing faculty provide QI leadership by ensuring that students, both undergraduate and graduate, are prepared to practice, understand

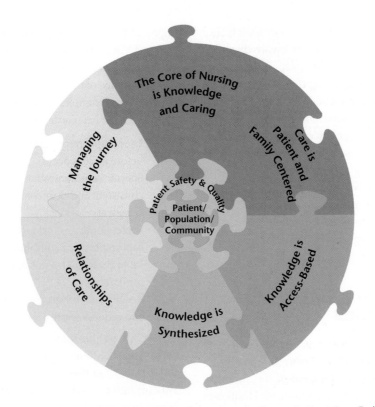

Figure 14-6 AONE Guiding Principles for the Role of the Nurse in Future Patient Care Delivery

and know how to apply information about CQI, utilize EBP and EBM, and engage in CQI during clinical experiences. The following sections discuss examples of some new initiatives that relate to CQI and nursing leadership focused on improving care.

The National Quality Strategy (NQS) is discussed in this text; however, in this chapter it is important to emphasize that the NQS is relevant to nurses and nursing care (Kennedy, Murphy, & Roberts, 2013). Nurses need to understand the strategy and integrate it into nursing education, practice, and research. The NQS has at its center the Triple Aim (better care, healthy people, affordable cost). Its priorities are (U.S. Department of Health and Human Services & Agency for Healthcare Quality and Research, 2017):

- Making care safer by reducing harm caused in the delivery of care
- Ensuring that each person and family is engaged as partners in their care
- Promoting effective communication and coordination of care
- Promoting the most effective prevention and treatment practices for the leading causes of mortality, starting with cardiovascular disease
- Working with communities to promote wide use of best practices to enable healthy living
- Making quality care more affordable for individuals, families, employers, and governments by developing and spreading new health care delivery models

After reviewing each of the priorities, it is clear that nurses and nursing care are involved in all of the priorities, but nurses must step up and engage as HCOs turn to integrating the NQS in their QI programs, as is recommended by the NQS and the HHS. In addition, we need more nursing leadership in all levels of health policy, and a critical example is the Trump administration's potential changes in healthcare delivery and reimbursement. Nurses need to advocate for quality care for all people; there should be no disparities in quality care. This requires knowledge of issues, keeping up-to-date with potential changes, providing professional input, and monitoring progress.

Transforming Care at the Bedside

The creation of Transforming Care at the Bedside (TCAB) is a result of the *Quality Chasm* reports (IOM, 2001). The development of this initiative began in 2003 through the Institute for Healthcare Improvement (IHI) in conjunction with the Robert Wood Johnson Foundation. The IHI is an effective initiative that provides multiple strategies for improving health care—its website provides excellent QI resources. "The goal is to make fundamental improvements in the healthcare delivery system that will result in safe and reliable care, vitality and teamwork, patient-centered care, and value-added care processes" (Martin et al., 2007, p. 445). In 2008, the TCAB program was implemented in 10 hospitals, starting in a hospital unit and then spreading throughout the hospital. The approach that was taken was to establish pilots in hospitals at the level of direct care, which could, after testing, have a greater impact on the entire organization. The current focus areas are safe and reliable care, vitality and teamwork, patient-centered care, and value-added care processes (Institute for Healthcare Improvement [IHI], 2017).

TCAB looks not only at innovative change, but also at the outcomes from the change. Did care improve? Was care monitored using indicators such as injury from falls, adverse events, readmission, voluntary turnover of RNs, patient satisfaction, and percentage of nurses' time in providing direct patient care? Examples of some of the innovative ideas that have been tested are (IHI, 2017):

- Use of rapid response teams to rescue patients before a crisis occurs
- Specific communication models that support consistent and clear communication among caregivers
- Professional support programs such as preceptorships and educational opportunities
- Liberalized diet plans and meal schedules for patients
- Redesigned workspace that enhances efficiency and reduces waste

TCAB has an impact on care delivery and nursing practice by introducing effective, innovative changes that can then be used in many hospitals. This initiative provides many opportunities for nurses to assume leadership in improving healthcare delivery—leadership can occur at the level of the staff nurse, the nurse manager, or other nurse administrative positions. The TCAB website provides information on the TCAB framework and current TCAB projects.

Magnet Recognition Program®

It is important that nurses assume active roles in determining the quality of care and the nurse's role in the process. Nurses run the risk of taking the blame for some of the problems that are found in acute care today. "Politics in healthcare may not end at the bedside, but it certainly begins there. It would be a tragedy if patients and family members blamed nurses for system failures. But the more nurses detach from their patients, the easier it becomes for the rest of us (consumers) to lose sympathy" (Kaplan, 2000, p. 25). The Magnet program, which offers a nursing professional practice model, is one way to address this issue. It is the "highest credential for nursing excellence and the leading source of successful nursing practices and strategies worldwide" (Robert & Finlayson, 2015, p. 8).

In 1981, researchers conducted a study that explored the issue of attracting and retaining nurses (McClure, Poulin, Sovie, & Wandelt, 1983). This study played a significant role in attempts to address the shortage at that time because it identified some methods for improving recruitment and retention of nurses. The researchers sought to identify factors or variables that have an impact on acute care hospitals in their staff recruitment and retention success. Stimulated by these results, the Magnet program was established in 1993 to be administered by the American Nurses Credentialing Center's (ANCC) Commission on the Magnet Recognition Program® (ANA & ANCC, 2014). Recognition is awarded to acute care hospitals and long-term care facilities. The program provides a "roadmap to achieve nursing excellence using the five model components and sources of evidence to drive organizational performance focused on improving the quality of patient care while lowering costs" (Robert & Finlayson, 2015, p. 12). The five model components are: (1) collaborative care practice; (2) transformational leadership; (3) culture; (4) evidence, research, and innovation; and (5) professional growth and development (ANA & ANCC, 2013a, 2013b, 2013c, 2013d, 2013e). The model and its components support the five healthcare professions core competencies, the Quality and Safety Education for Nurses (QSEN) competencies, and national initiatives to improve care such as the *Quality Chasm* reports, including *The future of nursing* report, *Healthy People 2020*, the NQS, and CMS QI efforts.

It is not an easy process to be awarded Magnet status. It requires commitment and time from HCO leadership, nursing leadership, and staff. Any size HCO that meets the standards may apply for Magnet status. "**Accreditation** as a voluntary process used to validate that an organization and

an approval body meet established continuing education standards. Recognition is a process used to evaluate an organization's adherence to excellence-focused standards" (Urden & Monarch, 2002, pp. 102–103). The Magnet program is a recognition program, not an accreditation program. Magnet HCOs must also successfully receive and maintain accreditation from The Joint Commission.

The first step for an HCO that wants to apply for Magnet status recognition is to complete a self-assessment using materials provided by the program. The HCO then has a better idea about where it stands and what needs to be improved before completing the application to achieve recognition. The recognition process does not focus solely on management; staff nurses must be involved in all steps of the process. After extensive sharing of information, an onsite survey is completed by the Magnet surveyors. Once recognition is obtained—and not all HCOs that apply receive Magnet status—the organization must maintain the expected standards, participate in the National Database of Nursing Quality Indicators® (NDNQI) (Press Ganey, 2017), and provide certain annual monitoring reports to ensure that the requirements for Magnet recognition continue to be met over time. Studies indicate that achieving recognition has a positive impact on Magnet HCOs, such as improving professional practice, clinical competence, and job experience—all of which influence staff retention rates (Aiken et al., 2008; Havens, 2001; Stone et al., 2006; Ulrich, Buerhaus, Donelan, Norman, & Dittus, 2007). Recognition is not permanent, however, and the HCO must apply for renewal. A website is maintained with current information about the Magnet program.

A hospital that has Magnet status also demonstrates a different form of management, focusing more on participative management in which staff members have input into decisions, with managers listening to staff, and typically using a decentralized structure, such as shared governance. This difference in management is evident in the role of the nurse executive and throughout all levels of nursing management, as well as in the overall organizational leadership's support of nursing. Effective leadership is present. Staff members feel the HCO nursing leaders understand their needs and provide resources and support for the work that staff perform daily—that is, the managers demonstrate transformational leadership. These hospitals have more nurses with BSN degrees because this is a Magnet requirement. Nurses are very active in committees, projects, and so on. EBP is actively pursued, and the hospitals are involved in nursing research. Clearly, staffing is of critical concern, and Magnet hospitals use innovative methods to respond to recruitment and retention issues and provide appropriate mix and levels of staffing per shift. Staff education is valued: There are opportunities for quality staff development, and staff members who want to pursue additional academic degrees are encouraged to do so. Promotion can occur through the management track, which is the most common method, but it also should occur through the clinical track. These HCOs typically demonstrate higher levels of quality of care, autonomy, a nursing model, mentoring, professional recognition, staff education and support for career development such as completing baccalaureate degree or a graduate degree, and respect of staff. They enable staff to practice nursing as it should be practiced.

Research in this area did not stop with the original 1981 study. Multiple studies that support the positive impact of Magnet recognition have been conducted. These HCOs have better outcomes—lower burnout rates, higher levels of job satisfaction, and higher quality of care—than non-Magnet HCOs (Laschinger, Shamian, & Thomson, 2001). Kramer and Schmalenberg, reexamined 14 Magnet hospitals and identified variables that are important in providing quality care (2002). These variables relate to nursing leadership demonstrated by formal leaders in management positions and by staff leaders, emphasizing transformational leadership and continue to be relevant today (pp. 53–55):

1. Working with other nurses who are clinically competent
2. Good nurse–physician relationships
3. Nurse autonomy and accountability
4. Supportive nurse manager–supervisor
5. Control over nursing practice and practice environment
6. Support for education
7. Adequacy of nurse staffing
8. Paramount concern for patients

There are now significant research results that indicate that Magnet HCOs tend to provide quality care that leads to positive outcomes for patients and better work environments for nurses (Aiken, 2002). As a result of the research on the Magnet program, 14 **Forces of Magnetism** were identified. These forces relate to the five components of the model and are used to evaluate an HCO and determine whether it can be designated as a Magnet HCO (ANA & ANCC, 2013a, 2013b, 2013c, 2013d, 2013e). Nurses who are considering new positions might use these variables or the forces to guide their job search, as the variables assist nurses in learning more about the HCO and help to assess whether the HCO has a positive workplace. If the HCO already has Magnet status, the forces should be present, but if not, the nurse applicant can still use the forces as a personal checklist. Less than 8% of HCOs reach Magnet recognition, but many more have Magnet-like characteristics that support quality care (Robert & Finlayson, 2015). The Magnet Program is not prescriptive and allows its recognized HCOs to be innovative as long as the expected criteria are met. The Forces of Magnetism represent the organizational elements of excellence in nursing care (ANA & ANCC, 2017):

1. Quality of nursing leadership
2. Organizational structure
3. Management style
4. Personnel policies and programs
5. Professional models of care
6. Quality of care

7. QI
8. Consultation and resources
9. Autonomy
10. Community and the HCO
11. Nurses as teachers
12. Image of nursing
13. Interdisciplinary (interprofessional) relationships
14. Professional development

Stop and Consider #8
Every nurse needs to be a leader in QI.

Moving the Profession
Forward: Students Are the Future of Nursing

In conclusion, we turn to the nursing report, *The future of nursing: Leading change, advancing health* (IOM, 2010) and assess the status of its recommendations. It is also important to emphasize that nursing leadership and development of leadership does not just apply to nurses but also to nursing students.

The Future of Nursing: Leading Change, Advancing Health

The future of nursing: Leading change, advancing health is a landmark report that addresses the need for nursing leadership. "By virtue of its numbers and adaptive capacity, the nursing profession has the potential to effect wide-ranging changes in the healthcare system. Nurses' regular, close proximity to patients and scientific understanding of care processes across the continuum of care give them a unique ability to act as partners with other health professionals and to lead in the improvement and redesign of the health care system and its many practice environments" (IOM, 2010, p. S-3).

Related to *The future of nursing* report, the Robert Wood Johnson Foundation conducted a Gallup poll in 2010 entitled "Nursing Leadership from Bedside to Boardroom" (Blizzard, Khoury, & McMurray, 2010). The purpose of the poll was to ask opinion leaders about their views of nursing leadership, particularly nurses' role and future and potential barriers. Past and current Gallop Polls on the image of nursing, as discussed in other content, typically indicate that the public views nurses as highly ethical and honest; however, this 2010 poll questioned why nurses continued to lag behind as leaders in the healthcare delivery system. The following were the key findings of this opinion poll about healthcare leadership and nursing (Blizzard, Khoury, & McMurray, 2010):

- Respondents rated doctors and nurses first and second out of a list of options for *trusted* information about health and health care.
- Government and insurance executives will have a great deal of influence in health reform in the next 5 to 10 years.
- Respondents perceived patients and nurses as having the least amount of influence in health reform in the next 5 to 10 years.
- Reducing medical errors and increasing the quality of care are two areas where nurses now have a great deal of influence in policy and management.
- Relatively few opinion leaders say nurses currently have a great deal of influence in increasing access to care, including primary care.
- Reducing medical errors, increasing quality of care, and promoting wellness top the list of areas in which large majorities of opinion leaders would like nurses to have more influence.
- Major barriers to nurses' increased influence and leadership were identified as not being perceived as important decision makers or

revenue generators compared with doctors, nurses' focus on primary care rather than preventive care, and nursing not having a single voice in speaking on national issues.

- Suggestions for nurses to take on more of a leadership role included making their voices heard and having higher expectations.

These results, which were identified in 2010 just as the ACA became law and *The future of nursing* report was completed, do not paint a positive picture of nursing leadership, but do identify some areas that require active nursing strategies to improve and develop leadership. Some of these elements have improved since 2010, but much more work is needed to develop nursing leadership.

The future of nursing report focuses on three nursing areas that need transformation: practice, education, and leadership (IOM, 2010). The leadership approach discussed is transformational leadership, with its emphasis on collaborative management. The report supports the leadership competencies discussed throughout this text. In particular, it supports interprofessional collaboration and QI by noting that it is important to learn "to be a full partner in a health team in which members from various professions hold each other accountable for improving quality and decreasing preventable adverse events and medication errors" (IOM, 2010, pp. 5–4). Leadership is needed among nurses who hold any position, and this need even extends to nurses who assume more entrepreneurial and business approaches.

In 2014, Sigma Theta Tau International (STTI) joined a global effort to improve nursing leadership. It formed the Global Advisory Panel on the Future of Nursing (GAPFON), whose purpose is to serve as a catalyst to stimulate partnerships and collaborations to advance global health outcomes (STTI & GAPFON, 2016). This initiative is directly related to the STTI theme, "Serve Locally, Transform Regionally, Lead Globally" (STTI, 2014). The focus is global nursing leadership, an important leadership for focus for the profession.

Susan Hassmiller, a nursing advisor to the Robert Wood Johnson Foundation, identified her vision for a 21st-century nursing workforce, which is related to the recommendations in *The future of nursing* report. This vision includes the following interconnected processes (Hassmiller, 2011):

- Develop nurse-led innovations
- Generate evidence
- Redesign education
- Embrace technology
- Diversify our workforce
- Expand scope of practice
- Foster interprofessional relationships
- Develop leadership at every level
- Be at the table

These are critical points that provide a guide for improving nursing leadership and engaging nurses in the healthcare delivery process. Furthermore, these points also apply to nursing leadership in healthcare policy development and implementation to improve health and health care.

Progress Report on The Future of Nursing: Leading Change, Advancing Health

In 2016, a critical progress report was published assessing the status of the recommendations from *The future of nursing: Leading change, advancing health* (IOM, 2010; National Academy of Medicine [NAM], 2016). Just as it is important to evaluate health care, it is also important to evaluate what the nursing profession accomplishes; thus, we turn to examining what has been done to reach the recommendations from the 2010 nursing report and how this affects nursing and its role in CQI (Pittman, Bass, & Hargraves, 2015). During the time from 2011 to 2016, including the passage of the ACA, there has been greater emphasis on CQI throughout the healthcare system. The Future of Nursing: Campaign for Action (the Campaign), which is a partnership with the Robert Wood Johnson Foundation and AARP, supports the recommendations of the 2010 report and provides a source of information and resources to assist the profession in implementing strategies to meet the recommendations (Campaign for Action, 2016).

The following content summarizes some of the key issues in the progress report by commenting on each of the *The future of nursing* recommendations and outcomes. As discussed in many chapters in this book, since 1999 and the first *Quality Chasm* reports, we have moved to a greater concern about quality, diversity and disparities, teams and interprofessional teamwork, cost, collaboration, care coordination, patient-centered care, and integration of the Triple Aim (better care, healthy people/healthy communities, affordable care) in our view of the healthcare delivery system. The progress report recommendations are related to all of these issues—even more so than in 2010 because there is now greater understanding of the quality care problems and greater initiatives to improve. The recommendations are noted in bold with commentary added and relevance to CQI described in italics (Finkelman, 2018, pp. 459–463; IOM, 2010):

1. **Remove scope of practice barriers:** In 2010, 13 states met the criteria for full practice authority, and since then, 8 more states have been added. Some states have made some changes but still do not fully meet the criteria. The CMS has expanded the scope of practice for CMS payment; however, medical staff membership and hospital privileges for APRNs continue to be based on state laws and business preferences rather than federal law. This outcome is not met with only 13 states improving since 2010, and more than 50% of the states do not meet the recommendation. *How does scope of practice affect CQI? It affects nursing practice—what nurses do. In the case of this report, the focus was on APRNs. What APRNs and also RNs can do in their practice is directed by state nurse practice acts. Scope of practice is part of each state's nurse practice act. The CMS as a federal program can determine*

what services and providers it will cover in its reimbursement payment system, but it cannot dictate state law. HCOs need to then ensure that all healthcare professions follow the requirements to meet the standards.

2. **Expand opportunities for nurses to lead and diffuse collaborative improvement efforts:** "The ACA provisions include development of new models of care to accommodate the large numbers of people previously without access to health insurance. These models focus on teamwork, care coordination, and prevention—models in which nurses can contribute a great deal of knowledge and skill" (NAM, 2016, p. 15). Some of these new models are accountable care organizations, nurse-managed clinics, and others. These new models support and assist in meeting this recommendation. Collaboration is a critical component of care today, and it is important to effective interprofessional teamwork, one of the healthcare professions core competencies identified in the *Quality Chasm* reports (IOM, 2003b). *Effective CQI requires care coordination and collaboration from many stakeholders—nonclinical and clinical, healthcare professional organizations, professional education programs, accrediting organizations, government agencies, and third-party payers. The new models provide new opportunities for nurses, and in the future, it is hoped other models will be developed—and nursing roles and responsibilities expanded.*

3. **Implement nurse residency programs:** At the time of the publication of *The future of nursing* report, there was concern about staff turnover and retention, and these continue to be concerns. The use of residency programs is one method that may reduce this problem, and the report focused on these programs for post-licensure RNs. The progress report notes that there is also need for this type of program for nurses transitioning to new settings and for APRNs.

In 2011, the National Council for State Boards of Nursing engaged in research about transition-to-practice programs (NCSBN, 2016b). Residency programs vary, but the progress report notes that they do have value in helping nurses develop competencies important to improving practice and self-confidence in practice. There is also need for similar programs focused on nurses in outpatient settings. This result indicates there has been some progress, although more programs are needed. These programs are costly to develop and implement. The American Association of Colleges of Nursing nurse residency accreditation provides a model and standards for nurse residency programs focused on baccalaureate graduates (BSN), although not all existing residency programs are accredited (AACN, 2016). *The programs can be particularly helpful in developing nurses to participate in CQI by including EBP, CQI, and EBM content and experiences.*

4. **Increase the proportion of nurses with a baccalaureate degree to 80% by 2020:** "Baccalaureate program enrollment has increased substantially since 2010: Entry-level baccalaureate enrollment increased from 147,935 in 2010 to 172,794 in 2014; accelerated baccalaureate enrollment increased from 13,605 to 16,935; and baccalaureate completion enrollment (so-called RN to bachelor of science in nursing [BSN]) increased from 77,259 to 130,345" (NAM, 2016, p. 6). There are other important improvements such as the number of 4-year nursing programs/BSNs increased, and more employers require their RNs to have minimum of a BSN degree. However, the progress report indicates a need to continue to focus on improving nursing education programs. Funding for degrees has been relatively flat, which is a barrier to increasing enrollment. *Leaders are needed in all types of healthcare settings to improve care. Education is needed to prepare competent nurses who can assume roles that include CQI activities,*

meeting the healthcare core competency related to QI (IOM, 2003b).

5. **Double the number of nurses with a doctorate by 2020:** The recommendation does not specify details as to type of doctorate and number per type (DNP, PhD in nursing, PhD in another field). Enrollment in total has increased 15% in 5 years. Major barriers are funding and number of faculty and their experience for these degree programs. This level of increase makes it difficult to meet this recommendation by 2020. *QI content should be part of all doctoral programs in order to develop more nursing leadership that understands QI and applies it in practice, education, and research.*

6. **Ensure that nurses engage in lifelong learning:** "Continuing education and competence have not kept pace with the needs of the increasingly complex, team-based health care system. Nurses and other providers will increasingly need to update skills for providing care in both hospital and community-based settings" (NAM, 2016, p. 7). *We need more data about CE, particularly about its impact on patient outcomes. As noted in other chapters, there have been greater efforts to understand and support interprofessional CE (IOM, 2009). In addition, we need to better understand the implications of the relationship between nurse certification and credentialing and lifelong learning and their impact on practice and patient outcomes, as well as on collaboration and leadership. Education, including lifelong learning, is discussed in other chapters, and it is critical for maintaining and developing knowledge and competencies. Lifelong learning should include content and experiences related to CQI because this is a rapidly changing area and one in which nurses must actively participate. If we expect staff to engage in interprofessional teams within the context of CQI and practice, interprofessional initiatives are particularly important.*

7. **Prepare and enable nurses to lead change to advance health:** There has been progress with the Campaign and development of the Interprofessional Education Collaborative supported by the Josiah Macy Jr. Foundation. In 2013, the Campaign noted that more work needs to be done to increase interprofessional collaboration. Leadership continues to lag—for example, the percentage of nurses who serve on hospital boards. In a 2011 survey of 1,000 hospitals, nurses held 6% of the positions and physicians 20%, and in 2014, physicians held the same percentage with nurse representation decreasing by 5%. This is not a positive outcome. There are, of course, many other types of leadership, and nurses are involved or need to be more involved in a variety of leadership situations. Hospital boards direct the vision and goals of hospitals, including CQI, and thus are important to nursing; however, other types of boards in the community and for other types of HCOs are just as important (Walton, Lake, Mullinix, Allen, & Mooney, 2015). Communicating the need for nursing leadership and what nurses can offer has progressed, but this effort has primarily focused on informing nurses. More needs to be done to inform other healthcare professionals, patients, families, and so on about the roles of nurses, and not just during the annual National Nurses' Week. *Changes in health care and in roles require that we consider QI implications and ensure that standards are met.*

8. **Build an infrastructure for the collection and analysis of interprofessional healthcare workforce data:** This book discusses measurement—how it works and barriers to success. The progress report notes similar concerns in assessing the outcomes of *The future of nursing* recommendations. Data must be collected and analyzed to drive decisions. As discussed earlier, the ACA included a provision to establish the National Healthcare Workforce Commission, which focused on all healthcare professions, including nursing. This was to be a resource for gathering workforce data and analysis. Many states have established their own workforce commissions; however, we also need a national perspective and one that includes all healthcare professions, and this is not yet sufficiently available. One workforce problem that *The future of nursing* report noted was nursing workforce diversity, and it continues to be a problem identified in the progress report. Some data about diversity in the nursing have been collected. The progress report, however, notes that a review of 5 years is not a sufficient time period to effectively evaluate these outcomes. The progress report notes, "African Americans make up 13.6 percent of the general population aged 20 to 40, and 10.7 percent of the RN workforce, 10.3 percent of associate's degree graduates, and 9.3 percent of baccalaureate graduates. The disparity is even greater for Hispanics/Latinos, who make up 20.3 percent of the general population aged 20 to 40, but only 5.6 percent of the RN workforce, 8.8 percent of associate's degree graduates, and 7.0 percent of baccalaureate graduates. Men make up just 9.2 percent of the RN workforce, 11.7 percent of baccalaureate nursing students, and 11.6 percent of graduates" (NAM, 2016, p. 9). Important focus points are recruitment, retention, and success in nursing education programs. Diversity needs to be a workforce priority. The progress report identifies barriers to data collection that need to be addressed: lack of consistent national indicators to provide consistent state-to-state data, lag time in data collection and reporting, lack of standardized databases, and need to use proxy measures to assess progress in meeting *The future of nursing* recommendations. The lack of a national infrastructure (the commission) to meet this recommendation continues to be a major problem. *Workforce data are also*

important to CQI. This information provides greater understanding of the current status of problems related to staffing levels and mix and competent staff (all healthcare professions, not just nursing). This information can then be used to develop strategies to address these problems, address problems with recruitment and retention as a component of ensuring quality care and reducing errors, and support funding for health professions education and identify improvements that might be needed in health professions education programs.

The progress report concludes with: "Continued work is needed to remove scope-of-practice barriers; pathways to higher emphasis on increasing diversity; avenues for continuing competence need to be strengthened; and data on a wide range of outcomes are needed—from the education and makeup of the workforce to the services nurses provide and ways in which they lead. A major and overarching need is for the nursing community, including The Campaign, to build and strengthen coalitions with stakeholders outside of nursing. Nurses need to practice collaboratively; continue to develop skills and competencies in leadership and innovation; and work with other professionals, as no one profession alone can meet the complex needs of the future of health care" (NAM, 2016, p. 16). Progress has been made, but not enough. Assessing some of the original report's recommendations using a 5-year time span is not sufficient time to determine if recommendations are met, but this is enough time to identify some weaknesses in reaching recommendations that require more effort.

If we are to develop nursing leadership and be more engaged, then we need to get involved in all aspects of healthcare change. As an example of change described by the National Academy of Medicine in a recent article about its initiative *Vital directions for health and health care*, the future will be one of interaction: "policy and practice in the nation's health, healthcare, and biomedical science communities" (Dzau, McClellan, & McGinnis, 2017). The initiative goals are highlighted in content throughout this text.

Student Leadership

Students need to begin developing their leadership skills while in their nursing educational program. This can be done by participation in student organizations, such as the National Student Nurses Association; working to be invited into STTI; or assuming leadership roles in courses and in other on-campus and off-campus activities. Developing leadership takes time, and every nurse needs leadership competencies to practice in today's complex healthcare system. Leadership development does not necessarily have to be done only in a nursing context—your involvement in campus activities and other organizations are all opportunities to develop leadership and learn more about yourself, communication, teamwork, handling conflict, and so on.

Moving forward implies change. Many people do not like change or do not feel comfortable with it. During an interview, the nurse leader Porter-O'Grady stated, "Our work isn't changing. Change is our work." He tells nurses, "If you looked at change like that, it wouldn't be an enemy" (Saver, 2006, p. 24). Patton, another nurse leader who served as president of the ANA, advised: "See opportunities instead of challenges" (Saver, 2006, p. 24). Nurses entering the profession have before them a healthcare delivery system in need of repair, as has been noted by many experts and reports. This challenge can be seen as an impossible task or as an opportunity for nurses to step up and assume new roles and expand old roles, if need be. Reforming the U.S. healthcare delivery system requires that nurses are educated; are competent in all five healthcare professions core competencies; provide quality nursing care; are able to communicate and collaborate effectively with others; use political skills; and advocate for patients, families, communities, and the nursing profession. Nurses need to base their decisions on EBP and EBM, whether they are in clinical practice, management, or education. They need to understand the possibilities that come with technology, participate in determining how technology can be used, and then use it effectively. Change should be based on data and analysis of data—for example, from nursing research. Data are also associated with CQI, another area in which nurses need to step up and participate so that they are among the healthcare professionals who drive QI, thereby, influencing how health care is provided. Last but not least, nurses of the future need to recognize that money drives most decisions. Understanding how money flows and how to communicate the value of nurses and nursing care are important nursing responsibilities.

Linda Burns-Bolton, vice president and chief nursing officer at Cedars-Sinai Medical Center, believes that in the future, "Nurses will get the evidence they need when they need it, get information for patients when they need it, deliver safe care, communicate with team members, engage with family members, and leave work feeling satisfied" (Saver, 2006, p. 25). Her view of the future really covers the key elements found in this text and the five core competencies (IOM, 2003b), but is not yet fully realized:

1. Provide patient-centered care
2. Work in interdisciplinary/interprofessional teams
3. Employ EBP
4. Apply QI
5. Utilize informatics

This text's content is an introduction to nursing as a profession; to the healthcare system; and, most importantly, to patients, their families, and communities. Nursing is a dynamic profession with multiple possibilities. A nurse can participate in many different nursing positions throughout the nurse's career. Some positions require additional education; others do not. As described in this chapter, nurses practice in many different settings. The future holds more change that will lead to new possibilities. You will have the responsibility as a nurse to participate actively in the profession to advocate for your patients (individuals, families, populations, communities) and demonstrate leadership in your practice.

Stop and Consider #9

As a nursing student, you need to begin developing leadership competencies now.

CHAPTER HIGHLIGHTS

1. There is much change occurring in nursing and in health care today.
2. Transformational leadership is the most effective leadership style. Transformational leaders are confident, self-directed, honest, loyal, and committed, and they have the ability to develop and implement a vision.
3. A leader may or may not hold a formal management position.
4. Nurses should influence how the healthcare delivery system works and be actively involved in healthcare delivery changes in all the clinical, management, or education positions that they may hold.
5. Nursing practice occurs in multiple settings, positions, and specialties.
6. Differentiated practice, shared governance, and collaboration are important elements of a successful professional practice model.
7. Legislation, regulation, and policy emphasize the need of nurses to work collaboratively with other stakeholders in shaping health policy through legislation and regulation.

(Continues)

CHAPTER HIGHLIGHTS (CONTINUED)

8. The economic value of nursing focuses on salaries and benefits, but it also needs to consider the value of nurses themselves and how the healthcare delivery system values nursing care.

9. Quality care requires a work environment focused on the need for a healthy, functional work environment.

10. Nurses need to assume active leadership roles in CQI.

11. The Magnet Recognition Program recognizes HCOs that provide quality nursing care or excellence in nursing care.

12. The goal of the TCAB program is to make improvements in the healthcare delivery system focused on direct care—"at the bedside."

13. *The future of nursing: Leading change, advancing health* (IOM, 2010) report has had a major impact on nursing education and practice.

14. The progress report for *The future of nursing: Leading change, advancing health* (IOM, 2010; NAM, 2016) indicates we still have much to do to meet the original recommendations.

15. Students have responsibility to develop leadership competency.

ENGAGING IN THE CONTENT

Discussion Questions

1. Why is leadership important in nursing? Your response should demonstrate knowledge of the differences between leadership and management.

2. Consider one of the issues in this chapter and conduct a literature review on an issue that interests you. Share your critique with classmates. How does the issue apply to leadership?

3. What is the Magnet Recognition Program? Why is it important?

4. Why should you as a student begin to work on your leadership competencies?

CRITICAL THINKING ACTIVITIES

1. What is a nursing professional practice model? Describe one type of model. Is one used in a clinical site where you have been? If so, what is it? How do the nurses demonstrate the model in their practice? What do you think about the model?

2. Visit YouTube on the Internet, and search for "nursing" or "nurses." What do you find? View one of the selections and critique the image portrayed. Discuss your findings in a team with classmates.

(Continues)

CRITICAL THINKING ACTIVITIES (CONTINUED)

3. In a team with your classmates, consider how the five core competencies might be used as a framework for a professional practice model. Describe your model in narrative form and graphically on large paper your instructor provides. Post it in the classroom. Each team should then explain its model.

4. After completing Critical Thinking Activity 3, each team should review another team's vision and decide which education, regulatory, and practice issues apply to the vision. What is the role of leadership?

ELECTRONIC REFLECTION JOURNAL

Develop your vision of the future of nursing. How does it compare with the "real world"? Save this vision and review it every 6 months while in school to see if your vision changes; then review it again after graduation as you enter into practice. You may find your vision of the future of nursing changes.

CASE STUDIES

Case 1

The CNL functions as a care coordinator either at the unit level or in a practice. For example, Ms. Apple heads up a busy practice in a cancer institute. As a CNL, she acts as a mentor to novice nurses while coordinating care and helping patients navigate the healthcare maze.

In one patient's case, Ms. Apple identified the need for transportation to and from radiation appointments. She also recognized financial counseling needs because the patient was no longer able to work, and her husband was on disability. Treatment plans needed to be explained, and teaching the patient about medications was necessary. A referral had been made to a radiation interventionist. The family needed knowledge about the problems and explanation about all aspects of care. The CNL pulled the interprofessional team together to ensure clear communication and the creation of an interprofessional plan of care.

CASE STUDIES (CONTINUED)

In some institutions, these positions are called nurse navigators; in others, CNLs, depending on the organization's structure and needs. The CNL, having expertise in interprofessional communication, financial management, and human relations, serves the patient and family to protect and ensure quality patient-focused care and promote safety. (Find out more about nurse navigators: Pruitt, Z., & Sportsman, S. (2013). The presence and roles of nurse navigators in acute care hospitals. *Journal of Nursing Administration, 43*(11), 592–596.)

Case Questions

1. Search the Internet to find HCOs that have CNL and nurse navigator positions. What can you learn about these positions?
2. Find nursing programs on the Internet that offer the CNL master's degree. Compare and contrast them.
3. How does these new positions apply or not apply to the five healthcare professions core competencies?

Case 2

You have taken a new position as a head nurse for a 30-bed unit. You have been working in the hospital for 7 years—for the first 4 years as a staff nurse and for the last 3 years as the assistant nurse manager on a surgical unit. However, the new position means you have to change units. The chief nursing officer arranged for you to have a mentor, another nurse manager, to help you as you transition to the new role and new unit. Before you meet with your mentor for the first time as a mentee, you consider the following questions.

Case Questions

1. What is your personal view of the transformational leadership style? Do you feel competent in applying this style? Why or why not? How might the leadership style of the previous nurse manager affect your transition to the position?
2. What should your unit assessment plan include as you assume your new role?
3. You have been told that the unit has an RN retention problem that has been increasing over the last 2 years. What more do you need to know about the problem?
4. The nursing department uses shared governance. How might this affect you and your new position?

Working Backward to Develop a Case

Write a brief paragraph that describes a case related to the following questions.

1. But if we want to be better leaders what should we do?
2. If you are not in a management position, I do not understand why this is important.
3. How might we use *The future of nursing* report and the follow-up progress report?

REFERENCES

Aiken, L. (2002). Superior outcomes for Magnet hospitals: The evidence base. In M. McClure & A. Hinshaw (Eds.), *Magnet hospitals revisited* (pp. 61–81). Washington, DC: American Nurses Publishing.

Aiken, L., Clarke, S., Sloane, D., Lake, E., & Cheney, T. (2008). Effects of hospital care environment on patient mortality and nurse outcomes. *Journal of Nursing Administration, 38*(5), 223–229.

Aiken, L. H., Clarke, S. P., Sloane, D. M., Sochalski, J., & Silber, J. H. (2002). Hospital nurse staffing and patient mortality, nurse burnout, and job dissatisfaction. *Journal of the American Medical Association, 288*(16), 1987–1993.

American Association of Colleges of Nursing. (2014, April). *Nursing shortage fact sheet.* Retrieved from http://www.aacn.nche.edu/media-relations/fact-sheets/nursing-shortage

American Association of Colleges of Nursing. (2016). *Nurse residency program.* Retrieved from http://www.aacn.nche.edu/education-resources/nurse-residency-program

American Association of Critical-Care Nurses. (2017). *The AACN synergy model for patient care.* Retrieved from https://www.aacn.org/nursing-excellence/aacn-standards/synergy-model

American Association of Nurse Practitioners. (2016). *American Association of Nurse Practitioners fact sheet.* Retrieved from https://www.aanp.org/all-about-nps/np-fact-sheet

American Hospital Association. (2002). *In our hands: How hospital leaders can build a thriving workplace.* Chicago, IL: Author.

American Nurses Association. (2014). *Workforce advocacy.* Retrieved from http://nursingworld.org/workforceadvocacy

American Nurses Association. (2016). *Nurse fatigue.* Retrieved from http://www.nursingworld.org/NurseFatigue

American Nurses Association, & American Nurses Credentialing Center. (2013a). *Magnet application manual for 2014.* Silver Spring, MD: Author.

American Nurses Association, & American Nurses' Credentialing Center. (2013b). *Structural empowerment: Criteria for nursing excellence, Magnet®.* Silver Spring, MD: Authors.

American Nurses Association, & American Nurses' Credentialing Center. (2013c). *Exemplary professional practice: Criteria for nursing excellence, Magnet®.* Silver Spring, MD: Authors.

American Nurses Association, & American Nurses' Credentialing Center. (2013d). *New knowledge, innovations, & improvements: Criteria for nursing excellence, Magnet®.* Silver Spring, MD: Authors.

American Nurses Association, & American Nurses' Credentialing Center. (2013e). *Transformational leadership: Criteria for nursing excellence, Magnet®.* Silver Spring, MD: Authors.

American Nurses Association, & American Nurses Credentialing Center. (2014). *Magnet Recognition Program® model.* Retrieved from http://www.nursecredentialing.org/magnet/programoverview/new-magnet-model

American Nurses Association, & American Nurses' Credentialing Center. (2017). *Announcing new model for ANCC's Magnet Recognition Program®.* Retrieved from http://www.nursecredentialing.org/Magnet

ModelBennis, W., & Goldsmith, J. (1997). *Learning to lead: A workbook on becoming a leader.* Reading, MA: Perseus Books.

Bertholf, L., & Loveless, S. (2001). Baby boomers and generation X: Strategies to bridge the gap. *Seminars for Nurse Managers, 9,* 169–172.

Blegen, M., Goode, C., Park, S., Vaughn, T., & Spetz, J. (2013, February). Baccalaureate education in nursing and patient outcomes. *Journal of Nursing Administration, 43*(2), 89–94.

Blizzard, R., Khoury, C., & McMurray, C. (2010). Nursing leadership from bedside to boardroom: Opinion leaders' perceptions. Robert Wood Johnson Foundation, *Nursing Research Network.* Retrieved from http://www.rwjf.org; full Gallup Poll report available at http://rwjf.org/files/ research/nursinggalluppolltopline.pdf

Boston, C. (1990). Differentiated practice: An introduction. In C. Boston (Ed.), *Current issues and perspectives on differentiated practice* (pp. 1–3). Chicago, IL: American Association of Nurse Executives.

Buerhaus, P., & Retchin, S. (2013). The dormant healthcare workforce commission needs congressional funding. *Health Affairs, 32*(11), 2021–2024.

Campaign for Action. (2016). *Campaign for action.* Retrieved from http://campaignforaction.org/

Cathro, H. (2013). A practical guide to making patient assignments in acute care. *Journal of Nursing Administration, 43*(1), 6–9.

Dzau, V., McClellan, M., & McGinnis, M. (2017). Vital directions for health and health care. Priorities from a National Academy of Medicine initiative. *Journal of American Medical Association, 317*(14), 1461–1470. Retrieved from http://jamanetwork.com/journals/jama/fullarticle/2612013

Fairman, J., Rowe, J., Hassmiller, S., & Shalala, D. (2010). Broadening the scope of nursing practice. *New England Journal of Medicine, 364*(3), 280–281.

Finkelman, A. (2016). *Leadership and management for nurses: Core competencies for quality care* (3rd ed.). Upper Saddle River, NJ: Pearson Education.

Finkelman, A. (2018). *Quality improvement. A guide for integration in nursing.* Burlington, MA: Jones & Bartlett Learning.

Friese, C., Lake, E., Aiken, L., Silber, J., & Sochalski, J. (2008). Hospital nurse practice environments and outcomes for surgical oncology patients. *Health Services Research*, 43(4), 1145–1163.

Gerke, M. (2001). Understanding and leading the quad matrix: Four generations in the workplace. *Seminars for Nurse Managers, 9,* 173–181.

Goffee, R., & Jones, G. (2000, September–October). Why should anyone be led by you? *Harvard Business Review,* 63–71.

Harden, S., & Kaplow, R. (Eds.) (2016). *Synergy for clinical excellence: The AACN synergy model for patient care.* (2nd ed.) Burlington, MA: Jones & Bartlett Learning.

Hassmiller, S. (2011). Vision for 21st century nursing workforce. Retrieved from http://thefutureofnursing .org/21stCenturyNursing

Havens, D. (2001). Comparing nursing infrastructure and outcomes: ANCC Magnet and non-Magnet CNEs report. *Nursing Economics, 19*(6), 258–266.

Hess, G. (2004). From bedside to boardroom: Nursing shared governance. *Online Journal of Issues in Nursing, 9*(1). Retrieved from http://www.nursingworld.org /MainMenuCategories/ANAMarketplace/ANA Periodicals/OJIN/TableofContents/Volume92004/No1 Jan04/FromBedsidetoBoardroom.aspx

Institute for Healthcare Improvement. (2017). *Transforming care at the bedside.* Retrieved from http://www.ihi .org/Engage/Initiatives/Completed/TCAB/Pages /default.aspx

Institute of Medicine. (2001). *Crossing the Quality Chasm.* Washington, DC: The National Academies Press.

Institute of Medicine. (2003a). *Leadership by example.* Washington, DC: The National Academies Press.

Institute of Medicine. (2003b). *Health professions education.* Washington, DC: The National Academies Press.

Institute of Medicine. (2004). *Keeping patients safe: Transforming the work environment of nurses.* Washington, DC: The National Academies Press.

Institute of Medicine. (2009). *Redesigning continuing education in the health professions.* Washington, DC: The National Academies Press.

Institute of Medicine. (2010). *The future of nursing: Leading change, advancing health.* Washington, DC: The National Academies Press.

Kaplan, M. (2000). Hospital caregivers are in a bad mood. *American Journal of Nursing, 100*(3), 25.

Katz, J. (2009). *Keys to nursing success.* (3rd ed.). Upper Saddle River, NJ: Pearson Education.

Kennedy, R., Murphy, J., & Roberts, D. (2013, September 30). An overview of the national quality strategy: Where do nurses fit? *Online Journal of Issues in Nursing, 18*(3). Retrieved from http://www.nursingworld.org /MainMenuCategories/ANAMarketplace/ANA Periodicals/OJIN/TableofContents/Vol-18-2013 /No3-Sept-2013/National-Quality-Strategy.html

Kerfoot, K., Lavandero, R., Cox, M., Triola, N., Pacini, C., & Hanson, M. (2006, August). Conceptual models and the nursing organization: Implementing the AACN synergy model for patient care. *Nurse Leader,* 20–26.

Kimball, B., Cherner, D., Joynt, J., & O'Neil, E. (2007). The quest for new innovative care delivery models. *Journal of Nursing Administration, 37,* 392–398.

Kovner, C., & Walni, S. (2010). Nurse managed health centers (NMHCs). Robert Wood Johnson Foundation. *Nursing research network.* Retrieved from http://www .rwjf.org

Kramer, M., & Schmalenberg, C. (2002). Staff nurses identify essentials of magnetism. In M. McClure & A. Hinshaw (Eds.), *Magnet hospitals revisited* (pp. 25–59). Washington, DC: American Nurses Publishing.

Laschinger, H., Shamian, J., & Thomson, D. (2001). Impact of Magnet® hospital characteristics on nurses' perceptions of trust, burnout, quality of care, and work satisfaction. *Nursing Economics, 19,* 209–219.

Lewis, H., & Cunningham, C. (2016). Linking nurse leadership and work characteristics of nurse burnout and engagement. *Nursing Research, 65*(1), 13–23.

Malone, B. (2001). Nurses in non-nursing leadership positions. In J. Dochterman & H. Grace (Eds.), *Current issues in nursing* (6th ed., pp. 293–298). St. Louis, MO: Mosby.

Martin, S., Greenhouse, P., Merryman, T., Shovel, J., Liberi, C., & Konzier, J. (2007). Transforming care at the bedside. *Journal of Nursing Administration, 37,* 444–451.

Martsolf, G., Fingar, K., Coffey, R., Kandrack, R., Charland, T., Eibner, C., . . . Mehrotra, A. (2016). Association between the opening of retail clinics and low-acuity emergency department visits. *Annals of Emergency Medicine.* Retrieved from http://www.annemergmed .com/article/S0196-0644(16)30998-2/pdf

McClure, M., Poulin, M., Sovie, M., & Wandelt, M. (1983). *Magnet hospitals: Attraction and retention of professional nurses*. American Academy of Nursing Task Force on Nursing Practice in Hospitals. Silver Spring, MD: American Nurses Association.

McHugh, M., Kelly, L., Smith, H., Wu, E., Vanak, J., & Aiken, L. (2012). Lower mortality in magnet hospitals. *Medical Care 51*(5), 382–388.

Murray, K., Yasso, S., Schomburg, R., Terhune, M., Beidelschies, M., Bowers, D., & Goodyear-Bruch, C. (2016). Journey of excellence: Implementing a shared decision-making model. *AJN, 116*(4), 50–56.

National Academy of Medicine. (2016). *Assessing progress on the IOM report The Future of Nursing*. Washington, DC: The National Academies Press.

National Council of State Boards of Nursing. (2016a). *National nursing database: A profile of nursing licensure in the US*. Retrieved from https://www.ncsbn.org/national-nursing-database.htm

National Council of State Boards of Nursing. (2016b). *Transition-to-practice*. Retrieved from https://www.ncsbn.org/transition-to-practice.htm

National Council of State Boards of Nursing. (2017). Highlights of the 2017 environmental scan. *Journal of Nursing Regulation, 7*(4), 4–14.

National Forum of State Nursing Workforce Centers. (2014). *About us*. Retrieved from http://nursingworkforce centers.org/AboutUs.aspx

National Nurse-led Care Consortium. (2016). *National nurse-led care consortium*. Retrieved from http://www.nncc.us/about-nurse-managed-care

Naylor, M., & Kurtzman, E. (2010). The role of nurse practitioners in reinventing primary care. *Health Affairs, 29*(5), 893–899.

Newhouse, R., & Mills, M. (2002). *Nursing leadership in the organized delivery system for the acute care setting*. Washington, DC: American Nurses Publishing.

Pittman, P., Bass, E., & Hargraves, J. (2015). The future of nursing. Monitoring the progress of recommended changes in hospitals, nurse-led clinics, and home health, and hospice agencies. *Journal of Nursing Administration, 45*(2), 93–99.

Press Ganey. (2017). *National database of nursing quality indicators®*. Retrieved from http://www.pressganey.com/solutions/clinical-quality/nursing-quality

Porter-O'Grady, T. (1999). Quantum leadership: New roles for a new age. *Journal of Nursing Administration, 29*(10), 37–42.

Rahn, D. (2016). Transformational teamwork. Exploring the impact of nursing teamwork on nurse-sensitive quality indicators. *Journal of Nursing Care Quality, 31*(3), 262–268.

Ritter-Teitel, J. (2002). The impact of restructuring on professional nursing practice. *Journal of Nursing Administration, 32*(1), 31–41.

Robert, N., & Finlayson, S. (2015). *Fundamentals of Magnet® toolkit*. Silver Spring, MD: American Nurses Association.

Robert Wood Johnson Foundation. (2014). An emerging blueprint for change. *Charting Nursing's Future, 22*, 8. Retrieved from http://www.rwjf.org/en/culture-of-health/2014/03/new_charting_nursing.html

Santos, S., & Cox, K. (2002). Generational tension among nurses. *American Journal of Nursing, 102*(1), 11.

Saver, C. (2006). Nursing—today and beyond: Leaders discuss current trends and predict future developments. *American Nurse Today, 10*, 18–25.

Siela, D. (2006, December). Managing multigenerational nursing staff. *American Nurse Today*, 47–49.

Sigma Theta Tau International. (2014). *About us*. Retrieved from http://www.nursingsociety.org/aboutus/Pages/AboutUs.aspx

Sigma Theta Tau International, & Global Advisory Panel on the Future of Nursing. (2016). *Global Advisory Panel on the Future of Nursing*. Retrieved from http://www.gapfon.org/

Smith, M. (1975). *When I say no, I feel guilty*. New York, NY: Bantam.

Stone, P., Larson, E., Mooney-Kane, C., Smolowitz, J., Lin, S., & Dick, A. (2006). Organizational climate and intensive care unit nurses' intention to leave. *Critical Care Medicine, 34*(7), 1907–1912.

Trinkoff, A., Geiger-Brown, J., Caurso, C., Lipscomb, J., Johantgen, M., Nelson, A., . . . Selby, V. (2008). Personal safety for nurses. In R. Hughes (Ed.), *Patient safety and quality: An evidence-based handbook for nurses* (pp. 473–502). Washington, DC: Agency for Healthcare Research and Quality. Retrieved from https://www.ncbi.nlm.nih.gov/books/NBK2661/

Trinkoff, A., Johantgen, M., Storr, C., Gureses, A., Liang, Y., & Han, K. (2011). Nurses' work schedule characteristics, nurse staffing and patient mortality. *Nursing Research, 60*(1), 1–8.

Ulrich, B. (2001). Successfully managing multigenerational workforces. *Seminars for Nurse Managers, 9*, 147–153.

Ulrich, B., Buerhaus, P., Donelan, K., Norman, L., & Dittus, R. (2007). Magnet® status and registered nurse views of the work environment and nursing as a career. *Journal of Nursing Administration, 37*(5), 212–220.

Urden, L., & Monarch, K. (2002). The ANCC Magnet Recognition Program®: Converting research findings into action. In M. McClure & A. Hinshaw (Eds.), *Magnet® hospitals revisited* (pp. 102–116). Washington, DC: American Nurses Publishing.

U.S. Department of Health and Human Services, & Agency for Healthcare Quality and Research. (2017). *About the national quality strategy.* Retrieved from https://www.ahrq.gov/workingforquality/about.htm

U.S. Department of Labor, & Bureau of Labor Statistics. (2013). *Economic news release.* Retrieved from https://www.bls.gov/news.release/ecopro.t08.htm

Walton, A., Lake, D., Mullinix, C., Allen, D., & Mooney, K. (2015). Enabling nurses to lead change: The orientation experiences of nurses to boards. *Nursing Outlook, 63*(2), 110–116.

Warshawsky, N., Havens, D., & Knafl, G. (2012). The influence of interpersonal relationships on nurse managers' work engagement and proactive work behavior. *Journal of Nursing Administration, 42*(9), 418–425.

Wasik, J. (2016, September 23). The doctor is in. In your house, that is. *The New York Times.* Retrieved from https://www.nytimes.com/2016/09/24/your-money/the-doctor-is-in-in-your-house-that-is.html

Wieck, K., Prydun, M., & Walsh, T. (2002). What the emerging workforce wants in its leaders. *Journal of Nursing Scholarship, 34,* 283–288.

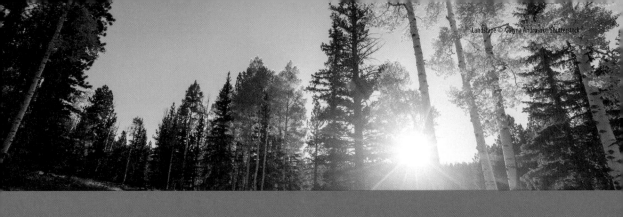

Appendix A

Quality Improvement Measurement and Analysis Methods

This appendix presents examples of QI measurement and analysis methods and information related to quality care. This information is applicable to your clinical experiences throughout your nursing program as you develop QI competency and leadership.

Definitions: Errors

- *Error:* Failure of a planned action to complete as intended or use of the wrong plan to achieve a goal. (Also search for this topic on the Institute for Healthcare Improvement website: http://www.ihi.org.)
- *Adverse event:* An injury resulting from a medical intervention, not due to the patient's underlying condition. It may or may not be due to an error and may or may not be preventable. If the adverse event is viewed as result of an error, then it is considered preventable. (Also search for this topic on the Institute for Healthcare Improvement website: http://www.ihi.org.)
- *Misuse:* An avoidable complication that prevents patients from receiving the full potential benefit of services.

- *Overuse:* Potential for harm that exceeds the possible benefit from a service.
- *Underuse:* Failure to provide a service that would have produced a favorable outcome for the patient.
- *Near miss:* Recognition that an event occurred that might have led to an adverse event. An error almost happened, but staff or the patient/family caught it before it became an error.
- *Active error:* An error that results from noncompliance with a procedure.
- *Omission:* Missed care should also be considered an error.
- *Common errors:* Falls, medication errors, development of pressure ulcers due to inadequate skin care, surgical errors such as wrong site, diagnosis (wrong diagnosis, incomplete diagnosis, and so on), wrong patient identification, lack of timely response, development of nosocomial infections,

wound infections, not washing hands, equipment failure, inappropriate use of restraints or used in unsafe manner, documentation errors or inadequate documentation, poor discharge planning or directions.

- *Sentinel event:* Unexpected events that happen to patients and that result in major negative outcomes such as an unexpected death or critical physical or psychological complication that can lead to major alteration in the patient's health. (Also search for this topic on the Institute for Healthcare Improvement website: http://www.ihi.org.)

Examples of High Risk for Errors and/or Reduced Quality Care

- *Working in silos:* Not working as a team or using poor communication; individuals or pairs working with little consideration of others who may be working on the same issue, with the same patient, and so on.
- *The Joint Commission Annual Safety Goals:* See the annual goals posted on the website: http://www.jointcommission.org/standards_information/npsgs.aspx.
- *Handoffs:* A handoff occurs when a patient experiences a change in provider or setting and there is a transfer of responsibility. (Also search for this topic on the Institute for Healthcare Improvement website: http://www.ihi.org.)
- *Medication reconciliation:* See the *Apply Quality Improvement* chapter. (Also search for this topic on the Institute for Healthcare Improvement website: http://www.ihi.org.)
- *Workaround:* Occurs when staff use a shortcut to get something done so they do not complete all the steps or substitute different steps in a process. This often happens when staff are behind; rather than figure out the problem they are experiencing, they use a workaround. (Also search for this topic on the Institute for Healthcare Improvement website: http://www.ihi.org.)

- *Health literacy:* See the *Provide Patient-Centered Care* chapter. Health literacy can affect errors—for example, if the patient does not understand the discharge directions or cannot read them, an error could occur.

Examples of Typical Errors or Concerns of Inadequate Quality Care

- *Hospital-acquired conditions (HACs):* See the *Healthcare Delivery System: Focus on Acute Care* chapter and the following websites:
  - Centers for Medicare & Medicaid Services, Hospital-Acquired Infections: http://www.cms.gov/Medicare/Medicare-Fee-for-Service-Payment/HospitalAcqCond/Hospital-Acquired_Conditions.html and http://www.cms.gov/Medicare/Medicare-Fee-for-Service-Payment/HospitalAcqCond/index.html.
- *Agency for Healthcare Research and Quality inpatient quality indicators:*
  - *Volume indicators/measures* are proxy, or indirect, measures of quality based on counts of admissions during which certain intensive, high-technology, or highly complex procedures were performed. They are based on evidence, suggesting hospitals that perform more of these procedures may have better outcomes for them.
  - *Mortality indicators/measures for inpatient procedures* include procedures for which mortality has been shown to vary across institutions and for which there is evidence that high mortality may be associated with poorer quality of care.
  - *Mortality indicators/measures for inpatient procedures* include conditions for which mortality has been shown to vary substantially across institutions and for which evidence suggests that high mortality may be associated with deficiencies in the quality of care.
  - *Utilization indicators/measures* examine procedures whose use varies significantly across

hospitals and for which questions have been raised about overuse, underuse, or misuse.

- *Primary and secondary data:* Primary data are data collected from firsthand experience; secondary data are collected by others.
- *Prevalence and incidence:* Prevalence is the proportion of the population that has a condition or risk factor. Incidence is the rate of occurrence.
- *Benchmarking:* Measuring quality across healthcare organizations based on same standards.
- *Report cards:* A published report that provides information about the quality of care for a healthcare organization or provider. (See examples at NCQA's website: http://reportcard.ncqa.org/portal/home .aspx and http://www.ncqa.org/Directories.aspx.)
- *Incident reports:* Healthcare organizations require that certain incidents, such as medication errors, are reported in written form using a standard form. This provides a record and helps in tracking errors for improvement.
- *Root-cause analysis (RCA):* A method used by many healthcare organizations today to analyze errors, supporting the recognition that most errors are caused by system issues and not individual staff issues. This in-depth analysis is intended to identify causes and then consider changes that might be required to reduce risk of reoccurrence. (Also search for this topic on the Institute for Healthcare Improvement website: http://www .ihi.org.)
- *Failure mode and effects analysis (FMEA):* A tool that "provides a systematic, proactive method for evaluating a process to identify where and how it might fail and to assess the relative impact of different failures in order to identify the parts of the process that are in most need of change" (Institute of Health Improvement, 2011). (Also search for this topic on the Institute for Healthcare Improvement website: http://www.ihi.org.)
- *Plan–do–study–act (PDSA):* A process that is used in planning; four steps are followed to reach effective results. (Also search for this topic on the Institute for Healthcare Improvement website: http://www.ihi.org.)

- *Employee surveys:* Written questionnaires used to get information from employees on a particular topic—for example, staff safety.
- *Patient/family surveys:* Written questionnaires used to get information from patients/families on a particular topic—for example, patient and/or family views of quality care and experience while hospitalized. A common standardized survey used by hospitals is offered by Press Ganey. (See the website: http://www.pressganey.com/index.aspx)
- *Flow charts and decision trees:* Methods used to describe a process so it can be clearly understood to improve the process or use to help identify when a process is not effective. (Search "decision trees" on Yahoo Images or Google Images.)
- *Patient safety indicators (PSI):* A set of indicators providing information on potential in-hospital complications and adverse events following surgeries, procedures, and childbirth. The PSIs were developed after a comprehensive literature review, analysis of ICD-10-CM codes, review by a clinician panel, implementation of risk adjustment, and empirical analyses. They can be used to help hospitals identify potential adverse events that might need further study, provide the opportunity to assess the incidence of adverse events and HACs using administrative data found in the typical discharge record, include indicators for complications occurring in hospitals that may represent patient safety events, and design area-level analogs to detect patient safety events on a regional level. (See the Agency for Healthcare Research and Quality for more information: http://qualityindicators.ahrq.gov /Modules/psi_overview.aspx.)
- *Interviews:* One-on-one collection of data that can be done in person or on telephone.
- *Observation:* Using staff or outside individuals to watch a procedure or work process and collect data on what occurs. This information is then used to track errors, improvement, and so on. An example would be to have observers watching staff to determine compliance with hand washing.

- *Quality measures:* Tools that help measure or quantify healthcare processes, outcomes, patient perceptions, and organizational structure and/or systems that are associated with the ability to provide high-quality health care and/or that relate to one or more quality goals for health care. These goals include safety, timely, efficient, effective, equitable, patient-centered (STEEEP) and timely care (Centers for Medicare and Medicaid Services [CMS]). (See more information at http://www.cms.gov/Medicare/Quality-Initiatives-Patient-Assessment-Instruments/QualityMeasures/index.html.)

- *Time-out:* During a procedure, the team may use a checklist to confirm the right patient, site, and procedure. If any staff member thinks there may be an error, that staff member can call a stop to any actions so that the correct information can be determined—for example, if the wrong site is identified and actions taken to ensure that care provided meets required outcomes.

- *Checklist:* A consistent method for ensuring that what needs to be done is done. The checklist is simple and requires limited, if any, training to use it. (Also search for this topic on the Institute for Healthcare Improvement website: http://www.ihi.org.)

- *Situation–background–assessment–recommendation (SBAR/ISBAR):* SBAR is a structured method of communication that is used to improve communication; commonly used with teams. See the *Work in Interprofessional Teams* chapter. (Also search for this topic on the Institute for Healthcare Improvement website: http://www.ihi.org.)

- *Rapid response team (RRT):* A team of critical care experts who can be called if there is concern about failure to rescue so as to respond quickly to complex and critical needs of patients. (Also search for this topic on the Institute for Healthcare Improvement website: http://www.ihi.org.)

- *Huddle:* This is a means by which a team gets together periodically during a shift to discuss critical issues. (Also search for this topic on the Institute for Healthcare Improvement website: http://www.ihi.org.)

- *Change of shift reports:* Clinical reports are done routinely, particularly in hospitals units, for bringing new staff coming on up-to-date regarding patient status. Such a report is also an opportunity to discuss quality and safety concerns for individual patients or for the unit or team as a whole.

- *Safety walkarounds:* Staff (usually management but can be other staff) walk through the unit or area of the healthcare organization and identify any safety concerns they may see that would apply to patients, families and visitors, and staff. This information is then used to plan improvement including prevention measures.

- *Crew resource management (CRM):* This is a communication method used in aviation to improve communication and decision making, providing a clear structure for the process. (Also search for this topic on the Institute for Healthcare Improvement website: http://www.ihi.org.)

- *Surveillance:* This is the ongoing assessment of patient status to identify problems and/or prevention of potential problems; nurses are primarily responsible for surveillance. Not doing surveillance may result in *failure to rescue.*

- *Universal protocol for preventing wrong site, wrong procedure, or wrong person surgery:* The Joint Commission established a procedure to prevent wrong-site, wrong-procedure, and wrong-person surgery errors. This procedure requires staff to utilize the following steps: (1) preprocedure verification, (2) site marking, and (3) use of time-outs. Any staff member may call a time-out if the staff member thinks there is a problem at any point during the procedure.

- *Early warning aystem (EWS):* A "physiological scoring system typically used in general medical–surgical units before patients experience catastrophic medical events" (Duncan & McMullan, 2012, p. 40). This is what triggers the use of the *rapid response team* to prevent *failure to rescue.*

- *Morbidity and mortality conferences:* M&M conferences are held in many hospitals on a routine basis to discuss patient care and outcomes.
- *Trigger points:* Clues that there may be an adverse reaction. Staff may use standardized lists of trigger points.
- *Electronic medical/health record:* Documentation is now most commonly done via electronic methods, which improve timely communication and usually have a positive impact on care. See the *Utilize Informatics* chapter.
- *Computerized physician/provider order-entry system (CPOES):* The CPOES is used to improve the process of physician ordering, usually reducing time and errors. It is commonly associated with electronic medical records. See the *Utilize Informatics* chapter.
- *Computerized decision support (CDS):* CDS offers providers an effective method to improve decision making and is usually associated with electronic medical records. See the *Utilize Informatics* chapter.
- *Use of other technology* (for example, smartphones, handheld computers)*:* Increased use of technology in healthcare delivery has assisted in improving timely communication that meets the need at the time. See the *Utilize Informatics* chapter.
- *Bar coding:* Bar coding is used routinely in medication administration and other times when identification of patient and action need to be ensured. See the *Utilize Informatics* chapter.
- *Safety primers (AHRQ):* See AHRQ's patient safety primers webpage (http://psnet.ahrq.gov /primerHome.aspx) for information on a variety of important safety concerns.

References

Duncan, K., & McMullan, C. (2012, February). Early warning. *Nursing 2012*, 38–44.

Finkelman, A. (2018). *Quality improvement: A guide for integration in nursing*. Burlington, MA: Jones & Bartlett Learning.

Institute for Health Improvement. (2011). *FMEA*. Retrieved from http://www.ihi.org/knowledge/Pages /Tools/FailureModesandEffectsAnalysisTool.aspx

Institute of Medicine. (2004). *Keeping patients safe*. Washington, DC: National Academies Press.

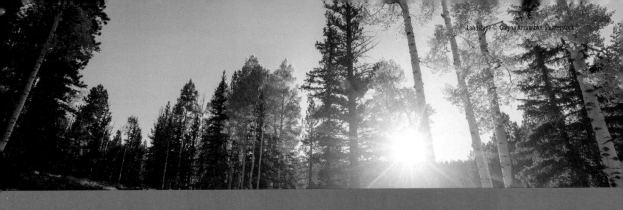

Appendix B

Staffing and a Healthy Work Environment

Staffing: What a New Nurse Needs to Know

When you search for your first job as a new graduate, it is critical that you inquire about staffing—who does the staffing plan, how far in advance is staffing done, which methods are used, how inadequate staffing areas are covered, and whether overtime is required. Nurses need information about staffing and the input they have in staffing.

American Nurses Association Staffing Principles

The American Nurses Association (ANA) staffing principles, which were reissued in 2010, support the need for adequate staffing to deliver quality patient care. Three underlying assumptions of these principles provide guidance for staffing decisions and are the major ethical concerns related to staffing:

1. Nurse staffing patterns and the level of care provided should not be based on the type of payer.

2. Evaluation of any staffing system should include quality of nurses' work–life outcomes as well as patients' outcomes.
3. Staffing should be based on achieving quality of patient care indices, meeting organizational outcomes, and ensuring that the quality of nurses' work life is appropriate.

Developing staffing schedules and then maintaining staffing as care is delivered are complex and time-consuming management activities. Nursing management uses different methods to determine the level of staff required, such as patient acuity assessment tools. Some states have legislated staffing requirement criteria. The following are some guides that nursing management uses to support staffing decisions:

- *Current Nursing: Scope and Standards of Nursing* (ANA)
- Appropriate scope and standards of specialty nursing practice
- Current state nurse practice act and scope of practice information (state board of nursing)

- Current *Code of Ethics with Interpretive Statements* (ANA)
- Copies of relevant facility policies and procedures (for example, staffing, floating, temporary staffing agency use)
- Copies of the current collective bargaining agreement/contract (if applicable)
- Copies of contracts with outside staffing agencies
- Information on competencies of agency staff
- *Bill of Rights for Registered Nurses* (ANA)

The ANA staffing standards are divided into three categories. First, the principles of the patient care unit focus on the need for appropriate staffing levels at the unit level. These standards reflect both the analysis of individual patient needs and aggregate patient needs, and the unit functions that are important in delivering care. The second category focuses on staff-related principles, such as the type of nurse competencies needed to provide the required care as well as role responsibilities. The third category involves institutional or organizational policies. These policies should indicate that nurses are respected, and they should state a commitment to meeting budget requirements to fill nursing positions. Competencies for all nursing staff (employees, agency, and so on) should be documented. A clear plan should describe how float staff are used and the required cross-training for these staff so that they are prepared to practice in multiple areas of care. Staff members need to know if they may be switched from one unit to another. There must be a clear designation of the adequate number of staff needed to meet a minimum level of quality care. The nursing model that is used has an impact on staffing.

The principles identify four critical elements that need to be considered when making staffing decisions (ANA, 2010, p. 23):

1. *Patients:* Patient characteristics and number of patients receiving care.
2. *Intensity of unit and care:* Individual patient intensity; across-the-unit intensity (taking into account the heterogeneity of settings); variability of care; admissions, discharges, and transfers; volume.
3. *Context:* Architecture (geographic arrangement of patient areas, size and layout of individual patient rooms, arrangement of entire patient care units, and so forth); technology (use of page systems, cellular phones, computers).
4. *Expertise:* Learning curve for individuals and groups of nurses; staff consistency, continuity, and cohesion; cross-training; control of practice; involvement in quality improvement activities; professional expectations; preparation; experience; and interprofessional teamwork.

Staffing Terminology

Nurse staffing includes not only RNs but also licensed practical nurses (LPNs)/licensed vocational nurses (LVNs) and unlicensed assistive personnel (UAPs). All of these staff members provide direct care. RNs and LPNs are licensed by the states in which they are employed. The state board of nursing in each state regulates state licensure. RNs assess patient needs, develop patient care plans, and administer medications and treatments, and they must meet the state's nurse practice act requirements. LPNs carry out specified nursing duties under the direction of RNs. Nurses' aides typically provide nonspecialized duties and personal care activities. Some states require that UAPs complete a certification program, at which point they are referred to as certified nurse assistants.

Hospitals and other healthcare organizations (HCOs) have written position descriptions for RNs, LPNs, and UAPs. These descriptions should be followed. They influence staffing because the descriptions identify what staff members may do, which in turn affects the staff mix. Nurse staffing is measured in one of two basic ways:

- Nursing hours per patient per day
- Nurse-to-patient ratio

Nursing hours may refer to RNs only; to RNs and LPNs; or to RNs, LPNs, and UAPs. It is important to know which staff category is identified by the nurse staffing measurement. *Nursing care hours* refers to the number of hours of patient care provided per unit of time or over the course of a specified time.

The term *full-time equivalent* is used to describe a position equal to 40 hours of work per week for 52 weeks, or 2,080 hours per year. One full-time equivalent can represent one staff member or several members; that is, a full-time equivalent can be divided (for example, two staff members each working half a full-time equivalent). Many nursing units employ part-time staff.

The *staffing mix* describes the type of nursing staff needed to provide care. This mix should be determined by considering the type of care needed and patient status, as well as the qualification and competencies needed to provide the care. In some cases, the staff must be RNs; in other situations, a mix of RNs, LPNs, and UAPs is needed, with the RN supervising. This issue is often a concern when the proportion of RNs is compared with other types of nursing staffing. Another factor that needs to be considered is the work level and work flow; for example, the typical time for discharges and admissions or the surgical schedule can make a difference as to when more or fewer staff members are needed (distribution of staff).

Scheduling

The shift, or typical pattern of time worked, is an important factor in scheduling. Some areas of care use multiple types of shifts, whereas others have only one type. Typical shifts are 8, 10, and 12 hours in length. More and more hospitals are using 12-hour shifts, and some schools of nursing are using 12-hour clinical rotations for students. Staff members often prefer the 12-hour shift because it allows for more days off (40 hours can add up quickly). However, there has been concern about 12-hour shifts and the resulting fatigue level that may lead to more errors (Geiger-Brown & Trinkoff, 2010; IOM, 2004; Montgomery & Geiger-Brown, 2010; Trinkoff, Johantgen, Storr, Gurses, Liang, & Han, 2011).

Trinkoff and colleagues (2011) examined the independent effect of work schedules on patient care outcomes. Their study surveyed 633 nurses in 71 acute care hospitals in two states. The results indicate that work schedule related significantly to patient mortality when staffing levels and hospital characteristics were controlled. Other concerns are increased risk of infections among staff who are fatigued and ergonomic stressors, accidents that result from driving home tired, and responsibilities at home that further increase nurses' fatigue (Geiger-Brown & Trinkoff, 2010; Worthington, 2001). More research needs to be done to determine the impact of shifts on fatigue and errors.

Split shifts are used to provide more staff at busy times of the day (such as 7:00–11:00 a.m. or later in the day). Part-time staff usually fill in during split shifts, and this has implications for consistency of care and quality with increased risk of errors. "Moving away from 12-hour shifts will require a real change in hospital culture" (Montgomery & Geiger-Brown, 2010, p. 148).

The staffing schedule can contribute to many negative results. Because staff usually do not get off on time, longer shifts can compound the problems associated with 12-hour shifts. For example, when staff work 10- or 12-hour shifts instead of 8-hour shifts, staying 1 hour past the end of their shifts can be very difficult. This is a frequent occurrence because some staff may be arriving late or not coming at all, and temporary coverage is needed until additional staff coverage is found. This makes a 10- or 12-hour shift much longer. In some HCOs, staff are required to rotate shifts so that they may switch back and forth from the day shift to the night shift. This can be hard for many nurses, although some like to work the night shift.

Scheduling is not easy and causes a lot of conflict among staff. Nurses invariably want more say in scheduling. Some organizations use computerized request systems so that staff can input their special staffing requests, and others do this in writing or orally. When staffing is posted is also of concern because staff need to make their personal plans. The procedures for schedule changes need to be known by all staff. The trend is for HCOs to develop staffing schedules centrally, although some may do it unit by unit. In addition, a non-nurse scheduler is more common today (Cavouras, 2006). This model has disadvantages because it may leave out or limit important input from nurse managers. However, "one of the most important reasons that people (nurse managers) leave hospital nursing is frustration with schedules and staffing" (Cavouras, 2006, p. 36), so it is important to find a balance. Scheduling must consider patient needs; staff competencies; individual staff issues such as days off, vacation time, sick leave, and so on; organization needs; legislative and regulation requirements; union requirements; shortage concerns; use of external sources for staff (for example, agencies); standards; and rising labor costs.

Patient classification systems may be used to assist with staffing levels. These computerized systems are used to identify and quantify patient needs, which can then be matched with staffing level and mix. It is thought that these systems are more objective because data related to patients and their needs are used to determine the number and type of staff required per shift.

Some organizations or patient care/clinical units use self-scheduling (Hung, 2002). With this system, guidelines are developed for the schedule. Staff members are then given a certain amount of time to fill in the schedule based on the guidelines. Individual staff members do need to consider the schedules that other staff members have already posted. When the designated time period is completed, the nurse manager (or a staff member who is responsible for completing the schedule) reviews it and makes any required changes or additions to ensure that staffing is adequate. This type of scheduling allows staff to feel more in control

of the staffing and to work with one another to come up with the most effective arrangement. It also reduces the time that the nurse manager or another scheduler might spend on staffing. More staff input and control over staffing usually results in greater staff satisfaction and less absenteeism, which leads to greater staff empowerment.

The schedule inevitably has holes—positions on the schedule for which there is no staff member assigned. What does the HCO do? One method HCOs use to fill holes in the schedule is to develop a float pool. This is a group of staff (RNs, LPNs, or UAPs) who may be moved from unit to unit based on need. These staff members need to be competent in the relevant area of care and should be flexible and able to adjust quickly to new environments. Float pool staff are HCO employees who are not assigned to a specific unit. Staff members who float need orientation and training related to the types of care that they are expected to provide.

When nursing shortages become a serious problem, hospitals increase the number of staff who are not permanent employees of the HCO but, rather, temporary employees. Agency nurses are nurses hired by a nursing agency; the agency then contracts with an HCO for specific types of staff to meet schedule requirements. Some hospitals contract with one supplemental staffing agency, whereas others contract with multiple agencies to meet their staffing needs. An agency nurse is paid by the agency (typically more than regular HCO staff), must be licensed, and should meet employee competency qualifications or any other criteria required by the HCO. Work assignments can be for one shift, for several days, or for weeks or months.

Another method for responding to incomplete schedules or lack of staff to fill all positions needed is the use of travelers. Travelers are nurses who work for an agency, but not a local agency. They are hired by the agency and then assigned to work at an HCO for a block of time (more than a few days and often several months). The nurse may come from anywhere in the United States. The agency pays the nurse's salary and benefits, and often moving, travel, and housing expenses are covered by the HCOs that use the travelers. Salaries are often very high for these nurses. Nurses can decline a specific assignment, and moving is required. Nurses might even be assigned a management position. Nurses who are employees of the HCO are often concerned about the pay difference; traveling nurses, as well as regular agency nurses, typically earn much more than the full-time employees, which can cause conflict. Travelers must meet the requirements to practice in the state and the HCO requirements.

All these nurses need orientation and should not be expected to just "get to work." It is not easy to change from one HCO to another because HCOs are not all the same. The nurse has to learn quickly to work with a new team. More experienced nurses are better at making this transition, and many of the traveling nurse agencies hire only experienced nurses. Although the fluctuations in the nursing shortage have decreased in some areas, when the shortage begins to increase again, which will occur when more nurses retire, there will be greater need again to use alternative staffing strategies.

Recruitment

Recruitment in nursing involves the recruitment of both nurses and nursing students. Some improvement has occurred in recruitment of nursing students, increasing supply. Recruitment is a critical function of HCOs—they must maintain sufficient staffing levels of competent staff. This requires a recruitment plan that is revised based on needs and a plan that includes input from management and staff. Clear position descriptions provide guidance to the types of staff needed.

Retention

After new staff are recruited, they need to be retained. HCOs want to avoid a situation in which staff do not stay in their positions—for example,

moving on to other jobs. Both new nurses and experienced nurses may change positions and employers. Nurse turnover is very costly. What are some of the costs and benefits of turnover? The following describe some of these costs that continue to be problems and related benefits (Jones & Gates, 2007):

Nurse Turnover Costs

- Advertising and recruitment
- Vacancy costs (for example, paying for agency nurses, overtime, closed beds, and hospital diversions when the emergency department must be closed)
- Hiring (review and processing of applicants)
- Orientation and training
- Decreased productivity (loss of staff who know routines)
- Termination (processing of termination)
- Potential patient errors; compromised quality of care
- Poor work environment and culture; dissatisfaction; distrust
- Loss of organizational knowledge (loss of staff who know the history of the organization and processes)

Nurse Turnover Benefits for the HCO

- Reductions in salaries and benefits for newly hired nurses versus departing nurses
- Savings from bonuses not paid to outgoing nurses
- Replacement nurses bringing in new ideas, reality, and innovations, as well as knowledge of competitors
- Elimination of poor performers (this is not guaranteed, it is merely hoped)

Creating a Healthy Work Environment: Retaining Nurses

Working in a healthcare environment can be a very positive experience, particularly if the environment is one in which staff are respected, communication is open, staff feel empowered and part of the decision-making process, staff safety and health are considered important, and staff feel that they are making a contribution. This, however, is not always the case. Staff experience stress, burnout, and conflict in the workplace. Some signs that students and staff should watch for in themselves, in others, and in organizations follow.

Personal Signs

- Irritability
- Lack of sleep or too much sleep
- Complaining about many aspects of work
- Unwillingness to help others
- Desire to just get the job done and leave
- Less enjoyment during personal time
- Dreading going to work
- High frustration with management
- Angry outbursts
- Gaining or losing weight
- Lack of energy

Attitude and behavior affect others, too—co-workers and family. Burnout is contagious because of this impact. Morale can decrease as staff members try to cope with their own stress and burnout. This affects productivity and the quality of care.

Organizational Signs

- Inadequate or confused communication
- Top-down decision making, leaving staff out
- Poorly planned change that is unsuccessful
- Increase in staff complaints

- Staff–management conflict
- Distrust of staff and staff distrust of management

References

American Nurses Association. (2010). *Utilization guide for the ANA principles for nurse staffing* (reissue). Silver Spring, MD: Author.

Cavouras, C. (2006). Scheduling and staffing: Innovations from the field. *Nurse Leader, 4*(4), 34–36.

Geiger-Brown, J., & Trinkoff, A. (2010). Is it time to pull the plug on 12-hour shifts? Part 1. The evidence. *Journal of Nursing Administration, 40*(3), 100–102.

Hung, R. (2002). A note on nurse self-scheduling. *Nursing Economics, 20*(1), 37–39.

Institute of Medicine. (2004). *Keeping patients safe: Transforming the work environment of nurses.* Washington, DC: The National Academies Press.

Jones, C., & Gates, M. (2007). The costs and benefits of nurse turnover: A business case for nurse retention. *Online Journal of Issues in Nursing, 12*(3). Retrieved from http://www.nursingworld.org/Main MenuCategories/ANAMarketplace/ANAPeriodicals /OJIN/TableofContents/Volume122007/No3Sept07 /NurseRetention.aspx

Montgomery, K., & Geiger-Brown, J. (2010). Is it time to pull the plug on 12-hour shifts? Part 2. Barriers to change and executive leadership strategies. *Journal of Nursing Administration, 40*(4), 147–149.

Trinkoff, A., Johantgen, M., Storr, C., Gurses, A. P., Liang, Y., & Han, K. (2011). Nurses' work schedule characteristics, nurse staffing, and patient mortality. *Nursing Research, 60*(1), 1–8.

Worthington, K. (2001). The health risks of mandatory overtime. *American Journal of Nursing, 101*(5), 96.

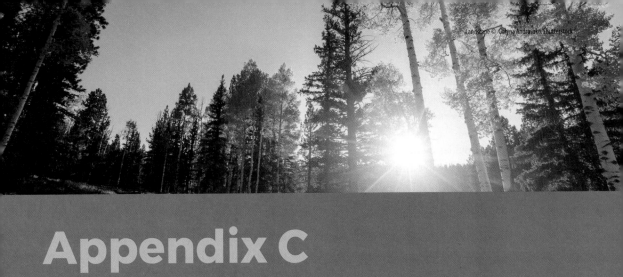

Appendix C

Getting the Right Position

Career Development—First Step: First Nursing Position

Career development is a responsibility of every nurse. This process really begins before graduation from a nursing program and completion of licensure requirements.

From Student to Practice: Reality Shock

Reality shock has been identified in nursing as the shock-like reaction that occurs when initial education comes in conflict with work-world values (Kramer, 1974). Another definition is "the incongruency of values and behaviors between the school subculture and the work subculture that leads to role deprivation or reality shock" (Schmalenberg & Kramer, 1979, p. 2). Benner (1984) identified five stages of competence: novice, advanced beginner, competent, proficient, and expert. The first three stages are affected by reality shock. Through the nursing education process, the novice nurse learns the rules for performance but has limited real-life clinical experience during

which to apply those rules and to expand clinical reasoning and judgment.

Getting your first job as an RN is a very important step in your career development. Even before graduation, you should take some time to begin a career plan. The plan will change over time, but having a plan provides a guide for personal professional decisions.

Tools and Strategies to Make the Transition Easier

Where to begin? You should begin by developing a résumé, composing a biosketch, and maintaining a professional portfolio. A résumé is a one- or two-page document that describes your career. It includes your name, contact information, credentials, education, goals and objectives, and employment and relevant experience (a résumé should be kept current and not be lengthy). The biosketch is a paragraph that provides a short summary of your work history and accomplishments. It should include your name, credentials, and education. It is a narrative rather than a list. Later, curriculum vitae can be developed. This is a more detailed accounting of information found in the résumé and includes publications, presentations, continuing education (CE), honors and awards, community activities, and grants.

The portfolio provides evidence of a person's competency. It is not always required for job applications, but sometimes it is, and in some positions, nurses are asked to maintain a portfolio for performance review. A portfolio is a collection of information that demonstrates experiences and accomplishments, such as committee work, professional organization activities, presentations, development of patient education material, awards, letters of recognition, projects and grants, and so on. The portfolio should include annual goals and objectives and review of outcomes, which should be updated annually.

A professional development plan, which is based on information found in your résumé and portfolio, lays out the direction you want to take with your career over the next year, 2 years, and 5 years. It should include a target time frame and strategies and activities to reach the goals. Self-assessment is a critical activity for any nurse, and this assessment helps you to further develop the career plan.

Interviewing for a New Position

Interviewing for a new position as a nurse should be taken seriously. The first step is setting up the interview. As the potential employee, you should find out the time of the appointment, the location, and the length of the interview. Will there be more than one interview on the same day? Will additional interviews take place later depending on whether the person is considered for the position? Will the interview be with one person or with a group and with whom? Do your homework; find out as much as possible about the healthcare organization (HCO) and people who will be at the interview, and think about the types of questions might be asked and how to respond to them. Wear business dress, look neat, and be prepared. Bring a copy of your résumé to all interviews and any other required documents.

Make sure you know how to get to the interview, and arrive early to allow yourself time to focus on the interview. Delays can happen when you least expect it, so planning to arrive early helps to prevent lateness.

During the interview, focus on the questions. Look the interviewer in the eye, take a moment to respond, and ask for clarification if you are unsure about the question. Share information about competencies and experiences—successes and challenges, and how you handled them. Ask the interviewer about the organization and the position.

When the interview is completed, thank the interviewer. Follow-up to thank him or her (in a letter or via email). Ask about the process—what comes next, when the decision will be made, and so on.

Exhibit C-1 suggests examples of questions to ask at an interview.

Determination of the Best Fit: You and a New Position

How does one choose a position and an organization for employment? It is not easy to know that the fit is a good one. First, know which type of nursing interests you and why. Second, based on what you know about the HCOs in the location where you want to work, focus on those organizations that most interest you. Today, the Internet is a resource for job hunting. Most HCOs, particularly hospitals, have websites. Explore them to learn about specific HCOs. Talk to people who may know about the HCOs that interest you.

Students often have clinical experiences in several HCOs, and they can use this opportunity to assess each organization. Do staff members seem happy working there? Does the HCO differentiate degrees in nursing and how? What is the quality of care? What are some of the negative aspects of the organization?

Salary and benefits are always an important factor. Potential employees should also consider driving distance, parking, schedules, and general work conditions. Asking about promotions and use of career ladders can yield helpful information,

Exhibit C-1 Examples of Questions to Ask during an Interview for a Hospital RN Position

- Do you have an opening on one of your _____ units in this hospital? For what shift?
- Would you hire a new BSN-prepared nurse to work in that unit? If not, why not?
- What is the position description for the job? (Ask to see it.)
- Which skills or knowledge (beyond basic preparation) would I need?
- How can I obtain these skills or knowledge?
- What are the opportunities for advancement in the unit?
- What is the culture of the unit?
- Is mandatory overtime; rotating shifts? (If so, ask more about this.)
- How is scheduling done? When is it done? What kind of notification of scheduling is given? Is there staff input into scheduling?
- Who is the nurse manager, and how long has the manager been in the position?
- What is the leadership style of the manager of the unit?
- What is the turnover rate of RNs in the unit and the healthcare organization?
- What is the relationship of RNs and physicians on the unit?
- Is a team concept practiced on the unit? If so, who are the members of the team?
- Is the hospital a Magnet hospital? (Even if the HCO is not a Magnet hospital, Magnet forces are a good guide for HCO characteristics to consider and to inquire about.)
- What orientation is provided? Are mentors provided for new staff (who and for how long)? What is the view of career development (staff education and academic)?
- What are the salary and benefits? (Typically not asked at the initial interview, but later when the HCO indicates an interest in hiring an applicant.)
- Does the HCO have a union? (If so, ask more about its function and membership.)

Reproduced from Milstead, J., & Furlong, E. (2008). *Handbook of nursing leadership: Creative skills for a culture of safety*. Sudbury, MA: Jones & Bartlett Learning.

along with how much support is given to staff for education (that is, orientation, staff development, CE, and academic degrees). Regarding education, a potential new employee should ask if tuition reimbursement is available and for whom and at which level. Is it difficult to get release time to attend classes, or is there flexible staffing to allow for this?

Nurses should also ask about staff turnover, use of supplemental staffing (agency, travelers), mandatory overtime, and change in nurse leaders. Organizations that experience high turnover in staff and nurse managers are organizations that are experiencing problems. Overreliance on supplemental staff indicates that the organization is having problems retaining nurses and developing strategies to cope with a nursing shortage. (Nursing shortages vary and may be HCO specific, local, or national.)

Is the HCO used for clinical experiences for nursing students? This usually means that the organization is interested in education, but it also means that staff members need to be willing to work with students. How is medical staff coverage handled? Are there medical students and residents? It is important to know who covers for medical issues because this has an impact on expectations of nursing staff and collaboration with others. Today hospitals are ranked locally, by state, and nationally. This information can be accessed through the Internet.

The HCO's top leadership, such as the chief executive officer (CEO), is an important person. The CEO signs off on the budget. If the CEO does not recognize the importance of nursing to the organization and to outcomes, this can have a negative impact on how nurses are treated, and it can affect such budget issues as the number of nursing positions, salaries and benefits, and funds for education.

Mentoring, Coaching, and Networking

Several methods are used in HCOs to support new staff, and mentoring is one of them. The mentor is more experienced and usually is selected by the staff nurse, but some HCOs assign new staff to mentors. The mentor acts as a role model and serves as a resource. Coaching is another method used for support, encouragement, and career development (for example, how to prepare for a promotion or change of career ladder level or to go back to school for a higher degree).

Networking is a less structured method. All nurses need to learn how to network or make connections with nurses and others who can help them. Professional organizations are good places to network and meet nurses who might provide guidance, support, and/or information. Nurses should keep contact information of potential connections even when they may not have a specific reason to make the contact; one never knows when this information may become important. Networking can also be done in non-healthcare settings that include people who may be helpful to know.

Career Ladder

Many HCOs today have developed career ladder programs for their nurses. The details of these career ladders vary from organization to organization. Typically, there are levels such as Clinician I, II, III, and so on. The first level is entry level. The levels describe the role and responsibilities, as well as the educational requirements for that position or level. This type of system provides clear criteria for promotion and an increase in salary that does not require moving to a management position, which in the past was the most common path for advancement. The career ladder structure recognizes that clinical work is important and deserves recognition. Nurses have to demonstrate that they meet the criteria for the level that they are requesting. This is the point at which a nurse might use a portfolio and mentor. In some HCOs, portfolios are required for promotion. Along with identified criteria, HCOs need clear procedures for staff members who want to apply for a change in level within the career ladder system.

Encouraging staff to participate in the career ladder offers positive outcomes for the organization, such as motivating staff to improve their competencies and increase their education level, increasing efforts to improve care, serving as an attractive recruitment strategy, and increasing retention. Performance improvement should be an active part of any nursing position. Through an active, positive performance improvement program, staff can use self-assessment and assessment from supervisors to further develop their career plans.

Going Back to School, Certification, and CE

Returning to school for another degree may not be your first thought after graduation and licensure, but when you develop a career plan, additional education should be considered. This decision should be based on your goals and timeline. You need to consider the best time to begin work on additional education. Competency is an important issue. Do you need more time to achieve competency and to further your development as a professional nurse before entering a graduate program or a specialty? Some specialties may require certain type of practice experience before entering a graduate program—for example, nurse anesthesia programs require practice experience in critical care. Entering into such specialties requires serious thought and planning. Additional education is most productive when you are competent at your current position level and practice effectively as a professional nurse. For many new graduates, achieving this level of competency takes time.

Certification is another way to expand competencies and education; however, it does require that you have a specified amount of experience before taking the examination. Thus you need to plan when to apply and obtain the required experience.

CE is a professional responsibility. Employers may provide educational experiences that also allow nurses to earn CE contact hours, or they may cover expenses for staff to attend CE programs outside the HCO. Many professional organizations offer CE programs, and some offer web-based programs. Many CE programs are offered via the Internet. Some states require that RNs earn a certain number of contact hours prior to relicensure. Certified nurses must meet CE requirements to continue their certification. CE is more effective if the content relates to the work that the nurse does and is in alignment with the nurse's professional goals. Nurses should keep a file of CE activities and update their records accordingly.

References

Benner, P. (1984). *From novice to expert, excellence and power in clinical nursing practice.* Menlo Park, CA: Addison-Wesley Publishing Company.

Kramer, M. (1974). *Reality shock: Why nurses leave nursing.* St. Louis, MO: Mosby.

Schmalenberg, C., & Kramer, M. (1979). *Coping with reality shock.* Wakefield, MA: Nursing Resources.

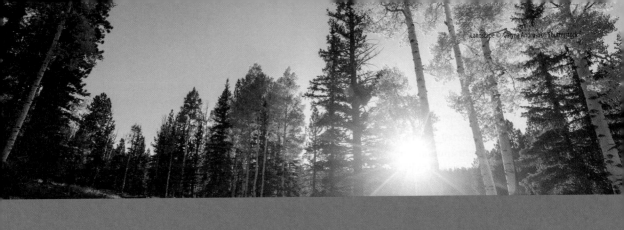

Glossary

Academic Health Center (AHC)   A medical center with acute care hospital and other services that is directly associated with medical, nursing, and other healthcare profession education institutions. Academic faculty usually serve in some of the key roles in the center. An AHC may include several hospitals such as acute care and pediatric.

academic nursing   A college of nursing associated with an AHC.

accelerated program   A nursing degree that is offered for students who have a non-nursing degree and want to obtain a nursing degree, which is typically a baccalaureate degree in nursing or may be combined with a master's degree. The program is offered at a faster pace.

accountability   An obligation or willingness to accept responsibility.

accreditation   The process by which organizations are evaluated on their quality, based on established minimum standards.

acute care   Treatment of a severe medical condition that is of short duration or at a crisis level.

acute illness   An illness of short duration with limited impact on the person.

advance directive   A legal document that allows a person to describe his or her medical care preferences.

Advanced Practice Registered Nurse (APRN)   A registered nurse with advanced education in adult health, pediatrics, family health, women's health, neonatal health, community health, or other specialties.

adverse event   An injury resulting from a medical intervention (in other words, an injury that is not caused by the patient's underlying condition).

advocacy   Speaking for something important (one of the major roles of a nurse).

advocate   A nurse who speaks for the patient but does not take away the patient's independence.

Affordable Care Act of 2010 (ACA)   This law was passed to revise healthcare reimbursement in the United States and to increase the number of persons who have access to health insurance.

alarm or alert fatigue   With the increasing use of alarms on equipment in health care and the frequency in which they are set-off in healthcare settings, staff may not respond to alarms as expected.

annual limit   A defined maximum amount that an employee/policy holder/patient would have to pay, and after that level is reached, he or she no longer has to contribute to the payment for care.

applied (or clinical) research   Research designed to find a solution to a practical problem.

apprenticeship A nursing program developed in England that provided on-the-job training and a formal education component.

articulation agreement A formal agreement between two or more institutions that allows specific programs at one institution to be credited toward direct entry or advanced standing at another.

assertiveness Confronting problems in a constructive manner and not remaining silent.

associate degree in nursing A degree offered as culmination of a 2-year program that includes some liberal arts and sciences curriculum but focuses more on nursing.

autonomy The quality or state of being self-governing; the freedom to act on what you know.

baccalaureate degree in nursing A degree from a 4-year nursing program in a higher education institution.

basic research Research designed to broaden the base of knowledge rather than solve an immediate problem.

benchmarking Measurement of progress toward a goal, taken at intervals prior to the program's completion or the anticipated attainment of the final goal.

bias A predisposition to a point of view.

blame-free environment An environment that encourages reporting of errors and focuses more on a systematic view of errors rather than individual causation.

breach of confidentiality Confidential information shared with others when it should not be shared.

breach of duty The proximate (foreseeable) cause or the cause that is legally sufficient to result in liability for harm to the patient; a breach of due care.

burnout A deterioration of attitude in which a person becomes tired, defensive, frustrated, cynical, bored, and generally pessimistic about the job; exhaustion of physical or emotional strength.

call-out In structured team communication, staff speak up and tell members of the team that something does not appear to be correct and ask for checks by the team to ensure correct care is provided.

care coordination Establishment and support of a continuous healing relationship, enabled by an integrated clinical environment and characterized by a proactive delivery of evidence-based care and follow-up.

care transition *See also* handoffs.

caregiver Someone who provides care to another; not a healthcare professional.

caring Feeling and exhibiting concern and empathy for others.

case management A system of management that facilitates effective care delivery and outcomes for patients through structured care coordination.

certification A process by which a nongovernmental agency validates, based on predetermined standards, an individual nurse's qualification and knowledge for practice in a defined functional or clinical area of nursing.

change agent Someone who engages deliberately in, or whose behavior results in, social, cultural, or behavioral change.

check-back *See also* **call-out**. In structured team communication, team members respond to call-out to ensure correct care is provided.

checklist A method used to ensure consistent steps are taken to ensure quality care is provided; the list is provided by the HCO for staff use (for example, prior to surgery).

chronic disease A disease that a person experiences long term that affects the person's quality of life.

clinical data repository An information warehouse that stores data longitudinally and in multiple forms, such as text, voice, and images.

clinical decision support systems (CDSS) Computerized system integrated into an electronic medical record system to provide immediate information that can influence clinical decisions.

clinical experience Practicum that occurs when students with faculty supervision provide care to patients for learning experiences.

clinical information system A method of data storage generally used at the point of care.

clinical judgment The process by which nurses come to understand the problems, issues, and concerns of patients; to attend to salient information; and to respond to patient problems in concerned and involved ways. It includes both conscious decision-making and intuitive response.

clinical protocols/pathways Written descriptions of how care is best provided for a specific patient population with specific problem(s).

clinical provider order-entry system (CPOES) A data-entry system that allows healthcare providers to input orders into a computer system rather than writing them.

clinical reasoning The nurse's ability to assess patient problems or needs and analyze data to accurately identify and frame problems within the context of the individual patient's environment. *See also* **clinical judgment.**

code of ethics A list of provisions that makes explicit the primary goals, values, and obligations of the nursing profession; published by the American Nurses Association.

coding system A set of agreed-upon symbols (frequently numeric or alphanumeric) that is used to change information into another form so that it can be better accessed and used.

collaboration Cooperative effort among healthcare providers, staff, and multiple organizations who work together to accomplish a common mission.

colleagueship Workplace relationships with common interests.

communication The exchange of thoughts, messages, or information.

community The people and their relationships that use common services and share specific space environment.

compassion fatigue The feeling of emotion that ensues when a person is moved by the distress or suffering of another, leading to a state of psychic exhaustion.

competency A behavior of a student or staff member is expected to demonstrate.

computer literacy Knowledge of basic computer technology.

concept/care map An innovative approach to planning and organizing nursing care.

confidentiality The responsibility to keep patient information private, except as required to communicate in the care process and with team members.

conflict A state of opposition between persons, ideas, or interests.

conflict resolution A process of resolving a dispute or disagreement.

consumer/customer The ultimate user of a product or service.

continuing education (CE) Systematic professional learning designed to augment knowledge, skills, and attitudes.

continuity of care "The degree to which a series of discrete events is experienced as coherent and connected and consistent with the patient's medical needs and personal context" (Haggerty, Reid, Freeman, Starfield, Adair, & McKendry, 2003, p. 1219).

continuous quality improvement (CQI) An organized approach to identify errors and hazards in care, and to improve care overall that emphasizes that this is an ongoing process.

continuum of care Care services available to assist an individual throughout the course of his or her disease.

coordination Proactive methods to optimize health outcomes.

copayment The fixed amount that a patient may be required to pay per service (doctor's visit, lab test, prescription, etc.).

coping The process of managing taxing circumstances.

corporatization Business; the business of health care.

counselor A person who gives guidance in a specific area of expertise or knowledge.

credentialing A process used to ensure that practitioners are qualified to perform and to monitor continued licensure.

critical thinking Purposeful, informed, outcome-focused (results-oriented) thinking that requires careful identification of key problems, issues, and risks.

culture The knowledge and values shared by a society or a group/organization.

culture of safety A work environment that does not focus on individual actions as cause for errors but, rather, considers impact of system factors, emphasizing a blame-free culture or just culture.

curriculum An integrated course of academic studies that describes the program's philosophy, level, and terminal competencies for students, or what they are expected to be able to accomplish by the end of the program.

dashboard A method, or part of electronic methods, to provide a quick view of data using key elements of concern.

data Discrete entities that are described objectively without interpretation.

data analysis software Computer software that can analyze data.

data bank A large store of information, which may include several databases.

data mining Locating and identifying unknown patterns and relationships within data.

database A collection of interrelated data, often with controlled redundancy, organized according to a scheme to serve one or more applications.

debriefing A method used to review a situation, incident, or experience immediately following; assists in identifying factors that support effective response and those that limit response (for example, faculty–student debriefing after simulation, healthcare team debriefs after a patient experiences a cardiac arrest).

deductible The part of the bill that the patient must pay before the insurer begins to pay for services.

delegatee The person to whom someone delegates a task.

delegation The transfer of responsibility to complete a task that is within the scope of the transferee's position.

delegator The person who assigns responsibility or authority.

dichotomous thinking Seeing situations as either good or bad, or black or white.

differentiated nursing practice A philosophy that focuses on the structuring of roles and functions of nurses according to education, experience, and competence.

diploma schools of nursing Nursing programs associated with a hospital that offer a nursing degree that is not offered through a college or university setting; typically 3 years in length.

direct care provider A healthcare provider who delivers care to a patient(s).

direct entry program *See also* **accelerated program**.

discrimination "Differences in care that result from bias, prejudices, stereotyping and uncertainty in clinical communication and decision-making" (IOM, 2002, p. 4).

disease management An approach to management of chronic diseases that emphasizes use of interprofessional teams with expertise in the specific disease, use of evidence-based clinical guidelines, clear descriptions of interventions and procedures and application of recommended timelines, patient support and education, and measurement of outcomes.

disease prevention Focuses on interventions to stop the development of disease, but also includes treatment to prevent disease from progressing further and leading to complications. The major levels of prevention are primary, secondary, and tertiary.

disparity An inequality or a difference in some respect.

distance education A set of teaching and/or learning strategies to meet the learning needs of students separate from the traditional classroom and sometimes from traditional roles of faculty (for example, an online course).

diversity All the ways in which people differ, including innate characteristics (for example, age, race, gender, ethnicity, mental and physical abilities, and sexual orientation) and acquired characteristics (for example, education, income, religion, work experience, language skills, and geographic location).

Doctor of Nursing Practice (DNP) A terminal degree that provides a clinical doctorate in nursing.

do not resuscitate (DNR) A form of advance directive that may be part of an extensive advance directive. This order means that there should be no resuscitation if the patient's condition indicates need for resuscitation.

educator A person who teaches others; typically a professional such as a nurse or teacher.

effective care The provision of services based on scientific knowledge (evidence-based practice) to all who could benefit, and refraining from providing services to those not likely to benefit (avoiding underuse and overuse).

efficient care Care that avoids waste, including waste of equipment, supplies, ideas, and energy.

electronic health record (EHR) An electronic record that provides a complete review of the person's health and medical care; person has access to it and can then be shared across healthcare providers.

electronic medical record (EMR) A medical record in a digital format.

email list A list of email addresses that can be used to send one email to all addresses at one time.

e-measurement The secondary use of electronic data to populate standardized performance measures.

empower To give power to another.

empowerment Having power or authority.

encryption Changing written information, especially patient information, into a code that protects the privacy of data for security purposes.

entrepreneur An innovator who recognizes opportunities to introduce a new process or an improved organization.

equitable care The provision of care that does not vary in quality because of personal characteristics such as gender, ethnicity, geographic location, and socioeconomic status.

error The failure of a planned action to be completed as intended or the use of the wrong plan to achieve an aim; errors are directly related to outcomes.

ethical decision making Ethical dilemmas that occur when a person is forced to choose between two or more alternatives, none of which is ideal.

ethical dilemma Occurs when a person is forced to choose between two or more alternatives, none of which is ideal.

ethical principles A standardized code or guide to behaviors for the nursing profession.

ethics A standardized code or guide to behaviors.

ethnicity A shared feeling of belonging to a group; peoplehood.

ethnocentrism The belief that one's group or culture is superior to others.

evidence-based management (EBM) Use of evidence such as research to support management decisions.

evidence-based practice (EBP) The integration of the best evidence into clinical practice, which includes research, the patient's values and preferences, the patient's history and exam data, and clinical expertise.

executive branch The branch of the U.S. government in charge of enforcing and executing the laws.

experimental study A type of research design in which the conditions of a program or experience (treatment) are controlled by the researcher and in which experimental subjects are randomly assigned to treatment conditions. This design must meet three criteria: manipulation, control, and randomization.

extended care The provision of inpatient skilled nursing care and related services to patients who require medical, nursing, or rehabilitative services.

failure to rescue (FTR) The inability to recognize a patient's negative change in status in a timely manner in order to prevent patient complications and to prevent major disability or death.

family Two or more individuals who depend on one another for emotional, physical, and/or financial support.

followers Members of a team.

for-profit An organization that must provide funds to pay stockholders or owners; this affects the availability of money for other purposes that have an impact on nurses and nursing.

Forces of Magnetism The identified effective descriptors of healthcare organizations that are designated as Magnet organizations by the Magnet Recognition Program®.

fraud A legal term that means a person deliberately deceived another for personal gain.

groupthink Occurs when all group or team members think alike. While all of the team members might be working together smoothly, groupthink limits choices, discourages open discussion of possibilities, and diminishes the ability to consider alternatives.

handoff A clinical situation (care transition) that occurs when the patient is passed from one provider or setting to another; increasing the risk for errors.

health The state of well-being; free from disease.

health disparity An inequality or gap in healthcare services that exists between two or more groups.

health informatics technology (HIT) Informatics that focuses on healthcare delivery.

Health Insurance Portability and Accountability Act of 1996 (HIPAA) A law that amended the Internal Revenue Code of 1986 to improve portability and continuity of healthcare information and ensure privacy of patient information.

health literacy The ability to understand and use health information.

health promotion Effort to stop the development of disease by emphasizing wellness; includes treatment to prevent a disease from progressing further and causing complications.

healthcare quality "The degree to which health services for individuals and populations increase the likelihood of desired health outcomes and are consistent with current professional knowledge" (IOM, 1990, p. 4).

healthcare report cards A report that provides specific performance data for an organization at specific intervals, with a focus on quality and safety.

healthy community A community that embraces the belief that health is more than merely an absence of disease.

Healthy People 2020 A federal initiative to improve the health of all citizens in the United States by establishing goals and leading indicators for communities to strive for; results are monitored and then used to adjust the initiative (goals and indicators).

home care The provision of healthcare services in the home.

hospice care A philosophy of care for managing symptoms and supporting quality of life as long as possible for the terminally ill.

hospital-acquired complications (HACs) Identification of complications that occur in the hospital that could have been preventable and the patient did not have on admission. The Centers for Medicare and Medicaid Services and some insurers have identified specific HACs that they will not cover in reimbursement.

hypothesis A formal statement in a research study describing the expected relationship or relationships between two or more variables in a specified population (the sample).

identity Sense of self as a professional nurse.

illness A sickness or disease of the mind or body.

incident report A method for documenting details about an incident in a healthcare organization such as a medication error, patient fall, and so on. Data are used to monitor quality care.

indicator A standard of aggregate performance measures used to monitor quality improvement.

indirect care provider A provider who does not provide direct care to a patient (for example, a laboratory technician who prepares a test but does not ever see the patient).

informatics An integration of nursing science, computer science, and information science to manage and communicate data, information, knowledge, and wisdom in nursing practice.

information (cognition) overload An "interpretation that people make in response to breakdowns, interruptions, interruptions of ongoing projects, or imbalances between demand and capacity" (Weick, 2009, p. 76).

information Data that are interpreted, organized, or structured.

information literacy The ability to recognize when information is needed and to locate, evaluate, and effectively use that information.

informed consent Permission required by law to explain or disclose information about a medical problem and treatment or procedure so that a patient can make an informed choice or informed consent with potential participants in a research study.

Institutional Review Board (IRB) An organization's (academic, healthcare) review of studies that may be conducted by employees and/or conducted in its organization to ensure that the study meets the requirements (for example, participant privacy and confidentiality; this is done by the IRB).

internship/externship A program that offers nursing students employment (typically during the summer) and includes educational experiences such as seminars, special speakers, and simulation experiences.

interoperability "The ability of a system to exchange electronic health information with and use electronic health information from other systems without special effort on the part of the user" (HHS, ONC, 2015a, p. 18).

interprofessional team-based care Care delivered by intentionally created, usually relatively small work teams in health care, who are recognized by others and by themselves as having a collective identity and shared responsibility for a patient or a group of patients (for example, rapid response team, palliative care team, primary care team, operating room team).

interprofessional teamwork The levels of cooperation, coordination, and collaboration characterizing the relationship between professions in delivering patient-centered care.

intuition Quick and ready insight.

invasion of privacy Occurs when individual providers or HCOs do not maintain patient privacy requirements (access to a person's body or behavior without consent) (for example, examining a patient in an area that is not private).

The Joint Commission A major nonprofit organization that accredits more than 20,500 healthcare organizations, including hospitals, long-term care organizations, home care agencies, clinical laboratories, ambulatory care organizations, behavioral health organizations, and healthcare networks or managed care organizations.

judicial branch The branch of the U.S. government that interprets and applies laws in specific cases.

knowledge An awareness and understanding of facts.

knowledge management A method for gathering information and making it available to others.

knowledge worker A person who is effective in acquiring, analyzing, synthesizing, and applying evidence to guide practice decisions.

leader One who has the ability to influence others; a role that nurses assume, either formally by taking an administrative position or informally as others recognize that they have leadership characteristics.

leadership The ability to influence others to achieve a common goal or outcome.

learning style A student's preferences for different types of learning and instructional activities; there are a variety of learning styles.

legal issues Questions and problems concerning the protections that make laws (U.S. Congress).

legislative branch The law-making branch of the U.S. government; made up of the Senate, the House of Representatives, and agencies that support Congress.

lifelong learning The need for healthcare professionals to continue with their professional learning throughout their careers.

living will A document that describes a person's wishes related to his or her end-of-life care needs.

lobbying Assembling and petitioning the government for redress of grievances.

lobbyist An individual paid to represent a special interest group, whose function is to urge support for or opposition to legislative matters.

long-term care A continuum of broad-ranged maintenance and health services delivered to the chronically ill, disabled, and the elderly.

macro consumer The major purchasers of care: the government and insurers.

Magnet hospital A hospital that demonstrates high levels of quality of care, autonomy, primary nursing care, mentoring, professional recognition, respect, and the ability to practice nursing; hospitals awarded this status meet specific standards, as determined by the Magnet Recognition Program®.

Magnet Recognition Program® A recognition program developed to support excellence in nursing services; program is administered by the American Nurses Credentialing Center's (ANCC) Commission on the Magnet Recognition Program®. HCOs and their nursing services must meet certain criteria, Forces of Magnetism, to be recognized as a Magnet organization.

malpractice An act or continuing conduct of a professional that does not meet the standard of professional competence and results in provable damages to a patient.

management A formal administrative position that focuses on four major functions: planning, organizing, leading, and controlling.

manager A person who holds a formal management or administrative position and who, in that position, focuses on four major functions: planning, organizing, leading, and controlling.

master's degree in nursing A graduate-level nursing degree of approximately 2 years with specialty focus (for example, advanced practice registered nurse or clinical nurse specialist).

meaningful use This government requirement focuses on use of certified electronic health record technology for the following purposes (HHS, Health-IT, 2014): improve quality, safety, efficiency, and reduce health disparities; engage patients and family; improve care coordination and population and public health; and maintain privacy and security of patient health information.

measure   A "standard used as a basis for comparison, a reference point against which other things can be evaluated" (HHS, AHRQ, 2014).

Medicaid   The federal healthcare reimbursement program that covers health and long-term care services for children, the aged, blind persons, the disabled, and people who are eligible to receive federally assisted income maintenance payments.

medical power of attorney   The right of a person given by another individual to speak for him or her if he or she cannot do so in matters related to health care. Also known as a durable power of attorney for health care or a healthcare agent or proxy.

Medicare   The federal health insurance program for people aged 65 and older, persons with disabilities, and people with end-stage renal disease.

mentor   A role model.

mentoring   Method used in healthcare organizations to support new staff; the mentor acts as a role model and serves as a resource.

micro consumer   The patients, families, and significant others who play a role in patient care and in the decision-making process.

microsystem   In healthcare delivery, a small group of people who work together on a regular basis to provide care to discrete subpopulations including the patients.

mindful communication   A process by which actively aware individuals engage in communication that is meaningful, is timely, and responds continually as events unfold.

minimum data set   The minimum categories of data with uniform definitions and categories; an example would be the Nursing Minimum Data Set.

missed nursing care   A type of error of omission when needed nursing care is delayed, partially completed, or not completed at all.

misuse   An event that leads to avoidable complications that prevent a patient from receiving the full potential benefit of a service.

moral disengagement   "The process that involves justifying one's unethical actions by altering one's moral perception of those actions" (Hyatt, 2016, p. 15, as cited from Bandura, 1999).

morals   An individual's code of acceptable behavior, which shapes one's values and is influenced by cultural factors and experiences.

National Database of Nursing Quality Indicators (NDNQI)   A system in which nursing data are collected to evaluate outcomes and nursing care.

National Quality Strategy (NQS)   A national initiative led by the U.S. Department of Health and Human Services to establish a national approach to healthcare quality with annual reports to Congress. The requirement to establish the NQS was part of the Affordable Care Act of 2010.

near miss   An event that occurred that could have led to an adverse event but did not.

negligence   Failure to exercise the care toward others that a reasonable or prudent person would have under the same circumstances; an unintentional tort.

networking   The cultivation of productive relationships for employment or business.

nomenclature   A system of designations (terms) elaborated according to pre-established rules; an example would be the International Classification for Nursing Practice.

not-for-profit   An incorporated organization whose shareholders or trustees do not benefit financially.

nurse licensure compact   An interstate licensure partnership that allows nurses to practice in adjacent states when licensed in one state. Clear requirements must be met by the individual nurses and the state boards of nursing in the compact.

nurse migration   The movement of nurses from one place to another, particularly globally; may affect number of nurses available in a country if too many move to another country, typically for better pay and working conditions.

nurse practice act   The act (law) that governs nursing practice in the state in which the nurse practices.

nurse residency   A special employment program that helps new RN graduates transition to practice in a structured program that provides content and learning activities, precepted experiences, mentoring, and gradual adjustment to higher levels of responsibility.

nursing The profession of a nurse.

nursing informatics (NI) The specialty that integrates nursing science, computer science, and information science to manage and communicate data, information, knowledge, and wisdom in nursing practice.

nursing process A systematic method for thinking about and communicating how nurses provide patient care; this includes assessment, diagnosis, planning, intervention or implementation, and evaluation.

occupational health care Health promotion, disease and illness prevention, and treatment; includes attention to the risks of illness and injury within the work environment.

organizational culture The values, beliefs, traditions, and communication processes that bring a group of people together and characterize the group.

organizational ethics Organizational concerns related to the beliefs, decision making, and behavior of the organization as an entity.

outcomes Measurable benefits of patient care.

outcomes research Research focused on determining the effectiveness of healthcare services and patient outcomes.

overuse The point at which the potential for harm from the provision of a service exceeds the possible benefit.

palliative care Care focused on alleviating symptoms and meeting the special needs of the terminally ill patient and the family.

patient advocacy Respecting patient rights and the patient and ensuring that the patient has the education to understand treatment and care needs.

patient-centered care (PCC) Identification of, respect, and care for patient differences, values, preferences, and needs; relief of pain; coordination of care; clear communication with and education of the patient; shared decision making; and continuous promotion of disease prevention and wellness.

personal health record (PHR) Computer-based health records that collect data over a lifetime; with permission of the patient, this record can be accessed easily by any provider who needs the information.

Peter Principle Occurs when someone is promoted beyond his or her leadership and management competencies required for a new position.

PICOT (patient–intervention–comparison–outcome–time) To ask a searchable and answerable question. The *P* (patient population) is specific and describes the population in terms such as age, gender, diagnosis, ethnicity, other. The *I* (intervention) relates to prognostic factors, risk behaviors, exposure to disease, clinical intervention or treatment, and so forth. The *C* (comparison intervention) can pertain to another treatment, no treatment, or other. The *O* (outcome) includes factors such as risk of disease, complications or side effects, or adverse outcomes. The *T* is the time, meaning the time involved to demonstrate the outcome.

plan–do–study–act (PDSA) cycle A systematic approach to planning and decision making.

policy A set course of action that affects a large number of people and is stimulated by a specific need to achieve certain outcomes.

political action committee (PAC) A private group that represents a specific issue or group and works to get someone elected or defeated.

political competence An understanding of the political process and how best to participate in the process.

politics The process of influencing the authoritative allocation of scarce resources.

population Group of people with something in common, such as a disease, age, ethnic group, where they live, and so on.

power The ability to influence decisions and have an impact on issues that matter.

practice model A framework used to guide practice.

practicum A course that includes clinical activities and stresses the practical application of theory in a field of study; also referred to as a "clinical."

preceptor An experienced and competent staff member (an RN or, for nurse practitioner students, possibly a nurse practitioner or physician) who has received formal training to function as a preceptor and who serves as a role model to guide student learning, serving as a resource for the nursing student.

prejudice Making assumptions or judgments about the beliefs, behaviors, needs, and expectations of other persons who are of a different cultural background than oneself because of emotional beliefs about the population; involves negative attitudes toward the different group.

prescriptive authority Legal authority granted to advanced practice nurses to prescribe medication.

primary care provider A healthcare provider who is the first contact for a patient at the entry point of care and who then may manage overall care for the patient; examples of providers are physicians and advanced practice registered nurses.

primary prevention Interventions used to stop development of disease; includes interventions that are used to maintain health before illness occurs. Health promotion is a critical component of primary prevention. Examples are teaching people (children and adults) about healthy diets before they become obese and encouraging adequate exercise (education about health and healthy lifestyles is an important intervention at this level).

private policy Policy created by nongovernmental organizations.

procedures A definite statement of step-by-step actions required for a specific result.

process Particular course of action intended to achieve a result.

professional ethics Generally accepted standards of conduct and methods in the nursing profession.

professional organization An organization that represents a professional group, such as nurses represented by the American Nurses Association.

professional socialization "Transition into professional practice is characterized by the acquisition of the skills, knowledge, and behaviors needed to successfully function as a professional nurse. This process involves the new nurse's internalization of the values, attitudes, and goals that comprise his or her occupational identity" (Young, Stuenkel, & Bawel-Brinkley, 2008, p. 105).

professionalism The conduct, aims, or qualities that characterize or mark a profession.

protocols Formal treatment plans focused on specific care needs and then applied to individual patients with changes made to meet individual patient needs.

provider of care A healthcare staff member who provides care to patients.

Public Health Act of 1944 This law consolidated all existing public health legislation into one law.

public policy Policy created by the legislative, executive, and judicial branches of federal, state, and local levels of government that affects individual and institutional behaviors under the government's respective jurisdiction.

qualitative study A systematic, subjective, methodological research approach; analysis of data that does not rely on statistics or mathematical equations.

quality Requirements that maintain high standards to meet expected outcomes.

quality improvement (QI) An organized approach to identify errors and hazards in care, and to improve care overall.

quantitative study A formal, objective, systematic research process that uses statistics for data analysis.

race A biological designation of a group.

randomized controlled trial (RCT) Often referred to as the gold standard in research designs, this is the true experiment in which there is control over variables, randomization of the sample with a control group and an experimental group, and an intervention(s) (independent variable).

rapid response team (RRT) A special team of staff with specific expertise related to assisting patients in critical condition; team is called by staff to a patient area, or in some cases, family may request that staff call for RRT support.

reality shock The reaction of students when they discover that the clinical experience does not always match the values and ideals that they had anticipated.

recognition A process used to evaluate an organization's adherence to excellence-focused standards (for example, the Magnet Hospital Recognition Program).

reflective thinking Creativity and conscious self-evaluation over a period of time.

regulation An official rule or order, based on laws, governing processes, practice, and procedures; in nursing, legal regulation governs licensure.

rehabilitation The restoration of, or improvement of, an individual's health and functionality.

reimbursement Payment for healthcare services.

research Investigation or experimentation aimed at the discovery and interpretation of facts about a particular subject.

research analysis The process of using methods to analyze and summarize results or data.

research-based doctorate A terminal degree that is focused on research (PhD).

research design A specific plan for conducting a study.

research problem statement A description of the topic or subject for a research study, which provides the context for the research study and typically generates questions that the research aims to answer.

research proposal A written document that describes recent, relevant literature on the problem area; describes the research topic/problem; and defines the processes or steps that will be followed to answer the research question(s); proposal is written before the study is conducted.

research purpose Identifies the potential uses of research results.

research question The interrogative statement that directs a research study.

researcher A person who systematically investigates and studies materials and sources to establish facts and reach conclusions.

resilience The ability to cope with stress.

responsibility Moral, legal, or mental accountability.

risk management (RM) Maintaining a safe and effective healthcare environment and preventing or reducing financial loss to the healthcare organization.

RN-BSN A nursing educational program for licensed nurses (RNs) who want to meet the requirements for a baccalaureate degree in nursing (BSN).

role Behavior oriented to the patterned expectation of others.

role transition Gradual development in a new role.

root-cause analysis (RCA) An in-depth analysis of an error to assess the event and identify causes and possible solutions.

rounds An organized method to observe and communicate between staff and patients; typically is done routinely, such as daily or per shift, but may also be done for special purposes in nonroutine time frame, such as safety rounds to check for safety concerns.

safety/safe care Freedom from accidental injury.

scholarship A fund for knowledge and learning.

scope of practice A statement that describes the who, what, where, when, why, and how of nursing practice.

scorecard A method used in quality improvement to document data and analysis providing a "rating or grade"; scorecards may be used internally or may be used to compare healthcare organizations.

secondary caregiver Assistant who helps home patients with intermittent activities such as shopping, transportation, home repairs, getting bills paid, emergency support, and so forth.

secondary prevention Interventions used to stop development of disease; includes interventions that are used to maintain health before illness occurs; occurs when a person is asymptomatic but after disease has begun. The focus here is on preventing further complications. Examples are breast cancer screening using mammography and blood pressure screening to diagnose hypertension.

security protections Methods used to ensure that information is not read or taken by persons not authorized to access it.

self-directed learning A process in which individuals take the initiative, with or without the help of others, in diagnosing their learning needs, formulating learning goals, identifying human and material resources for learning, choosing and implementing appropriate learning strategies, and evaluating learning outcomes.

self-management (of care) The systematic provision of education and supportive interventions to increase patients' skills and confidence in managing their own health problems, including regular assessment of progress and problems, goal-setting, and problem-solving approaches.

sensemaking Making sense of a problem; it is part of using critical thinking and clinical reasoning and judgment.

sentinel event An unexpected medical event that results in death or physical or psychological harm, or the risk thereof.

shared governance A management philosophy, a professional practice model, and an accountability model that focuses on staff involvement in decision making, particularly in decisions that affect their practice.

simulation Replication of some or nearly all essential aspects of a clinical situation as realistically as possible.

situation-background-assessment-recommendations (SBAR) A systematic communication method that is used to improve communication of critical information about a patient that requires immediate attention and action.

social policy statement A statement that describes the profession of nursing and its professional framework and obligations to society; published by the American Nurses Association.

Social Security Act of 1935 The act that established the U.S. Medicare and Medicaid programs—two major reimbursement programs—and also provided funding for nursing education through amendments added to the law.

software Computer programs and applications.

standard A reference point against which other things can be evaluated and that serve as guides to practice.

standardized terminology A collection of terms with definitions for use in informational systems databases.

status A position in a social structure with rights and obligations.

STEEEP® Description of critical characteristics of care delivery: safe, timely, effective, efficient, equitable, and patient-centered care.

stereotype The process by which people use social groups (for example, gender and race) to gather, process, and recall information about other people; also known as labeling.

stress A complex experience felt internally that makes a person feel a loss or threat of a loss; bodily or mental tension.

stress management Strategies used to cope with stress to alter bodily or mental tension; reducing the negative impact of stress, improving health, and developing health-promoting behaviors.

structure The environment in which services are provided; inputs into the system, such as patients, staff, and environments.

surveillance Purposeful and ongoing acquisition, interpretation, and synthesis of patient data for clinical decision making.

system The coming together of parts, interconnections, and purpose.

systematic review (SR) A summary of evidence typically conducted by an expert or a panel of experts on a particular topic; uses a rigorous process to minimize bias for identifying, appraising, and synthesizing studies to answer a specific clinical question and draw conclusions about the data gathered; different methods may be used depending on the type of review such as integrative review or meta-analysis.

team A number of persons associated in work or activity.

team leader The person who leads the team.

teamwork Work done by several associates, with each doing a part but all subordinating personal prominence to the efficiency of the whole.

telehealth The use of telecommunications equipment and communications networks to transfer healthcare information between participants at different locations.

telenursing The use of telecommunications technology in nursing to enhance patient care.

tertiary prevention Interventions used to stop development of disease; includes interventions that are used to maintain health before illness occurs; occurs when there is disability and the need to maintain or, if possible, improve functioning.

theory A body of rules, ideas, principles, and techniques that applies to a particular subject.

therapeutic use of self The nurse's use of his or her personality consciously and in full awareness in an attempt to establish relatedness and to structure a nursing intervention.

time management Strategies used to manage and control time productivity.

timely care Meeting the patient's needs; providing high-quality experiences and improved healthcare outcomes when needed.

training Activities and instruction intended to foster skilled behavior.

transformational leadership This approach emphasizes a positive work environment, recognition of the importance of change and using change effectively, rewarding staff for expertise and performance, and development of staff awareness. Transformational leaders create vision and mission statements with the staff to guide the work of the organization and are described as honest, energetic, loyal, confident, self-directed, flexible, and committed.

translational research This research may be (1) the application of discoveries generated in the laboratory and in preclinical studies to the development of trials and studies in humans and (2) research aimed at enhancing the adoption of best practices in the community. A common use is to determine comparative effectiveness of prevention and treatment strategies.

Triple Aim Major goals or aims of healthcare delivery: Improve the health of the population; enhance the patient experience of care (including quality, access, and reliability); and reduce, or at least control, the per capita cost of care.

types of power Legitimate (formal), referent (informal), informational, expert, reward, and coercive power.

underuse Failure to provide a service that would have produced a favorable outcome for the patient.

unlicensed assistive personnel (UAP) Healthcare workers who are not licensed to perform nursing tasks but are trained and often certified.

utilization review/management (UR/UM) Evaluating necessity, appropriateness, and efficiency of healthcare services for specific patients or in patient populations.

vulnerable population A population (group of people with something in common) at risk for medical or other problems such as lack of funds, housing, and so on, who may not be able to effectively care for themselves. Examples of these populations are children, the elderly, those with mental illness or other disabilities, and prisoners.

whistleblowing This action occurs when a person who works for an organization that is committing fraud and abuse reports these activities to legal authorities, sharing extensive information that would be difficult for the authorities to obtain on their own. The False Claims Act protects whistleblowers.

wisdom The appropriate use of knowledge to solve human problems; understanding when and how to apply knowledge.

wraparound services Services that offer social and economic interventions, preferably within the healthcare provider setting to better ensure that full services are provided for complex patient needs.

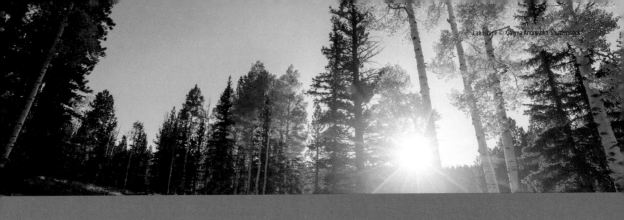

Index

Note: Page numbers followed by *f* and *t* denotes figures and tables respectively.